Women's Health: Childbearing

Women's Health

Edited by
Lois J. Sonstegard, Karren Mundell Kowalski, and Betty Jennings

Volume 1: **Ambulatory Care**
Volume 3: **Illness and Crisis in Childbearing**

Volume 2 | Women's Health: Childbearing

Edited by

Lois J. Sonstegard, R.N., M.S.N., F.A.A.N.
Project Director for Perinatal Nursing
School of Nursing
University of Minnesota
Minneapolis, Minnesota

Karren Mundell Kowalski, R.N., M.S., F.A.A.N.
Doctoral Student
Department of Sociology
University of Colorado
Boulder, Colorado

Betty Jennings, R.N., C.N.M., M.S.N.
Assistant Professor, School of Nursing
Clinical Instructor, Department of Obstetrics and Gynecology
School of Medicine
University of Colorado Health Sciences Center
Denver, Colorado

Grune & Stratton
A Subsidiary of Harcourt Brace Jovanovich, Publishers
New York   London
Paris   San Diego   San Francisco   São Paulo
Sydney   Tokyo   Toronto

Library of Congress Cataloging in Publication Data

(Revised for volume 2)
Main entry under title:

Women's health.

 Bibliography
 Includes indexes.
 Contents: v. 1. Ambulatory care—v. 2. Childbearing.
 1. Gynecological nursing. 2. Women's health services.
3. Women's health and hygiene. I. Sonstegard, Lois.
II. Kowalski, Karren. III. Jennings, Betty. [DNLM:
1. Ambulatory care—Nursing texts. 2. Gynecology—
Nursing texts. 3. Genital diseases, Female—Nursing.
WY 156.7 W8717]
RG105.W648 1982   362.1'088042   82-11933
ISBN 0-8089-1501-0 (v. 1)
ISBN 0-8089-1508-8 (v. 2)

Grune & Stratton, Inc.
111 Fifth Avenue
New York, New York 10003

Distributed in the United Kingdom by
Grune & Stratton, Inc. (London) Ltd.
24/28 Oval Road, London NW 1

Library of Congress Catalog Number 82-11933
International Standard Book Number 0-8089-1508-8

Printed in the United States of America

This book is dedicated to our families:

our parents

who nurtured us into adulthood,

our husbands, Lou, Walt, and Glenn

who have worked
to create relationships that encourage us to grow as individuals as well
as professional women,

and our children, Kyle, Nathan, Liv, and Devin

for whom we hope to create a more humanistic world.

Contents

Acknowledgments

Nearly fifty years of combined clinical experience in nursing serve as the basis of our perspective and philosophy of maternal–child nursing. We have worked and lived in such faraway places as Tunisia, West Germany, Viet Nam, and Japan as well as in rural America and large metropolitan areas. Our relationships with childbearing women in various cultures and socioeconomic groups have greatly influenced us. Although our obstetrical roots are in the traditional practices of the early 1960s, we have tried to be good observers and to listen to women and their families. These women have helped to shape our philosophy, our attitudes, and ultimately this book. We are exceedingly grateful for their patience in teaching us and their perseverance in helping us to understand what childbearing in America can be.

For their efforts in encouraging us to undertake this task, we would like to recognize Barbara E. Bishop, Mitzi Duxbury, Ingeborg Mauksch, Virginia Paulson, and Edith Walker. For their invaluable critical reviews of the manuscript, we thank Sally Yeomans, C.N.M., M.S., Watson A. Bowes, M.D., Brenda Canedy, Ph.D., and Glenn T. Foust, M.D. We particularly appreciate the assistance of friends and family members Joanne Gottschalk-Washburn, Judith Hyland, Carol Judd, and Phyllis Larson, who helped assemble the final manuscript.

From the first draft to the finished product numerous women functioned in the timeless role of secretary. The work could never have been completed without them. Our contributors have had the patience and endurance of saints, for which we are grateful. Finally, we want to thank each of our husbands and children for their love, their understanding, and their humor.

L.S., K.K., B.J.

Foreword

The focus of many childbearing families today is on their participation in the joy of childbirth; they expect it to be a positive physical, psychological, social, and emotional experience. The loss of mother or baby is not even considered a possibility by most. Such expectations are due in part to the advance of technology. Some healthy babies born today would not even have been conceived in previous years.

Yet despite such advances, many women who experience normal pregnancies object to the routine application of technology in the management of their childbearing. They want knowledgeable, skillful attendance by professionals who will use their senses of sight, hearing, and touch as well as their knowledge and expert clinical judgment first, resorting to the use of technology only as it becomes necessary.

Books available today for the advanced practitioner of nursing tend to focus on the latest technological advancements and their application in patient care. This book, however, conveys the art as well as the science of providing care and supervision of the pregnant, laboring, and birthing woman, her newborn, and her family. Care of the normal, low-risk woman and her baby is specifically highlighted; the use of technology is minimized.

Risk assessment is a pervasive theme, acknowledging that risk status is susceptible to change at any time. While high-risk women and newborns benefit greatly from complex technological care, the childbearing women and their newborns discussed in this book benefit from the personalized, individualized, expert care described.

Each of the editors of this book is committed to extensive, high-quality care of the low-risk childbearing woman, her newborn, and her family. Each continues to work to create a better environment in which to accomplish the goal of optimal pregnancy outcome for every family. This book reflects the commitment of the editors to a team approach in the care of the childbearing woman, as is evidenced by the inclusion of contributors who are nurses, nurse-midwives, nutritionists, neonatologists, psychologists, and child psychiatrists.

The role of the nurse, as described herein, is that of primary care provider, nursing-care coordinator, patient advocate, and agent of change. Important advances in improving pregnancy outcome for all will be made, in a cost-effective manner, as nurses become more widely involved in managing the care of healthy women experiencing normal pregnancy. Nursing roles are uniquely suited to focusing on preventive health measures, continuity of care, and screening and referring higher-risk women and newborns for care by other health team members.

Nurses practicing in the field of women's health care—particularly childbearing—and students preparing for specialized roles in the field will value *Women's Health: Childbearing*. It is an important resource book for those seeking unique, expert clinical guidance, a review of the most current literature in the field, and a challenge to develop new knowledge that will result in higher standards of care.

Colleen Conway, Ph.D., C.N.M., F.A.A.N.

Preface

The birth of each child changes a family constellation or begins the formation of a new family. During 1980, there were 3,598,000 live births in the United States.[1] This represented a four percent increase in births over 1979. The 1980 birth rate was 16.2 live births per 1000 population[1] and represented a three percent higher rate than in 1979. The National Center for Health Statistics observed that this increase in the birth rate was the result of the increased number of women of childbearing age as well as an increase in the actual rate of childbearing. They predicted that the birth rate would continue to increase by one percent each year until 1985.[1] Thus it would seem that families will continue to grow and establish themselves. An important concern then is how health care providers might best assist families in general, and more specifically the childbearing family.

The National Institute of Child Health and Human Development declared in 1968 that optimal health care for mothers and children was a national priority. This resulted in a great proliferation of literature and research in an attempt to decrease maternal, fetal, and neonatal mortality. Tremendous interest was generated in preventive and health promotional care for the childbearing family.

What has been the impact of this emphasis on preventive care? Examination of various studies conducted since 1968 provides useful information. For example, using infant birthweight as a proxy measure, Sema Taffel found a positive relationship between the number of prenatal visits and pregnancy outcome.[2] Marital status, level of education, and age of the pregnant woman have all been found to influence the decision to seek prenatal care. Other factors found to affect pregnancy outcome are the interval between pregnancies, the socioeconomic and nutritional status of the pregnant woman, her dietary habits, and her physical and emotional health prior to pregnancy.

Many of these factors can be addressed through active consumer education programs and careful patient counseling. Some require that health care providers become actively involved in the political arena in order to obtain legislative and financial support necessary to provide preventive health care to the childbearing family. With today's emphasis on cost containment, individual responsibility for one's own health, and faltering government programs, it has become more important than ever that the health care provider continuously be appraised of the health and well-being of all childbearing families and act as an advocate on their behalf.

Women's Health: Childbearing is intended to critically examine those factors that will enhance pregnancy outcome. The focus is on the healthy woman, her pregnancy, labor and delivery, and baby. The management and care of the woman or fetus at risk during pregnancy have been omitted from this volume. It is our belief that health care providers need to gain a firm understanding of the normal, healthy pregnancy before they can examine the dynamics of the compromised pregnancy. The challenge of caring for the healthy childbearing family lies in preventing potential perinatal complications, avoiding family disruption, and promoting the family's health as members integrate pregnancy, labor, birth, and the newborn into their lives.

Part 1 of this volume deals with the prenatal development of the family. The chapters are intended to provide the reader with an understanding of those factors that may positively or negatively influence the parent–infant relationship as it evolves and develops. Pregnancy, the birth process, and family relationships are discussed, with the primary concern being the ultimate emotional and physiological adjustment of an individual family.

---

[1]National Center for Health Statistics. (1981). Births, marriages, divorces and deaths for 1980. *Monthly Vital Statistics Report, 29*(12), 1–11.

[2]Taffel, S. (1978). *Congenital anomalies and birth injuries among live births.* United States Department of Health, Education and Welfare, pp. 1–14.

Part 2 discusses the needs and concerns of families during the antepartal period. The essential elements of prenatal care are addressed as well as aspects of nutritional assessment and counseling. Parental concerns for childbirth preparation are also discussed in relation to recent research findings.

Part 3 deals with the health care of families through labor and birth. The needs of the laboring and birthing woman are discussed, examining both the psychological and physiological requirements. Two chapters on birth emergencies are included. Of course, it is always hoped that pregnancy will proceed without complication, but crises may occur for which the attendant must be adequately prepared. The complications discussed center on emergency delivery and infant resuscitation. The last two chapters in this section examine various alternatives to the traditional birth settings and the health care needs of the mother and newborn immediately following birth.

Part 4 addresses the many concerns and needs of the family following the birth of the infant. Two chapters provide a theoretical framework for nursing care to the childbearing family postpartum and through the first year following birth. Another addresses educating the childbearing couple for parenting. The remaining chapters are devoted specifically to the infant: a systematic approach for assessing the baby's health and well-being; the impact of the infant on the family (and vice versa) and factors that facilitate family development; and infant nutrition, both by breast- and bottle-feeding.

A number of personal and professional commitments form the philosophy of this book:

• The majority of women who seek health care are essentially well. Too few textbooks and other resources sufficiently cover the range of health and its manifestations. Too few books appreciate the forces that affect women's lives and thus their health. Too few books discuss women in the context of their social network. Health is multifaceted and complex, and there is much still to be learned about healthy women.

• Nurses who provide health care for women must understand and internalize feminist values in order to provide high-quality health care for women.

• Women's health care is equally concerned with physical, social, physiological, and political issues. Traditional health care has isolated disease from the rest of life, ignoring the needs of the healthy and imposing unnecessary hardships on women and their families. Modern health care for women must include aspects of life that extend beyond the home, clinic, or hospital.

• To achieve the high levels of education and skill that are necessary for providing quality care, nurses require excellent advanced educational opportunities as well as outstanding role models. Nurses also must inform the public, legislators, and policy developers of the unique and vitally important contributions that nursing makes to health care delivery.

Many outstanding clinicians, scholars, researchers, and teachers have contributed to this text. Most of them are nurses, the notable exceptions being individuals who have contributed immeasurably in other ways to the health care of women and their families. Because the contributors are all experts in their fields, we asked them to discuss their subjects as they chose, and we have made every effort to retain their unique perspectives. The authors have extensively drawn on and referred to research that relates to their subjects and have sometimes identified areas where more research is needed. It is hoped that further important research will result from the coverage in this book.

Women's Health: Childbearing is the second in a series of books that examine the clinical aspects of women's health care. Written for practicing nurses and nurses engaged in graduate education, *Women's Health* challenges nurses to pay close attention to the issues of health as well as illness within the health care delivery system.

L.S., K.K., B.J.

Contributors

Cathryn L. Anderson, C.N.M., M.S., M.P.H.
Doctoral Student, Department of Maternal–Child Health, School of Hygiene and Public Health, Johns Hopkins University, Baltimore, Maryland. Formerly Assistant Professor, School of Nursing, University of Colorado Health Sciences Center, Denver, Colorado

Carmela Cavero, C.N.M., M.S.
Clinical Director, Nurse Midwifery Group of Fresno, Fresno, California; and Assistant Clinical Professor, University of California, San Francisco, California

Rosemary Cogan, Ph.D.
Associate Professor of Psychology, Texas Tech University, Lubbock, Texas

Libby Lee Colman, Ph.D.
Psychologist, Sausalito, California

Margaret A. Emrey, C.N.M., M.S.
Nurse Consultant, Maternal and Child Health, California Department of Health Services, Berkeley, California

Joan E. Hoffmaster, C.N.M., M.S.
Improved Pregnancy Outcome Project, Texas Department of Health, Lubbock, Texas

Robert J. Harmon, M.D.
Associate Professor of Psychiatry (Child), School of Medicine, University of Colorado; Adjunct Assistant Professor of Psychology, University of Denver, Denver, Colorado; and Adjunct Assistant Professor, School for Social Work, Smith College, Northampton, Massachusetts

Betty Jennings, R.N., C.N.M., M.S.N.
Assistant Professor, School of Nursing, and Clinical Instructor, Department of Obstetrics and Gynecology, School of Medicine, University of Colorado Health Sciences Center, Denver, Colorado

Patricia J. Johnson, R.N., M.S.
Arizona Certified Neonatal Nurse Practitioner and Director, Extended Role Programs, Good Samaritan Medical Center, Phoenix, Arizona; and Nursing Coordinator, Neonatal Nurse Practitioner Program, College of Nursing, University of Arizona, Tucson, Arizona

Marcia Gruis Killien, R.N., Ph.D.
Lecturer, Perinatal Nurse Specialist Program, Department of Parent and Child Nursing, University of Washington, Seattle, Washington

Karren Mundell Kowalski, R.N., M.S., F.A.A.N.
Doctoral Student, Department of Sociology, University of Colorado, Boulder, Colorado. Formerly Associate Professor, School of Nursing, University of Colorado; Coordinator, Maternal–Child Continuing Education Grant; and Director, Women's Health Care Nurse Practitioner Program, Denver, Colorado

Betty Lia-Hoagberg, R.N., Ph.D.
Clinical Director of Parent–Child Nursing Services (Maternity/Pediatrics/NICU), Hennepin County Medical Center, Minneapolis, Minnesota

Lula O. Lubchenco, M.D.
Professor Emeritus, Department of Pediatrics, Division of Perinatal Medicine, University of Colorado Health Sciences Center, Denver, Colorado

Ramona T. Mercer, R.N., Ph.D., F.A.A.N.
Associate Professor, Department of Health Care Nursing, University of California, San Francisco, California

Laura Duckett Newton, M.S., R.N.
Assistant Professor, School of Nursing, University of Minnesota, and Doctoral Student in Educational Psychology, University of Minnesota, Minneapolis, Minnesota

Allison Singleton Parsons, M.S., R.D.
Fort Collins, Colorado

Carol Jean Poole, C.R.N., M.N.
Coordinator, Satellite R.N. Baccalaureate Program, The Swedish Hospital Medical Center, Seattle, Washington

Reva Rubin, C.N.M., M.N., M.S.
Professor and Director, Graduate Programs in Maternity Nursing, University of Pittsburgh, Pittsburgh, Pennsylvania

Part 1 | Prenatal Development of the Family

MANY FACTORS affect the health and well-being of families. Currently, consumer demands and a proliferation of literature aimed at educating the consumer, along with psychosocial research, require that we address ourselves more than ever to how pregnancy, the birth process, the time immediately following birth, and various family factors influence the ultimate emotional and psychological adjustment of an individual family. A new expectation for the professional has been expressed. Various research findings have provided great insight into those factors that may facilitate family development. Studies of maternal–infant attachment processes have indicated the importance of physical contact. Thus, no longer is it acceptable for family members to be separated, no longer is it acceptable to leave a baby alone in an incubator until someone deems the temperatures stable, no longer are women routinely sedated and unable to participate in their own birth experiences, and no longer do structured feeding rituals dominate a mother and her new baby.

Chapter 1 of this book explores the psychological experiences of pregnancy; in particular it examines the effect of pregnancy on a woman's psychological and emotional well-being and discusses the adjustments that pregnancy necessitates. Chapter 2 explores the research on maternal–infant attachment and lays the foundation for understanding those factors that facilitate a positive relationship between mother and infant.

Chapter 1

Psychology of Pregnancy

Libby Lee Colman

PREGNANCY is a psychosomatic event that occurs with equal power in the mind and body. Thus, the mind can create physical symptoms, such as occur in false pregnancies among men and women, and the physiological changes can profoundly affect the mind (most dramatically seen when schizophrenia goes into remission for the duration of the pregnancy).

This chapter will look at some of the psychological meanings that pregnancy can carry and at the emotional activity generated by those meanings in people who are involved in a pregnancy. The emphasis will be on the conscious and unconscious meanings of pregnancy in and between individuals in a family. These meanings result from a complex interaction between physiological changes that affect mood, sociological forces that impose role changes, and psychological transformations that occur while attempting to integrate the dramatic new forces with an ongoing sense of self.

The dynamics of pregnancy for a particular woman are influenced by her characteristic psychological coping mechanisms; her stage of pregnancy; her current life stresses; her stage in the life cycle; the symbolic meanings pregnancy carries for her; and the relationships within her family. Each of these topics will be discussed separately in this chapter. The last section will deal briefly with the use of counseling in pregnancy.

CHARACTERISTIC COPING MECHANISMS

Certain people who have trouble in the childbearing year have been psychologically marginal for a long time; they have characteristically had trouble coping with life, especially at times of stress or change. Any psychological difficulty can become more extreme under pressure. Thus, pregnancy, childbirth, and the presence of an infant can contribute to a physical or mental weakening or breakdown.

It is hard to predict whether a given individual will feel better or worse in the childbearing year. Some disturbed women do very well, while some apparently well-adjusted women decompensate (Brown & Shereshefski, 1972; Shereshefski & Yarrow, 1973). Some women who feel anxious during pregnancy feel much

Portions of this chapter have appeared in a slightly different form in Colman, L. (1978). Delayed childbearing: A descriptive study of twelve women having their first baby after the age of thirty. Unpublished Ph.D. dissertation for Wright Institute, Berkeley, Ca.

The theory of psychological merger is discussed at greater length in Colman, A., & Colman, L. (1975). *Love and Ecstasy.* New York: Seabury Press; and Colman, L., & Colman, A. (1974). Pregnancy as an altered state of consciousness. *Birth and the Family Journal, 1,* 7–11.

better when they are able to hold and care for their baby. Conversely, some who are euphoric during pregnancy are unable to cope after the birth.

It is helpful to know something about a woman's prepregnancy psychology and her ability to cope with stress in order to evaluate her status during pregnancy and make predictions about her adjustment to childbirth and parenting. Unfortunately, such information is not always available. Pregnancy must generally be dealt with as a real event happening in the present. This makes it difficult to separate difficulties that have been created by the pregnancy from ones that were already present in the woman's psychological makeup and in her relationships. The problem is compounded by the characteristic psychological state of pregnancy. Many investigators have described emotional swings, unexplained crying, and disturbing dreams that seem to be usual in pregnancy but would be taken as symptoms of a disturbance at other times (Bibring, 1959; Colman & Colman, 1977; Shereshefski & Yarrow, 1973).

Some women have a truly happy and unconflicted pregnancy, and move smoothly through the postpartum period. They could safely be said to have been ready for the experience and well adapted to the realities of becoming a mother. These women generally have a positive image of what it means to be a mother, are eager to assume the additional responsibilities, have experience with babies, and have good relations with a loving and supportive family, especially the child's father (Colman, 1978). They are optimistic and happy because of a realistic evaluation of their life situation.

It is important to recognize, however, that not every woman who has a smooth pregnancy is truly without conflict. There is the "sunny pregnancy syndrome," characterized by a euphoric pregnancy that leads to a severe postpartum letdown. In these cases it seems as though the pregnant woman has failed to do the psychological "work" of pregnancy. Instead of experiencing the turmoil implicit in the transformation from "person" to "parent," she lives with a fantasy of herself as a pregnant woman or a blissful, perfect mother. This fantasy, often accompanied by a regressive identification with the fetus, may make pregnancy a happy time, but it can rarely survive the strains of mothering, as illustrated by the following case study.

Case 1

Barbara was the image of a healthy, happy expectant mother throughout her pregnancy. When she came for psychotherapy two months after her baby was born, she was deeply depressed and suicidal. She said, "When I looked at the baby, it was like something inside of me just broke. I tried to

hold him, but he just wasn't cuddly. I always thought I'd be a perfect mother, but he wouldn't let me take care of him."

In retrospect, Barbara's family and friends could recall that she had sometimes seemed unnaturally happy during the pregnancy. They suspected that the marriage was in trouble, but no one, least of all Barbara herself, had guessed that she might have trouble with mothering, especially since this was her second child. She had been able to cling to her image of herself as a perfect mother as long as she had only one little girl to care for; the arrival of her second child shattered her self-concept and her ability to cope.

The psychological work of pregnancy is to prepare for parenthood, to get oneself ready to accept a child into the family. This is an inner task as well as an outer task. It requires reevaluating personal identity as well as taking practical steps to be ready to care for an infant. It also requires getting past the fantasy of being the perfect mother and into the practical acceptance of personal strengths and limitations. Sometimes this entails painful confrontations.

Case 2

Jennifer came for help because she was six months pregnant and suicidal. She described a loving husband and much-wanted pregnancy. Everything had been going well, but she had become increasingly anxious. She had no apparent reason for the anxiety but was overwhelmed with thoughts of death and schemes for killing herself.

As she talked about her history, it rapidly became apparent that she had rejected her mother at an early age and had made an adult adjustment that she perceived as the antithesis of her mother's. Once she felt the baby move inside her and realized that she was not only going to have a baby, but was going to become a mother herself, she found the situation intolerable. She literally decided that it would be better to kill herself and her baby than to risk becoming like her own mother.

Pregnancy gives a woman nine months to work on the transformation of her deepest sense of self and to work out new patterns if the old ones are unacceptable. It is this work that underlies the introspection that has so often been found to characterize pregnant women. Shereshefski and Yarrow describe the state:

> Much of the need for aloneness concerns itself with the matter of looking ahead—daydreaming, weaving fantasies about the infant, seeing themselves in the new role of mother. The women were in the process of giving up much that had been meaningful in the past and at the same time reorganizing their psychological resources to look toward the future. This was work for the woman at this period of her life: relinquishing her hold on an earlier phase of her life, to some extent mourning the

loss of the old self, and looking to the new phase and tasks ahead—work of the pregnancy period that seemed meaningful and necessary to many of the women. Possibly it yielded dividends in adaptability during the time of waiting and, later, in achievement of psychological readiness to meet maternal responsibilities.*

This psychological work of pregnancy is harder for some people than for others. Some women need to do more than others. An individual who shows no sign of upheaval or change may not be preparing herself. This may be as true for a man as a woman. A professional should ask, Why is this person acting as though nothing is happening?

It occasionally turns out that an individual dares not experience pregnancy as real because she is very afraid that something may go wrong. She does not really believe that she is going to have a baby at all. This may be because she, or women close to her, have lost babies at term, and she must wait to see a healthy baby before she risks forming an attachment to the idea of a child.

STAGES OF PREGNANCY

Pregnancy has been defined as a developmental stage with an expectable progression (Caplan, 1957). Certain emotional concerns are more characteristic of one stage than of another. In other words, the psychological work changes as pregnancy progresses.

It is normal and expectable for a woman at first to think of pregnancy as an event in her own body. She may not conceptualize the baby at all. This is understandable, as the first signs of pregnancy are all body changes: sensitive nipples, enlarged breasts, thickened waistline, perhaps nausea. None of these changes are experienced as due to the presence or development of the fetus.

The psychological task of this early phase of pregnancy is generally to recognize and acknowledge the pregnancy, incorporating it as a real fact of life, and to begin appropriate plans for the future (which may mean getting an abortion rather than moving on to the subsequent stages of pregnancy). Women who have delayed pregnancy for several years, either by choice or because of fertility problems, may have used the time to prepare for the idea of having a baby and may incorporate the idea faster than those who get pregnant without careful planning (Bing & Colman, 1980). In practice,

the psychological work of pregnancy often begins when a couple stops using contraceptives. Where it does, the concerns will not be related to body changes but may manifest themselves as a preoccupation with health (especially diet and exercise) or with a reevaluation of the parental generation.

The first perceptible movement of the fetus is a significant event for most women. In the early months, they may be haunted by a feeling that the baby is dead. Once they feel movement, this fear is generally allayed. The woman begins to differentiate the baby from her own inner organs. She knows it is hers, but not her. This comes as a gradual awareness, not as a sudden discovery. For most women, the baby becomes increasingly real as the pregnancy progresses, although some perfectly healthy women continue to think only of the pregnancy and not of the baby until as late as the eighth or ninth month.

The baby becomes increasingly differentiated, personalized, and even individuated as the mother begins to perceive the baby's unique habits of sleep and wake, feels elbows and feet, and knows where the head is. This is important preparation for the inevitable separation that occurs at birth and beyond.

The word *postpartum* literally means "after the separation." The physical separation takes place at birth, although even that is not as complete as the term suggests. When there is continued contact between mother and child, birth becomes a transitional moment rather than an abrupt separation.

It is most satisfying to talk of the dynamics of the childbearing year as continuous, but the actual experience often seems discontinuous. Pregnancy and postpartum require different coping styles. Some women are good at one stage but have trouble with another. Each event builds on the experience of the preceding phase. A situation that is expectable and appropriate at one stage may be a sign of trouble at another. For example, a disbelief in the separate reality of the baby is expectable in the first four months of pregnancy, common in the middle period, and not too disturbing even at the end of pregnancy. If it continues postpartum, however, it can be a sign of severe pathology and can prevent the mother from being able to care for her infant. Similarly, anxiety about labor is appropriate in the last six weeks of pregnancy, but when it is acute in the first trimester, it hints that the woman is using this event in a special way. She may have reason to fear it because of events in her past, such as a previous difficult birth or the knowledge of traumatic births in women close to her. She may also be focusing on the birth as a single event on which to place all her anxiety about

---

*From Shereshefski, P., & Yarrow, L.J. (1973). *Psychological aspects of a first pregnancy and early postnatal adaptation.* New York: Raven Press. With permission.

becoming a mother and, in the process, ignoring all the other issues of pregnancy.

The progress of pregnancy should be toward a realistic appraisal of the woman's support system. This often occurs through a process of reevaluating her relationships with the important people in her life, especially her mother and the father of the baby (Colman & Colman, 1977). A rather fantastic and idealistic image of what will happen often gives way to a more realistic picture of what is likely to happen. Thus, pregnancy is more than just an event in itelf; it is also a preparation for the future.

CURRENT LIFE STRESSES

Pregnancy is an expectable life crisis; as such, it brings certain expectable stresses to the people who participate in it. Holmes and Rahe (1967) devised a chart of life changes, called the Social Readjustment Rating Scale, that assigns points for the degree of stress created by various life situations. In it, they assume that every change, positive or negative, creates stress. Their list ranges from 100 points for death of spouse to eleven points for minor violations of the law (e.g., traffic tickets). They say that a person with a total score of over 300 points in a single year has an eighty percent chance of a significant illness within two years.

Pregnancy is assigned 40 points on the Social Readjustment Scale. Gaining a new family member through birth or adoption receives 39 points. This means that a person who has just had a baby starts out with a remarkably high score for the year. It is easy to accumulate enough additional stress points to be at high risk for illness, since it is rare for a child (especially a first child) to be born without other changes occurring at the same time. Parenthood often precipitates new career directions in both parents. Women often take a leave of absence or quit a job entirely when they become mothers, while men frequently take on an extra job or seek a promotion when they know they are becoming fathers. It is also extremely common for a family to move either before or after a baby is born. Moving is worth 25 points; a major change in financial state is worth 38; a major change in responsibilities at work is worth 29. Some further changes are forced by the presence of a baby: a major change in the usual type and/or amount of recreation (nineteen points) and a major change in sleeping habits (16 points). Holmes and Rahe estimate that people with 150–299 Life Change Units run a fifty percent chance of getting sick in the near future.

Change is inherently stressful, and pregnancy is a process of change that entails deep psychological reorganization. The security of one's former self may seem to break apart while a new structure of personal identity is being created. This may be a realistic preparation for new life demands, but it is also a great deal of upheaval. Individuals who are subjected to other major changes at the same time may be expected to have trouble coping.

STAGE IN THE LIFE CYCLE

Pregnancy should be expected to have radically different meanings for a teenager than for a woman in her thirties. Socially, the twenties are often thought of as the most appropriate time to have a baby, although the thirties are also increasingly seen as appropriate, even for a first child. The woman's experience of her pregnancy will be affected by her sense of it as either appropriate and conflict-free, or as inappropriate and conflictual.

Absolute age is not the only factor that determines the individual's stage in the life cycle. It is important to keep in mind the stage of psychological development, which may be ahead of or behind the average for any age. Some 18-year-olds are ready to move away from their family of origin and direct their energy to their new family; some 35-year-olds remain so emotionally invested in their parents that they cannot believe in themselves as competent adults. The individual case will rarely conform to the general rule, but some patterns can be expected to reflect absolute age.

A 15-year-old in our society is appropriately still dependent on her parents. Even without pregnancy, she can be expected to be struggling with issues of maturity and may doubt her own adult competence. Society at large would not blame her for feeling unready to set up a household away from her parents. The main support system for a pregnant teenager will probably be her family of origin. She may have few peers in a comparable situation, and even if she has a husband, she is not likely to have had much time to develop a secure and trusting relationship with him.

At 21, a woman may still be struggling with issues of maturity and may still doubt her own competence, but she is likely to be able to set up a household separate from her parents. She may still be extremely dependent on them and may feel conflicts of allegiance between the family of her childhood and the family in which she herself is a parent, but these are feelings that she will probably be ready to resolve.

By 30, many women have already worked through their separation from their parents (especially from their mothers), and may have even entered a phase of reconciliation in which they are secure in their individuality and are not afraid of becoming dependent on their families for help during pregnancy or in the postpartum period. Older women are also more likely to have had time to establish a more intimate and long-term relationship with the baby's father. Since the childbearing year is a time that a woman needs both physical and emotional support, it becomes a time when dependency needs are stronger than usual. An older woman may be able to let people take care of her without fearing regression into a childish role.

Like a young teenager, a woman at the end of her childbearing years may have very few peers in her situation, but she is very different from the teenager in all other regards. A 40-year-old woman can rarely expect to find her own mother ready or able to play a role in caretaking. Her isolation may become a problem, but it is more likely that the pregnancy has been an active and conscious choice and that the woman is using it as a "last chance" to create a baby and become a mother.

The contrasting experience of two women of different ages when they had their first child is highlighted by the following cases.

Case 3

Sally was a 17-year-old high school student when she became pregnant. Her boyfriend married her, and she continued to attend school. The pregnancy was extremely uncomfortable for her, especially because she felt that "everyone" (especially her parents) now knew about her sex life. She was extremely labile and cried much of the time. She and her young husband lived with her parents. When she was in the final trimester, she switched to a special school for pregnant teenagers.

Once the baby was born, Sally found life wonderful. She loved the baby and enjoyed playing with it. Her mother was around to help much of the time. In addition, she found a neighborhood woman who took the baby in while Sally returned to high school.

While Sally found pregnancy a nightmare, she found motherhood a delight. She had a lot of help and support and was amazed to find that she was really good with the baby.

Case 4

Jane was a 32-year-old social worker when she became pregnant. She had wanted a child for years, but she felt she should wait until everything was "perfect." She wanted to make sure that she and her husband had "time to get to know one another" and she wanted to be financially secure. When these goals were achieved and she finally felt "ready," she stopped using contraceptives and became pregnant soon afterwards.

Jane's pregnancy was a delight. She felt special, more alive and radiant. She continued to work and felt that everyone was envious of her condition.

After the baby was born, Jane took a nose dive. Suddenly, she didn't feel perfect. When the baby cried, she couldn't always stop it. Her husband was working long hours and often became irritable when the baby fussed in the evenings. Her friends from work stopped visiting. She missed her work and felt guilty every time she thought about leaving the baby.

While pregnancy did not disrupt life for Jane, motherhood changed everything. She lost her former way of life and did not have much support for her new way of life. Her parents were far away; her husband and her friends did not know or care much about baby care; she found herelf lonely and bored. Worst of all, she found that she could not be the perfect mother, even after she had planned everything so carefully. She, like many women her age, felt an intense conflict between her desire to be a good mother and her desire to continue her career with minimal disruption. Sally felt none of this conflict, for she had no expectation of being a good mother and did not have a career.

Pregnancy, like every crisis, triggers a reevaluation of the question Who am I? A woman must integrate a sense of herself as a mother with her prior identity. This process will be radically affected by the nature of that prior identity. Someone still in the flux of adolescence is already working on issues of creating an adult identity. Motherhood becomes part of that process. Someone who has already established a fixed sense of herself as an adult will need to open herself up again to a new level of change. Her prior adult adjustment must give way to a new situation.

Such popular books as *Passages* (Sheehy, 1974) and *The Seasons of a Man's Life* (Levinson et al., 1978) have raised our awareness of the expected changes of adult development. They focus on the identity changes that occur when moving from one phase of life to another. However, they put little emphasis on the developmental transformations caused by family life. There is a need for more work on understanding the role of parental experience on personal identity (Daniels & Weingarten, 1977).

SYMBOLIC MEANINGS OF PREGNANCY

Pregnancy has important symbolic values in every culture. The exaggerated sexual organs of the childbearing are among the earliest known artifacts created in the stone age. The mysteries of fertility and the creation of life are at the center of most religions. Even men, who conspicuously lack a womb and childbearing organs, have wondered at the miracle of birth and have tried to find a way to create a child themselves. Zeus gave birth to Athena from his own head; Pygmalian created a statue so lifelike that it became an ideal woman (George Bernard Shaw chose the name *Pygmalion* for his play about a professor who transformed a cockney flower girl into an elegant beauty); Dr. Frankenstein constructed his famous monster; and today, there are men trying to create babies in test tubes. Psychoanalyst Karen Horney has suggested that civilization, predominantly the product of creative acts by men, is sublimation for their inability to give birth to a human being (Horney, 1967).

In the twentieth century, as in all ages, pregnant women are subject to special taboos and rites throughout the world. The specific beliefs reflect the underlying values of the society (Mead, 1935; Mead & Newton, 1967). Thus, the Arapesh of New Guinea have a culture that relies on close cooperation between men and women. Appropriately, father and mother share in the care of an infant, even before it is born. They see it as the product of the father's sperm and the mother's menstrual blood. They believe that it is important for the parents to make love frequently early in the pregnancy, to help the baby grow. The father is, in essence, "feeding" it. When the pregnancy is well established, they initiate a taboo on sexual activity for both parents. Neither can have sexual intercourse from mid-pregnancy until the child is weaned several years later (Mead, 1935). In contrast, the Mundugumor have a society characterized by hostility and distance between the sexes. The pregnant and breast-feeding woman is sexually taboo, but the father suffers no such restraints. If he can afford to, he takes a new wife rather than suffer any inconvenience from the pregnancy.

In our own technological society, we use the medical care system to express the specialness of the childbearing year. There are few other times when a healthy individual receives so much constant attention from modern technology as during pregnancy and birth. This reflects the society's faith in medical science. Individuals and subcultures in the United States who do not share the larger society's values seek alternatives that reflect their views of the meaning of pregnancy and birth. Some use birth to make a political statement in rebellion against "the establishment"—for example, by having their babies at home with the assistance of lay midwives. Some seek to return birth to the hands of women. Most who choose alternative care systems are simply trying to create an environment in which they will feel safe. Many people feel safe in the hands of "experts" who

"know best." Others hesitate to yield control to anyone else. Pregnancy and birth are a time of transformation. It is important that people trust their caretakers when they make the passage.

The meaning that pregnancy holds for a woman may radically shape her experience. This section will explore some of the more common meanings that pregnancy and birth can hold and the effects of these meanings.

The Ultimate Creative Act

Pregnancy is the ultimate symbol of—or, more pragmatically, the concrete example of and model for—all other forms of creativity. The act of conceiving and gestating a human being within one's body is a miracle beyond comprehension. Other creative acts pale beside it.

The concept of pregnancy as a creative act is generally very positive and even exhilarating. Sometimes, however, it can be disturbing. Some women experience a conflict between their desire to be passively, biologically creative and their desire to be more actively, productively creative. They feel the pull toward the biological creativity as a regression away from career success. This may be threatening to their sense of themselves as competent individuals in the work world.

Perhaps the people with most conflicts surrounding pregnancy as a creative event are artistic men (Colman & Colman, 1981). It is the one thing they cannot do. It is not unusual for writers, artists, and other men who have devoted their lives to creativity to feel ambivalent and even impotent in the face of a pregnancy. This has aptly been called "womb envy."

Birth and Rebirth

Pregnancy obviously creates a life for the infant, but it also can be seen as creating a new life for all members of the family. It is not unusual for a woman to get pregnant when she is open for a change. When the yearning for a new life for herself is particularly strong in a woman, she may find it easier to create that new life through a pregnancy than through another form of change. Thus, women often get pregnant when they are about to graduate from high school, college, or graduate school; when they are bored with a job; when they feel like moving; or when they are becoming dissatisfied with a relationship.

Case 5

Stacy was 31 years old. Her first child had been born nine months after her marriage in her first year out of college. Her second child was born two years later. At 29, when both children were in school, Stacy began training as a dental technician. She was on the brink of graduation and about to face the challenge of her first real job when she found herself unexpectedly pregnant. Although disappointed that she would now devote another five years to child care, Stacy was also deeply relieved to be able to return to a pattern that she understood and to defer the movement into a new life phase.

It is obvious that Stacy could have continued with her work plans and found an alternative child care system, but she chose to return to full-time parenting. For women like Stacy, pregnancy and mothering are secure identities that can give life meaning. Pregnancy can be used to avoid the exploration of other aspects of self.

The reverse can also be true: the experience of having created a new life for herself may make it possible for a woman to get pregnant. This is the phenomenon that seems to occur for women who are unable to conceive, adopt a child, and then conceive a child in addition.

Case 6

Connie was a businesswoman who had tried to get pregnant with her first husband while she was in her twenties. She did not conceive right away, but she did realize that the relationship was not a good one. She resumed using contraceptives, got a divorce, and moved to another city. Several years later, at the age of 32, she remarried, stopped using contraceptives, but still did not conceive. She was by then a corporate vice-president. After two years of trying to get pregnant, her gynecologist told her that she would never conceive. Her reaction to the news was to quit her job and start a business of her own, one that she specifically described as being "more creative" than anything she had done before. During the week that she moved into her new office, her gynecologist confirmed what she had begun to suspect: she was at last pregnant.

Connie's story reflects the way in which a pregnancy can be the manifestation of a real readiness for a new life style. As she said in her ninth month: "When I see you next time, I may not even recognize you; I may forget everything about my former life."

The hope for a "new life" is both real and illusory. It is clear that things are different after the baby is born, but this difference is not necessarily magical. Families who are optimistic about parenting and who are truly ready to incorporate change can find the postpartum an exciting time. Occasionally, however, the new life may seem discontinuous with the past. A woman, in particular, may find it almost impossible to integrate her sense of herself as a mother with her sense of herself as a competent adult.

Case 7

Fran had taken a six-month leave of absence to have her child but did not really expect to return to work. To her surprise, she did not like staying at home, so she returned to work. "Coming back to work was almost like starting a new job. I was a different person, I was Mary's mommy coming back to work, and I was becoming Fran Funston again and not Mary's mommy."

A woman who has a positive image of mothers and mothering may have an easier time feeling good about the new life that has been created for herself as well as for her child.

A Rite of Passage into Adulthood

Some women see pregnancy as the ultimate initiation into womanhood. It may be sought or avoided as a symbol of becoming an adult.

Case 8

Patty came to therapy because she was depressed after her father's death. The week that she started treatment, she also learned that she was pregnant. A single woman with ten years of successful contraceptive use behind her, Patty had been careless about inserting her diaphragm. She elected to have an abortion. In the period before the abortion, Patty felt "plugged up" and "blocked." She could not get in touch with her feelings about her father, though she was very close to her feelings about her mother, who had died eight years earlier. She also made a clear connection between the man who had impregnated her and her father.

Immediately after the abortion, Patty was elated; she was at last "unplugged." She mourned for her father but also talked about the "new life" she was going to make for herself, a life that would be adult and independent and creative for the first time. She felt that pregnancy had signaled her movement into adulthood.

Although Patty's case was complicated by her fantasies about her father's role in her pregnancy, the fact that the two events coincided in her life was not an accident. Patty felt that she had experienced herself as "Daddy's girl" and had been unable to grow up as long as he was alive. With his death, she could at last try her wings as an adult. She literally killed off "his" infant and started over. Another woman, Lori, stated the same assumption during her pregnancy: "I think becoming a mother is tantamount for me to becoming a woman, working through giving up the child in me and becoming a woman."

When a woman has an abortion or gives her baby up for adoption, she may be unconsciously rejecting "the child in me." Since a fetus is often experienced as a part of the self, it may never be fully objectified, particularly if the mother never knows or cares for the infant. But by symbolically "giving up" the "child in me," a woman does not necessarily become a competent adult. This is a rejection of childishness and, perhaps, a false vision of the nature of maturity. A person operating from this dynamic may need extra help in the early postpartum period in recognizing that the child is not just a symbol of her own regressive impulses but also has an external reality of its own. She may have to learn to take care of its needs; she may also have to learn that even mothers can relax and have fun.

Case 9

Lori (quoted earlier) wanted to "give up the child in me and become a woman," but she had more trouble than she anticipated. She became extremely regressed around the time of birth and acknowledged that she had always enjoyed getting sick and being waited on. It was a time to lie back and be nostalgic. But she was so absorbed in her own experience that she did not have much interest in the baby. At the same time she felt worthless and asked her husband, "Now that I've given you a son, will you abandon me?" She became so fatigued at two weeks' postpartum that she described it as "a numbness of just not being there. It's scary, like being dead."

Lori experienced giving birth as a death—the death of "the child within her." She spent her postpartum period trying to return to life and eventually "found herself" by returning to work full time. Only then did she feel that she had come back to life; it was like "my past life that I had managed to salvage."

Proof of Womanhood

Childbirth, rather than pregnancy, is often chosen as the moment of passage, the proof of womanhood. This is an understandable focus, for childbirth is a single, dramatic event rather than a prolonged period of development. Unfortunately, childbirth is an initiation rite that can only partially be controlled. A woman who has decided to base her evaluation of her worth as a woman on her passage through the birth experience may have trouble dealing with unavoidable complications. She may experience herself as a failure because of a cephalopelvic disproportion or may go in the opposite direction and be disappointed that her labor was too short and too easy to provide the suffering necessary to mark an initiation.

It is safe to assume that every woman has an agenda for childbirth. The most common agenda is probably to get through it as easily as possible and have a healthy baby at the end. However, not all people have an adaptive agenda. When childbirth is conceptualized as an initiation rite, some women feel they need to suffer. Others feel just the opposite, that a "real" woman will experience no pain. Sometimes a birthing woman wants to prove to her caretakers, especially her partner,

that they can never take care of all her needs. Other women want to show their partners how much they must suffer.

If a woman fails in her agenda, she may feel compelled to try to repeat the experience. Sometimes a woman is satisfied with her mode of childbirth at the time, but later goes through changes that leave her with something new to prove. In such a situation, she may become pregnant to experience the birth more than to have a baby.

Case 10

Susan had moved directly from her father's home to that of her first husband. She had two children in her early twenties. In her early thirties, she felt the urge to become independent. She became a feminist, and by the time she was 34 she had left her husband and had trained to be a nurse. Within six months, however, she became pregnant with a man she hardly knew. They decided to marry and keep the baby (it would be his first). For Susan this was an opportunity to "do it right," which meant without medication and without the overdependence on men and medicine that she had had in her earlier experiences. To her surprise, however, she spent most of her pregnancy yearning for the protective arms of her first husband.

Susan, like many women, had two agendas, one conscious (to prove her maturity and competence) and the other unconscious (to be protected by a strong, loving man).

Birth is a powerful event; it also results in a baby that requires care. A woman who has unresolved issues related to the birth may have trouble getting on with the job of parenting (Affonso, 1977).

A Symbol of Sexuality

The need to prove one's fertility is a deep, if not always rational, impulse in both men and women. It is based on the need to reproduce, a need that is as crucial for the survival of the race as the need to eat and excrete. This desire for immortality can be expressed through art; its fundamental manifestation is through having a baby.

The desire for fertility is essentially sexual but not necessarily erotic. Pregnancy is tied up with feelings about erotic sexuality. It is the explicit evidence of sexual activity and involves the transformation of the sex organs. Few people pass through the childbearing year with their sexuality unchanged. Some find themselves far more erotic than usual (Bing & Colman, 1978). Many others find themselves abstaining from sexual contact for long periods. Many societies place sexual taboos on the childbearing couple or at least on the full-term and postpartum mother (Ford & Beach, 1970). Our own culture has a deeply ingrained image of the new mother as pristine and asexual. This madonna image denies erotic impulses and makes it difficult for a woman to feel sexy and maternal at the same time.

Many women feel that they become more comfortable with their bodies and more open in their sexuality as a result of having a baby (Masters & Johnson, 1966). They feel that the extreme physical changes and the physical intimacy of both the birth itself and the care of an infant make them less self-conscious about body parts. The idea that sexual activity can create a baby adds magic and pleasure to the sex act for some people.

An Expression of the Relationship with the Mother

Women often get pregnant in response to unconscious feelings about their own mothers, or even their daughters (Morgan, 1979; Nilsson, et al., 1971).

A teenager may get pregnant with the clear intention of giving the baby to her mother. This may be related to her own guilt about leaving home. She wants to get free from her parents and yet is afraid to leave her mother with no one to care for. The baby is intended as a guilt offering to the mother. Such daughters rarely check with their mothers to learn whether they really want to take care of an infant. It is generally the daughter's need to feel that the mother is safely at home protecting an infant rather than the mother's need to have a baby that motivates these pregnancies. A young mother who has been counting on her mother's help may be shocked to learn, either during the pregnancy or after the baby is born, that her mother has her own life to lead and prefers outside employment to child care.

Daughters occasionally become pregnant when they learn that their mothers are menopausal, as though to give a gift to the mother—or, in a more hostile vein, to prove that they are now the potent generation. The reverse also occurs: a mother becomes pregnant when her daughter begins to menstruate. In such a case, the older generation is proving that it is not yet ready to yield power to the younger generation. When such competitiveness is unspoken, it may manifest itself through the teenaged daughter refusing to help the mother.

The blurring boundaries between mother and daughter may be most extreme in psychotic or borderline cases, but the same feelings can occur in normal individuals. There is a certain appropriateness in the younger generation taking over the childbearing func-

tion from the older generation. In healthy families, it is done with the blessing rather than with the envy of the elders.

Pregnancies that are used as statements to another person rarely work out well for the expectant mother and seldom please the other person. This is true whether it is a daughter flaunting her sexuality at her mid-life mother, a mother showing up her pubescent daughter, or a wife defying her unwilling husband.

An Expression of the Relationship with the Husband

Pregnancy can be a very healthy and wonderful expression of the union between a man and a woman. When a woman becomes pregnant with the willing participation of a man, the partners can experience it as a creation of their own new life, as the movement into a new phase, as the completion of their sexual life together.

Sometimes, however, women get pregnant "for" their men in the way they get pregnant "for" their mother or daughter. Sometimes a woman does not particularly want a child herself but uses her womb to create it for her partner. Occasionally, the husband wants the baby more than the wife and will assume full care of it. More frequently, however, the woman finds herself assuming all the burdens of parenting even though she was not the one who wanted the baby. Understandably, this situation produces conflict and frustration in the mother.

Even when a man does assume full responsibility for a baby, a woman can experience deep conflicts. She may feel pushed out of her "rightful" role as a mother. Both partners may experience profound sexual and identity confusion when this occurs.

The most common reason to get pregnant "for" a man is to cement the relationship or to attempt to change an independent, uncaring man into a more family-oriented man. The romantic fantasy of a woman who feels out of touch with her man and hopes that by having his baby she will attract his attention and bind him to her is one of the most familiar stories of pregnancy.

A Trap

While unwanted pregnancies have always been thought of as something to be avoided, especially by single women, the ability to actually avoid or terminate a pregnancy has not been widespread until this generation. The pronatalism of the 1950s was followed by a streak of antinatalism in the late 1960s and through the 1970s. Many women who came of age in this era—and particularly women who felt that their own mothers' lives had been ruined by childbearing and mothering—see pregnancy as the ultimate trap (Colman, 1978). Even when they carefully delay pregnancy until they are ready, and even when they consciously make the choice to become a mother, they still often feel the conflict inherent in their condition. They are so used to associating pregnancy and mothering with all that is negative in the female condition that they have trouble enjoying the condition or finding anything positive about themselves. Like Lori, quoted earlier, they may experience the childbearing year as discontinuous with their usual sense of self. They may express a fear of dying, of suffocating, of smothering, or of strangling. This may remain an anxiety throughout the pregnancy and may become more acute in the postpartum-period. It seems to be resolved by returning to work after the baby is born. The feeling seems to be an expression of the loss of freedom combined with a fear of being drawn inevitably into the stereotypical role of a self-sacrificing, dependent, housewife-mother.

Support groups and child care courses are particularly valuable for women who have trouble feeling comfortable about themselves in the role of mother. Instructors and group leaders can become important models of women who recognize the difficulties of raising children but who are still able to experience joy in mothering.

RELATIONSHIP WITHIN THE FAMILY

The symbolic meanings discussed in the preceding sections carry implications for the experience of the childbearing year. A symbolic statement made through the act of conception will pervade a woman's experience during the pregnancy and with the baby. Yet such meanings do not occur in a vacuum and are not exclusive to women. They occur in a family unit and can also be experienced by men, grandparents, and children.

The meaning of pregnancy is often related to an experience of blurred boundaries between the individual members of a family. Thus, a woman gets pregnant because her mother wants a baby; a man thinks that he is the one who is carrying the fetus; a child experiences him- or herself as the fetus in the mother's womb. These are tendencies in all people. When we are in close relationships with other people, we become empathic with them: we know how they feel, and we share their

experience; we almost feel at one with them (Colman & Colman, 1975).

The experience of union between family members can be exciting and wonderful for individuals who feel safe and who are reasonably comfortable with their own ego boundaries. A temporary rush of identification with another member of the family can be a positive experience. For people who have never achieved secure separation or who have found that merger with another was a dangerous experience, it can be a problem.

Pregnancy is a time when members of a family are particularly susceptible to boundary confusion. Pregnancy is the result of a sexual union and the emotional union that is called "love" (Colman & Colman, 1974). This produces the genetic union of two individuals into one new person. Furthermore, the hormonal changes of pregnancy probably predispose a woman to experiencing empathy and caring for others (Newton, 1973). The experience is dominated by the singular phenomenon of one human being actually living inside of another. The fetus is often in the minds of other members of the family as dramatically as it is in the body of the expectant mother.

There are problems inherent in the overidentification of one member of the family with another. If a mother cannot differentiate between herself and her infant, she will have trouble acting like a caretaking adult (Pugh et al., 1963). If she "becomes" the infant, she may regress to the point that she needs "babying," and will need help discovering the mother half of the dyad within herself.

It is appropriate to have only a faint boundary between a mother and her fetus and even between a mother and her infant. The theory of bonding is based on an assumption of the powerful linkage. We are learning more and more about the dangers of disrupting this bond too precipitously. Mothers and infants seem to benefit from growing into their separateness gradually. It is becoming apparent that the physical and emotional closeness between mother and infant is a healthy part of the childbearing process (Mahler, 1968). It does not necessarily lead to overprotective parenting or to prolonged symbiosis. The mother who is secure in her union may be able to move more comfortably into the subsequent stages of physical and emotional separation from her growing child.

All of us began in symbiotic dyad with our mothers. We may have had another primary caretaker, but that person then became the other half of our initial dyad until we developed an awareness of others around us and, eventually, an awareness of our own separate existence. Because these were our psychological origins, we are all capable of returning to a state of union with others (Benedek, 1970; Nilsson et al., 1971).

The experience of pregnancy can reactivate the sense of merger with the mother. It often feels to a pregnant woman as though she is not the "real" mother. That other woman who was the original mother suddenly becomes very important; if the original mother has been rejected as an inadequate or a cruel person, the experience of union with her can be extremely frightening.

The experience of merger with the mother can also be a strong and supportive element in a woman's adjustment to becoming a mother. It can give her confidence in her maternal role and help her feel secure and cared for while she is taking care of her infant—as long as the younger woman is not afraid of being destroyed or supplanted by the older woman.

The husband–wife relationship superficially appears to be quite different from the mother–child relationship. In our society, it does not begin with a symbiotic situation in which one is totally dependent on the other. Nor is it based on an assumption of ever-decreasing dependence. Nevertheless, the marital bond is very profound. The cultural ideal of "romantic love" is as strong as the ideal of "mother love." The couple is seen as a social unit, but it often becomes a psychological unit as well. Through sexuality, the partners can achieve a physical bond as intimate and profound as that between mother and infant.

When two mature adults marry (especially, if they marry after a period of living together), they often subscribe to the notion that they are separate individuals. Evidence of a blurring of the ego boundaries between them can be experienced as frightening. Nevertheless, such blurring can occur, especially during pregnancy. It is manifested most directly by men who develop physical symptoms when their wives are pregnant. This intimacy takes the form of sympathetic morning sickness, weight gain, headaches, and abdominal cramps in "pregnant" men. Occasionally a man will overidentify with the pregnant woman and lose touch with himself as a man, but generally the close identification between the man and the woman is a positive and enriching part of the marriage.

Parenting places new stresses on a marriage, perhaps especially for a marriage that has been based on equality and comradery. Few couples can achieve equal roles in parenting. The heavily biological nature of pregnancy, birth, and lactation exaggerate the differences between the sexes. Men often feel impotent in the face of such conspicuously superior equipment for parenting. Furthermore, most men have not been socialized to expect to participate fully in the care of an infant. Husband and wife may feel estranged from each other and jealous of the baby if they are not careful to express how they are feeling about their respective situations. Too often, each feels overburdened and isolated. It is a particularly important time for open communication and cooperation.

Pregnancy initiates the need to develop a new identity for the family as a whole as well as for the individuals within it. This is not necessarily a smooth process. While there are so many intimate dyads (mother–fetus; husband–wife; wife–mother; husband–mother; husband–father), there are also many opportunities for rivalry. A man who sees his wife absorbed with the fetus or the infant may simultaneously wish he were the baby, wish he were the wife, and feel like a rejected outsider. Other members of the family can feel equally estranged. All family members may be subject to mood swings and depression, as well as joy and elation, during the childbearing year.

COUNSELING IN THE CHILDBEARING YEAR

Extra attention to psychological matters can significantly affect the outcome of pregnancy. This has been demonstrated by at least two ambitious studies that compared an experimental group, who received psychological testing and interviews, with a control group, who received routine perinatal care. In both studies, the experimental group had significantly less illness and depression than the controls (Kumar & Robson, 1978; Shereshefski & Yarrow, 1973).

On the basis of her experience in a large study, Shereshefski recommends supportive counseling during pregnancy. The lability and access to dreams that are characteristic of pregnant women have caused some psychotherapists to see pregnant women as quite disturbed (Bibring, 1959). This may be misleading. Crisis theory suggests that this openness is part of a life transition and in the service of growth and change rather than a sign of great psychological fragility. Counseling that is directed toward insight as well as support can help an individual search for an answer to the question Who am I? The openness to a new answer to that old question is appropriate preparation for the new identity that must be established as part of the process of accepting a new member into the family.

Some women feel that they are "breaking down" or

"going crazy" because of the rapid mood changes, irrational outbursts, sudden obsession with their mothers, impatience with their husbands, disturbing dreams, and fears that the baby will be born deformed. These anxieties can be very disturbing. Counseling can reassure a woman of her normalcy and at the same time explore the reasons for the disturbing thoughts. Insight into the reasons for experiencing upheaval and insecurity can be of great benefit to the expectant mother; it gives meaning to an otherwise chaotic experience. Counseling can help a woman anticipate the future, integrate the past, and maintain some sense of continuity throughout a period that too often feels discontinuous with the rest of her life.

A woman who has lost or rejected her own mother is a particularly appropriate candidate for counseling, for she is seeking a new identity without an immediate model to draw from. In our rapidly changing society, almost every woman might be said to be doing the same. Support groups are particularly helpful, both during pregnancy and in the postpartum.

Couple and family work is also beneficial during the childbearing year. This chapter has emphasized the psychodynamics of pregnancy for the pregnant woman, but the dynamics may be even more disturbing for the expectant father, and he is so seldom recognized as passing through a significant transition that it may be even more difficult for him to find support at this time.

The Role of the Nurse

Because of their regular contact with women during the prenatal and postnatal visits, female nurses may be in particularly good positions to provide meaningful support and reassurance during pregnancy. They can have an important positive effect on women and their families simply by being attentive and accepting negative as well as positive feelings.

Women are often more emotionally dependent and needy in the childbearing year than at other times. This makes them particularly likely to turn to professionals for help and support. Pregnant women often make a positive transference to a particular nurse. This means simply that the nurse will become very important to the patient because of traits that the patient projects onto the nurse rather than because of any real perception of the nurse as a person. Professionals are understandably flattered and excited by this transference, which makes them the very models of competent, caretaking adults. They feel as wise and good as the patient thinks they are. The problem inherent in the situation is that since the transference comes from the needs of the patient as

much as from the objective characteristics of the caregiver, it is subject to sudden and irrational shifts. A patient with particularly strong dependency needs may expect the nurse to take care of everything and may cling to each casual remark as though it were a sacred truth. A patient who has been rejected or abandoned in the past may start out idealizing the nurse but may rapidly project her previous experience onto the present situation and accuse the nurse, in various ways, of not taking enough care of her. The nurse may feel bewildered by the hostility she feels from someone who seemed to adore her just a few weeks before.

Case 11

Ellen had elected to deliver in an alternative birth center with a midwife and to use a childbirth educator as labor coach. She and her husband were both unemployed and spent much of their time in bars. Their relationship was highly unstable; both knew that he was not the father of the child. When she went into labor, Ellen remained calm and collected. Her husband and several friends came with her to the hospital. The labor coach arrived soon afterwards. Everything seemed to be progressing normally at first. The friends were affable and supportive; the husband was attentive. Ellen seemed controlled and cooperative. She simply never dilated beyond 8 cm. As the hours went by, the crowd began to disperse. Eventually, there was no one left except the husband and the labor coach. The midwife checked on the progress from time to time, and staff nurses were continuously available. Ellen began demanding more and more attention from all of them.

After more than twenty-four hours in continuous attendance and during a lull in the labor, the labor coach left to check in with her own family and to eat. Ellen immediately went into hard labor. Her husband, the nurses, and the midwives all rushed to her assistance, but nothing could make her comfortable. An obstetrical resident (male) was called in. As soon as she saw him, Ellen calmed down. She was transferred to a traditional delivery room and soon gave birth without undue difficulty to a normal child.

There was probably nothing that the husband, the labor coach, the nurses or the midwives could have done to change the outcome of Ellen's labor. She needed to test their devotion, but she never really expected them to be able to help her. While consciously hostile toward authority, on an unconscious level Ellen really believed that only the physician, the symbol of institutional authority, would be able to help her. She re-created her life script as an abandoned child reared in a series of foster homes. As usual, the mother and fathers who were "supposed" to take care of her could not give her enough.

When caught in the web of a script like Ellen's, good

intentions and sincere interest are not enough to help the professional provide health care. The patient's unconscious dynamics may place severe limitations on the professional's ability to help.

The childbearing year is filled with anxiety, but also with optimism. Although the nurse would like to play a role in alleviating anxiety and facilitating the birth of a healthy, contented baby to a happy family, it is important to recognize that this is not always possible. The nurse's work situation generally places restrictions on the amount of time she can spend with each patient. Even if blessed with an unlimited amount of time and energy, there may be some patients who have deep-seated needs that cannot be met in an obstetrical setting.

The nurse performs the vital function of meeting the patient and assessing her emotional and physical status. She can provide reassurance and support and can do as much counseling as her expertise and time allow. She can be particularly helpful in specific trouble areas related to objective situations and can thus often be an effective counselor in sexual matters simply by providing some factual information. Anxiety and even family conflicts can often be alleviated through simple educative techniques.

It is important for the nurse to be sensitive to the difference between expectable anxiety created by the present life situation, which can generally be dealt with in an obstetrical setting through information and reassurance, and more disturbed patterns that reflect a deeper level of trouble with life in general, and are not alleviated by information or reassurance. It is not always easy to tell the difference between the two. When she feels herself being drained by a seemingly unlimited needfulness, a nurse may feel inadequate; it is more likely that this feeling is in response to the patient's disturbance. The best counseling tool that a professional may develop is a sense of when to refer a patient to another setting for additional help.

REFERENCES AND ADDITIONAL READINGS

Affonso, D. (1977). Missing pieces: A study of postpartum feelings. *Birth and the Family Journal, 4,* 159-164.

Benedek, T. (1970). The psychobiology of pregnancy. In P. Antony & T. Benedek (Eds.), *Parenthood.* Boston: Little, Brown.

Bibring, G. (1959). Some considerations of the psychological process of pregnancy. *Psychoanalytic Study of the Child, 14,* 113-121.

Bibring, G. (1961). A study of the psychological processes in pregnancy and the earliest mother-child relationship. *Psychoanalytic Study of the Child, 16,* 9-72.

Bing, E., & Colman, L. (1978). *Making love during pregnancy.* New York: Bantam.

Bing, E., & Colman, L. (1980). *Having a baby after thirty.* New York: Bantam.

Breen, D. (1980). *The birth of a first child.* New York: Methnen.

Brown, W. (1979). *Psychological care during pregnancy and the postpartum period.* New York: Raven Press.

Brown, W., & Shereshefski, P. (1972). Seven women: A prospective study of postpartum psychiatric disorders. *Psychiatry, 25,* 139-159.

Caplan, G. (1957). Psychological aspects of maternity care. *American Journal of Public Health, 47,* 25-31.

Caplan, G. (1960). *Emotional implications of pregnancy and the influences on family relationships in the healthy child.* Cambridge, Ma.: Howard University Press.

Colman, A. (1969). Psychological state during first pregnancy. *American Journal of Orthopsychiatry, 39,* 788-797.

Colman, A. (1971). Psychology of a first baby group. *International Journal of Group Psychotherapy, 21,* 74-83.

Colman, A., & Colman, L. (1975). *Love and ecstasy.* New York: Seabury.

Colman, A., & Colman, L. (1977). *Pregnancy: The psychological experience.* New York: Bantam.

Colman, L. (1978). Delayed childbearing: A descriptive study of twelve women having their first baby after the age of thirty. (Unpublished Ph.D. dissertation, Wright Institute, Berkeley, Ca.).

Colman, L., & Colman, A. (1981). *Earth father/sky mother.* Englewood Cliffs, N.J.: Prentice-Hall.

Colman, L., & Colman, A. (1974). Pregnancy as an altered state of consciousness. *Birth and the Family Journal, 1,* 7-11.

Daniels, P., & Weingarten, K. (1977). Now or later? The timing of parenthood in adult life. (Unpublished monograph, Center for Research on Women, Wellesley, Ma.).

Ford, C.S., & Beach, F.A. (1970). *Patterns of sexual behavior.* New York: Harper & Row.

Holmes, T., & Rahe, R., (1967). The Social Readjustment Rating Scale. *Journal of Psychosomatic Research, 11,* 213-218.

Horney, K. (1967). *Feminine psychology.* New York: Norton.

Kumar, R., & Robson, K. (1978). Neurotic disturbance during pregnancy and the puerperium: Preliminary report of a prospective survey of 119 primiparae. In M. Sandler (Ed.), *Mental illness in pregnancy and the puerperium.* New York: Oxford University Press.

Levinson, D., et al. (1978). *The seasons of a man's life.* New York: Knopf.

Mahler, M. (1968). *On human symbiosis and the vicissitudes of individuation.* New York: International Universities Press.

Masters, W.H., & Johnson, V.E. (1966). *The human sexual response.* Boston: Little, Brown.

Mead, M. (1935). *Sex and temperament in three primitive societies.* New York: Morrow.

Mead, M., & Newton, N. (1967). Cultural patterning of perinatal behavior. In S. Richardson & A. Guttmacher (Eds.), *Childbearing: Its sociological and psychological aspects.* Baltimore: Williams & Wilkins.

Morgan, E. (1979). The relationship of the primpara to her mother. (Unpublished Ph.D. dissertation, California School of Professional Psychology, Berkeley, Ca.).

Newton, N. (1973). The interrelationship between sexual responsiveness, birth, and breast feeding. In J. Zubin & J. Money (Eds.), *Contemporary sexual behavior: Critical issues in the 1970s.* Baltimore: Johns Hopkins University Press.

Nilsson, A., Uddenberg, N., & Almgren, P.E. (1971). Parental relations and identification in women with special regard to paranatal emotional adjustment. *Acta Psychiatrica Scandinavia, 47,* 77–153.

Pugh, T.F., Jerath, B.K., Schmidt, W.M., & Reed, R.B. (1963). Rates of mental illness related to childbirth. *New England Journal of Medicine, 268*(22), 1224–1228.

Sandler, M. (1978). *Mental illness in pregnancy and the puerperium.* New York: Oxford University Press.

Sheehy, G. (1974). *Passages.* New York: Dutton.

Shereshefski, P., & Yarrow, L.J. (1973). *Psychological aspects of a first pregnancy and early postnatal adaptation.* New York: Raven Press.

Chapter 2 | Parent–Infant Attachment

Ramona T. Mercer

U NTIL THE LATE 1960s, almost all research on attachment focused on either the development of or the behavioral characteristics of the attachment process of infants. Studies of mother–infant interactions concentrated on the relationship between sensory stimulation or deprivation and infant development. These studies did not focus on the development of parental ties that motivate and commit parents to two decades of supportive, nurturant care for a child. Although the enduring and profound effect of the mother–infant relationship on human personality development has been accepted since Freud's work, it was not until Kempe (1962) and his colleagues coined the term battered child syndrome, that widespread attention was turned to studying the attachment process in parents. Even then, research focused more on maternal than on paternal attachment.

Bowlby (1953) probably represented the thinking of the time in observing that the father had value "as the economic and emotional support of the mother." Authorities generally acknowledged that the child's most important relationship during the early years was with the mother. With the changing social and economic climate, in which women have sought fulfillment in roles apart from mothering, fathers have had the opportunity to assume more active roles in parent-

ing. Thus, in the 1970s the father's role became the focus of much more research.

This chapter presents some of the major theorists' views of the attachment process. The emphasis is on the parents, but the infant's role and the challenge to nurses are also discussed.

DEFINING ATTACHMENT

Object Relationships and Dependency

Attachment behaviors were first defined in terms of the infant's fear of loss of the mother as the primary attachment figure (Freud, 1959), and in terms of the loss or absence of a tie to a primary mothering person, as occurred in early institutions for infant care (Freud & Burlingham, 1944; Provence & Lipton, 1962). Attachment has been used synonymously with the terms *object relationship* and *object choice*. The terms come from the psychoanalytic views of the infant at birth as being unable to differentiate *self* from *other*, and as driven by internal tensions, such as hunger, to seek gratification through oral means. Through oral satisfaction (feeding and sucking), an infant gradually perceives a mother as a separate object and becomes dependent on her.

Attachment has also been used synonymously with *dependency* by some social-learning theorists for whom the secondary drive explains the beginning of the mother–infant relationship. (Primary drives include sex and feeling; secondary drives include human relationships.) Through dependency on the mother for gratification of all needs, an infant becomes oriented to her via her response. Bowlby (1958) noted that attachment and dependency are two different phenomena; although physiological dependency and psychological attachment are related, they are not the same. Bowlby (1977) later elaborated on this differentiation: dependency, unlike attachment, is not specifically related to maintaining proximity. It is not directed toward a specific individual, is not necessarily associated with strong feelings, and does not imply an enduring bond.

Attachment research has referred to a social process of human infants and of nonhuman animals of all ages. Attachment is an emotionally laden relationship with special motivational properties. Gewirtz (1972) noted that attachment research has combined psychoanalytic, ethological, and cognitive concepts to study the emotional dependency of animals that develops after prolonged contact with their mothers, often during the critical period following birth; dependency research has been used largely in the framework of learning theories. Gewirtz (1972) referred to attachment and dependency as parts of a reciprocal learning process that "serve as one explanation of many of the diverse [stimulus–response] phenomena commonly termed 'love'" (p. 157). As such, attachment and dependency are not age-specific but "may refer to behavior systems connoting reciprocal, dyadic patterns between any two people (child and adult, children, or adults)" (p. 142). According to Gewirtz, dependency relationships exert control over many of an individual's responses by discriminating and reinforcing stimuli exerted by a class of persons through their common physical and behavioral characteristics; in attachment relationships, only one particular person exerts this control over an individual's response.

Not only have the terms object relationship, dependency, and attachment been used interchangeably, they have also been used to refer to a developmental process, the outcome of that process, and both process and outcome at the same time (Gewirtz, 1972). Rosenthal (1973, pp. 201–202) argued that mother–infant interaction should be viewed as attachment itself rather than as a function of attachment.

> Attachment is not a "thing" resulting from an interaction between mother and infant but rather a characteristic of some patterns of interaction between mother and infant itself.

Lamb (1974, p. 382) countered that

> the hallmark of attachment is that it is an enduring affectional and specific bond, and the emphasis must be on the bond, not on the specific behaviors which mediate the attachment...[for behaviors] are certain to differ when comparisons are attempted between two or more mother–infant dyads.

Sroufe and Waters (1977) have observed that attachment behaviors do not remain constant across all situations but are influenced by the social context.

The continuous reciprocal interplay between two partners is an important part of the attachment process. Yarrow and Pederson (1972) identified two major factors in infant attachment that seem applicable in all attachment dyads: first, it is a contingent relationship (i.e., one partner responds to the other's signals with a high degree of sensitivity), and second, a quantity and quality of social stimulation occurs within the relationship. Therefore, the cognitive and social development of an individual reflects capacities and abilities for attachment.

Ainsworth (1964) included affective, cognitive, and interactional behavioral components in defining attachment, and specified that attachment implied affection and discrimination through specificity to a person. These affective, cognitive, and interactional behaviors were included in the components of maternal attachment as defined by Robson and Moss (1970, p. 977):

> the extent to which a mother feels that her infant occupies an essential position in her life...feelings of warmth or love, a sense of possession, devotion, protectiveness, and concern for the infant's well-being, positive anticipation of prolonged contact, and a need for a pleasure in continuing transactions.*

Bowlby (1977, p. 201) has referred to the attachment theory as

> a way of conceptualizing the propensity of human beings to make strong affectional bonds to particular others and of explaining the many forms of emotional distress and personality disturbance, including anxiety, anger, depression, and emotional detachment to which unwilling separation and loss give rise.

ATTACHMENT AS A PROCESS

Attachment, as used in this chapter, might be defined as a "process in which an affectional and emotional commitment or bonding to an individual is formed and

---

*From Robson, K.S., & Moss, H.A. (1970). Patterns and determinants of maternal attachment. *Journal of Pediatrics, 77* (6), 976–985. With permission.

is facilitated by positive feedback to each partner through a mutually satisfying experience" (Mercer, 1977, p. 16). Close proximity and a contingent relationship are assumed in this definition—positive feedback through a mutually satisfying experience depends on the closeness and sensitivity of the partners toward each other. Emotional commitment or bonding insures a long-term relationship in which continuity and proximity are valued; the attached parties feel anxiety or loss when these values are threatened.

The definition of attachment includes three concepts that merit emphasis. First, attachment is a *process*— that is a progressive or developmental course involving change over time. The process is rarely instantaneous; changes, both affective and cognitive, occur in both partners gradually. No single event will necessarily stop the process or prevent its occurring. Some factors may make the process more difficult, may prolong it, or may delay the initiation of it, but the nature of the attachment process makes it possible for attachment to occur despite some negative feedback or a negative occurrence.

Second, attachment is facilitated by *positive feedback* to each partner. Positive feedback includes the social, verbal, and nonverbal responses, either real or perceived, that indicate acceptance of one partner by the other. An infant's grasp around a father's finger, even though the action may be accidental and reflexive, means "I love you" to the father. An infant's fleeting, involuntary smile means "I like you as a parent" to an anxious mother.

Third, attachment occurs through a *mutually satisfying experience.* Thus, if a mother is in severe pain or is physically exhausted, she needs a lot of help in order to enjoy interacting with her infant. Likewise, if her baby is vomiting copious amounts of mucus and not feeding well, it will be difficult for the mother to enjoy or feel competent in her feeding experience. In such situations, manipulation of the environment has the potential to enhance or detract from mother–infant interaction.

THE TIE LINKING FAMILY MEMBERS

Although Bowlby (1953) described fathers as providers of emotional support for mothers, he noted (1958) that even though attachment is mother oriented, an infant can become attached to others. In cultures where infants have more than one caretaker, they become attached to persons other than their mothers (Yarrow & Pedersen, 1972). Fox (1977), in his research in kibbutzim in Israel, found that infants were attached both to their primary caretaker and to their mothers. The infants protested

equally to separation from either one. Therefore, we can assume that an infant in a family attaches to the father and to siblings as well as to the mother, although the attachment may differ both qualitatively and quantitatively for each dyad.

Turner (1970) has noted that some pairs of dyads in families are more bondable than others, depending on the mutual gratification or decision making attributed to the persons within the family unit. He described two kinds of bonds linking family members: identity bonds and interaction, or crescive, bonds. Identity bonds reinforce or improve an individual's self-concept, and the bonded individuals are linked through shared or complementary qualities. Interaction or crescive bonds develop more slowly, as individuals form irreplaceable links. Both identity and crescive bonds fall within the definition of attachment used in this chapter.

Heard (1978) viewed the family as a homeostatic system of individuals at differing stages of development who share mutual goals of terminating a specific form of proximity-seeking attachment behavior and promoting exploratory behavior. The attachment dynamic is not only the fundamental educative relationship between children and parents; it also serves to help regulate the physical distance and social interaction between the members of a family. Family members, for example, promote exploratory behavior of a toddler or an adolescent when they encourage autonomy and independence.

Infant Attachment

Researchers view infants as active instigators in the parent–infant attachment process. Although their interactional attachment behaviors increase with cognitive and physical development, infants exert a powerful influence on their caretakers from birth; they play a large role in creating their own environments through innate behavioral responses (Aleksandrowicz & Aleksandrowicz, 1975; Bennett, 1971; Haar et al., 1964; Yarrow 1963). Infant personality characteristics of autonomy and adaptability seem to result from underlying functions or rudimentary adaptive mechanisms rather than from environmental influences (Aleksandrowicz & Aleksandrowicz, 1976). These characteristics create quite different physical environments in the same home or nursery. For example, a visually alert, easily consolable infant becomes endeared to a caretaker and thereby gains more stimulation and caretaker contact. An irritable infant with a short attention span, who resists being held, will soon be labeled as unpleasant and will be avoided as much as possible by caretakers.

Infant Behavioral Styles

An infant may facilitate or inhibit parental attachment through behavioral style or temperament, social responsiveness, physical ability and appearance, and gender. The match or fit of a particular infant with the temperament, desires, and goals of the parents plays a large part in early attachment behaviors. When parents are faced with an infant who departs dramatically from their fantasies, the attachment process is delayed because they must resolve their feelings of disappointment or loss before attaching to their infant.

In a study of thirty firstborn children and their mothers during the infants' first 3 months of life, Moss (1968) found that, except for vocalization, the infants' states (including crying, fussing, active awake, passive awake, and sleeping) showed some stability over this period, although the 3-month-old infants cried less and were awake for longer periods. Mothers held their 3-month-old less than when they were newborns, and showed a decided increase in affectionate behavior toward 3-month-olds who smiled and vocalized more. Initially, maternal behavior was greatly influenced by the infants' behavioral responses; as the mothers became more competent in their skills and sensitive to infant cues, however, the infants exerted less control over them. Mothers held their male infants longer than their female infants both at 3 weeks and at 3 months, but a decrease of thirty percent holding time was observed at age 3 months for both sexes. Male infants were more fussy, irritable, and active awake at the beginning of the study and at the end, although their irritability had lessened by the age of 3 months. Richards et al. (1976), pointed out that eighty-three percent of 14,116 male infants born at eighteen teaching hospitals during 1973 were circumcised. These data indicate that gender differences may really be "circumcision" differences, since research has demonstrated that male infants exhibit prolonged wakefulness and crying after circumcision, and that behavioral differences according to gender were insignificant when females were compared to uncircumcised males.

Thomas and Chess (1977) evolved nine categories of infant temperament or behavioral style that may be assessed by clinicians in determining parent–infant fit:

- Infant activity level
- Rhythmicity or regularity
- Approach or withdrawal
- Adaptability to new or altered situations
- Threshold of responsiveness
- Intensity of reaction
- Quality of mood
- Distractability or attention span
- Persistence

Much can be learned about infant social behavior and personality by using the Brazelton Neonatal Behavioral Assessment Scale (1973), preferably on the third day of life. The scale is helpful in determining such factors as response to stimuli, motor maturity, cuddliness, consolability, defensive movements, peaks of excitement, irritability, activity, tremulousness, amount of startle, lability of states, self-quieting activity, and smiles. All of these may facilitate or inhibit parental attachment. The Carey Survey of Temperamental Characteristics (Carey, 1970) is helpful in identifying infant temperament at age 5 months and may reflect temperament later. McInerny and Chamberlain (1978) found that infants with "difficult" and "intermediate high" temperaments at 6 months of age were also more difficult for parents and more aggressive at 2 years of age.

Cultural and economic factors play a role in reinforcing or discouraging infant states and behavioral styles. For example, a mother with several children in a small apartment might encourage quiet play and reinforce passive behavior, whereas a mother with household help who lives in a large home with a large yard might encourage active play and exploration activities.

Lewis and Wilson (1972) found that maternal response differed between middle and lower socioeconomic classes. Middle-class mothers vocalized when their infants vocalized, and touched and held the infants when they cried; lower-class mothers tended to hold their infants fifty percent more than did middle-class mothers, to touch their infants when they vocalized, and to vocalize to their infants when they fretted. It was not the frequency of vocalization, but what it was used for, that made a difference. Lewis and Wilson suggested that the style of response of the middle-class mothers might lead to more representational thought through distancing; touching is less of a distancing response.

Infants' behavioral styles have been found to be consistent across situations (Osofsky & Danzger, 1974; Thoman, 1975)—for instance, infants who are alert and respond to auditory cues also tend to look at their mothers much of the time during feedings or when they are being held.

Attachment-Facilitating Behaviors

Bowlby (1958) was the first to use the term *attachment behaviors* for behaviors that promoted proximity of infant to caretaker. He identified such species-specific behaviors as sucking, clinging, following, crying, and smiling. Activation of these attachment behaviors depends on both internal and external sources; some behaviors occur only in the presence of particular external conditions or stimuli such as caretaker vocalization or cuddling. Such conditions serve as social releasers for both the activation and the termination of attachment behaviors. An infant must be equipped with an appropriately balanced repertoire of responses for activation of attachment behaviors. Richards (1971) emphasized that a wide range of infant behaviors brings mothers into proximity—for example, choking, hiccuping, and changes in movement or breathing patterns.

Serafica (1978) added to proximity an additional goal of attachment behavior: contact, or the experiencing of the caretaker. An infant can experience a mother's presence by sensorimotor operations (patting the mother's face or by perceptual operations (recognizing visual appearance or voice). Later the mother can be experienced through conceptual-symbolic operations (recognizing objects as being personal belongings of the mother).

Ainsworth (1964) also catalogued infant attachment behaviors that were exclusive of feeding behaviors: differential crying, smiling, and vocalization; visual–motor orientation toward the mother; crying when the mother leaves; following; scrambling; burying the face; exploration from a secure base; clinging; lifting arms or clapping hands in greeting; and approach through locomotion. Differential refers to an infant's responding to his or her mother rather than to others, and these differential infant responses have been observed to be potent facilitators of maternal attachment.

Harper (1971) grouped mammalian offspring's behaviors that facilitate caretaker response into three categories: triggering, orienting, and sensitizing. An infant who cries only when hungry or wet triggers a positive parental response; an infant who cries for long periods without ceasing triggers feelings of inadequacy in parents that may soon be projected to their infant. While feeding, an infant gazes into the mother's eyes and fondles her breast or body with a tiny hand; this behavior orients a mother to pay particular attention to her infant's face or hands. Through this unique interplay, both members of the dyad develop a tie with the other as each becomes sensitized to the other and benefits from mutually pleasurable interaction.

At birth infants trigger parental response by gazing at their parents during the period of alertness that usually occurs during the first hour or two of life. Although this initial alertness may be due to the endogenous adrenalin secreted in response to the stress of labor and delivery, parents perceive it personally. The helpless appearance of their infant's uncoordinated physical movements may also evoke early parental response (Bell, 1974). Visual alertness is later evoked by maternal care (Korner and Thoman, 1970) and by soothing activities such as placement on the mother's shoulder (Korner & Grobstein, 1966; Korner & Thoman, 1970). Brazelton (1974) observed lethargic infants with symptoms of dysmatur-

ity at birth who became alert to voice, handling, and motor adjustments and who maintained their alert states after ten days of frequent breast-feedings and placement in an upright position on their mothers' hips. Robson (1968) has noted that visual alertness and eye-to-eye contact are potent facilitators of maternal attachment during the first six months of life. Following and fixation are among the first acts of the infant that are both intentional and subject to his or her control. Vision is the only modality that, by closure of the eyelids, gaze aversion, and pupillary constriction and dilation, is constructed as an "on–off" system that can easily modulate or eliminate external sensory input.

An infant's orienting responses can facilitate mother–infant synchrony in feeding so that both infant and mother are sensitized to the optimal feeding situation. Call (1964) observed anticipatory approach behavior in infants as early as their fourth feeding. For example, one mother, who fed her infant while lying down, very skillfully and rapidly inserted a large portion of her areola and nipple into the infant's mouth. The infant's adaptation was to open his mouth widely when brought next to his mother's body in a lying position. Early sensitivity to the mother's breast pad (MacFarlane, 1975) suggests that olfaction plays an important role in infant behavior. MacFarlane (1975) observed that 5-day-old infants turned toward their mothers' breast pads more often than toward clean breast pads, and at 6 days old they showed a preference for their own mother's breast pads over other women's breast pads.

Infants may trigger and orient parental response through movements as well as through vocalization. Condon and Sander (1974) observed that infants moved in synchrony with adult speech patterns as early as the first day of life. Perhaps parents who say that their infant knows them at birth have been talking to the infant during pregnancy and orienting the infant to their speech patterns.

Attachment-Inhibiting Behaviors

Just as positive infant behavioral response facilitates parental attachment, opposite behaviors may inhibit parental attachment. Infants who avert their gaze from a parent, who stiffen when held, who do not adapt to feeding style, who are irritable, and who exhibit little self-consolation, are difficult for fatigued and frustrated parents who have been kept awake for several nights to love. Behavioral styles communicate. When an infant molds to the mother's body, the action says "I love you." When an infant resists cuddling, the action says "I don't like you" even if this behavior is simply the particular infant's behavioral style. Richards (1971) asserted that infant behavioral patterns influence maternal behavior on a minute-to-minute basis. In addi-

TABLE 2-1   Infant behaviors affecting parental attachment

Facilitating Behaviors	Inhibiting Behaviors
Visually alert; eye-to-eye contact; tracking or following of parent's face	Sleepy; eyes closed most of the time; gaze aversion
Appealing facial appearance; randomness of body movements reflecting helplessness	Resemblance to person parent dislikes; hyperirritability or jerky body movements when touched
Smiles	Bland facial expression; infrequent smiles
Vocalization; crying only when hungry or wet	Crying for hours on end; colicky
Grasp reflex	Exaggerated motor reflex
Anticipatory approach behaviors for feedings; sucks well; feeds easily	Feeds poorly; regurgitates; vomits often
Enjoys being cuddled, held	Resists holding and cuddling by crying, stiffening body
Easily consolable	Inconsolable; unresponsive to parenting, caretaking tasks
Activity and regularity somewhat predictable	Unpredictable feeding and sleeping schedule
Attention span sufficient to focus on parents	Inability to attend to parent's face or offered stimulation
Differential crying, smiling, and vocalization; recognizes and prefers parents	Shows no preference for parents over others
Approaches through locomotion	Unresponsive to parent's approaches
Clings to parent; puts arms around parent's neck	Seeks attention from any adult in room
Lifts arms to parents in greeting	Ignores parents

From Gerson, E. (1973). *Infant behavior in the first year of life.* New York: Raven Press. Copyright © 1973. With permission.

tion, an infant's behavior also influences a mother's attitude, which then reflects a bias in her interactions with the child. In infants aged 6 weeks, 3 months, and 6 months Gerson (1973) found that a mother's confidence correlated with her pediatrician's rating of her infant's functioning in terms of feeding behavior, adjustment to routine, and overall integration. In turn, the infant's adjustment at the age of three months (adjustment including tension, mood, affective stability, irritability, and vulnerability to ease of recovery from stress) correlated with the mother's confidence in her ability. Infant behaviors affecting the attachment process are summarized in Table 2-1.

Parent Attachment

People fall in love differently with different people; attachment is a selective process. A secundigravida may have difficulty imagining how she will have enough love for two children until she works through the differences in the children and the differences in relationships (Jenkins, 1976). Both facilitating and inhibiting factors affect the parents' ability to become attached

to their first, and to each subsequent infant. For each parent the process may be similar, yet the resulting attachment may be qualitatively different.

Paternal Attachment

The increase in dual-career families (both heads of the household pursuing careers and maintaining a family life together) has resulted in more dual-parenting families. Current research suggests more similarities than differences between paternal and maternal behavior.

First contact with his newborn has been shown consistent from father to father and has been characterized by the same sequence of behaviors that has been observed in mothers. McDonald (1978) studied the behavior of seven fathers in a homelike environment in which the fathers had unrestricted contact with their newborn infants. The fathers' interactions with their infants were videotaped, and their behaviors independently coded by trained observers. Seven paternal behaviors—four distal and three contact—were predominant during the first nine minutes following birth. Hovering was the most pervasive distal behavior;

it accounted for eighty-one percent of the father's activity during the first three minutes with his infant. Hovering was characterized by the father's bending from the waist over his infant with his face in a frontal position. The father spent seventy-seven percent of the first three minutes looking at their infants. McDonald described this intense gazing as being *lock on.* When the fathers were not touching their newborn infants, they directed their arms, hands, and fingers toward the newborn; this was called *pointing behavior.* The fathers maintained face-to-face positions with their infants in as closely a vertical axis as was possible. The en face position as observed in mothers could not always be maintained since only one parent's face could usually be on the same vertical plane as the infant's.

The fathers' contact behaviors were uniform, and the progression similar to that observed in mothers. First, each father made initial contact with his fingertips. Each father then moved to more extensive finger and palm contact. The behavior of these fathers in an unrestricted birth environment suggests that the distal and contact behavior observed could be species-specific. Further research with different groups of fathers in different cultures is warranted to explore whether this behavior is characteristic of all human fathers.

Greenberg and Morris (1974) studied two groups of first fathers. One group had contact with their newborns in the delivery room, and the second group had first contact with their newborns shortly following the birth, when nursing personnel showed them their infants. Both groups of fathers indicated strong feelings of involvement with their infants. Ten fathers in each group of fifteen indicated that they felt their infants were "all theirs" immediately, and twenty-nine of the thirty fathers were pleased with the sex of their infants. The researchers chose the term *engrossment* to mean more than involvement; when a father became engrossed, his infant had assumed great importance for him and had increased his sense of self-esteem and worth. Leonard (1976) observed similar emotional responses in fifty-two fathers soon after their infants' births. These feelings reflect the identity bonds described by Turner (1971). Early contact (proximity) seemed to encourage engrossment. The sensory modalities that led to a father's engrossment included visual awareness, tactile awareness, and perception of distinct characteristics and of his infant as perfect. Normal infant reflex activity and behavior also enhanced paternal engrossment. Fathers were especially impressed by infant eye contact and grasp reflex, which they interpreted as responsiveness to them personally.

Fein (1976) found that men felt both gratified and burdened during the first weeks after their infants' birth. These feelings were affected by the extent to which a father perceived himself to be excluded or included in family life. More men felt more included than excluded and exhibited strong identification with their infants: "I sense that I identify with him some, and so in cuddling him, I care for parts of myself" (p. 55). Nineteen of the thirty-two fathers studied by Fein experienced much pride in their infants. Factors that affected postpartum adjustment included preparation for parenting (only three fathers had had extensive experience caring for children), the baby's health (one couple whose baby was colicky reported feelings of rage, guilt, desperation, and exhaustion), support from families, support from work (flexibility in working hours was usually lacking), and agreement about roles (couples who were at odds about family roles had a difficult time postpartum).

Although mothers may spend more time than fathers in feeding and caretaking activities, they do not differ in their caretaking competence or in their sensitivity to an infant's cues (Parke & Sawin, 1976). On the basis of their research, Parke and Sawin concluded that when fathers have the opportunity to become involved with their newborns, they are interested in them, are as nurturant as mothers, and can be capable and competent in caretaking skills. Reiber (1976) observed that women directed men's involvement in child care activities; if a woman wanted her husband involved, he agreed he would be.

Redina and Dickersheid (1976) found that fathers of 5-to-6-month-old children were more involved in social activities—playing with the child, for example—rather than physical caretaking. Fathers spent more time in visual interaction than in any other activity; they watched their infants even while the mothers fed or held the babies. Infant characteristics such as sex, developmental status, or temperament had little effect on fathers' interactions. Richards et al. (1977) also found that of eighty fathers whose infants were delivered at home, a majority played with their children regularly, but only a minority took regular responsibility in caretaking; they rarely changed diapers or bathed their infants.

Lamb and Lamb (1976) found that fathers of 7-to-13-month-old infants played with them differently than did mothers and held them for different reasons. Mothers engaged in more conventional games and used toys to stimulate their children. Fathers were more likely to play physically vigorous games that were unusual and unpredictable and that the infants most enjoyed. Infants were judged to be attached to both parents, but to experience qualitatively different interactions with each. Toward a child's first birthday, parents began to feel responsible for the development of commonly perceived sex-appropriate behaviors; fathers withdrew dramatically from interaction with their daughters and were more than twice as active with their sons.

Knox and Gilman (1974) studied the first year of fatherhood through use of 260 mailed questionnaires. Of 102 fathers responding, fifteen percent reported feelings of love for their babies, and eighty-five percent reported extreme happiness in addition to love. Although these fathers reported love and happiness, twenty-five percent of the sample also said they sometimes wished they could return to the time before their babies were born.

According to all research reports, men have the same potential to become attached to infants and to care for them as do women. Different types of behavior occurs, however, probably because of continued sexual stereotyping of gender roles. Further research is needed regarding qualitative differences between father–infant and mother–infant interaction.

Maternal Attachment

Multiple factors affect maternal attachment: early life experiences, events during pregnancy and the perinatal period, and current life events. Early life events that affect maternal attachment might include temporary or permanent separation from one or both parents before the age of 11 (Frommer & O'Shea, 1973), childhood deprivations or illness, death or illness of prior children (Barbero, 1975), genetic background, cultural background, relationships with the infant's father or with her own parents, (de Chateau, 1977), and experiences with previous pregnancies (Klaus & Kennell, 1982). Events occurring during pregnancy that might affect maternal attachment include a woman's protracted emotional or physical illness, and deaths or major illnesses of close family members (Barbero, 1975). Whether the pregnancy was desired is also an issue that affects maternal attachment (Robson and Moss, 1970). During the perinatal period complications of labor and delivery, acute illness of mother or infant, prematurity, congenital defects or diseases (Mercer, 1974, 1977a, 1977b), parity, postnatal adaptation, and infant's sex, state, and development (de Chateau, 1977) are all factors that can affect maternal attachment. Current life events that have an impact include marital strains, mental or medical illness, alcoholism, use of drugs, financial crises (Barbero, 1975), personal and social isolation,

low self-esteem, and parent–child role reversal (Helfer, 1974).

Many of these factors are essentially unalterable by health care professionals. Factors that are alterable include the quality of the postpartum care provided and the behavior of doctors, nurses, other hospital personnel, and perhaps hospital policies—for example, the practice of enforced separation of mother and infant (Klaus & Kennell, 1982). Intensive psychological and supportive help for parents with low self-esteem and no friends or support system can help them learn to relate and interact with others (Blumberg, 1974).

The attachment process is unique for the mother in that she experiences the event both psychologically and physiologically. During pregnancy a woman agrees to have her body used by another human being; this kind of intimate nurturance is not possible for anyone else for this particular child. After quickening, the assurance that there is indeed a child growing within her, a woman begins binding-in to her infant (Rubin, 1975). The giving of oneself that occurs during pregnancy is profound and reflects what Deutsch (1945) has described as a feminine quality of masochism of the highest order. No one except the mother gives to this extent. Through giving and relating to the fetus, postquickening attachment begins.

Rubin (1977) described binding-in and maternal identification as two of the major developmental and interdependent changes that occur over the three trimesters of pregnancy and the two trimesters following delivery of a child. Binding-in occurs via a mother's identification of her infant, mother's and family's claiming of the infant, and polarization. Polarization is a process in which a mother separates from the oneness of the mother–infant unit and identifies her infant as an individual in his or her own right (Rubin, 1977). Bibring (1965) described polarization as the development of the ability "to love the child as an independent being with his own individual personality though there will exist a deeper bond with him as he remains forever part of herself" (p. 25).

The Sensitive Period Klaus et al. (1970) first suggested the existence of a sensitive period for mother and infant after they studied maternal behavior during first postnatal contact. They observed an orderly progression of maternal behavior that began with fingertip touch on the infant's extremities and progressed to palmar contact on the trunk within four to five minutes. (Rubin [1963] had earlier suggested that this progression occurred over a period of three to five days.) They also observed that eye-to-eye contact was very important for the mothers. Visual taking-in is an important part of a mother's identifying her infant.

Cannon (1977) tested the time for reaching these stages of maternal touch. She studied twenty-four mothers who interacted with twelve dressed and twelve undressed infants and found that the number of minutes the mothers took to reach stage two (fingertip touching proceeding to the trunk) was significantly lower for the mothers of undressed infant. Mothers of undressed infants reached stage four (complete enfolding with entire arms and holding the infant's body against her body) in a mean of 2.8 minutes, and the mothers of dressed infants reached the stage in a mean of 5.2 minutes. Six primiparas and six multiparas were in each of the dressed and undressed groups; no significant differences were found.

In a study comparing fourteen mothers who had extended contact with their infants following birth and for sixteen additional hours to fourteen mothers who had routine physical contact with their infants during hospitalization, Klaus et al. (1972) verified the importance of the first postpartum days for maternal attachment. After one month the mothers who had had extended contact demonstrated more fondling and en face behaviors and scored higher on extended contact scores. These differences in the group with extended contact were also observed at one year (Kennell et al., 1974). After two years mothers who had had extended contact used different verbal patterns; they asked more questions, used more adjectives, and gave fewer commands to their children (Ringler et al., 1975).

Research by de Chateau (1976) suggests that the first postpartum hour is a very sensitive period. He found differences in attachment behaviors between twenty primiparous women who had had skin-to-skin and suckling contact during the first postpartum hour and twenty women whose routine had not included this contact. The early-contact mothers demonstrated more holding, encompassing, looking, and smiling behaviors. These differences were apparent both at thirty-six hours and at three months postpartum.

Imprinting and the Critical Period Imprinting is used largely to refer to attachment behaviors of the young of animals or fowl. Sears (1972, p. 14) supports using the term for nonhumans only: "There is…a certain looseness about both chronological age and objects that distinguishes human attachment formation from the more precise imprinting seen in geese." Kennell et al. (1975, p. 88) defined the sensitive period as "that time after delivery when the mother forms, or begins to form, a special attachment to her infant," and

noted that the maternal sensitive period differs from imprinting in that "there is not a point beyond which the formation of an attachment is precluded." They add that while the maternal sensitive period is an optimal time for mother–infant attachment behaviors, it is not the only time for attachment to develop.

Caldwell (1962, p. 230) reviewed the use of the term *critical period* for the study of human infant attachment behavior and found that the term was used in two ways:

> a critical period beyond which a given phenomena will not appear (i.e., a point in time which marks the onset of total indifference, or resistance, to certain patterns of stimulation); and a critical period during which the organism is especially sensitive to various developmental modifiers, which, if introduced at a different time in the life cycle, would have little or no effect (i.e., a period of maximum susceptibility).*

Caldwell suggests that it is dangerous to emphasize a critical period for infant attachment too strongly because of the wide range of individual differences. The same advice seems appropriate for adult attachment.

Premature Infants Studies of mothers of premature infants, and retrospective studies of children who have been abused, strongly support the idea that the early postpartal days are a sensitive period. Thus, the needs of parents who experience unavoidable situations imposing early separation must be considered. Salk (1970) found seventy-seven percent of the women who did not have prolonged postpartum separation from their infants held their infants on the left side of their chests over their hearts, while women who experienced prolonged separation (i.e., did not hold the baby during the first twenty-four hours postpartum) showed no preference in the way they held their infants. Leifer et al. (1972) compared three groups of mothers at one week and at four weeks after giving birth: one group had premature infants and the women were allowed only visual contact with their infants, a second group had premature infants also, but they were allowed to enter the intensive-care nursery and do caretaking tasks, and a third group had full-term infants and full contact with the infants.

Mothers of full-term infants smiled at their infants and held them closer to their bodies than did mothers of prematures. No differences were observed in the attachment behaviors of the two groups of mothers of

---

*From Caldwell, B.M. (1962). The usefulness of the critical period hypothesis in the study of filiative behavior. *Merrill-Palmer Quarterly, 8,* 229–242. With permission.

premature infants; however, two of the mothers in the group with only visual contact relinquished custody of their infants when their marriages ended in divorce. Seashore et al. (1973) reported that self-confidence was lower in primiparous mothers who had not had early contact and caretaking experience with their premature infants than in primiparous mothers who had been allowed early contact. The multiparous mothers were not affected by contact or lack of contact except in cases in which they initially had low self-confidence.

A woman's self-image and body image are threatened by a premature birth because her body does not perform as it should to carry a baby to term. Being barred from the nursery and from caretaking tasks would conceivably lower a woman's self-esteem even more. The identification and claiming process might also be slower for the mother of a premature because of the premature infant's less attractive body image and reduced capacity to function. In such a case, it is more difficult for her to identify the infant with herself and her loved ones.

Fanaroff et al. (1972) observed that mothers of prematures who did not seek proximity (i.e., visit or call the nursery) as often as three times in two weeks later exhibited more disorders of mothering (i.e., failure-to-thrive infants, incidents of abuse, or desertion). To develop criteria for mother–child bonding, Minde et al. (1978) studied eighteen mother–infant pairs in which each infant weighed less than 1501 g at birth. Infants were observed both alone and with their mothers, during nursery visits and during at-home interviews at one, two, and three months following discharge from the hospital. The length of the mothers' nursery visits and the number of caretaking behaviors increased from early to later visits and remained consistent in rank order for the women over time. Caretaking behaviors were highly intercorrelated, and mothers fell into groups of consistently high, medium, or low interactors with their infants. Those mothers who were high interactors visited and telephoned the nursery more often and stimulated their infants more often at home. The converse was also true, low interactors visited and called the nursery less and stimulated their infants less. The attachment patterns that the women in this study experienced seemed connected to the patterns they experienced with other adults (Leifer et al., 1972). For example, in the low-interaction group of mothers, all but one lacked the support of her spouse. Five of the women in the low-interaction group did not have any friends with whom they could share their concerns. In contrast, women in the high-interaction group all enjoyed good relationships with their husbands. Husbands accompanied these women on more than half of the visits to the infants. All the women in the high-interaction group also had many friends.

Infants of less than twenty-nine weeks' gestation did not respond to any type of maternal stimulation; however, those beyond twenty-nine weeks' gestation opened their eyes significantly more often when their mothers touched them. The researchers observed that during the first two visits to the nursery the mothers were hesitant to interact with their infants but spent the time looking at them.

Harper et al. (1976) observed that parental anxiety increased as the quantity and quality of the contact they were allowed with their infants in the intensive care nursery increased. A high correlation was found between parental anxiety and the seriousness and extent of an infant's illness. Ninety percent of the ninety-one parents under study performed at least one of the nurturing activities allowed; while mothers performed more nurturing activities than fathers, the differences were not significant. The high level of parental anxiety and participation in nurturing activities suggests that parent–infant attachment had occurred in the intensive care nursery where parents were allowed to remain any time except during emergency resuscitations or major diagnostic procedures.

The Early Months Robson and Moss (1970) studied fifty-four primiparous women and their infants from an antepartum interview through three months postpartum. To determine the mothers' feelings toward their infants the researcher asked three questions: When did you first experience positive feelings and love toward your baby? When did your baby first become a person to you? When did your baby first seem to recognize you? They found that the women responded vaguely and impersonally about their infants for the first four days postpartum. Twenty-four percent of the women elected to room in, but the attachment process was not accelerated for these women. The mothers' responses differed dramatically from the research of Greenberg and Morris (1974) on fathers of newborns. Perhaps fathers are more inclined to early attachment because they do not suffer bodily insult giving birth or because the lack of threat to their intimate selves makes it possible for them to be more objective.

Robson and Moss also observed that the women they interviewed felt tired and insecure during the first three to four weeks at home, and many felt that it had been easier to feel more warmth toward their infants when they were together in the hospital. Shereshefski et al. (1973) reported intense and unanticipated fatigue, disorganization, and feelings of inadequacy among fifty-two primiparous mothers during the early weeks. These data support Rubin's (1977) thesis that until a woman's intactness and wholeness are assured at the completion of involution, it is difficult for her to feel good about herself and to see her infant as whole and complete.

During the first month after giving birth, the majority of mothers in the Robson and Moss study did not experience an intense attachment to their infants. Four to six weeks after the birth was a transitional period; the infants began responding with more socialization behaviors—for example, smiling, following with eyes, and general responsiveness. By the end of three months the majority of mothers felt strongly attached to their infants. The authors observed both early and late attachers in their sample. Seven mothers were early attachers; they had had a strong desire for an infant and had idealized images of their infants. Of the nine late attachers, six had strongly ambivalent feelings about having a baby. One had an infant who was later found to be brain damaged; another had an infant who was inconsolable for the first ten days of life; another woman was highly anxious. Three of the mothers were considered detached and unreactive after three months. Robson and Moss concluded that an infant's ability to exhibit adult social relationship characteristics was of central importance to the development of attachment in mothers and that infant eye contact may, like the smiling response, suppress maternal anger.

For her study of eleven mothers, Gottlieb (1978) defined attachment as the growth of positive feelings toward the infant, a desire to possess, to prolong, and to seek contact with the infant, and pride in and love for the infant. Gottlieb observed a discovery process that was activated by the mother's need to turn "the baby" into "my baby." This discovery, described earlier by Rubin (1977) as *polarization,* involves identifying, relating, and interpreting. *Identifying* is a mother's work of determining her infant's physical characteristics and actions; *relating* is her linking infant behavior with familiar events, persons, objects, or the ideal child of her fantasies; *interpreting* is the meaning that a mother gives to her infant's actions and needs. Identifying preceded relating and interpreting; the latter two enhanced the infant's significance to the mother. Qualitative changes in the identifying process evolved over the first four weeks; this discovery process was the key in the development of the bonding system. Gottlieb identified a complementary system of facilitators that directed women's energies toward discovery: positive input, personalized contact between mother and infant, and the mother's physical well-being. An antagonistic system of inhibitors competed with the mother's energies: negative input, depersonalized contact between mother and infant, and the mother's physical distress or discomfort.

Kennedy's (1973) observations of the maternal–infant acquaintance process were similar to Gottlieb's. Kennedy described a positive acquaintance process in which a woman perceived her baby's attitude toward her as positive (positive feedback): in turn she felt positive toward her baby and was encouraged to seek more knowledge about the infant through observation and interaction. If the woman perceived her baby's attitude toward her as negative, she reciprocated with feelings of irritation and annoyance toward her infant. Kennedy observed that within the first two weeks after birth negative maternal feelings were translated into aggressive acts such as yelling, shaking, and being rough with the infant. A key element in the acquaintance process was a woman's ability to trust herself, her social support system, and her infant.

COMPONENTS OF PARENTAL ATTACHMENT

Commonly observed components of the attachment process as it occurs in parents may be grouped as (1) favorable preconditions for attachment and (2) identification and claiming of the infant as partner. The latter is facilitated by the former.

Favorable Preconditions for Attachment

The favorable preconditions for attachment to begin and progress without untoward difficulty are

- A parent's emotional health (including the ability to trust another person)
- A social support system encompassing mate, friends, and family
- A competent level of communication and caretaking skills
- Parental proximity to the infant
- Parent–infant fit (including infant state, temperament, and sex)

Without skilled help and intervention, attachment can fail to proceed or may be seriously hampered if any of these factors is missing or awry.

The ability to form love ties to another person is learned as an infant. Work with mothers who have abused their children has indicated that these women often did not have warm, nurturant care as children and did not learn mothering behaviors as children; they were often abused themselves (Cohler et al. 1976; Frommer & O'Shea 1973). Harlow's (1958, 1962, 1977) forty years of experimental research with monkeys demonstrated that infant monkeys who had no physical contact with their mothers from birth were neurotic, did not mate, and did not know normal heterosexual behavior. When forced to mate and become pregnant, they battered and abused their infants.

A woman's self-image and her ability to function physically are crucial to her ability to trust herself in caring for another individual. Failure to deliver an infant vaginally may inhibit a woman's ability to relate to her infant (Marut, 1978; Mercer, 1977a; Marut & Mercer, 1979). Women who have undergone Cesarean births after having given birth vaginally report that a Cesarean birth deprives them of the feelings of euphoria they experienced with earlier births and that, for the first day or two, they do not have enough energy to care about their babies; pain and immobility preempt their energies and thoughts.

Several research reports have noted the importance of supportive mates and friends to the attachment process. Sears et al. (1957) observed that wives who had low respect for their husbands did not express high feelings of warmth for their children.

Since identification and claiming of the partner is dependent on communication skills, such skills cannot be overlooked. Identification and claiming occur through visual, tactile, auditory, verbal, and olfactory modes; information derived through these modes is perceived and translated into emotions and further interactions. Sensitivity to cues, or "reading the infant," is one of the most important challenges for a parent, and parents who acquire this skill enjoy feelings of competence and confidence in their caretaking abilities. The identification and claiming process is enhanced through nurturant caretaking, which is essential for the dependent infant's survival. Studies of rooming-in (Greenberg et al., 1973; Schroeder, 1977) have shown that proximity to her infant and the opportunity to perform caretaking tasks enhance a woman's feelings of maternal competence.

All attachment research documents the importance of proximity to the partner. As a tie is formed, proximity is valued more highly; anxiety, grief, and disturbed emotional behavior are observed when proximity of attached persons is threatened. Parents who are not anxious or upset about infants in the intensive care nursery have not yet begun the attachment process.

Identification and Claiming of the Infant as Partner

One cannot love a stranger; identification and claiming of the partner is an inextricable factor in attachment. The identification of the infant is differentiating the infant as an individual; motivation for mothering is born in relating the infant to one's family tree and in interpreting infant behaviors. The positive feedback that comes through the infant's socialization responses—either real or imagined—provides nourishment for the parent–infant relationship. Parents use all of their senses, and delight in discovering their infant's remarkable repertoire of behaviors and abilities. Parental behaviors affecting the attachment process are summarized in Table 2-2. Behaviors described in the table as inhibiting can be a signal that a parent is experiencing difficulty with the attachment process.

The real infant, as opposed to the desired or fantasied infant, is the one on whom all the parents' hopes and dreams rest. If parents are disappointed for any reason, the attachment process is delayed. Attachment also proceeds more easily when infant adaptation to the parents' environment is easy and when an infant's innate personality and behavioral style are not greatly at odds with those of the parents.

SELECTED TOOLS FOR ASSESSING PARENT–INFANT ATTACHMENT

Some tools for assessing parental attachment have been constructed to facilitate screening for at-risk parents. In assessing parent–infant attachment, knowledge of alterable as well as unalterable factors is important to nurses. The need for continuity and long-term follow-up of families is inherent in the assessment of the parent–infant attachment process. Because of the nurse's long-term intimate contact with childbearing clients, especially during parturition, many tools for assessment of parental attachment have been proposed by nurses.

Levels of Maladaptive Maternal Behavior

Porter (1973) identified three levels of maladaptive maternal behavior and related them to a mother–infant environmental interactional framework. Level I, Maternal Adaptation Stresses, is experienced to some extent by all mothers. It is characterized by perplexity, insecurity, increased anxiety, chronic fatigue, and an irritable

TABLE 2-2 Parental behaviors affecting infant attachment

Facilitating Behaviors	Inhibiting Behaviors
Looks; gazes; takes in physical characteristics of infant; assumes en face position, eye contact	Turns away from infant; ignores infant's presence
Hovers; maintains proximity; directs attention to, points to infant	Avoids infant; does not seek proximity; refuses to hold infant when given opportunity
Identifies infant as unique individual	Identifies infant with someone parent dislikes; fails to discern any of the infant's unique features
Claims infant as family member; names	Fails to place infant in family context or to identify infant with family member; has difficulty naming
Touches; progresses from fingertip to fingers to palmar to encompassing contact	Fails to move from fingertip touch to palmar contact and holding
Smiles at infant	Maintains bland countenance or frowns at infant
Talks to, coos, or sings to infant	Wakes infant when sleeping; handles roughly; hurries feeding by moving nipple continuously
Expresses pride in infant	Expresses disappointment, displeasure in infant
Relates infant's behavior to familiar events	Does not incorporate infant into life
Assigns meaning to infant's actions and sensitively interprets infant's needs	Makes no effort to interpret infant's actions or needs
Views infant's behaviors and appearance in positive light	Views infant's behavior as exploiting, deliberately uncooperative; views appearance as distasteful, ugly

infant. Level-I behavior is due to a lack of knowledge about infant care, unrealistic expectations of self and infant, or the lack of societal support.

Level II, Psychosocial Stress, is characterized by vacillation in attachment behaviors; alternating acceptance and rejection of the infant. Causes are psychosocial situations that include marital problems, financial and housing problems, mother–infant separation, infant characteristics, cultural influences, or unwanted pregnancy.

Level III, Affective Deprivation Stresses, represents the most severe, global rejection of the infant. The mother is developmentally unready for mothering. This level is characterized by negative attachment behavior, distorted perception of infant behavior, unrealistic childrearing ideas, increased preoccupation with and concern for self, inability to understand the infant's needs, and concern about "spoiling" the infant. Etiological factors include parental history of affective deprivation (e.g., early abuse or neglect, foster placement, maladaptive pattern with own mother, or other severe emotional trauma).

Porter cautions that if nurses do not establish priorities for nursing care with families in which nursing can make a difference, many salvageable cases may not be

helped. She proposes long-term studies of nursing intervention in mother–infant maladaptation cases as an aid in identifying and determining the impact of nursing skills.

Porter's levels of maladaptive maternal behavior are particularly helpful for screening-nurses. The nursing role in handling level-I stresses is one of counseling, supportive care, helping the client to utilize available resources, and role modeling. Level-II stresses present some situations that the nurse cannot necessarily alter; however, the nurse's continuing relationship with the family is invaluable in providing continuity of care. The nurse can also collaborate with others involved in the family's care and can make referrals to such professionals as social workers, physicians, psychological counselors, or community services. Porter cautions that nurses must recognize their limited ability to deal with level-III stresses and to refer clients to proper psychological counseling or to appropriate community agencies. It remains important, however, for the nurse-client relationship to continue in order that the client's health needs be met. If others are focusing on the woman's immature emotional state, the nurse may be the only one focusing on such physical concerns as birth control, diet, and follow-up medical care.

TABLE 2-3 Mothering behaviors

Adaptive Behaviors	Maladaptive Behaviors
Feeding	
Offers appropriate amount and/or type of food to infant	Provides inadequate type or amount of food for infant
Holds infant in comfortable position during feeding	Does not hold infant, or holds in uncomfortable position during feeding
Burps baby during and/or after feeding	Does not burp infant
Prepares food appropriately	Prepares food inappropriately
Offers food at comfortable pace for infant	Offers food at pace too rapid or slow for infant's comfort
Infant stimulation	
Provides appropriate verbal stimulation for infant during visit	Provides no, or only aggressive, verbal stimulation for infant during visit
Provides tactile stimulation for infant at times other than during feeding or moving infant away from danger	Does not provide tactile stimulation or only that of aggressive handling of infant
Provides age-appropriate toys	No evidence of age-appropriate toys
Interacts with infant in a way that provides for infant's satisfaction	Frustrates infant during interactions
Infant rest	
Provides quiet or relaxed environment for infant's rest, including scheduled rest periods	Does not provide quiet environment or consistent schedule for rest periods
Ensures that infant's needs for food, warmth and/or dryness are met before sleep	Does not attend to infant's needs for food, warmth, and/or dryness before sleep
Perception	
Demonstrates realistic perception of infant's condition in accordance with medical and/or nursing diagnosis	Shows unrealistic perception of infant's condition
Has realistic expectations for infant	Demonstrates unrealistic expectations of infant
Recognizes infant's unfolding skills or behavior	Has no awareness of infant's development
Shows realistic perception of own mothering behavior	Shows unrealistic perception of own mothering
Initiative	
Shows initiative in attempts to manage infant's problems including actively seeking information about infants	Shows no initiative in attempts to meet infant's needs or to manage problems; does not follow through with plans
Recreation	
Provides positive outlets for own recreation or relaxation	Does not provide positive outlets for own recreation or relaxation
Interaction with other children	
Demonstrates positive interaction with other children in home	Demonstrates hostile-aggressive interaction with other children in home
Mothering role	
Expresses satisfaction with mothering	Expresses dissatisfaction with mothering

TABLE 2-4 Infant behaviors

Adaptive Behaviors	Maladaptive Behaviors
Sleeping	
Receives adequate sleep for normal growth—at least 16 hours each day without restless sleep patterns or prolonged crying at nap or bedtime after other needs have been met	Receives inadequate sleep for normal growth—less than 16 hours each day; shows restless sleep patterns and/or prolonged crying at nap or bedtime
Feeding	
Actively seeks food offered	Resists food offered
Effectively sucks and swallows food	Does not suck effectively
Demonstrates pleasurable relief after eating	Remains fussy after adequate amount of feeding—no pleasurable relief
Response to environment	
Demonstrates active response to environment by exploring or reaching-out behavior	Seems apathetic to environment
Vocalizing	
Demonstrates vocalizations when alert if developmentally ready	Makes infrequent or no vocalizations during visit although developmentally ready
Smiling	
Demonstrates smiling behavior if older than 2 months	Does not demonstrate smiling behavior during visit
Cuddling	
Cuddles when held	Resists being held or stiffens when held

Categories of Maternal and Infant Behavior

Harrison (1976), in working with failure-to-thrive families, identified eight categories of adaptive and maladaptive mothering behaviors (Table 2-3), and six categories of adaptive and maladaptive infant behaviors (Table 2-4). For work with failure-to-thrive families, Harrison suggests a master nursing-care plan that can be adapted to individual cases if it is kept in mind that the suggestions in the plan are for beginning long-term intervention.

Neonatal Perception Inventories

Clark (1976) reported her use of the Neonatal Perception and Degree of Bother Inventories developed by Elsie R. Broussard (1971). The Neonatal Perception Inventories measure a woman's concept of her own baby and of an average baby on the first or second postpartum day and at one month after birth. Dissonance between a woman's perceptions of an average infant and of her own infant can be recognized with the tool; an infant who is perceived as below average is at risk for later psychological problems (Broussard & Hartner, 1970, 1971). Therefore, infant behaviors that a woman views as below average may be explored with her. If her expectations are unrealistic, teaching about normal infant behavior may be helpful. Using newborn assessment procedures modified from the Brazelton Behavioral Assessment Scale—for example, Clark's tool (Clark & Affonso, 1979)—at a mother's bedside is helpful in acquainting a mother with her infant's uniqueness.

Attachment Measurement in a Clinical Setting

Cropley et al. (1976) devised a tool for measuring maternal attachment in a clinical setting during the neonatal period (Figure 2-1). The tool measures maternal identifying behaviors, locating behaviors (baby's position in mother's social system), modalities of interaction, and caretaking behaviors. It does not reflect

Patient's name _____ Delivery date _____ Today's date_____

Circle points
for observed
behavior

I. **Identifying Behaviors:** The mother's observing or inquiring about her infant to gain
knowledge of infant's appearance, wholeness, and state of function
  A. Appearance and function
    1. Makes reference to sex of the infant, e.g., "He's going to be a football
       player," or gets infant a sex-linked toy   +1
    2. Makes reference to size of the infant, e.g., "She's so little"   +1
    3. Inspects or reviews baby's body features (hair, fingers face, feet, and other
       parts of body)   +1
    4. Asks questions or makes statements pertaining to wholeness of the infant,
       e.g., "Is he all right?" or "Well, he has all ten toes"   +1
    5. Verbally questions or comments on body functions of baby, e.g., "Look,
       she's wet," or "Look at him move!"   +1
         I-A Score (total circled points)   ___
  B. Appraisal of infant's condition
    6. Asks no questions about baby's condition   0
    7. Makes unrealistic statements (optimistic or pessimistic) regarding baby's
       condition, e.g., saying skin looks better when it looks worse   –1
    8. Asks brief questions about baby's condition, e.g., "How's he eating?" or
       "How much weight has he gained?"   +1
    9. Asks realistic questions or makes realistic comments about infant's con-
       dition with specific reference to such things as skin, scalp, eyes, face,
       circumcision, and cord in the normal newborn; or IV, monitor, bilirubin
       lights, and physical symptoms (e.g., jaundice or color) in the high-risk infant   +2
   10. Verbal statements by mother that denote her awareness of changes in the
       baby's condition, e.g., "She is breathing more slowly today," or "His skin
       doesn't look as dry today"   +3
         I-B Score (total circled points)   ___

II. **Locating Behaviors:** Cognitively determining the baby's position within the sphere
of her significant social system
  A. Verbally associates infant with an animal or animal characteristics   0
  B. Associates infant with inanimate object   0
  C. Associates infant's characteristics with human characteristics, e.g., "He looks
     like an old man," or "She looks more like a real baby now"   +1
  D. Associates infant's characteristics with other family members, e.g., "She has her
     daddy's big feet," or "She looks just like her sister"   +2
       II Score (*Do not total:* record *highest* circled score)   ___

III. **Modalities of Interaction:** The method through which the mother begins to relate to
her baby, using visual, verbal, and tactile behaviors
  A. Verbal contact
    1. Mother talks or sings to baby   +1
    2. Mother uses infant's given name when talking to baby   +1

FIGURE 2-1   Maternal attachment tool. (From Cropley, C., Lester, P., & Pennington, S. (1976). Assessment tool for measuring
maternal attachment behaviors. In L.K. McNall & J.T. Galeener (Eds.), *Current practice in obstetric and gynecologic nursing*
(Vol. I). St. Louis: The C.V. Mosby Co. With permission.) *(Continued on pp. 33 and 34.)*

B. Visual contact
    3. Establishes position en face   +1
    4. Talks about baby's opening eyes; verbally encourages this   +1
    5. Stimulates infant to open eyes by shading them from the light, changing position, and other maneuvers   +1
C. Tactile-kinesthetic contact
    6. Touches extremities or head   +1
    7. Extends touch to trunk of baby's body   +2
    8. Fingertip touch   +1
    9. Finger touch (stroking)   +1
    10. Palm contact   +2
    11. Draws infant to trunk of her body (body contact)   +1
    12. Snuggles baby to shoulder with cheek-to-cheek contact   +2
    13. Spontaneous movements initiated by mother·to increase her contact with baby, e.g., patting, kissing, cuddling, rocking, playing, and soothing   +1
        III Score (total circled points)   ___

IV. **Caretaking Behaviors:** Activities of mother aimed at supporting and protecting infant to foster child's optimal growth and development
A. Participation in care
    1. No participation in baby's care   0
    2. Holds infant but performs no care tasks   +1
    3. Recognizes infant's needs but leaves solution up to nurse, e.g., "Oh, the baby's wet"   +2
    4. Communicates baby's need to nurse and asks if she can do the task, e.g., "She's wet; can I change her?"   +3
    5. Performs isolated aspects of care such as changing diapers and feeding baby but needs encouragement from staff   +4
    6. Recognizes baby's needs and performs appropriate interventions, e.g., bathing, changing, and giving medication   +5
        IV-A Score (*Do not total:* record *highest* circled score)   ___
B. Planning home care
    7. Makes no reference to baby's discharge or to care that infant will require at home   0
    8. Refers to baby's eventual discharge or the care that infant will require at home   +1
    9. Asks questions in preparation for infant's discharge, e.g., "What kind of soap should I use?" or "When is the best time to give the bath at home?"   +2
    10. Makes reference to preparing for discharge actively, e.g., "We've just finished her room," or "I bought everything but the bottles today"   +3
        IV-B Score (*Do not total:* record *highest* circled score)   ___

        Scores for each section: I-A ____
        I-B ____
        II   ____
        III   ____
        IV-A ____
        IV-B ____

FIGURE 2-1 (*continued*)

Total Maternal Attachment Score	

Length of visits by mother to hospitalized infant
  1. None
  2. 1–15 minutes
  3. 16–30 minutes
  4. 31–60 minutes
  5. 61–120 minutes
  6. Over 2 hours
	____
	
	____

Frequency of visits by mother to hospitalized infant
  1. None
  2. Once a day
  3. Twice a day
  4. Three times a day
  5. More than three times a day
	____

Frequency of calls to hospital by mother
  1. None
  2. Once a day
  3. Twice a day
  4. Three times a day
  5. More than three times a day
	____

anything about a mother's emotional or physical condition, and does not attempt to assess the father's involvement with parenting or his support of the mother.

Delivery Room Screening

Screening tools for use in the delivery room are helpful so that nurses know the extent of initial parent–infant interactions and of parental responses to their newborns. Choi (1976) devised a screening tool for assessing parent–infant relationships in the delivery room and during the postpartum period (Figure 2-2). The Choi tool measures both mother and father contact with the infant in the following areas: sight, touch, talking, calling infant by name, and acceptance of child's sex.

Rising (1974) constructed a form for recording thirty-five responses by the mother during the fourth stage of labor (Figure 2-3). Maternal verbal and nonverbal responses are circled, and other significant information is obtained. This tool would be helpful in large hospitals in which intrapartal nurses are with the mother during the first postpartum hour. (See Chapter 10 for further information on the immediate post-delivery period.)

Assessment of Parenting Abilities

Bishop's (1976) guide to assessing parenting abilities is particularly helpful in that it assesses a mother's (or primary caretaker's) emotional and physical state, available support systems, and current level of parenting. Nurses who care for women during the postpartal period will find Bishop's hints particularly helpful. For *physical assessment,* Bishop recommends noting blood pressure, hemoglobin or hematocrit levels, pain of any intensity or duration, bleeding of any type, acute or chronic infections or any other medical problems, amount of sleep, weight in relation to height, medications, and woman's general appearance (e.g., clearness of eyes, posture).

For *emotional assessment,* Bishop recommends observation of listlessness, body language, level of understanding (which if less than it was antepartally, suggests depression), how mother was treated as a child, and cleanliness of the house (a scrupulously clean house is a danger signal). Both personal and professional support systems should be assessed. In assessing mothering skills Bishop uses Morris's *Criteria for Motherhood* and Rubin's *touch progression.* Morris (1966) has described mother–infant unity as satisfactory when a mother finds pleasure in her infant and in doing

	Mother	Father
Pregnancy: Planned Unplanned Wanted Unwanted		
Antepartal Reaction to Pregnancy		
Early weeks _____		
After quickening _____		
Late pregnancy _____		
Behavior and Reaction During Labor and Delivery		
( ) ( )		
Cooperative Uncooperative		
Parental Contact with Infant in Delivery Room		
Sight		
Touch		
Verbal		
Calls infant by name		
Acceptance of child's sex		
Postpartum Parental Contact		
Date		
Greeting to baby		
Eye contact		
Movements to and about baby		
Touching, caressing		
Caregiving skills		
Infant response		
Maternal concerns		
Paternal concerns		

FIGURE 2-2 Screening tool for assessing the parent–infant relationship. (From Choi, M.W. (1976). The significance of birth and the immediate postpartum period. Reprinted with permission of the publisher of PEDIATRIC NURSING, Vol. 2, No. 4, (July/August) 1976.)

tasks for the child, understands her infant's emotional states and comforts the infant accordingly, reads the infant's cues for new experiences, and senses infant fatigue level. Morris also enumerates several examples of negative responses to infant behaviors and notes that such responses indicate maladaption.

Assessment of Attachment as a Process

The tools and guides we have discussed, while helpful as screening devices, do not examine attachment as a process per se. Collaboration with other nurses and health professionals should be planned when screening suggests potential problems; assess-ment of the process of attachment requires the observations of many people. Nurses should also keep in mind that as an infant develops, the mother's interactional role with the infant changes.

Table 2-5 summarizes reports that focus on the process of attachment and on the changing tenor of mother–infant interactions over the first year of life. Behaviors have been grouped into two periods—the *turning-on* period and the *hooking* period. The turning-on period includes the first two and a half months of an infant's life, which includes an early sensitivity period, and the hooking period refers to the rest of the period of infancy, during which an infant becomes mobile and socially expressive.

Patient's name_____

Please circle appropriate responses:

Verbal Responses

1. Calls baby by name
2. Calls baby affectionate terms
3. Comments on beauty of baby and on realistic defects
4. Voices unhappiness over sex of baby
5. Calls baby "it"
6. Uses unhappy or scolding inflections
7. Asks husband or nurse if baby is all right
8. Talks about baby
9. Answers in monosyllables
10. Complains of difficult labor and delivery
11. Doesn't talk about baby
12. Requests that baby be taken to nursery
13. Seeks considerable support for own discomfort

Nonverbal Responses

1. Looks, reaches out to baby
2. Hugs, touches baby
3. Smiles at baby
4. Kisses baby
5. Undresses baby
6. Doesn't touch baby
7. Doesn't look at baby
8. Pushes baby away
9. Tenses face, arms
10. Sleepy, not drug induced
11. Turns away from baby
12. Turns away from husband, nurse, visitor
13. Positive eye contact, emotional feeling with husband
14. Unresponsive to husband, nurse, visitor
15. Cries unhappily
16. Holds husband's hand
17. Breast-feeds baby

First comments made in delivery room by mother about baby

_____

Visitor with mother during fourth stage_____

Involvement of husband or visitor_____

Problems with baby_____

Subjective opinion of response of mother   Parity _____

_____   Age_____

Analgesia within last four hours _____   Marital status_____

Anesthesia_____   Feeding method_____

Complications_____   Service_____

Significant social history_____   Race_____

_____

Behavior of baby

    Crying: None   Periodic   Almost continuous

    Affect: Difficult to arouse   Dozes   Eyes open

               Very alert

FIGURE 2-3 Form for recording responses of the mother during fourth-stage labor. (From Rising, S.S. (1974). The fourth stage of labor: Family integration. *American Journal of Nursing, 74*(5), 873. With permission.)

TABLE 2-5 Attachment process—First year of parenthood

Source	Turning-On Period	Hooking Period
Robertson (1972)	*0–8 weeks:* Mother aware of baby's affective status and able to respond to it; feels and expresses pleasure in having baby and in mothering activities; normal heightened anxiety of this period used in service of baby	*2½–5 months:* Infant has repertoire of accomplishments: hand–mouth movements, finger play with mother's help; infant differentiates mother from others; communication exchanged *6–12 months:* New movements initiated by baby or elicited by mother perfected with her help; infant derives pleasure from new skills—plays with mother; skills directed from communication with mother outward to environment
Sander (1962)	*0–2½ months:* Meshing of mothering activities with baby cues; learning to "read" baby's signals	*2½–5 months:* Alteration of stimulus–response *5½–9 months:* Infant more active, mother more passive *9–15 months:* Infant sees mother as person who meets needs; takes initiative to manipulate mother
Klaus et al. (1970)	*First contact with infant:* Touch progression, fingertip progression from extremities to trunk to massaging, encompassing palmar contact on trunk; en face position	
Robson & Moss (1970)	*0–4 weeks:* Maternal fatigue and insecurity; brief, intermittent feelings of love for infant *4–6 weeks:* Maternal sense of physical well-being and confidence; perception of infant increases feelings of rapport and intimacy *6–9 weeks:* Infant recognizes mother as person	*3 months:* Infant irresistible; pangs of conscience on leaving infant with sitter; strongly attached
Bromwich (1976)	*Level 1:* Mother enjoys being with infant *Level 2:* Mother is sensitive observer of infant; reads cues accurately; is responsive to them *Level 3:* Mother engages in a quality and quantity of interaction with infant that is mutually satisfying and provides opportunity for development of attachment and beginning system of communication likes in both familiar and new situations and at new levels of infant's development	*Level 4:* Mother demonstrates awareness of materials, activities, and experiences suitable for infant's stage of development *Level 5:* Mother indicates new play activities and experiences based on same principles as activities suggested to or modeled for her *Level 6:* Mother independently generates a range of appropriate activities; experiences infant's
Rubin (1977)	*0–6 weeks:* Involution—maternal fatigue, hostility to body image; polarization—mother sees infant as individual through identifying and claiming process	
Gottlieb (1978)	*0–4 weeks:* Discovery process—identifying, relating, interpreting	

THE ROLE OF NURSES IN FACILITATING PARENTAL ATTACHMENT

Nurses have great potential to help parental attachment through providing a supportive environment and caring for mother, father, and infant (Figure 2-4). To affect the alterable preconditions for parental attachment, nurses function in an advocacy role for parents and their rights, and they make judgments about situations that can be altered to increase mother–infant proximity without risk to mother or infant. Thus, nurses provide an environment conducive to mutually satisfying parent–infant interactions. Nurses in a hospital setting also identify potential or actual problem areas and collaborate with social workers, physicians, public health nurses, or nurse practitioners who will be seeing clients after their discharge from the hospital. Nurses can aid the attachment process by bolstering parents' self-confidence. They lend ego-support as parents assume parenting tasks, and provide the opportunity for a mother to review her parturition experiences and to integrate them into her self-system. Pediatric nurses and pediatricians were found to be equally accepted by parents and equally effective in reducing postpartal anxiety and depression (Kleinberg, 1977).

Nurses need to have accurate, comprehensive information about a client's emotional, physical, and social state; if the patient's records do not have the necessary data, some direct, nonthreatening questions are helpful. Because of the importance of a mother's having learned love and trust in her own childhood, two questions are particularly salient in regard to a wom-

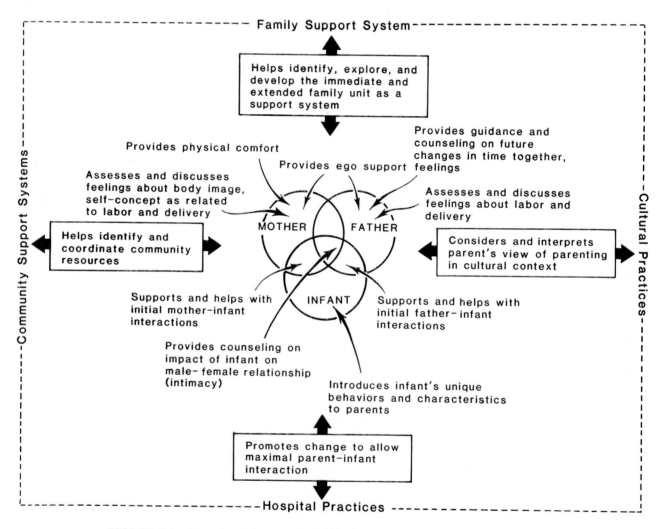

FIGURE 2-4 The role of the nurse in facilitating parental attachment to the infant.

an's emotional state: What was your childhood like for the first ten years? (Did you live with both parents? Happily? Emotional or physical problems?) What happened when you misbehaved or didn't do as your parents told you? (Emotional or physical abuse as child?)

A woman's adaptation during pregnancy is important because her attachment for her infant begins then. Therefore, the following questions are important: Was your pregnancy planned? When did your baby first move in utero? What was it like when you first felt your baby move? (If a woman does not remember when fetal movement first occurred, she was not very emotionally involved.) Any physical or medical complications that arise during pregnancy are usually among the first data recorded and are easily available, but the nurse may need sensitive questioning to discover what the emotional impact may have been.

The physical state of a new mother is usually well known to the intrapartal or postpartal nurses involved in her care; however, determining a woman's feelings about her body image and helping her express these feelings is as important to her emotional state as determining hemoglobin and hematocrit is to her physiological state.

Cultural expectations have an influence on a woman's self-concept; some women have related that their mothers viewed them as weak if they took analgesia or anesthesia when they had not. Some women who had to have Cesarean births have reported that other women looked down on them and suggested they were not able to "take" labor and delivery.

Ascertaining whom the mother has to help her when she goes home is important and can be followed by asking how she feels about the arrangement. In cases where the helper is her mother or mother-in-law, a woman may have ambivalent feelings and be in need of support in emphasizing that the helper is to help with household chores while infant care remains in the new mother's domain. In some cases, the new father may not perceive that his mate needs help, while the woman perceives that she does. This difference of opinion may reflect a lack of empathy and perhaps a lack of support and sensitivity in other areas as well. Other questions that are helpful in determining a woman's social situation are: Do you know other women with young children? Do you intend to return to work and if so, when? What day care is available to you? In the case of very young, immature mothers, teaching has to be on a level with their cognitive understanding. An assessment of cognitive and emotional maturity is therefore important. A nurse needs to discover who the young

woman has to help her: Does she have a mother or surrogate mother if she still needs one?

Promoting proximity of mother and infant is perhaps one of the greatest and most exciting challenges for nurses. The following may be helpful in promoting mutually satisfying mother–infant interactions:

- Giving the mother pain-relief medication well in advance of feedings, so that she has optimal relief during infant feedings.
- Staying with the new mother until she feels comfortable undertaking a task alone.
- Letting her watch a nurse perform a task before she attempts it herself. (The nurse, in this case, should be careful not to make the task look too easy and not to finish too quickly; it is less devastating to a new mother if the infant's foot or hand gets in the nurses way, too.)
- Being sensitive to fatigue levels. (The mother in her euphoric state may not realize her fatigue.)
- Pursuing changes in hospital rules and regulations until they allow for unlimited parent–infant interaction, sibling visits, and continued presence of the mother's support person during labor, delivery, and the postpartum period.

Parental attachment, the tie that binds parents to their child so that they lovingly and willingly provide physical, emotional, and social support for the ensuing twenty years, deserves more careful study. Parental commitment, which must endure through the stresses and vicissitudes of family life, is an extraordinary challenge.

Based on an understanding of the theoretical formulations about parent–infant attachment, nurses can provide care that facilitates family development. Because many aspects of the perinatal period have an impact on the long-term emotional and physiological adjustment of families, measures that enhance parent–infant attachment serve to strengthen the family unit and thus contribute to the health of family members.

REFERENCES AND ADDITIONAL READINGS

Ainsworth, M.D. (1964). Patterns of attachment behavior shown by the infant in interaction with his mother. *Merrill-Palmer Quarterly, 10,* 51–58.

Aleksandrowicz, M.K., & Aleksandrowicz, D.R. (1975). The molding of personality: a newborn's innate characteristics in interaction with parents' personalities. *Child Psychiatry and Human Development, 5,* 231–241.

Aleksandrowicz, M.K., & Aleksandrowicz, D.R. (1976). Precursors of ego in neonates. *Journal of the American Academy of Child Psychiatry, 15*(2), 257–267.

Barbero, G. (1975). Failure to thrive. In M.H. Klaus, T. Leger, & M.S. Trause (Eds.), *Maternal attachment and mothering disorders: A round table.* New Brunswick, N.J.: Johnson & Johnson Baby Products.

Bell, R.Q. (1974). Contributions of human infants to caregiving and social interaction. In M. Lewis & L.A. Rosenblum (Eds.), *The effect of the infant on its caregiver.* New York: Wiley.

Benedik, T. (1949). The psychosomatic implications of the primary unit: Mother–child. *American Journal of Orthopsychiatry, 19,* 642–654.

Bennett, S. (1971). Infant–caretaker interactions. *Journal of the American Academy of Child Psychiatry, 10,* 321–335.

Bibring, G.L. (1965). Some specific psychological tasks in pregnancy and motherhood. In *First International Congress of Psychosomatic Medicine and Childbirth.* Paris: Gauthier-Villars.

Bishop, B. (1976). A guide to assessing parenting capabilities. *American Journal of Nursing, 76*(11), 1784–1787.

Blumberg, M.L. (1974). Psychopathology of the abusing parent. *American Journal of Psychotherapy, 28*(1), 21–29.

Bowlby, J. (1953). *Child care and the growth of love.* New York: Penguin.

Bowlby, J. (1958). The nature of the child's tie to his mother. *International Journal of Psychoanalysis, 39,* 350–373.

Bowlby, J. (1977). The making and breaking of affectional bonds I. Aetiology and psychopathology in the light of attachment theory. *British Journal of Psychiatry, 130,* 201–210.

Brazelton, T.B. (1973). *Neonatal behavioral assessment scale.* Philadelphia: Lippincott.

Brazelton, T.B. (1974). *Does the neonate shape his environment?* Perinatal Reprint Series. White Plains, N.Y.: National Foundation March of Dimes.

Bromwich, R.M. (1976). Focus on maternal behavior in infant intervention. *American Journal of Orthopsychiatry, 46*(3), 439–446.

Broussard, E.R., & Hartner, M.S.S. (1970). Maternal perception of the neonate as related to development. *Child psychiatry and human development, 1*(1), 16–25.

Broussard, E.R., & Hartner, M.S.S. (1971). Further considerations regarding maternal perception of the first born. In J. Hellmuth (Ed.), *Exceptional Infant. II.* New York: Brunner/Mazel.

Cairns, R.B. (1972). Attachment and dependency: A psychobiological social-learning synthesis. In J.L. Gewirtz (Ed.), *Attachment and dependency.* New York: Wiley.

Caldwell, B.M. (1962). The usefulness of the critical period hypothesis in the study of filiative behavior. *Merrill-Palmer Quarterly, 8,* 229–242.

Call, J.D. (1964). Newborn approach behavior and early ego development. *International Journal of Psychoanalysis, 45,* 286–293.

Cannon, R.B. (1977). The development of maternal touch during early mother-infant interaction. *Journal of Obstetric, Gynecologic, and Neonatal Nursing, 6*(2), 188–194.

Carey, W.B. (1970). A simplified method for measuring infant temperament. *Journal of Pediatrics, 77*(2), 188–194.

Choi, M.W. (1976). The significance of birth and the immediate postpartum period. *Pediatric Nursing, 1*(4), 8–13.

Clark, A.L. (1976). Recognizing discord between mother and child and changing it to harmony. *MCN: The American Journal of Maternal Child Nursing, 1*(2), 100–106.

Clark, A.L., & Affonso, D.D. (1979). *Childbearing: A nursing perspective.* Philadelphia: Davis.

Cohler, B.J., Grunebaum, H.U., Weiss, J.L., Hartman, C.R., & Gallant, V.H. (1976). Child care attitudes and adaptation to the maternal role among mentally ill and well mothers. *American Journal of Orthopsychiatry, 46*(1), 123–134.

Condon, W.S., & Sander, L.W. (1974). Neonate movement is synchronized with adult speech: Interactional participation and language acquisition. *Science, 183,* 99–101.

Cropley, C., Lester, P., & Pennington, S. (1976). Assessment tool for measuring maternal attachment behaviors. In L.K. McNall & J.T. Galeener (Eds.). *Current practice in obstetric and gynecologic nursing. I.* St. Louis: Mosby.

de Chateau, P. (1976). The influence of early contact on maternal and infant behavior in primiparae. *Birth and the Family Journal, 3*(4), 149–155.

de Chateau, P. (1977). The importance of the neonatal period for the development of synchrony in the mother-infant dyad—A review. *Birth and the Family Journal, 4*(1), 10–22.

Deutsch, J. (1945). *The psychology of women* (Vol. II). New York: Grune & Stratton.

Fanaroff, A.A., Kennell, J.H., & Klaus, M.H. (1972). Follow-up of low birth weight infants—The predictive value of maternal visiting patterns. *Pediatrics, 49*(2), 287–290.

Fein, R.A. (1976). The first weeks of fathering: The importance of choices and supports for new parents. *Birth and the Family Journal, 3*(2), 53–58.

Fox, M. (1977). Attachment of kibbutz infants to mother and metapelet. *Child Development, 48,* 1228–1239.

Freud, S. (1959). *The complete psychological works of Sigmund Freud* (standard ed., Vol. 20). (J. Strachey, trans.). London: Hogarth Press.

Frommer, E.A., & O'Shea, G. (1973). Antenatal identification of women liable to have problems in managing their infants. *British Journal of Psychiatry, 123,* 149–156.

Gerson, E.F. (1973). Dimensions of infant behavior in the first half year of life. In P.M. Shereshefski & L.J. Yarrow (Eds.), *Psychological aspects of a first pregnancy and early postnatal adaptation.* New York: Raven Press.

Gewirtz, J.L. (1972a). Attachment, dependence, and a distinction in terms of stimulus control. In J.L. Gewirtz (Ed.), *Attachment and dependency.* New York: Wiley.

Gewirtz, J.L. (1972b). On the selection and use of attachment and dependence indices. In J.L. Gewirtz (Ed.), *Attachment and dependency.* New York: Wiley.

Gottlieb, L. (1978). Maternal attachment in primiparas. *Journal of Obstetric, Gynecologic, and Neonatal Nursing, 7*(1), 39–44.

Greenberg, M., & Morris, N. (1974). Engrossment: The newborn's impact upon the father. *American Journal of Orthopsychiatry, 44*(4), 520–531.

Greenberg, M., Rosenberg, I., & Lind, J. (1973). First mothers rooming-in with their newborns: Its impact upon the mother. *American Journal of Orthopsychiatry, 43*(5), 783–788.

Gregg, C.L., Haffner, M.E., & Korner, A.F. (1976). The relative efficacy of vestibular-proprioceptive stimulation and the upright position in enhancing visual pursuit in neonates. *Child Development, 47,* 309–314.

Haar, E., Welkowitz, J., Blau, A., & Cohen, J. (1964). Personality differentiation of neonates: A nurse rating scale method. *Journal of the American Academy of Child Psychiatry, 3,* 330–342.

Harlow, J.F. (1958). The nature of love. *American Psychologist, 13,* 673–685.

Harlow, J.F. (1962). The heterosexual affectional system in monkeys.

American Psychologist, 17, 1–9.

Harlow, J.F. (1977). The need for mother-love. J. Greenberg (rep.), *San Francisco Sunday Examiner and Chronicle, This World,* Oct. 2, pp. 28–29.

Harper, L.V. (1971). The young as a source of stimuli controlling caretaker behavior. *Developmental Psychology, 4*(1), 73–88.

Harper, R.G., Consepcion, S., Sokal, S., & Sokal, M. (1976). Observations on unrestricted parental contact with infants in the neonatal intensive care unit. *Journal of Pediatrics, 89*(3), 441–445.

Harrison, L.L. (1976). Nursing intervention with the failure-to-thrive family. *MCN: The American Journal of Maternal Child Nursing, 1*(2), 111–116.

Heard, D.H. (1978). From object relations to attachment theory: A basis for family therapy. *British Journal of Medical Psychology, 51,* 67–76.

Helfer, R. (1974). Relationship between lack of bonding and child abuse and neglect. In M.H. Klaus, T. Leger, & M.A. Trause (Eds.), *Maternal attachment and mothering disorders: A round table.* New Brunswick, N.J.: Johnson & Johnson Baby Products.

Hunter, R.S., Kilstrom, N., Kraybill, E.N., & Loda, F. (1978). Antecedents of child abuse and neglect in premature infants: A prospective study in a newborn intensive care unit. *Pediatrics, 61*(4), 629–635.

Jenkins, P.W. (1976). Conflicts of a secundigravida. *Maternal–Child Nursing Journal, 5*(2), 117–126.

Kempe, C.H. (1962). The battered-child syndrome. *Journal of American Medical Association, 181,* 17–24.

Kennedy, J.C. (1973). The high-risk maternal–infant acquaintance process. *Nursing Clinics of North America, 8*(3), 549–556.

Kennell, J.H., Jerauld, R., Wolfe, H., Chesler, D., Kreger, N.C., Maclpine, W., Steffa, M., & Klaus, M.H. (1974). Maternal behavior one year after early and extended postpartum contact. *Developmental Medicine Child Neurology, 16,* 172–179.

Klaus, M.H., Kennell, J.H., Plumb, N., & Zuehlke, S. (1970). Human maternal behavior at the first contact with her young. *Pediatrics, 46*(2), 187–192.

Klaus, M.H., Jerauld, R., Kreger, N.C., Maclpine, W., Steffa, M., & Kennell, J.H. (1972). Maternal attachment importance of the first postpartum days. *New England Journal of Medicine, 286*(9), 460–463.

Klaus, M.H., & Kennell, J.H. (1982). *Parent–infant bonding.* St. Louis: Mosby.

Kleinberg, W.M. (1977). Counseling mothers in the hospital postpartum period: A comparison of techniques. *American Journal of Public Health, 67*(7), 672–674.

Knox, D., & Gilman, R.C. (1974). The first year of fatherhood. *Family Perspective, 9*(2), 31–34.

Korner, A.F., & Grobstein, R. (1966). Visual alertness as related to soothing in neonates: Implications for maternal stimulation and early deprivation. *Child Development, 37,* 867–876.

Korner, A.F., & Thoman, E.B. (1970). Visual alertness in neonates as evoked by maternal care. *Journal of Experimental Child Psychology, 10,* 67–78.

Lamb, M.E. (1974). A defense of the concept of attachment. *Human Development, 17,* 376–385.

Lamb, M.E., & Lamb, J.E. (1976). The nature and importance of the father–infant relationship. *The Family Coordinator, 25*(4), 379–385.

Leifer, A.D., Leiderman, P.H., Barnett, C.R., & Williams, J.A. (1972). Effects of mother–infant separation on maternal attachment behavior. *Child Development, 43,* 1203–1218.

Leonard, S.W. (1976). How first-time fathers feel toward their newborns. *MCN: The American Journal of Maternal Child Nursing, 1*(6), 361–365.

Lewis, M., & Wilson, C.D. (1972). Infant development in lower-class American families. *Human Development, 15,* 112–137.

Lozoff, B., Brittenham, G.M., Trause, M.A., Kennell, J.H., & Klaus, M.H. (1977). The mother–newborn relationship: Limits of adaptability. *Journal of Pediatrics, 91*(1), 1–12.

Macfarlane, A. (1975). Olfaction in the development of social preferences in the human neonate. In *Ciba Foundation Symposium 33, Parents-Infant Interaction.* New York: Elsevier.

Marut, J.S. (1978). The special needs of the cesarean mother. *MCN: The American Journal of Maternal Child Nursing, 3*(4), 202–206.

Marut, J.S., & Mercer, R.T. (1979). A comparison of primiparas' perceptions of vaginal and cesarean births. *Nursing Research, 28*(5), 260–266.

McDonald, D.L. (1978). Paternal behavior at first contact with the newborn in a birth environment without intrusions. *Birth and the Family Journal, 5*(3), 123–132.

McInerny, T., & Chamberlin, R.W. (1978). Is it feasible to identify infants who are at risk for later behavioral problems? *Clinical Pediatrics, 17*(3), 233–238.

Mercer, R.T. (1974). Mothers' responses to their infants with defects. *Nursing Research, 23*(2), 133–137.

Mercer, R.T. (1977a). *Nursing care for parents at risk.* Thorofare, N.J.: C.B. Slack.

Mercer, R.T. (1977b). Postpartum illness and acquaintance–attachment process. *American Journal of Nursing, 77,* 1174–1178.

Mercer, M.T. (1980). Teenage motherhood: The first year. Part I. The teenage mother's views and responses. Part II. How their infants fared. *Journal of Obstetric, Gynecologic, and Neonatal Nursing, 9*(1), 16–27.

Minde, K., Trehaub, S., Corter, C., Boukydis, C., Celhoffer, L., & Martow, P. (1978). Mother–child relationships in the premature nursery: An observational study. *Pediatrics, 61*(3), 373–379.

Morris, M.G. (1966). Psychological miscarriage: An end to mother love. *Trans-Action, 3*(2), 8–13.

Moss, H.A. (1968). Sex, age, and state, as determinants of mother-infant interaction. In S. Chess & A. Thomas (Eds.), *Annual Progress in Child Psychiatry and Child Development 1968.* New York: Brunner/Mazel.

Osofsky, J.D., & Danzger, B. (1974). Relationships between neonatal characteristics and mother–infant interaction. *Developmental Psychology, 10*(1), 124–130.

Parke, R.D., & Sawin, D.B. (1976). The father's role in infancy: A reevaluation. *The Family Coordinator, 25*(4), 365–371.

Porter, C.P. (1973). Maladaptive mothering patterns: Nursing intervention. *American clinical sessions, ANA, 1972 Detroit.* New York: Appleton-Century-Crofts.

Provence, S., & Lipton, R.C. (1962). *Infants in institutions.* New York: International Universities Press.

Reiber, V.D. (1976). Is the nurturing role natural to fathers? *MCN: The American Journal of Maternal Child Nursing, 1*(6), 366–371.

Rendina, I., & Dickerscheid, J.D. (1976). Father involvement with first born infants. *The Family Coordinator, 25*(4), 373–378.

Richards, M.P.M. (1971). Social interaction in the first weeks of human life. *Psychiatria Neurologia, Neurochirurgia, 74,* 35–42.

Richards, M.P.M., Bernal, J.F., & Brackbill, Y. (1976). Early behavioral differences: Gender or circumcision? *Developmental Psychology, 9*(1), 89-95.

Richards, M.P.M., Dunn, J.F., & Antonis, B. (1977). Caretaking in the first year of life: The role of fathers, mothers' social isolation. *Child: Care, Health, and Development, 3,* 856-859.

Rieser, J., Yonas, A., & Wilkner, K. (1976). Radial localization of odors by human newborns. *Child Development, 47,* 856-859.

Ringler, N.M., Kennell, J.H., Jarvella, R., Navojosky, B.J., & Klaus, M.H. (1975). Mother-to-child speech at two years—Effects of early postnatal contact. *Journal of Pediatrics, 86*(1), 141-144.

Rising, S.S. (1974). The fourth stage of labor: Family integration. *American Journal of Nursing, 74*(5), 873.

Robertson, J. (1972). Mothering as an influence on early development. *Psychoanalytic Study of the Child, 17,* 245-264.

Robson, K.S. (1968). The role of eye-to-eye contact in maternal-infant attachment. In S. Chess & A. Thomas (Eds.), *Annual progress in child psychiatry and child development 1968.* New York: Brunner/Mazel.

Robson, K.S., & Moss, H.A. (1970). Patterns and determinants of maternal attachment. *Journal of Pediatrics, 77*(6), 976-985.

Rosenthal, M.K. (1973). Attachment and mother-infant interaction: Some research impasse and a suggested change in orientation. *Journal Child Psychology and Psychiatry, 14,* 201-207.

Rubin, R. (1961). Basic maternal behavior. *Nursing Outlook, 9*(11), 683-686.

Rubin, R. (1963). Maternal touch. *Nursing Outlook, 11*(11), 828-831.

Rubin, R. (1975). Maternal tasks in pregnancy. *Maternal-Child Nursing Journal 4*(3), 143-153.

Rubin, R. (1977). Binding-in in the postpartum period. *Maternal-Child Nursing Journal, 6*(2), 67-75.

Salk, L. (1970). The critical nature of the post-partum period in the human for the establishment of the mother-infant bond: A controlled study. *Diseases of the Nervous System, 31*(Suppl.), 110-116.

Sander, L.W. (1962). Issues in early mother-child interaction. *Journal of American Academy of Child Psychiatry, 1,* 141-166.

Sander, L.W. (1964). Adaptive relationships in early mother-child interaction. *Journal of American Academy of Child Psychiatry, 3,* 231-264.

Schroeder, M.A. (1977). Is the immediate postpartum period crucial to the mother-child relationship? *Journal of Obstetric, Gynecologic, and Neonatal Nursing, 6*(3), 37-40.

Schroeder, M.A., Macoby, E.E., & Levin, H. (1957). *Patterns of child rearing.* New York: Harper & Row.

Sears, R.R. (1972). Attachment, dependency, and frustration. In J.L. Gewirtz (Ed.), *Attachment and dependency.* New York: Wiley.

Seashore, J.J., Leifer, A.D., Barnett, C.R., & Leiderman, P.H. (1973). The effects of denial of early mother-infant interaction on maternal self-confidence. *Journal of Personality and Social Psychology, 26*(3), 369-378.

Serafica, F.C. (1978). The development of attachment behaviors: An organismic-developmental perspective. *Human Development, 21,* 119-140.

Shereshefski, P.M., Liebenberg, B., & Lockman, R.F. (1973). Maternal adaptation. In P.M. Shereshefski & L.J. Yarrow (Eds.), *Psychological aspects of a first pregnancy and early postnatal adaptation.* New York: Raven Press.

Sroufe, L.A., & Waters, E. (1977). Attachment as an organizational construct. *Child Development, 48,* 118-199.

Stratton, P.M. (1977). Criteria for assessing the influence of obstetric circumstances on later development. In T. Chard & M. Richards (Eds.), *Benefits and hazards of the new obstetrics.* Philadelphia: Lippincott.

Sugarman, M. (1977). Paranatal influences on maternal-infant attachment. *American Journal of Orthopsychiatry, 17*(3), 407-421.

Thoman, E.B. (1975). Sleep and wake behaviors in neonates: Consistencies and consequences. *Merrill-Palmer Quarterly, 21*(4), 295-314.

Thomas, A., & Chess, S. (1977). *Temperament and development.* New York: Brunner/Mazel.

Turner, R.H. (1970). *Family interaction.* New York: Wiley.

Winnicott, D.W. (1970). The mother-infant experience of mutuality. In E.J. Anthony & T. Benedek (Eds.), *Parenthood: Its psychology and psychopathology.* Boston: Little, Brown.

Part 2 | Prenatal Family Needs and Concerns

HEALTH AND WELL-BEING are dependent on knowledge and information of healthful habits and practices. Education for quality childbirth, parenting experiences, and prenatal care are essential aspects of quality living.

The chapters in this section deal with various aspects of childbearing health. Chapter 3 examines those elements essential to providing quality prenatal care to families including antepartal screening and physiological assessments. Chapter 4 addresses the nutritional requirements of pregnant women. Nutrition assessment tools are discussed, as are suggestions for nutritional counseling. Principles for ascertaining a wom-

an's nutritional status are explored, recognizing that there are many different dietary choices based on individual preference, religious beliefs, and cultural practices. Chapter 5 deals with education for childbirth and parenthood. Emphasis is placed on the provision of responsible education.

Education provided to families must focus on the strengths and needs of the individual family members, supporting them and encouraging them. The recognition of these strengths may allow families to develop further and to gain the self-confidence necessary for the demanding tasks of childbearing and child-rearing

Chapter 3 | Essentials of Prenatal Care

Marcia Gruis Killien
Carol Jean Poole
Betty Jennings

THE PRENATAL PERIOD involves complex phys-iological changes and emotional adjustments for the pregnant woman. These changes affect not only the woman but also her family and the significant others in her social environment.

The growth of the fetus and accompanying physical changes that occur during the forty weeks of gestation are relatively predictable. The feelings and behaviors that accompany these changes, however, may be more diverse, dependent on the unique situation and charac-teristics of the individual woman. Through early and continuous prenatal health care, the pregnant woman and her family can be assisted in successfully adapting to pregnancy changes. Health care includes the on-going assessment of the expectant mother's physical and emotional health, assessment of fetal development and well-being, education for health maintenance during pregnancy, and guidance in preparing for labor, delivery, and the postpartum period. While the primary goal of prenatal care is to assure a healthy mother and baby, an equally important goal is to promote an optimal physical and emotional experience for the expectant family. Achieving this goal is dependent on the sensitivity of the practitioner to the unique needs of the couple.

Pregnancy is a normal physiological process. How-ever, the process imposes stress upon the body to which both the woman and fetus must adapt. The fetus is particularly vulnerable during the earliest stages of pregnancy when organogenesis is occurring. The woman's health status at the beginning of pregnancy and her health habits, such as cigarette, alcohol, or drug use, can have an impact on the developing baby. Ideally, a woman will be in an optimum state of health and free of exposure to harmful substances prior to conception. This is not always the case, however. Thus, health care, if not begun preconception, should begin as soon as pregnancy is suspected.

The pregnant woman of today has many options for the type of care she receives during her pregnancy. Increasingly, prenatal care is being provided by an interdisciplinary team including an obstetrician, nurse-midwife, nurse, nutritionist, and social worker. Each of these professionals offers a unique service to the preg-nant woman, and their cooperative efforts can facilitate a more optimal pregnancy experience for the woman

TABLE 3-1 Clinical diagnosis of pregnancy

Gestation (weeks)	Sign	Symptom
4–6	Softening of the cervix (Goodell's sign)	Amenorrhea or "missed period"
5–6	Softening of the cervical-uterine junction (Laden's sign)	
6	Compressibility of lower uterine segment (Hegar's sign)	Urinary frequency, nausea, vomiting
	Bluish violet appearance of vagina and cervix (Chadwick's sign)	
6–8	Dilation of breast veins	Breast tenderness
	Pulsation of uterine arteries in lateral fornices (Osiander's sign)	Constipation, fatigue, leukorrhea
7–8	Flexing fundus or cervix (McDonald's sign); uterus softened and enlarged asymmetrically (globular rather than pear-shaped)	
12–14	Detection of fetal heart tones with Doppler unit	
16	Uterine souffle bilaterally above symphysis (same rate as mother's pulse)	Skin pigmentation, i.e. chloasma or linea nigra
16–18	Fetal movement; ballottement of fetus	Quickening
18	Auscultation of fetal heart tones	
24	Palpable fetal outline	
24–26	Braxton Hick's contractions	Contractions

From Roberts, J. Antepartum module. College of Nursing, Department of Maternal-Child Nursing, Nurse-Midwifery Program, University of Illinois Medical Center, Chicago, 1975. With permission.

and her family. This approach can also result in better utilization of health care personnel. Often the nurse practitioner or midwife is the primary health provider for the woman with an uncomplicated pregnancy while the obstetrician provides care to the high-risk patient. In each situation the nurse and physician need to work together to meet the woman's needs for physical care, emotional support, and information.

INITIAL PRENATAL CARE

The nature of the first visit between the nurse and the pregnant woman will be determined to some extent on the phase of the pregnancy process that the woman is in. She may be seeking confirmation of a suspected pregnancy, or she may be seeking further prenatal care for a confirmed pregnancy. While women seek initial prenatal care at different stages of pregnancy, ideally the first visit is as early in the pregnancy as possible. Regardless of the stage of pregnancy, the purposes of the initial prenatal visit include the following:

- Diagnosis (or confirmation of diagnosis) of pregnancy and establishment of the expected due date or expected date of confinement (EDC)
- Assessment of the individual needs of the client for care (including an initial assessment of risk status)
- Establishment of a mutually satisfying contract for ongoing care or initiation of an appropriate referral

Diagnosis of Pregnancy

The first step in health care delivery during the antepartum period is confirmation of the pregnancy. Whether the pregnancy has long been planned or comes unexpectedly, there is still a time of uncertainty. Many of the signs of early pregnancy are so well known that most women suspect the pregnancy first themselves and then seek confirmation from other women or from health professionals. Some women seek medical confirmation as soon as they suspect they are pregnant while others choose to wait until later in the pregnancy.

It is important to detect the pregnancy early if a

woman desires a voluntary termination of pregnancy or if an ectopic or other pregnancy complication is suspected. Whenever possible women should be tested for a possible pregnancy prior to having any kind of x-rays.

The diagnosis of pregnancy is based on the presence of particular signs and symptoms (Table 3-1). Physical signs and symptoms are traditionally divided into three categories: presumptive, probable, and positive. The presumptive signs of pregnancy are those the patient can identify herself. All are factors that could be caused by processes other than pregnancy. Women who are in touch with their bodies, i.e., are aware of changes their bodies go through normally, such as breast tenderness prior to menstruation, and women who have been pregnant before are usually quicker to notice the symptoms and to relate them to a possible pregnancy. *Presumptive signs* include cessation of menses, breast changes, nausea and vomiting, discoloration of the mucosa and skin of the vulva and vagina, quickening, changes in pigmentation of the skin, urinary disturbances, and fatigue. *Probable signs* of pregnancy include enlargement of the abdomen, changes in size, shape, and consistency of the uterus, cervical changes, Braxton Hicks contractions, ballottement, outlining the fetus through palpation, and pregnancy tests. *Positive signs* of pregnancy include outlining the fetus through ultrasound or x-ray, hearing and counting fetal heart tones, and palpating fetal movements during an examination.

The presence or absence of these signs is determined by a thorough interview and history, physical examination, and laboratory tests. If the woman is suspected of being in the early stages of pregnancy, general procedure includes a brief interview followed by a pregnancy test. The interview is aimed at establishing the presence of the presumptive signs of pregnancy. The woman should be asked why she thinks she is pregnant and what physical changes she has experienced. She should be specifically asked about the following signs.

Cessation of Menses When a healthy woman with a history of regular menses skips a period, pregnancy should be suspected. This is not a reliable indication until at least ten days after the day the period was due. Cessation of menses occurs because chorionic gonadotropin secreted by the trophoblast stimulates the corpus luteum to continue producing estrogen and progesterone. Continued production of these hormones maintains the endometrium and suppresses ovulation. If the corpus luteum is removed during the first two months

of pregnancy (by ovariotomy) the pregnancy will terminate (Landau, 1976).

In adolescent girls or women with a history of irregular periods, cessation of menses is not a reliable sign of pregnancy. Also, lactating women may not menstruate, and if reliable contraception is not used, a pregnancy may occur prior to return of menses. Absence of menses may also be related to emotional tension, environmental changes, chronic disease, or participation in endurance sports.

Conversely, it is not unusual for women to have small amounts of bloody discharge during pregnancy. Speert and Guttmacher (1954) studied 225 women who did not abort; they reported that macroscopic vaginal bleeding occurred between conception and the 196th day following the last menstrual period in 21.8 percent of the women. For eight percent the bleeding occurred during the first forty days. Vaginal bleeding was found three times more often in multiparas than in primigravidas. These factors make determination of a woman's expected due date difficult to base on menstrual history alone.

Breast Changes During pregnancy, many changes occur in the breasts. Women frequently describe breast tingling and tenderness during the first weeks of pregnancy. The breasts increase in size due to increased hormonal stimulation.

Nausea and Vomiting Some degree of nausea and vomiting occurs in about half of all pregnancies. The nausea occurs most frequently in the morning, hence it is called *morning sickness*. However, some women experience it at other times or throughout the day. For most women the symptom begins about the time of the first missed menstrual period and disappears at the end of the first trimester.

The etiology of nausea and vomiting is unknown. There are several theories mentioned in discussing the symptom. Women who have excessive nausea and vomiting have been found to have higher titers of chorionic gonadotropin in their urine and serum (Reid et al., 1972). These titers are elevated beyond the normal increases found in early pregnancy. However, some clinicians feel that the high titer may be a result of dehydration rather than an increase in the amount of hormone secreted.

Another theory is that women who experience nausea and vomiting are having trouble adjusting to the quantities of estrogen present during pregnancy. This theory is supported by the fact that estrogen overdosage causes nausea and vomiting in nonpregnant women. (Reid et al., 1972)

It has also been suggested that the pregnant woman may react to the products of conception as to a foreign body. At the same time liver glycogen metabolism may be altered by the demands of the new conceptus. Supporters of this theory explain that by the twelfth week the mother becomes desensitized to the conceptus and glycogen metabolism compensation has occurred (Sites, 1972). With these adjustments the nausea and vomiting disappears.

Traditionally, nausea and vomiting have been considered psychosomatic conditions. The symptom was felt to be due to ambivalence toward the pregnancy, social or economic stresses, fear of labor and delivery, or a variety of other life stresses. Although these factors may be related to the incidence of nausea and vomiting, research shows that except in the condition of hysteria there is no sustenance to the belief that the patient who has nausea and vomiting has a greater incidence of psychiatric difficulties than other pregnant women (Reid et al., 1972).

Nausea and vomiting may also have cultural implications. Of 475 Native American women, only fourteen percent experienced nausea and vomiting. There was not even a word for "morning sickness" in their vocabulary (McCammon, 1951). Erickson (cited in Ferreia, 1969) noted that when a group of Mexican villagers who had previously had no experience with "morning sickness" moved to California they began to display the syndrome.

The presence of nausea and vomiting may be related to the outcome of pregnancy. Brandes (1967), in studying 7027 pregnant women, found that absence of nausea and vomiting was correlated with a higher abortion rate and higher neonatal and infant mortality rates.

Urinary Disturbances During the early months of pregnancy the uterus places pressure on the bladder, resulting in urinary frequency. This symptom disappears as the uterus displaces the abdominal organs and rises out of the pelvic cavity during the third month. When this symptom is evaluated, it is necessary that signs of urinary tract infection also be assessed.

Fatigue Another common symptom experienced by pregnant women is fatigue, the cause of which is unknown. In fact, little attention has been paid to this symptom; most literature mentions that fatigue occurs along with nausea and vomiting during the first trimester, but it is not discussed further. It has been

suggested that the increased levels of progesterone may be a factor, since progesterone in high doses can cause somnolence and the hormone has occasionally been used as an anesthetic agent (Quilligan, 1977).

Fatigue is usually present during the first trimester of pregnancy. After this period, the woman frequently experiences a feeling of well-being with increased amounts of energy until the third trimester, when fatigue may reoccur.

Women differ in the extent to which they experience and report these early signs of pregnancy. While these signs do provide a clue to the diagnosis of pregnancy, laboratory tests provide stronger evidence.

Laboratory Tests

Pregnancy tests can be divided into three main categories: biological, immunological, and hormonal. Biological and immunological tests depend on the presence of human chorionic gonadotropin (HCG), found in the plasma and urine of pregnant women. HCG is detectable as early as two weeks by some tests and after four weeks' gestation by most pregnancy tests. HCG peaks at six weeks and the peak persists until the twelfth week. Low levels of HCG are present after the sixteenth week.

Biological Tests Biological tests depend on the reaction of an animal's sex organs to HCG present in the urine of the woman being tested. The rat ovarian hyperemia test is considered to be the most satisfactory test of this type. The biological tests are accurate, but they are also expensive, time-consuming, and necessitate animal wastage.

Immunological Tests The most frequently used immunological test is the latex inhibition slide test. This is easily done in the patient care setting, and requires only minutes to perform. This test is based on the principle of antigen–antibody response. Rabbit serum containing antihuman chorionic gonadotropin antibodies will produce agglutination of latex particles that have been coated with HCG. If urine from a pregnant woman is mixed with the rabbit serum antibody, agglutination does not occur when the HCG coated latex particles are added. This is because the serum antibody has already combined with the urine HCG and is not available to agglutinate with the latex particles. Thus, a positive pregnancy test appears smooth; the negative test appears granular or agglutinated.

False-positive or false-negative tests are very common. Problems arise from the fact that there are immunological and biological similarities between the HCG formed by the trophoblast and the luteinizing hormone secreted by the pituitary. In almost all assay tests the luteinizing hormone cross-reacts with the antibody to HCG, producing a false-positive test. False-positives can occur whenever (1) an interfering substance (protein) neutralizes the HCG antiserum, (2) damage occurs to the carrier particles causing dissociation of HCG from the particles, or (3) there is a deterioration of the antiserum (Cabrera, 1972). Very early in pregnancy a false-negative test may occur due to the small amount of HCG being produced by the trophoblast.

Pregnancy diagnosis can also be made by immunoassay of serum HCG, which is so sensitive as to detect pregnancy one to two weeks after conception. This test is performed by a specially equipped laboratory. The antibodies used are specific to HCG, do not cross-react with luteinizing hormone, and greatly diminish false-positive tests. Immunoassay is especially helpful when early pregnancy diagnosis is critical (Beers, 1979).

Hormonal Tests The third type of pregnancy test also differentiates anovulatory amenorrhea from early pregnancy. If a patient receives progesterone tablets daily for two to five days, bleeding will occur one to fifteen days after the hormone is stopped if the woman is not pregnant and the endometrium is adequately primed with estrogen. False-positive tests may occur in cases of traumatic amenorrhea or ovarian failure. Because reliable immunological and biological tests are available and because of the risk of fetal exposure to exogenous hormones, this type of pregnancy test is not recommended (Beers, 1979; Pritchard & MacDonald, 1980).

It is important that health practitioners not rely on laboratory tests alone. The patient should be examined at frequent intervals until the pregnancy can be positively determined.

Pelvic Examination

Early signs of pregnancy can also be detected during a pelvic examination. These signs include changes in the size, shape, and consistency of the uterus, and changes in the appearance of the vaginal mucosa.

Uterine and Cervical Changes The pregnant uterus enlarges throughout the pregnancy. During the first few weeks, substantial growth occurs in the anterioposterior diameter of the uterus. Later it becomes almost globular; changing as it grows from a pear-shaped organ to a spherical one. The size of the uterus can also be palpated on bimanual examination. Increased size of the uterus, consistent with suspected gestation, is a probable sign of pregnancy.

Changes in uterine consistency also occur. During pregnancy, the uterus changes from firm to doughy, elastic, or soft. About the sixth week after the last period, the junction of the corpus and the cervix in the region of the uterine isthmus becomes so soft that on bimanual examination, the examiner seems to feel nothing. This is known as *Hegar's sign* and is a very useful indicator of pregnancy. It cannot be considered a positive sign since occasionally the walls of a non-pregnant uterus are soft enough to exhibit Hegar's sign.

By the second month of pregnancy the cervix also shows changes in consistency. It becomes soft, resembling the consistency of the lips rather than cartilage. This change is known as *Goodell's sign.*

Vulval and Vaginal Changes During pregnancy, increased vascularity causes the vulva and vagina to change in color from pink to dark bluish or purplish red. This sign, noted during vaginal examination, is called *Chadwick's sign.* Chadwick's sign may occur in any condition causing pelvic congestion.

Additional changes that support a positive diagnosis of pregnancy occur later in pregnancy. These signs will be detected during the ongoing assessment that occurs throughout pregnancy.

Emotional Responses to Pregnancy Diagnosis

Before proceeding with plans for prenatal care it is important for the nurse to assess the woman's response to the diagnosis of pregnancy. A positive diagnosis of pregnancy has considerable psychological impact on the woman and her family. Whether the pregnancy was planned or is unexpected, desirable or unwanted, the woman first faces the task of accepting the pregnancy as a reality, not just a possibility. It is this acceptance that enables her to make decisions about continuing or terminating the pregnancy, seeking health care, and reordering her life to incorporate the pregnancy.

Most women respond to the diagnosis of pregnancy with ambivalence. In a study of primiparas, Caplan (1957) found that while many women were happy about being pregnant, eighty percent admitted to feeling disappointed and anxious. Rubin (1970) hypothesized that pregnancy evokes questions in the areas of the woman's sense of personal identity (Pregnant...who, me?) and in her sense of time within life (Pregnant ...now?)

Even if the pregnancy was planned, there is usually some element of surprise and disbelief at actually having conceived. The discovery of pregnancy can bring special feelings of excitement and anticipation, especially if the pregnancy is desired by the woman and her loved ones. The proof of the ability to conceive often brings increased self-esteem, due to an affirmation of sexual identity for both the woman and her partner.

While early physical symptoms such as nausea or breast tenderness may help the pregnancy seem more real, there are few obvious signs to assist the woman in "feeling pregnant." Outwardly, she looks and seems much the same to herself and to those around her. Her ambivalence may be increased by the nausea and fatigue of early pregnancy.

Along with accepting the reality of pregnancy, women often feel that now is not the "right time" to be pregnant. The woman must begin to question how she can accommodate the baby into her life. Career plans, finances, or needs of other children are examined; feelings of conflict are common for both the woman and her partner.

Thus, the discovery of pregnancy evokes both positive and negative emotional responses. It is important for the health care practitioner to help the woman and her partner explore their emotional responses to the diagnosis of pregnancy. The couple may need counseling and support if they are uncertain about continuing the pregnancy. If they decide not to continue the pregnancy, referral for pregnancy termination should be made as soon as possible. Support is also important for the woman who remains pregnant. She and her family need reassurance that feelings of conflict and ambivalence are common and natural. Sharing feelings of joy about pregnancy is acceptable; sharing doubts is more difficult. If the couple can share their concerns with each other at this time, it can form the framework for meaningful communication throughout pregnancy. The nurse should facilitate this communication as part of promoting optimal health during pregnancy.

Initial Assessment

Once the pregnancy has been confirmed, a complete prenatal assessment is indicated in order to assess risk and establish a plan of care. This assessment includes an interview and history, a complete physical examination, and laboratory tests.

Assessing Risk

One of the purposes of the first visit is to assess the needs of the woman for care during pregnancy and to identify those women who are at risk for problems and need special care. Between one-third and one-half of the women who will subsequently develop problems during their pregnancy can be identified at their first prenatal visit (Quilligan, 1981). However, Nesbitt (1969) found that fifty percent of maternal complications occurred in women classified as low risk at the first prenatal visit, illustrating the need for careful ongoing risk assessment throughout pregnancy.

The limitations of time, personnel, and resources make it necessary for medical professionals to classify patients into risk categories so that the patients at highest risk can be given appropriate intensive care.

Roberts (1977) defined the individual at high risk as being one who has a greater than average chance of developing a disease or other pathological condition, or whose chances of survival are low. In obstetrics the purpose of risk assessment is to determine "the likelihood of a poor outcome at any point along the perinatal continuum" (Hobel, 1978).

The goal of care for the high-risk individual is to prevent pathology from occurring or, if that is not possible, to provide the best possible medical management of the problem. There are many prenatal factors (genetic, environmental, nutritional, medical, and psychosocial) that increase risk during pregnancy.

The extent to which the nurse in a specialized role utilizes other health professionals in managing clients at risk depends on his or her own skill, knowledge and experience, the resources available within the setting, and the availability of specialized health care services. A moderate or high-risk situation often involves a cooperative approach between the specialized nurse, the physician, and other health professionals.

Several tools have been devised to calculate and designate risk status. The most effective tools are simple enough to use easily in the prenatal setting and are able to accurately classify the patent into the proper risk category. The forms on the second and fourth pages of Figure 3-1 are an antepartum risk tool from the Washington State Regional Perinatal Program Standardized Record. It allows medical personnel to calculate an antepartum risk score from information taken at the initial history and physical examination. In addition, it provides opportunity for an ongoing risk assessment throughout the antepartum period.

The Interview and History

The prenatal interview is an essential part of nursing practice. The information obtained is used to identify the various psychosocial influences on the pregnant woman and her family, to validate and supplement data gathered from the physical examination, and to ascertain the expectations of the woman for care during pregnancy. The interview and history are also used to obtain the family history and to evaluate the woman for past, existent, and potential health problems.

The interview should be conducted in a setting that allows for privacy and limits distractions and interruptions. The atmosphere should be one that demonstrates interest and caring for the patient and establishes mutual trust, confidence, and respect. The client has a right to know what to expect from the health professionals, to be assured of confidentiality, and to be encouraged to be an active participant in her own care.

The goal of the initial interview is to gain understanding of the woman and her family. Such an understanding is essential to providing optimal care throughout pregnancy. While total assessment cannot be accomplished in a single visit, the conduct of this first visit may well determine if the woman will return for further care.

Patient Profile

The patient profile provides information about the woman's background. This information should be included in the patient's record and used to avoid needless repetition of questions by other members of the health team. The patient profile includes the following information:

- *Age*
- *Marital status:* Length of marriage? Husband's name? Age? Occupation?
- *Family composition:* Who lives in the household? Relationships of household members? Responsibilities for housework, food selection and preparation? Significant others not in household?
- *Housing:* Adequate housing arrangements?
- *Finances:* Who is responsible for family income? Adequate income?
- *Educational and employment background:* Highest grade completed? Currently employed? Plans for continued employment during pregnancy? Typical work responsibilities?
- *Workplace:* Exposure to noxious substances, hazards, environmental stress?
- *Ethnic and religious background*

The woman's age may be indicative of the resources (physical, emotional, social) she has with which to deal with pregnancy. Physiologically, the woman is most able to adapt to the demands of pregnancy in her late teens through her mid-twenties. Young women, especially those under age 17, may be at high risk. Risk potential increases with advancing maternal age. Genetic defects such as trisomy 21 (Down's syndrome) are more prevalent in women over 35 years old. Amniocentesis is recommended as a routine diagnostic procedure for any woman of this age (Pritchard & MacDonald, 1980). Other complications including hydatidiform mole, placenta previa, twinning, and low birthweight infants have also been associated with advanced maternal age (Pritchard & McDonald, 1980). On the other hand, the woman's age may be indicative of her maturity and extent of life experiences, both of which can aid her in adjusting to pregnancy and parenthood. *Pregnancy After Thirty-Five* (McCauley, 1976) is a useful resource for older women who are contemplating pregnancy.

Information about the woman's marital status and other family relationships can suggest the amount and type of support available to her during pregnancy. Adjusting to a recent marriage in addition to pregnancy increases the stress with which she must deal. Finding out who lives in the household provides clues as to the types of responsibilities the woman has for housework, care of younger or older family members, and food preparation. This information is useful when making recommendations about nutrition and rest during pregnancy. Suggesting diet changes will only be effective if the person who buys and prepares the food is included in teaching. Counseling the pregnant woman about increasing rest periods must take into account the demands of other family members for time and attention, as they are also affected by the pregnancy and their responses to the woman and her pregnancy can either facilitate her adjustment or increase her stress. Supportive relationships have been found to decrease the woman's risk for pregnancy complications (Nuckolls et al., 1972).

Data about the father of the baby should be considered when assessing risk. The socioeconomic status of the family, often reflected by the father's occupation, is related to the incidence of prematurity and infant mortality. Paternal influences on pregnancy outcome are speculative at this point. There is some evidence that older age of the father is related to an increased incidence of stillborn infants and congenital abnormalities. Chronic alcoholism and diabetes mellitus in the father may also have an adverse affect on fetal development (Babson et al., 1980). The woman's partner may be one of the most significant influences on her attitude about the pregnancy. His response to the pregnancy should be assessed, as well as his goals and desires for involvement in the pregnancy and birth.

The adequacy of both housing and finances indicate the woman's material resources. A living arrangement

DATE		AGE	ADDRESS			CITY, STATE, ZIP CODE	MARITAL STATUS		RACE	RELIGION
							M S SEP D W LW			

OCCUPATION		SOCIAL SECURITY NO.	PHONE (HOME/WORK)		FATHER OF BABY	OCCUPATION (His)	HIS WORK PHONE	PLANNED PREG.
								☐ YES
								☐ NO ☐ BUT OK

LMP		☐ NORMAL ☐ ABNORMAL	LNMP	EDC		REFERRED ☐ YES ☐ NØ	BY WHOM		REASON	

GRAVIDA	PARA		ABORTIONS			DEATHS		LIVING CHILDREN	MENARCHE				# DAYS	REG.	IREG.
	TERM	PRETERM	SPONT	ELEC	ECTOPIC	FETAL	NEONATAL				DURATION			☐	☐
											INTERVAL ▶			☐	☐

✓ IF POSITIVE	PRESENT PREGNANCY HISTORY		✓ IF POSITIVE	GYNECOLOGIC HISTORY	
		DESCRIBE POSITIVE HISTORY	ORAL CONTRACEPTIVES C̄ IN 30 DAYS LMP ☐ YES ☐ NO		DESCRIBE POSITIVE HISTORY
	NAUSEA/VOMITING				
	BLEEDING			INFERTILITY	
	URINARY SYMPTOMS			GYN DISORDERS	
	VAGINAL DISCHARGE			GYN SURGERY	
	DRUGS / MEDS			SEXUALLY TRANSMITTED INFECTIONS	
	SMOKE / ETOH				
	INFECTIONS / FEVER			PRIOR BIRTH CONTROL	
	PREGNANCY TEST				

PREVIOUS PREGNANCIES

NO.	DATE	LENGTH GESTATION IN WKS	LABOR HRS.	TYPE OF DELIVERY	TYPE OF ANESTHESIA	SEX · WT.	COMPLICATIONS - PREGNANCY, LABOR, DELIVERY, POST PARTUM OR INFANT

✓ IF POSITIVE	MEDICAL HISTORY		✓ IF POSITIVE	PHYSICAL EXAMINATION	DATE:	
		DESCRIBE POSITIVE HISTORY			DESCRIBE POSITIVE FINDINGS	
	HEENT			HEENT/TEETH		
	CARDIOVASCULAR			SKIN		
	RESPIRATORY			NECK		
	GASTROINTESTINAL			LUNGS		
	GENITOURINARY			BREASTS		
	METABOLIC			HEART		
	NEUROPSYCHIATRIC			ABDOMEN		
	INFECTIOUS DISEASE			NEURO		
	TRANSFUSIONS			EXTREMITIES		
	OPERATIONS			PELVIS-(EXT. GENITALIA)		
	ALLERGIES			VAGINA		
	OTHER	☐ ✓ IF ALL ITEMS ABOVE ARE NEGATIVE		CERVIX		
				UTERUS (SIZE, ETC.)		
				ADNEXA		
				RECTUM	☐ ✓ IF ALL ITEMS ABOVE ARE NEGATIVE	

✓ IF POSITIVE	FAMILY HISTORY	
	DIABETES	
	CONGENITAL ANOMAL	
	HYPERTENSION	
	RENAL DISEASE	
	TWINS	
	OTHER	☐ ✓ IF ALL ITEMS ABOVE ARE NEGATIVE

PELVIMETRY

PUBIC ARCH_____ BI-ISCHIAL _____ CM

SIDE WALLS_____ SPINES _____ SS NOTCH____FB

DC_____ cm SACRUM_____COCCYX_____

CONCLUSION: ☐ ADEQUATE   ☐ BORDERLINE   ☐ CONTRACTED

X_____ M.D.

UNIVERSITY OF WASHINGTON HOSPITALS
HARBORVIEW MEDICAL CENTER · 223-3074
UNIVERSITY HOSPITAL · 543-3270
SEATTLE, WASHINGTON

PRENATAL RECORD

UH 0108 REV. JAN. 81   2-81-113   PAGE 1 OF 4

FIGURE 3-1   Prenatal record sheet. (From the University of Washington Hospitals, Harbor View Medical Center, Washington State Regional Prenatal Care Program, Seattle Washington. With permission.) *(Continued on pp. 53-55.)*

LAB DATA

BLOOD TYPE	RH		IF RH NEGATIVE: ANTIBODY TITER			DIABETIC SCREEN (28-32 WKS)	
HCT	32 WK HCT		INITIAL	28 WKS	36 WKS	GTT	RESULTS
						FAST	
RUBELLA ☐NEG	SEROLOGY		SICKLE CELL PREP			30'	
TITER ☐POS	☐NEG ☐POS		☐ NEG	☐ POS		60'	
PAP:	UA		URINE CULTURE			120'	
						180'	
PPD/TINE	G C SCREEN ☐NEG ☐POS		OTHER			DATE	

PRENATAL MEDS — SEE SIDE 4 TO CODE RISK

MEDICATION	DOSE	RISK

PRENATAL ☐C̄ FOLATE VITAMINS ☐S̄ FOLATE   IRON: ☐NONE ☐DAILY ☐BID ☐TID

OTHER HEALTH PROFESSIONALS INVOLVED IN CARE (I.E. CONSULTING PHYSICIAN, PHN., SOC. WORK & NUTRITIONIST.   PHONE

ASSESSMENTS/PROBLEMS

1.
2.
3.
4.
5.
6.
7.
8.

EDUCATIONAL ASSESSMENT

PREFERRED/PLANNED METHOD OF LEARNING ☐ READING ☐ CASSETTES ☐ 1:1 ☐ CLASSES ☐ FILMS

CLASSES ☐ HOSPITAL-PREPARED ☐ HOSPITAL-REGULAR SERIES ☐ CEA ☐ BRADLEY ☐ PEP ☐ RED CROSS

INSTRUCTOR: _____

☐ TOUR   ☐ PHN REFERRAL:

PATIENT PREFERENCE

SMOKER ☐ YES ☐ NO

IF YES, L&D SMOKING POLICY REVIEWED ☐

SUPPORT PERSON IN L&D ☐ YES ☐ NO

IF YES:

☐ BOTTLE ☐ BREAST   NAME _____ RELATIONSHIP

PATIENT EDUCATION ✓ WHEN COMPLETED

	INIT.		INIT.
☐ NUTRITION		☐ L&D PROCEDURES	
☐ EXERCISE		☐ WARNING SIGNS	
☐ BREAST/BOTTLE		☐ SIGNS OF LABOR	
☐ BREATHING/RELAXATION		☐ ANALGESIA/ANESTH.	

BIRTH PLANS ☐ YES ☐ NO

IN CHART ☐ YES ☐ NO

REVIEWED BY:

FAMILY PLANNING

☐ BTL   ☐ PAPERS SIGNED

☐ OTHER:

NEWBORN PLANS

☐ ROOMING IN POLICY EXPLAINED

TYPE DESIRED:

☐ Optional c̄ demand breast feeding

☐ Optional s̄ demand breast feeding

☐ 24 HOUR

BABY'S PHYSICIAN:

SPECIAL CONCERNS

FETAL ASSESSMENT PROFILE

GESTATIONAL AGE	30		32		34		36		38		40		42	
DATE (Place under appropriate gestation)														
ANTEPARTUM FHR TESTING														
NST														
CST														
FETAL MOVEMENT INDEX														
ULTRASOUND														
BPD														
TIUV														
HEAD/ABDOMEN RATIO														
AMNIOTIC FLUID ANALYSIS														
L/S														
△ OD @ 450 mu														
CHLOROFORM EXTRACTION														
ESTRIOL (E3)														

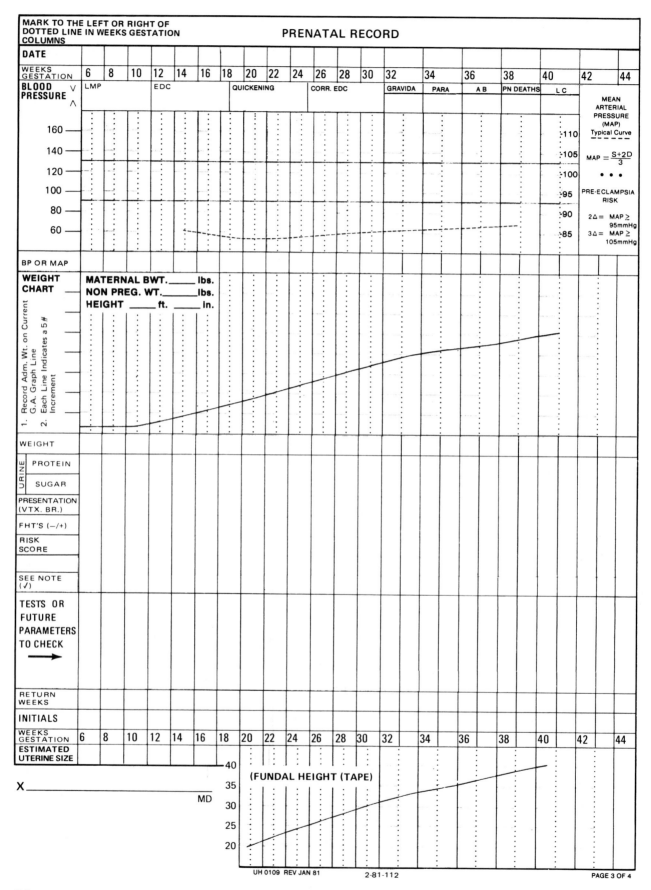

MARK TO THE LEFT OR RIGHT OF DOTTED LINE IN WEEKS GESTATION COLUMNS

PRENATAL RECORD

DATE																				
WEEKS GESTATION	6	8	10	12	14	16	18	20	22	24	26	28	30	32	34	36	38	40	42	44

BLOOD PRESSURE ∨ ∧

LMP   EDC   QUICKENING   CORR. EDC   GRAVIDA   PARA   A B   PN DEATHS   L C

160
140
120
100
80
60

110
105
100
95
90
85

MEAN ARTERIAL PRESSURE (MAP)
Typical Curve - - - -

$MAP = \dfrac{S+2D}{3}$

• • •

PRE-ECLAMPSIA RISK

$2\triangle = MAP \geq 95mmHg$
$3\triangle = MAP \geq 105mmHg$

BP OR MAP

WEIGHT CHART

MATERNAL BWT. _____ lbs.
NON PREG. WT. _____ lbs.
HEIGHT _____ ft. _____ in.

1. Record Adm. Wt. on Current G.A. Graph Line
2. Each Line Indicates a 5# Increment

WEIGHT

URINE — PROTEIN

SUGAR

PRESENTATION (VTX. BR.)

FHT'S (−/+)

RISK SCORE

SEE NOTE (✓)

TESTS OR FUTURE PARAMETERS TO CHECK →

RETURN WEEKS

INITIALS

WEEKS GESTATION	6	8	10	12	14	16	18	20	22	24	26	28	30	32	34	36	38	40	42	44

ESTIMATED UTERINE SIZE

X _____ MD

40
35
30
25
20

(FUNDAL HEIGHT (TAPE)

UH 0109 REV JAN 81   2-81-112   PAGE 3 OF 4

54

RISK	PATIENT PROFILE
2	AGE < 17 OR AGE > 34
3	DRUG ABUSE OR ADDICTIVE BEHAVIOR
2	BINGE DRINKING (5 DRINKS/SESSION)
1	SOCIAL DRINKING (2 DRINKS/DAY)
	SMOKING: ≥ 1 PACK/DAY (2); ≥ ½ PACK/DAY (1)
1	EDUCATION ≤ 9TH GRADE
1	CROWDED LIVING CONDITIONS
1	LOW SOCIO-ECONOMIC STATUS (IE., ADC, WELFARE)
1	OVERWEIGHT } SEE WEIGHT CHART @ BOTTOM OF PAGE
1	UNDERWEIGHT } RIGHT HAND SIDE
1	SMALL STATURE (≤ 5')
	OTHER_____ (SPECIFY)

	PRESENT PREGNANCY
	BLEEDING (RISK 2-5 BASED ON ASSESSMENT)
	MEDICATIONS:_____THERAPEUTIC/ADDICTIVE
5	RUBELLA (1ST TRIMESTER)
1	1ST PRENATAL VISIT ≥ 20 WKS. GESTATION
	X-RAY_____ (SPECIFY & ASSIGN RISK)
	OTHER_____ (SPECIFY & ASSIGN RISK)

	GYNECOLOGIC HISTORY
1	PAST UTERINE SURGERY (NON-CESAREAN)
2	UTERINE OR CERVICAL MALFUNCTIONS
1	SEXUALLY TRANSMITTED INFECTION (Rx) ☐ GENITAL HERPES ☐ GC ☐ SYPHILIS
1	INFERTILITY (≥ 2 YRS)
	OTHER_____ (SPECIFY & ASSIGN RISK)

	OBSTETRICAL HISTORY
2	ELDERLY PRIMIGRAVIDA (≥ 35)
1	PRIMAGRAVIDA (IF, YES, DISREGARD REST)
2	MULTIPARITY (5 OR MORE ≥ 20 WKS)
2	REPEATED SPONTANEOUS ABORTIONS (≥ 3)
5	INCOMPETENT CERVIX
2	MIDFORCEP OR DIFFICULT DELIVERY
1	INFANT (≥ 9 #)
3	LBW/SGA INFANT (< 10% WT. FOR DATES OR < 2500 GM @ 37 WKS)
	PREMATURE (< 37 WEEKS) (PREMATURE x1=3; x2=4; x3=5)
3	PERINATAL DEATH (STILLBORN OR DEATH 1ST 28 DAYS)
1	CONGENITAL ANOMALIES
2	SURVIVING BIRTH DAMAGED INFANT(S) p̄ 1ST 28 DAYS OF LIFE
2	PREVIOUS ANTEPARTUM HEMORRHAGE
2	PREGNANCY INDUCED HYPERTENSION (OTHER THAN 1ST PREG.)
5	RH SENSITIZATION PREV. PREG. WITH PREV. FETAL/NEONATAL RX
	PREVIOUS C-SECTION (1) LOW TRANSVERSE
	(3) CLASSICAL (2) UNKNOWN (2) LOW VERTICAL
1	≤ 12 MOS. FROM MONTH OF LAST DELIVERY TO MONTH OF CONCEPTION
	OTHER_____ (SPECIFY & ASSIGN RISK)

	MEDICAL HISTORY
	CARDIOVASCULAR
2	ANEMIA (Hgb ≤ 9.5/HCT < 30)
2	ASYMPTOMATIC HEART DISEASE
4	SYMPTOMATIC HEART DISEASE
3	THROMBOEMBOLISM
3	HYPERTENSION (≥ 140/90)
	RESPIRATORY
2	CHRONIC PULMONARY DISEASE
	GENITOURINARY
3	RENAL DISEASE (EXCL. ACUTE PYLONEPHRITIS X 1)
	METABOLIC
5	DIABETES MELLITUS — INSULIN
1	DIABETES MELLITUS — NON-INSULIN
2	OTHER ENDOCRINE PROBLEMS (SCORE ONLY IF SERIOUS)
	NEUROPSYCHIATRIC
1	EMOTIONAL OR PSYCHIATRIC PROBLEMS
	INFECTIOUS DISEASE
1	HEPATITIS
	OTHER_____ (SPECIFY & ASSIGN RISK)

	FAMILY HISTORY
1	DIABETES (PARENTS OR SIBS)
1	INHERITABLE DEFECT
	OTHER_____ (SPECIFY & ASSIGN RISK)

	PHYSICAL EXAM (ASSIGN RISK 0-5)
	OTHER_____ (SPECIFY)

	PELVIMETRY
1	ABNORMAL PELVIS

		HOW TO ASSIGN RISK TO A FACTOR
	TOTAL HISTORY AND PHYSICAL EXAM SCORE ◄	1-2 - LOW RISK
		3-4 - MEDIUM RISK
☐ CHECK HERE IF NO RISK FACTORS NOTED		5 - HIGH RISK

UH 0109 REV JAN 81 BACK   2-81-112

CODE	RISK	ABUSED/ADDICTIVE DRUGS
0260	3	ALCOHOL (6 DRINKS/DAY)
0270	2	ANTIDEPRESSANT
		I.E. SPEED, RITALIN
0280	2	HALLUCINOGENS, I.E. LSD
0290	2	NARCOTICS
		I.E. HEROIN, METHADONE
0300	1	PYSCHOTROPHIC HERBS
		I.E. MARIJUANA
0310	2	SEDATIVES/HYPNOTICS

RECORD DRUG ➡

CODE	RISK	MEDICATIONS/DRUGS
		ANALGESICS
0010	2	SALICYLATES
		ANTIBIOTICS
0020	2	AMINOGLYCOSIDES (I.E. STREPTOMYCIN)
0030	4	CHLORAMPHENICOL
0040	2	FLAGYL
0050	2	NOVOBIOCIN
0060	1	SULFA
0070	2	TETRACYCLINE
0080	2	TRIMETHOPRIM (I.E. BACTRIM, SEPTRA)
		ANTICOAGULANT
0090	4	COUMADIN TYPE
		ANTICONVULSANT
0100	3	DILANTIN
		ANTIDIABETIC
0110	3	ORAL
		ANTIHYPERTENSIVE
0120	3	HEXAMETHONIUM
0130	3	PROPRANOLOL
0140	3	RESERPINE
0150	3	THIAZIDE DIURETICS
		ANTINAUSEA
0160	2	TIGAN
		CHEMOTHERAPEUTIC
0170	5	METHOTREXATE
0180	3	CORTICOSTEROIDS
		SEX STEROIDS
0190	5	DES
0200	4	19—NOR-PROGESTINS
0210	4	TESTOSTERONE
		THYROID DRUGS
0220	2	IODIDES
0230	5	RADIOACTIVE IODINE THERAPY
0240	3	THIOURACILS
0250	3	ERGOTS

CIRCLE, ADD TOTAL AND TRANSFER TO PRESENT PREGNANCY COLUMN

CAUTION IS INDICATED IN THE USE OF ANY OF THE ABOVE MEDICATIONS. (If used during pregnancy, add to risk score, page 3.)

MED. FRAME IDEAL NON-PREGNANT WTS.
Height (without shoes) add one inch
Weight (with shoes)

HEIGHT	NORMAL	10% UNDER	20% OVER
4'10''	97	87	118
4'11''	100	89	121
5'0''	103	92	129
5'1''	106	95	125
5'2''	109	97	132
5'3''	111	99	135
5'4''	116	104	141
5'5''	121	108	147
5'6''	125	112	151
5'7''	131	115	156
5'8''	133	119	161
5'9''	137	123	166
5'10''	141	126	171
5'11''	144	131	175
6'0''	149	133	180

DESIRED WEIGHT GAIN

3 LBS 1st TRIMESTER   = 3
3 LBS /MO 12-36 WKS   =18
1 LB/WK 36th WK-TERM = 4
              25 lbs

N.E. Wisconsin Perinatal Program (Adjusted to Women ≥ 18 Yrs. Old)

X_____ M.D.

that allows for some privacy may enable the woman to get needed rest. Does the present living situation have adequate space for the addition of the baby? The woman can begin to plan for this space during her pregnancy. Many couples move during pregnancy or soon after delivery. While such a move may provide more adequate living arrangements, a move can disrupt supportive relationships and cause both physical and emotional stress. If necessary, moving early in pregnancy may be advantageous so that new social ties can be established before the baby arrives.

Financial worries can be an additional source of stress, and need to be considered when counseling about diet, clothing, and activity so that suggestions are realistic for the woman's financial situation. Referral to other social services for assistance may be indicated.

Knowing the educational and work background of the expectant couple can be helpful in individualizing teaching and counseling approaches. The mother's education may be an indicator of the type of environment she will provide for her child. College women have half as many low-birth-weight infants as those with a grade school education (Babson et al., 1980). This may be related to better pregnancy planning, living conditions, or nutrition and other health practices.

An occupational health history is an important component of the patient profile, since the employment situation and exposure to environmental factors and substances may affect the woman's health and that of her unborn child. Once hazards and stressors are identified, an assessment of risk is possible and anticipatory guidance may be provided for the woman through the remainder of her pregnancy (Greenberg, 1980; *Guidelines on Pregnancy and Work,* 1977; Stetlman, 1977). The effect of the pregnancy on educational and vocational goals should be ascertained. Did the pregnancy disrupt plans? Is the woman concerned about the effect the baby will have on her future goals? Planning for child care following the birth should begin during pregnancy.

Beliefs and practices specific to pregnancy, childbirth, and childrearing are common in every cultural group; to effectively provide health care for others, the practitioner needs to acknowledge her or his own biases. Cultural beliefs about dietary practices and activity during pregnancy should be incorporated into the prenatal care.

Prenatal History

The history includes subjective data gathered by interview. These data are important in identifying the woman's potential risk for problems during pregnancy.

At the initial visit detailed information should be documented in the following areas:

Reason for Visit (Chief Complaint) Usually this information relates to the signs and symptoms of pregnancy, including amenorrhea, frequency of urination, breast changes, nausea, fatigue, and possibly a positive pregnancy test.

Menstrual History Data include the date of menarche, characteristics of the menstrual cycle (i.e., length of cycle, duration, and amount of flow), menstrual disorders, and symptoms associated with menstruation and usual treatment of discomfort. The date of the last menstrual period and its characteristics should be particularly noted. These dates are valuable in estimating the woman's expected date of delivery (EDC). The EDC is computed utilizing Naegel's rule. Three months are substracted and seven days added to the first day of the last normal menstrual period. Since this formula is based on a twenty-eight-day cycle, some people suggest that additional days should be added or substracted to the EDC for each day that the woman's cycle is of longer or shorter duration than twenty-eight days. The merits of this approach are not documented. It seems it might be useful when the length of the usual menstrual cycle varies markedly from the twenty-eight-day average.

It is important, though often difficult, to establish when the last *normal* period occurred. Women may have some bleeding believed to be associated with implantation of the fertilized ovum, and may assume this bleeding to be the menstrual period. Usually this bleeding is of shorter duration than is characteristic of the woman's regular menstrual period. However, bleeding may also be due to a threatened abortion. The EDC may be calculated from the previous menstrual period and other indices of pregnancy duration utilized to determine a more accurate EDC. It is important to inform the woman that the EDC is only one estimate of the due date, and not to be interpreted as an accurate prediction of when she will deliver the baby. Jensen et al. (1979) stated that only four percent of women deliver on their predicted EDC. The actual time of labor onset may vary two weeks either way.

Family Health History Because of the hereditary nature of many health conditions, a complete family history is essential to planning prenatal care. Of particular concern is family history of multiple pregnancy, cardiovascular disease, diabetes mellitus, renal disease, congenital abnormalities, genetic disorders, blood dyscrasias, and emotional problems. If there is a

TABLE 3-2 Pregnancy risk factors associated with medical and surgical history

High-Risk Factors	Moderate-Risk Factors
Moderate to severe chronic hypertension	Mild chronic hypertension
Moderate to severe renal disease	Mild renal disease
Severe heart disease (class II to IV, or a history of congestive heart failure)	Mild heart disease (class I)
	History of mild hypertensive states of pregnancy
Diabetes (class B to F)	History of pyelonephritis
Previous endocrine ablation	Diabetes (class A)
Abnormal cervical cytology	Family history of diabetes
Sickle-cell disease	Thyroid disease
Drug addiction or alcoholism	Positive serology
History of tuberculosis or PPD test revealing a diameter of more than 1 cm	Excessive use of drugs
Pulmonary disease	Emotional problems
Malignancy	Sickle-cell trait
Gastrointestinal or liver disease	Epilepsy
Previous cardiac or vascular surgery	

From Babson, S., Benson, R., Pernoll, M., & Benda, G. (1980). *Management of high-risk pregnancy and intensive care of the neonate* (ed. 4). St. Louis: The C. V. Mosby Co., pp. 18–19. With permission.

positive history of any one of these, additional evaluation (i.e., amniocentesis or genetic counseling) may be warranted.

Past Health Status Some conditions can adversely affect pregnancy; similarly, pregnancy can aggravate an existing or previously resolved health problem. Of particular concern are *chronic diseases* such as diabetes, heart disease, or hypertension, any of which require careful supervision throughout the pregnancy; and *acute problems* such as infections that occurred early in pregnancy and may have adversely affected the developing fetus (Alford et al., 1975; Nahmais, 1974; Sever, 1978; Waterson, 1979).

Factors from the client's medical and surgical history can identify a high or moderate risk for pregnancy difficulty, as shown in Table 3-2. A history of blood transfusions, allergies, and drug sensitivity should also be obtained and documented on the client's record. If there is a positive history of any of these conditions, it is important to document the dates of occurrence of the problem, treatments utilized, and any residual effects.

Past Obstetric History Previous childbearing experiences can significantly influence the course of the present pregnancy: the information has predictive value in suggesting potential complications, and can

positively or adversely shape the woman's expectations for the current pregnancy. Information to be discussed includes maternal experiences during pregnancy, labor and delivery, and the puerperium; fetal and neonatal complications; and growth and development of the children to date. Pertinent areas to explore include

- Number and dates of past pregnancies
- Duration of pregnancies: full-term deliveries (note date of delivery, birthweight of infant); preterm deliveries (note cause if known, birthweight and gestational age of infant, infant complications); postterm deliveries (note if labor induced or spontaneous, gestational age of infant at birth, fetal or infant complications)
- Abortions: gestation attained, cause of spontaneous abortions if known, method used for voluntary terminations
- Pregnancy experiences: type of complications (i.e., diabetes, bleeding, toxemia) and treatment, general experience with pregnancy
- Labor and delivery experience: onset spontaneous or induced (note reason for and method of induction if known), length of labor, complications, anesthesia used and attitude towards anesthesia, place of birth, type of delivery (vaginal, Cesarean)

TABLE 3-3 Pregnancy risk factors associated with obstetric history

High-Risk Factors	Moderate-Risk Factors
Previously diagnosed genital tract anomalies: incompetent cervix, cervical malformation, and/or uterine malformation	Previous premature labor, low-birth-weight infant (less than 2500 g), or abortion
Two or more previous abortions	One excessively large infant (more than 4000 g)
Previous stillborn or neonatal loss	Previous operative deliveries (i.e., Cesarean section, midforceps delivery, breech extraction)
Two previous premature labors or low-birth-weight infants (less than 2500 g)	Previous prolonged labor or significant dystocia
Two excessively large previous infants (more than 4000 g)	Borderline pelvis
Maternal malignancy	Previous severe emotional problems associated with pregnancy or delivery
Uterine leiomyomas (5 cm or more or submucus in location)	Previous uterine or cervical operations
Ovarian mass	Primigravida
Parity of eight or more	Parity of five to eight
Previous infant with isoimmunization	Involuntary infertility
History of eclampsia	Prior ABO incompatibility
Previous infant with known or suspected genetic or familial disorders, and/or congenital anomaly	Prior fetal malpresentation
Previous infant requiring special neonatal-infant care or birth-damaged	History of endometriosis
Medical indications for termination of a previous pregnancy	Pregnancy occurring three months or less after last delivery

From Babson, S., Benson, R., Pernoll, M., & Benda, G. (1980). *Management of high-risk pregnancy and intensive care of the neonate* (ed. 4). St. Louis: The C. V. Mosby Co., pp. 17–18. With permission.

- Postpartum experience: problems (i.e., bleeding, infection, emotional difficulties), course of recovery
- Fetal and neonatal complications: type of problems and treatment, condition of infant at birth, stillbirths, multiple births
- Living children: course of growth and development, current health status

Factors from the woman's obstetric history can also be classified as having high or moderate risk potential, as seen in Table 3-3.

Sexual History Pregnancy may result in changes in sexuality, and may precipitate sexual problems. Information from the woman's sexual history can be utilized to provide sensitive counseling in this area during and following pregnancy. Areas to be explored include the age of entry into sexual activity, usual frequency of sexual relations, libido, sexual preference, the woman and her partner's satisfaction with sexual practices and experiences, and areas of sexual concern or difficulty. The number of sexual partners should also be known so that the risk of developing a sexually transmitted disease during pregnancy can be determined. Many

individuals have misconceptions about the safety of continuing sexual relations during the pregnancy (Ellis, 1980). The couple should be reassured that, during a normal pregnancy, sexual activity can continue without fear of harming the mother or the baby. The range of sexual response during pregnancy should be explained so that the couple understands that the differences they may be experiencing are normal. Some women experience increased sexual enjoyment and interest during pregnancy; this can cause concern because it is a change from usual patterns.

Contraceptive History The woman's contraceptive history should be reviewed. The methods she has used and her satisfaction with them; her pattern of contraceptive use (sporadic, consistent) can be utilized in planning for contraception following delivery. The couple's goals for family size and spacing can be explored.

Status of Current Pregnancy At the initial visit, in-depth information about the woman's health status in relation to her present pregnancy should be gathered.

Not only does this information aid in identifying any pathological conditions that may exist, it also establishes guidelines for evaluating changes throughout the pregnancy.

When gathering these data, the nurse should first seek to confirm the diagnosis of pregnancy by reviewing the symptoms the woman is experiencing (i.e., gastrointestinal symptoms, urinary tract symptoms, fatigue). The meaning of the pregnancy to the woman should be assessed at this time. Is the pregnancy planned or unplanned? How do the woman and her partner feel about the pregnancy at this time?

Additional data should be solicited to ascertain if there are any conditions that might cause problems for the mother or fetus. An open-ended question—such as What has this pregnancy been like for you so far? can be useful in identifying problems or concerns the mother might have. For instance, the presence of abdominal pain or bleeding should be noted as warning signs of a threatened abortion or placental abruption. Questions should be continued as pregnancy progresses, since such symptoms as bleeding, edema, headaches, dizziness, and visual disturbances could be signs of placenta previa, cervical abnormality, or developing preeclampsia.

The nurse should investigate the woman's general health habits and lifestyle patterns that may affect or be altered by the pregnancy. These include

- Prescribed medications
- Self-medication
- Use of alcohol, tobacco, recreational drugs, coffee, tea, and soft drinks
- Exercise and activity patterns
- Usual social and recreational patterns
- Sleep patterns
- Immunization record

It is sometimes helpful to ask the woman to describe a typical day, and from this identify the frequency of some of the above health habits. It is important to know *how* these patterns have been altered by the pregnancy and how the woman feels about those changes. This review can be useful in indicating areas for patient counseling to promote optimal health practices during pregnancy.

Physical Examination

A thorough physical examination at the initial prenatal visit is indicated to establish the diagnosis and stage of pregnancy, to gather baseline information, and to detect any abnormalities that may be present. The physical examination provides objective data to supplement or confirm those gathered during the patient interview. Any areas of concern or potential problems identified during the interview should be given particular attention at this time.

The physical examination should follow the patient interview and its purposes and procedure should be explained to the client. It provides the opportunity for teaching and counseling, and for familiarizing the woman with her own body and the changes that will occur during pregnancy. She may or may not wish to be accompanied by her partner, friend, or family member during the examination. The examination should take place in a setting that insures privacy and comfort. The client will need to be disrobed and should have a gown and/or drapes available for warmth and privacy during the examination.

The initial data to be gathered include vital signs such as temperature, pulse, respirations, and blood pressure; both nonpregnant and present weight; and height. These data should be recorded in such a way that patterns of change throughout the pregnancy can easily be seen (i.e., on a graph). An example of such a graph is shown on the third page of Figure 3-1. On this graph, the lines indicate optimal blood pressure ranges, weight gain patterns, and uterine growth curves. By comparing similar findings for the patient against these norms, the nurse can easily recognize deviations.

Some women seek care only when they are pregnant, so it is important to include a complete assessment of the eyes, ears, nose, throat, teeth, thyroid, breasts, heart, lungs, abdomen, genitalia, extremities, and neurological status. Particular importance should be placed on the examination of the breasts, abdomen, and pelvis.

Breast Examination

The purpose of the breast examination is to note normal breast changes of pregnancy and to detect any breast abnormalities. Since pregnancy may seriously aggravate breast cancer, any suspicious findings should be evaluated by a specialist immediately. Procedures for the breast examination are discussed in detail in "The Breast," *Women's Health: Ambulatory Care.*

During pregnancy, the breasts increase in size. The superficial veins of the breasts become engorged and are visible under the skin. The nipples become larger, increase in pigmentation and become more erect. After fourteen to sixteen weeks, colostrum, a thick, yellowish fluid, may be expressed from the nipples. The areolae also enlarge and become more pigmented. The increase in pigmentation is most notable in brunettes and dark skinned women. Changes in pigmentation of the breasts are thought to be the result of increased melanocyte stimulating hormone produced by the anterior lobe of the pituitary, and increased amounts of estrogen and progesterone. Sebaceous glands, called *Montgomery's tubercles* or *follicles,* hypertrophy and become more apparent.

Skin Changes

In addition to those of the breasts, other pigmentation changes occur. *Cholasma,* also known as *melasma* or the *mask of pregnancy,* consists of areas of splotchy and irregular hyperpigmentation appearing on the forehead, cheeks, temples, and upper lips. Estrogen and progesterone are felt to be primarily responsible for cholasma, which occurs most frequently in brunettes. The mask usually disappears after the pregnancy.

Preexisting moles (nevi) and freckles darken during the pregnancy, and may increase in size and number. A dark line known as the *linea nigra* forms between the umbilicus and the symphysis pubis. It will lighten after the pregnancy is over but usually does not disappear. Vascular spiders (telangiectasia) may appear on the breasts, face, neck, chest, and arms as a result of increased estrogen and increased vascular permeability and proliferation.

Abdominal Examination

The abdomen is examined with the client in a recumbant position. This procedure will be more accurate and comfortable if the woman has emptied her bladder prior to the examination.

The abdomen should be inspected for scars, striations, and contour. The height of the fundus of the uterus is then palpated. Uterine enlargement usually begins six to eight weeks after the last normal menstrual period and can be detected on abdominal exam after the thirteenth week of pregnancy. The abdominal enlargement is more pronounced in multiparas than in primigravidas due to the loss of muscle tone following previous pregnancies. The height of the fundus is measured with a flexible (nonstretch) tape from the top of the symphysis pubis to the top of the fundus, at the midline. This measurement should be recorded in such a way that subsequent measurements can easily be compared for evidence of normal fetal growth.

Measurement of fundal height is one way of estimating the length of gestation. Accuracy of fundal measurements are dependent on the consistency of both the examiner and the measurement techniques.

By about the thirtieth week of gestation, the outline of the fetus and presentation can be detected utilizing Leopold's maneuvers (Exhibit 3-1).

EXHIBIT 3-1   Procedure for Leopold's Maneuvers

- Facing the patient's head, palpate the uterine fundus with the palms of both hands to ascertain the part of the fetus that is located in the upper part of the uterus. If the fetal head is in this region it will feel smooth, hard, round, and moveable. In contrast, the breech will feel large, nodular and irregularly shaped.
- Next, with one hand on each side of the uterus, palpate the uterus to detect the fetal spine and small parts of the fetus. A firm continuous resistance (spine) on one side and small, irregular parts (knees, feet, arms) on the other side should be felt. If the fetus is in a transverse lie, the fetal head or breech will be palpated instead.
- Finally, facing the client's feet, with one hand on each side of the uterus, palpate the lower uterine segment to determine which part of the fetus occupies this region. After the thirty-eighth week of gestation, the presenting part of the fetus may become engaged. Engagement can be detected by palpating for presence and mobility of the lower part of the fetal head in the lower uterine segment (Varney, 1980).

During the abdominal examination, fetal heart tones are auscultated. The heart beat is most easily heard in the region of the fetal back, which can be detected through the previous maneuvers. It can be heard with a fetoscope at approximately twenty weeks' gestation, and earlier (ten to fourteen weeks) with a Doptone (Doppler unit). Hearing the fetal heartbeat is an additional parameter utilized in estimating fetal gestational age. It also aids in confirming the reality of the baby to the expectant mother. It is essential, for assuring that the fetus is alive and well and for determining gestational age, that the fetal heart rate be definitely distinguished from the mother's. This can best be done by palpating the mother's pulse while listening to the fetal heart tones.

After the fifth lunar month, active fetal movements can be felt by the examiner. This is considered a positive sign of pregnancy. When the movements first become apparent they may be faint flutters, but later they become very brisk. Contraction of the intestines or abdominal wall muscles may produce similar sensations but an experienced examiner should be able to differentiate them.

Pelvic Examination

The pelvic examination provides information about the presumptive and probable signs of pregnancy. Such laboratory tests as the cytological (Pap) smear and gonococcal culture are important to complete early in pregnancy. Chadwick's sign may be noted, and signs of vaginitis or cervical abnormalities should be evaluated, treated, and referred as appropriate. (See "Physical Assessment" for specifics of the pelvic examination, as well as "Sexually Transmitted Diseases and Vaginitis" and "Conditions of the Cervix" in *Women's Health: Ambulatory Care.*)

After completion of the speculum examination of the cervix, the uterus is palpated bimanually. Goodell's, Laden's, Hegar's and Osiander's signs may be noted (see Table 3-1). The uterus should be outlined, noting position, shape, size, mobility, and consistency. Bimanual evaluation of uterine size is an essential component of assessing the gestation of the pregnancy. The uterus, ovaries, and rectum should be examined for any irregularities.

Pelvimetry

At some point during the prenatal period, adequacy of the pelvic diameters for delivery is usually estimated. This may be done at the initial prenatal visit or delayed until the third trimester, when measurement may be more accurate and comfortable for the patient because pelvic tissues are more relaxed and pliable. There may be value in repeating the examination just prior to term to evaluate the fetopelvic relationships and detect any disproportion that may indicate a need for special management during labor.

The value of clinical pelvimetry is a controversial matter. The diagnosis of fetopelvic disproportion is based not only on the diameters of the pelvis, but also on the size, position, presentation, attitude, and gestational age of the fetus, and on the strength of uterine contractions during labor. Thus, some clinicians prefer to let the patient have a trial labor rather than base labor management decisions on clinical pelvimetry. If, however, the patient is of short stature (possibly indicating inadequate pelvic bone growth) or has had an injury to the pelvis, pelvimetry may reveal obvious deficiencies in the adequacy of the pelvis for a vaginal delivery.

The procedure for pelvimetry outlined in Exhibit 3-2 is used to assess the three major planes of the pelvis: the inlet, midplane, and the outlet (Varney, 1980). The procedure should be carefully explained to the patient. Often the pressure that she experiences during the procedure is greater than expected.

Laboratory Tests

A variety of laboratory tests should be done at the first prenatal visit and should be repeated periodically or when indicated. Data obtained will aid the practitioner

---

EXHIBIT 3-2 Procedure for clinical pelvimetry

• With the examining fingers in the vagina, evaluate the width of the subpubic arch in fingerbreadths (two fingerbreadths usually indicates a normal subpubic angle of 90°) and the length and inclination of the symphysis.

• Proceed either left or right and palpate the side walls of the pelvis to determine whether they are straight, convergent, or divergent. This determination is made by following a line from the point of origin of the widest transverse diameter of the inlet downward to the inner aspect of the tuberosity. The normal gynecoid pelvis has straight or parallel sidewalls.

• Continue down and back until the ischial spines are reached. Estimate the interspinous distance (the average is 10.5 cm) and note if the spines are blunt, prominent, or encroaching. Blunt spines are typical of the gynecoid pelvis.

• Outline the sacrosciatic notch and determine its width in fingerbreadths. The length of the sacrospinous ligaments should be evaluated as short, average (at least two fingerbreadths), or long.

• Sweep the fingers down the sacrum, noting whether it is straight, curved or hollow; inclined forward or backward. Note whether the coccyx is tilted anteriorly or posteriorly; fixed or moveable. A curved sacrum and mobile coccyx are normal for the gynecoid pelvis.

• Measure the diagonal conjugate with the examining fingers directed upward at an acute angle toward the upper sacrum; with the longest finger touching the sacral vertebrae, "walk up" the sacrum to reach the sacral promontory. Then raise the finger from the other hand to mark off the point on the examining hand that touches the symphysis. This distance should be measured after withdrawing the examining hand. The diagonal conjugate is normally 12.5 cm (Oxorn, 1980). If the diagonal conjugate is greater than 11.5 cm, it is assumed that the pelvic inlet is adequate for delivery (Pritchard & MacDonald, 1980). The obstetric conjugate (anteroposterior diameter of the pelvic inlet) is estimated by subtracting 1.5–2.0 cm from the diagonal conjugate measurement.

• The transverse diameter of the pelvic outlet is measured by the distance between the ischial tuberosities. This measurement can be made with a Thom's pelvimeter, or estimated by placing a closed fist between the protrusions of the ischial tuberosities. The usual distance is 10.5 cm, but a distance of over 8 cm is considered normal (Pritchard & MacDonald, 1980). These measurements are recorded along with a summary conclusion that the pelvis is adequate, borderline, or contracted. This conclusion should be viewed as tentative, however, until labor ensues, and the relationships between the fetal size at term, powers of labor, and pelvic capacity are demonstrated. At that time, further evaluation by roentgenograms may be indicated.

TABLE 3-4 Causes of anemia during pregnancy

Acquired	Hereditary
Iron deficiency anemia	Thalassemia
Anemia caused by acute blood loss	Sickle-cell anemia
Anemia caused by infection	Sickle cell–hemoglobin C disease
Megaloblastic anemia	Sickle cell–thalessemia disease
Acquired hemolytic anemia	Homozygous hemoglobin C disease
Aplastic or hypoplastic anemia	Other hemoglobinopathies
	Hereditary hemolytic anemia without hemoglobinopathy

From Pritchard, J., & MacDonald, P. (1980). *Williams obstetrics* (ed. 16). New York: Appleton-Century-Crofts, p. 713. With permission.

in determining the types of intervention needed during the prenatal period.

Blood

Red Blood Count, Hematocrit, Hemoglobin The red blood count, hematocrit, and hemoglobin levels should be determined at the first prenatal visit. The hematocrit and hemoglobin should be tested again between the thirty-second and thirty-sixth weeks of pregnancy. In populations with a predelection for anemia earlier evaluation may be advisable. Earlier identification of anemia allows for therapeutic correction prior to delivery.

In the nonpregnant adult woman the red blood count is 4.0–5.5 million/mm³, the hematocrit 37–47 percent, and the hemoglobin 12–16 g/100 ml. Total body iron ranges from 3.0 to 3.5 g with more than sixty percent of the iron contained within the circulating hemoglobin and ten to thirty percent stored in the bone marrow, liver, and spleen.

During pregnancy, the blood volume increases about forty-five percent. This volume increase starts during the third month of gestation and reaches its peak early in the third trimester. The expanded volume amounts to approximately 1000–1500 ml in a single fetus pregnancy. During pregnancy, total red blood cell volume and hemoglobin mass increase by about thirty percent. This increase begins at three months' gestation and

TABLE 3-5 Iron requirements during pregnancy

Need	Amount
Maternal normal daily losses	200 mg
Fetoplacental unit	300–450 mg
Maternal blood volume	250–550 mg
Delivery losses	250 mg
Lactation	0.1–1 mg/day

peaks early in the third trimester. The red blood cell increase amounts to approximately 250–450 ml (Pritchard & MacDonald, 1980). Due to a greater increase of plasma volume over red cell mass, the hematocrit falls during pregnancy. This fall is considered to be a physiological anemia.

Anemia Anemia occurs frequently during pregnancy. The most common causes are presented in Table 3-4.

IRON DEFICIENCY ANEMIA The most common type of anemia found in pregnancy is iron deficiency anemia because many women become pregnant with inadequate stores.

Iron requirements during pregnancy depend on the size of the woman and her developing fetus. Table 3-5 shows the average iron requirements for pregnancy, delivery and lactation. The iron required by the full-term pregnancy ranges from 800 to 1200 mg. Women whose iron stores or iron intake during pregnancy do not meet the requirements will become anemic. Even for women with adequate iron stores at the onset of pregnancy, depletion to some extent is expected. After a pregnancy, up to two years may be required to replenish iron stores (Levin & Algazy, 1975).

Prevention of iron deficiency anemia is possible if a woman begins pregnancy with sufficient iron stores. During the first twenty weeks of pregnancy, an iron, protein, and nutrient rich diet probably will meet her pregnancy needs. From the twentieth week on, few women can absorb the necessary 5–8 mg of iron per day from dietary sources without supplemental iron. Initiation of supplemental iron near the beginning of the second trimester may be ideal. Approximately 60 mg of absorbable iron per day is recommended for all pregnant women. This is often administered as a prenatal multiple vitamin with iron. Preparations vary so it is important to consult the product information for the elemental iron available (Carr, 1974; McFee, 1973). It is appropriate to reevaluate the hematocrit and hemoglobin at the beginning of the third trimester and again near term (thirty-six weeks' gestation) to identify those women who may demonstrate anemia. Four to six weeks is a reasonable length of time to expect correction of a mild anemia. Iron should be continued for a period of time after birth and throughout lactation to aid in replenishing iron stores for all women.

If the hemoglobin falls below 11 g/100 ml or the hematocrit approaches 30 percent, the pregnant woman requires an evaluation of the cause of anemia. The woman should be instructed not to take her iron the morning of drawing the blood as oral iron preparations can elevate serum iron for several hours after ingestion. A morning specimen is recommended because of diurnal fluctuation in circulating iron, with lower levels in afternoon and evening hours. Hemoglobin, hematocrit, red cell count and peripheral smear, reticulocyte count, white cell count, and differential should be obtained (Carr, 1974). If the woman is black and has not been screened for sickle cell disease, hemoglobin electrophoresis, which specifically identifies her hemoglobin, or at least a screening test should be performed.

Diagnosis of iron deficiency anemia is made by the presence of low serum iron (less than 60 $\mu g\%$), and the percentage of iron saturation of the serum transferrin (Fe/TIBC). When saturation is 16 percent or less with an elevated TIBC, the diagnosis of iron-deficiency anemia can be made with confidence. (With sufficient iron stores, the Fe/TIBC ratio ranges from 25 to 35 percent). Subnormal saturation percentages can exist in other conditions such as chronic infection, chronic inflammatory disease and malignancy. Usually in these cases the TIBC is low-normal or depressed (Carr, 1974; McGee, 1973).

Treatment for iron-deficiency anemia is iron. However, the woman with iron-deficiency anemia may have a poor nutritional pattern, and a complete dietary review is in order. If her nutrition has been inadequate, she should be encouraged to follow a diet high in protein and other essential nutrients. It is important that hemoglobinopathy not exist when embarking upon treatment of anemia with iron. Because anemia may result from abnormal destruction of red blood cells, iron may actually have accumulated and be present in toxic amounts, although with the increased demands for iron in pregnancy this is unlikely. Certainly these women need evaluation and care by a high-risk team.

The recommended iron dosage for treatment of iron deficiency anemia is 100–180 mg of elemental iron per day (Carr, 1974; Danforth & Holly, 1977; McFee, 1973). Iron compounds vary as to their elemental or absorbable iron. Product information will clarify the amount present in each product. Ferrous sulfate, 300 mg, supplies 60 mg of elemental iron. Three tablets daily are recommended. Gastrointestinal irritation (nausea, vomiting, or diarrhea) are frequent complaints with iron ingestion. Iron needs increase appreciably with growth of the fetus, so therapy is particularly important after the twentieth week of gestation. Thus, if iron preparations exaggerate nausea in the first trimester, the dosage may be safely reduced until the nausea subsides. Taking the medication in three divided doses with meals is recommended to minimize gastric irritation. There is some evidence that ingestion of iron with milk decreases absorption. Ingestion with meat meals, or perhaps with vitamin C may enhance absorption (Carr, 1974). Constipation is another side effect of iron ingestion for some women (see p. 76).

Evaluation of the pregnant anemic woman's response to iron can be done in a number of ways. If, after two weeks of therapy, there is an increment of 0.2 mg% of hemoglobin, therapy is continued with the expectation that the patient will progress to nonanemic levels (Carr, 1974). The retriculocyte count will rise in one week and the hemotological values will return to normal in four to six weeks (McFee, 1973). For those women whose anemia does not respond to iron therapy by a 5-point rise in hematocrit (McFee, 1973) in four to six weeks, further evaluation is in order. The use of parenteral iron has the advantage of delivering the total estimated required dose in a contracted period of time (McFee, 1973). Blood transfusions may be in order in severe iron deficiency anemia associated with cardiac insufficiency and pathological hypovolemia (Pritchard & MacDonald, 1980).

FOLIC ACID DEFICIENCY ANEMIA   Dietary deficiency of folic acid is another possible cause of anemia for women, particularly during pregnancy. The actual incidence of true megaloblastic anemia is conjectured to be very low in the United States. Foods rich in folic acid are yeast, leafy vegetables, liver, fruits, grains, nuts, eggs, cheese, and milk. True megaloblastic anemia may be discovered in women who are very poorly nourished. However, twenty to twenty-five percent of women in this country may show early evidence of folic acid deficiency in late pregnancy (McFee, 1973).

Folic acid is a necessary nutrient; 50–100 μg per day are required when not pregnant. Because of the growing fetus, rapid growth of maternal tissues, and decreased gastrointestinal absorption, folic acid needs during pregnancy are increased to 150–300 μg per day.

An additional 60 μg per day are required during lactation. Folic acid requirements are increased even more when there is twin pregnancy, a hemoglobinopathy, a malabsorptive state such as sprue, an infectious process, and when taking anticonvulsant drugs (e.g., Dilantin) (Levin & Algazy, 1975).

Folic acid is an essential coenzyme necessary for DNA synthesis. As a result, many cells of the body can be adversely affected when a severe deficiency exists. There may be leukopenia and thrombocytopenia, which may lead to risk of hemorrhage at birth (Levin & Algazy, 1975). There is some evidence that spontaneous abortion, placental abruption, and congenital malformation may be increased in folate deficient women (McFee, 1973).

Folate stores are primarily in the liver and are normally sufficient for six weeks. Eighteen weeks of a folic-acid-deficient diet are necessary before megaloblastic anemia becomes apparent (Levin & Algazy, 1975). Laboratory tests to evaluate folic acid deficiency include serum or erythrocyte folate concentration, urinary formiminoglutamic acid excretion, the number of leukocytes with hypersegmented nuclei (lobe average), and bone marrow biopsy showing megaloblastic changes. When severe anemia exists, thorough evaluation must exclude the presence of megaloblastic anemia. Otherwise it is generally recommended that pregnant women receive folic acid supplements to prevent a deficient state. When a woman has iron deficiency anemia, folate deficiency often coexists. For women in both of these categories, 1 mg of folic acid per day, usually included in the prenatal vitamin, is considered both preventive and therapeutic (McFee, 1973; Levin & Algazy, 1975).

SICKLE CELL ANEMIA AND HEMOGLOBIN C   Pregnancy is a convenient time to do sickle cell screening on all black women. In the United States, 1 in 12 of all blacks have the sickle cell trait. The incidence of sickle cell anemia is 1 in 540. The incidence in pregnant women is much less due to the fact that many women with the actual anemia die before reaching childbearing age. Pregnancy adds a great burden to the woman with sickle cell anemia as it usually becomes more intense.

In a population where hemoglobinopathies are common, it is wise to do a hemoglobin electrophoresis routinely. This test identifies abnormal hemoglobin present in red blood cells in sickle cell disease, thalassemia, and other hemoglobinopathies (e.g., hemoglobin C or E disease). Because of the high degree of morbidity and mortality resulting from these hemoglobinopathies, women with any of these conditions should be cared for by high-risk obstetrical teams during pregnancy.

White Blood Count   In the nonpregnant woman, the white blood count ranges between 5,000 and 10,000/mm^3. During pregnancy the count can increase to 15,000/mm^3. Elevations beyond these ranges may indicate an infectious process. More information should be elicited from the patient, as white blood count elevation alone is not sufficient evidence to assume infection.

Blood Typing and Atypical Antibodies   Every pregnant woman should have a blood test to determine her blood type and Rh factor. A maternal-fetal blood incompatibility may occur when the woman is Rh-negative and her partner is Rh-positive, or when her type is O and her partner's type is A, B, or AB. The resulting condition in the fetus is erthroblastosis fetalis (EBF) or hemolytic disease of the newborn.

All women should also be screened for atypical antibodies during the first prenatal visit and again in the third trimester (32 weeks). If antibodies are present, further assessment must be made. The most well-known antibody that causes EBF is associated with an Rh-negative mother. Other antibodies, those formed in response to antigens such as C, c, E, e, Kell (K), Duffy, M, and Kidd, have also been found to cause hemolytic disease (Zipursky, 1981).

Antibody titers (in Rh-negative women) should be checked at the first visit, the twenty-eighth week, the thirty-second week, and the thirty-sixth week. In the presence of a positive Rh antibody titer the woman should be referred for care to a high-risk obstetrical team. Unsensitized women (those with negative Rh antibody titers) should be offered Rh immune globulin at the twenty-eighth week of pregnancy. This prevents sensitization in the two percent of women who would become sensitized during pregnancy or immediately postpartum before Rh immune globulin is given. If the father is known to be Rh-negative, eliminating the possibility of sensitization of the women during this pregnancy, prenatal Rh immune globulin is not indicated. Those women who receive prenatal Rh immune globulin require no further Rh antibody testing during this pregnancy (Bowman, 1978). These women are given Rh immune globulin postpartum if they deliver an Rh-positive infant.

Rubella   A rubella titer must be determined at the beginning of prenatal care to ascertain the presence or absence of immunity. If a woman has a negative titer, her fetus is at risk should she develop rubella during the first trimester. She should attempt to avoid young children who have not been vaccinated against rubella during this period. If an infection does occur during the first three months of pregnancy, termination is usually recommended. If the antibody titer is negative, plans should be made for immunization postpartum. Rubella immunization should not be given during pregnancy.

Blood Sugar Women having a positive family history of diabetes, obesity, recurrent infections, previously large for gestational age babies or poor obstetrical history (frequent spontaneous abortions or previous loss after age of viability) should be screened for blood glucose at the first antepartum visit and again toward the end of the second trimester. Some clinicians recommend that all women be screened at the end of the second trimester when the greatest challenge occurs to maternal insulin production.

The postprandial blood sugar is the most common and convenient laboratory test. Women can be instructed to eat a meal or drink a solution containing 100 g of carbohydrates following an eight-hour fast. Some authorities suggest a high carbohydrate diet for three days preceding the fast (Schneider, 1978). Drinking the solution is simpler, and possibly less prone to error. However, the meal is more nutritious and the woman may feel better, as drinking the glucose solution sometimes causes nausea.

Two hours after the 100-g carbohydrate meal or solution is ingested, a blood specimen is drawn. The blood sugar value should be 140 mg/100 ml of blood or less. If the blood sugar is higher, the woman will require further evaluation, usually in the form of an oral glucose tolerance test.

Serology A serologic test for syphilis is required by all states. (See "Sexually Transmitted Diseases and Vaginitis," *Women's Health: Ambulatory Care,* for tests available.) If the disease is detected prior to the twelfth to sixteenth week of gestation, the mother can be treated and there is relative assurance that there will be no fetal damage. In areas where syphilis is prevalent, the serology should be repeated during the seventh month of pregnancy. Women found to have syphilis during pregnancy require consultation with someone knowledgeable about infectious disease in pregnancy and possibly complete management by high-risk obstetrical team.

Urine

Bacteria Urinary tract infections occur more frequently during pregnancy because of physiological changes in the urinary tract. Treatment of bacteriuria is necessary to prevent complications during pregnancy and subsequent chronic renal disease.

Bacteriuria refers to bacteriologically significant amounts of bacteria in the urine, which usually is sterile. A standard was established by Kass in 1957 to mean at least 100,000 colonies of organisms per milliter in three successive, fresh, clean catch, midstream specimens of urine. The first culture with 100,000 colonies/ml is eighty percent indicative of significant bacteriuria, the second is ninety-one percent indicative (Rees, 1978) and the third is ninety-five percent indicative. When urine is obtained by catheterization, 100,000 colonies/ml in the first urine specimen means a probability of ninety-five percent of true bacteriuria. Urine obtained by suprapubic aspiration is either found to be sterile or to contain significant bacterial growth. In the latter case, bacteriuria is confirmed (Andriole, 1975).

BACTERIURIA Four to almost seven percent of women have asymptomatic but detectable bacteriuria at the first prenatal visit. Twenty to forty percent of women with untreated bacteriuria in early pregnancy develop acute, symptomatic pyelonephritis with fever, dysuria, and flank pain in later pregnancy. Treating asymptomatic bacteriuria in pregnancy eliminates ninety percent of pyelonephritis in pregnancy. Twenty to fifty percent of women with symptomatic urinary tract infection in pregnancy deliver prematurely. Thus, the relationship between bacteriuria, even asymptomatic, and subsequent pyelonephritis in pregnancy and premature delivery gives significance to screening and treating pregnant women for bacteriuria (Andriole, 1975).

Symptomatic urinary tract infection includes the broad categories of cystitis, pyelonephritis, and clinical pyelonephritis. *Cystitis* is defined as an inflammatory condition of the urinary bladder and may be bacterial or nonbacterial. Classic symptoms are dysuria, particularly at the end of urination, frequency, and urgency. There are few systemic symptoms associated with cystitis, and women with cystitis can usually be treated on an ambulatory basis. *Pyelonephritis* can be acute or chronic and is defined as an inflammatory condition of the renal substance and renal pelvis. *Clinical pyelonephritis* is used to describe patients with suspected or confirmed urinary infection who also have fever and loin pain or tenderness (Rees, 1978). Pregnant women with pyelonephritis usually require hospitalization and intravenous antibiotic therapy.

An appropriate protocol for frequency of screening for bacteriuria during pregnancy is shown in Figure 3-2.

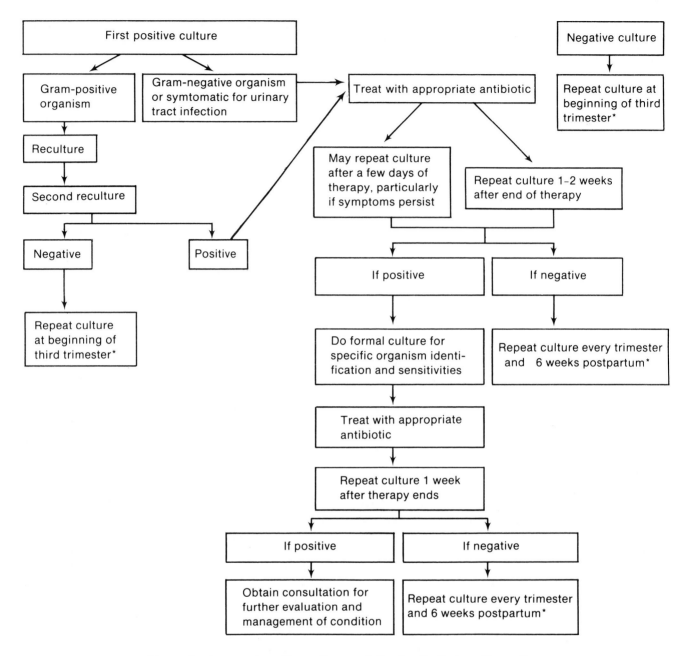

*Treat all subsequent positive cultures as following the first positive culture.

FIGURE 3-2 Screening of pregnant women for asymptomatic bacteriuria at initial prenatal visit.

Screening is accomplished by collecting a clean catch midstream specimen, which requires careful instruction of the woman. Separation of the labia minora, careful single-stroke washing of the vestibule (avoiding Benzalkonium solutions and soaps containing pHiso-Hex because of their antimicrobial effect in the collected urine), and midstream collection into a sterile container facilitate an uncontaminated specimen

(Andriole, 1975). The appropriate culture media needs to be inoculated within one hour or the urine specimen kept refrigerated at 4°C until it can be innoculated. Otherwise, urinary pathogens can multiply rapidly enough to give a false-positive result (Rees, 1978).

Catheterization should be used as infrequently as possible, since a single catheterization carries a four to six percent risk of introducing infection (Andriole,

1975). It is always in the best interest of the women to use catheterization only when immediate uncontaminated urine culture results are of paramount importance. Suprapublic urine aspiration is another means of obtaining an uncontaminated specimen. Some recommend suprapublic aspiration over catheterization to reduce the risk of introducing infection (Andriole, 1975; Rees, 1978).

Formal or plate culture results may yield the number of colonies per mililiter or give colony counts of specific organisms with their related sensitivities to specific drugs. Less specific culture techniques, called *dipinoculum techniques,* are suited to health care sites where full laboratory facilities are unavailable. A glass or plastic slide coated with various agars is dipped into fresh urine and replaced in a self-contained unit. After incubation in room air or at body temperature, the density of colonies can be determined by a photographic standard supplied with the method. Preliminary identification of the organism can be made from the selective agar. For those patients with symptoms or significant bacteriuria, more specific laboratory tests can be performed. This method is simple, inexpensive, and accurate (Andriole, 1975; Rees, 1978).

Microscopic examination of urine is sometimes used in conjunction with urine culture methods. This is a rapid and inexpensive screening procedure, which may be used while awaiting culture results. A drop of uncentrifuged urine can be examined with the high dry lens of a microscope. The presence of even a few bacilli in the urine strongly suggests a colony count of at least 100,000/ml. Certainly, false-positive results could be caused by contamination. False-negative results can result from simply missing bacteria in that particular specimen. (Andriole, 1975) A negative microscopic examination may be sufficient reason to await culture results before beginning antibiotics for urinary tract infection when signs and symptoms are equivocal.

Interpretation of laboratory results is based on differentiation of contaminated urine (from skin, mucus membrane) versus urine containing bacteria. Bacteriuria is ninety-five percent probable if three clean catch, midstream urine cultures yield 100,000 colonies/ml. If the colony count is less than 10,000 bacteria/ml, there is a ninety-eight percent probability that the patient does not have urinary infection. Ninety-five percent of women who have between 10,000 and 100,000 colonies of bacteria on the first specimen will not demonstrate bacteriuria in a second specimen (Andriole, 1975).

Most bacteria causing urinary tract infections in the previously healthy woman are of the type found in the bowel and sometimes vagina. These gram-negative organisms are *Escherichia coli* and related paracolon species, *Klebsiella, Proteus* species and *Bacillus pyocyaneus* (Nesbitt, 1977). These organisms are usually sensitive to sulfa drugs (sulfisoxazole), nitrofurantoins, or broad-spectrum antibiotics. Nitrofurantoins (e.g., Macrodantin, Eaton) may lead to hemolytic anemia in women who have G6PD (glucose-6-phosphate dehydrogenase) deficiency. Perhaps two percent of black women are homozygous for this sex-chromosome-linked enzyme deficiency. Arbitrary use of this drug in black women may be contraindicated. Sulfa drugs (Gantrisin, Roche) should be avoided in the third trimester of pregnancy because of the possibility of inducing hyperbilirubinemia in the newborn. This drug competes with unconjugated bilirubin for albumin binding sites in the fetus. Tetracycline should not be given during pregnancy. It may discolor the deciduous teeth of the child and may create hepatotoxicity in the mother. Chloramphenicol may depress bone marrow, causing fetal blood dyscrasias. Streptomycin, kanamycin, and gentamicin may be ototoxic and nephrotoxic. Ampicillin does not appear to be harmful to the fetus and, except for maternal hypersensitivity, seems safe to use in pregnancy (Andriole, 1975; Rees, 1978; Pritchard & MacDonald, 1980)

If the initial positive culture specifically identifies the invading organisms and the drugs to which they are sensitive, the appropriate drug can be given. If a screening culture is the basis for treatment and one of the drugs that usually eradicates infection (sulfisoxazole, nitrofurantoins, ampicillin) is used, a culture and sensitivity should be obtained a few days after initiating therapy (see Figure 3-2). The drug will be appropriately altered if the causative organism is still present. Some would eliminate this interval culture if the woman's symptoms were cleared by treatment. One to two weeks after treatment is completed another culture is obtained (a screening culture is satisfactory). If bacteriuria persists, cultures, sensitivities, and treatment are repeated. During pregnancy, cultures should be repeated at least each trimester and at the six-week postpartum examination. For nonpregnant women, cultures at repeated intervals (three and then six months) will guard against reinfection (Andriole, 1975). Women who have recurrent urinary tract infections when not pregnant and those who have upper urinary tract infections when pregnant need additional medical evaluation. Intravenous pyelogram and cystoscopic studies to ascertain normal urinary tract anatomy may be in order (Ledger, 1981).

When women are under treatment for urinary tract infections, certain measures will facilitate a favorable response to therapy. All medication should be taken. Less than a complete course of therapy may make organisms resistant to a particular drug. Large volumes of fluids should be consumed. This will literally help flush out infection. Rest and adequate nutrition are appropriate to help the body heal and recover.

For women who are susceptible to urinary tract infections or who experience recurrent bouts of cystitis, certain measures will help abate relapses:

- Maintain an adequate daily intake of fluid.
- Urinate regularly (three-hourly) and completely empty the bladder.
- Take care to cleanse the genitalia regularly; wipe from front to back and avoid rectal contamination of the vaginal introitus with sexual activity.
- Try to minimize trauma to the bladder and urethra from sexual intercourse by experimenting with various positions and adequate lubrication (artificial if necessary).
- Avoid oils, salts, and disinfectants in bath water.
- Avoid aerosol vaginal deodorants (Rees, 1978).

Glucose, Protein, and Ketones Dipstick tests for glucose and protein should be done at each prenatal visit. In a nonpregnant woman there should be no glucose present in the urine. During pregnancy, however, glucosuria is not necessarily pathological. There is an increase in glomerular filtration without an increase in tubular reabsorptive capacity for filtered glucose. Even though glucosuria is common during pregnancy, the possibility of diabetes mellitus should not be ignored. Women having glucosuria should be evaluated for abnormal glucose metabolism. Slight albuminuria may be insignificant or may indicate serious trouble. Physiological albuminuria occurs after chilling, cold baths, and severe physical or mental exertion. When the precipitating cause is removed, the albuminuria disappears. Physiological albuminuria will be present during the day but not at night (Squier, 1972). Albuminuria may also result from previous kidney disease or that due to pregnancy.

Whenever a finding of 1+ protein or greater occurs, the possibility of preeclampsia, urinary tract infection, abnormal kidney function, or a contaminated urine specimen should be considered. In most settings, trace protein is usually considered to be contamination by vaginal secretions. A clean catch midstream urine specimen may be obtained for screening. If albuminuria is a pattern (more than 1+ on two visits) the woman may require renal function studies, and physician consultation would be appropriate.

The routine evaluation for presence of ketones in the urine is beneficial. Some women become ketonuric when pregnant if they are eating with insufficient frequency or quantity. As ketonuria is a state to be avoided in pregnancy, identifying its presence is important. These women need to be careful to eat more frequently and in sufficient quantity.

Routine Urinalysis Except for glucosuria, pregnancy does not alter a routine urinalysis, which can provide significant clues to urinary disturbances such as chronic kidney damage or bladder infection. It is not necessary to use urinalysis as a screening device since the dipstick and bacteria screen can pick up early signs of problems.

Cervical Studies

Cytologic Screening Pregnancy presents an excellent opportunity for early detection and treatment of cervical carcinoma. (See "Physical Assessment" and "Conditions of the Cervix," *Women's Health: Ambulatory Care,* for further discussion of the Pap smear.)

Neisseria gonorrhea Screening for gonorrhea is an important part of the initial antepartum visit. This smear can be done at the same time as the Pap smear. There is an increasing incidence of the disease in this country, and if a woman has a history of gonorrhea or is from a group where the incidence is high (poverty or adolescent, for instance), the culture should be repeated during the third trimester. It is extremely important that the disease be treated prior to delivery to prevent neonatal eye infection. (See "Sexually Transmitted Diseases and Vaginitis," *Women's Health: Ambulatory Care,* for further discussion of gonorrhea.)

Tuberculosis Skin Testing

Pregnancy is a good time for a routine screening for tuberculosis. Since 1950 one to three percent of pregnant women have had tuberculosis (Schneider, 1978). The Mantoux, Tine skin test, and purified protein derivative (PPD) are recommended means of screening during pregnancy.

The practitioner must be certain that the woman has not had a previous positive skin test. A second positive skin test could potentially cause severe sloughing of the skin in the area tested. A woman with a positive skin test needs careful evaluation of the status of her disease. If a roentgenogram of the woman's chest is done, care should be taken to shield the abdomen due to the effect of radiation on fetal growth and development. If possible, even x-ray with a shielded abdomen should be avoided in the first trimester of pregnancy.

Conclusion of Initial Visit

The initial visit should be concluded by reviewing the results of the history and physical assessment with the client and determining an ongoing plan for prenatal care. Specific concerns of the mother should be addressed and health maintenance education initiated. Usual areas of counseling at this time include diet, smoking, drug use, exercise, and sexual activity. If medications such as vitamins or iron have been prescribed, their proper use should be explained. Specific suggestions for relief of common pregnancy discomforts should be given, and a plan for return visits should be agreed on with the client. The pregnant woman should be told what she might expect during the interval between visits and should be informed about any signs or symptoms (i.e., bleeding) for which she should seek immediate care. Referral for prenatal classes or other special care can also be made at this time.

INTERVAL PRENATAL ASSESSMENT

The frequency of subsequent prenatal visits will be determined from the initial and ongoing assessment of the pregnant woman's needs. The American College of Obstetricians and Gynecologists recommends that the normal, low-risk patient should be seen at least every four weeks for the first twenty-eight weeks of pregnancy, every two weeks until the thirty-sixth week, and weekly thereafter.

It is often beneficial for the woman to return two weeks after the initial visit to discuss laboratory results and to reinforce and continue prenatal teaching and counseling. This visit is also a good time for the woman's partner or significant other to accompany her, meet the nurse, and be included in assessment and plans for care. At this time, the woman may be referred to early pregnancy classes or other resources. It is also helpful to see the client at the twentieth week of gestation to gather data about fetal heart tones, uterine size, and quickening as further estimates of gestational age.

Interval History

The expectant mother's current health status and any changes since the initial visit should be reviewed; included should be physical discomforts and changes, emotional changes, and alterations in lifestyle or social situations that may affect the pregnancy experience.

The experiences of the woman's partner or other significant individuals in her life should also be explored. Health practices such as diet, exercise, and rest should be assessed and appropriate feedback offered. The client's prenatal record should be updated to include data gathered at each visit. Problems or concerns identified on previous visits should be followed up and reassessed.

It is helpful for the health care provider, as well as for the pregnant woman herself, to keep a list or diary of questions, concerns, and significant occurrences between visits. If the client reports any new problems or concerns, these should be explored in depth and appropriately charted according to a problem oriented medical record format. Data to be collected should include (1) the nature of the symptom or event; its onset, course, and duration, as well as any precipitating events; (2) factors in the woman's situation, history, or patient profile that are relevant to the problem; (3) measures taken to alleviate or cope with the problem, and the results of those measures.

Ongoing Physical Assessment

At each subsequent prenatal visit the following areas should be assessed.

Weight

Weight gain during pregnancy is an indicator of fetal growth and maternal nutrition and health. It is important to assess both the amount and pattern of weight gain during pregnancy. The pattern should be regular, with the major increase of weight occurring during the second half of pregnancy. Weight gain should not exceed 0.9 kb (2 lb) in one week or 2.25 kg (5 lb) in one month. If gain is less than or greater than desired, cause should be determined and an appropriate plan of management formulated.

Blood Pressure

Changes in blood pressure may be noted during pregnancy; while cardiac output increases by twenty-five to fifty percent, peripheral resistance decreases by approximately thirty-five percent (Shaver, 1979). These changes result in a slight decline in arterial blood pressure. Systolic pressure often does not change significantly although diastolic pressure falls 10–15 mm Hg. Any rise in blood pressure, therefore, becomes a matter of concern.

Blood pressure measurements at each visit should be compared with the reading from the initial prenatal visit. If the blood pressure is elevated, have the woman

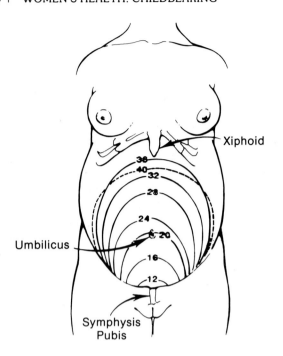

FIGURE 3-3 Approximate height of fundus during pregnancy (see Table 3-6 for further explanation). (Redrawn from the Medical University of South Carolina, School of Nursing, Nurse-Midwifery Program, 1975. With permission.)

rest for fifteen to twenty minutes and then remeasure; the elevation may have been caused by stress or excitement. A blood pressure reading of 140/90 or a rise of 30/15 from the woman's baseline reading is considered suggestive of a pathological condition. Such an elevation should be evaluated in conjunction with data on edema, weight gain, and proteinuria to predict developing preeclampsia or hypertensive disorders.

A woman may also be screened for risk of preeclampsia by use of the *roll-over test* (Marshall & Newman, 1977). This test is used to screen women in the twenty-eighth to thirty-second week of pregnancy who have no medical illnesses such as chronic hypertension, diabetes, or renal disease. The woman is placed in the left lateral position and her blood pressure taken. Within one to two minutes, the woman is turned supine and another blood pressure recorded. A rise of 15 mm Hg diastolic blood pressure is considered a positive test for preeclampsia risk.

Blood pressure in late pregnancy, similar to cardiac output, is influenced by posture. Readings are lower when lying down; hypotension may be noted when the woman is supine, due to pressure of the uterus on the inferior vena cava. This lowered blood pressure may

cause the woman to feel faint or dizzy when lying on her back, thus, the supine position is to be avoided during the latter half of pregnancy.

Edema

Physiological edema, not detectable by observation, is normal in pregnancy, resulting from storage of approximately 2.5 liters of extra water in the interstitial space.

Clinical edema of the lower extremities, particularly late in the day, is also common during late pregnancy, due to the effects of progesterone and estrogen on kidney function, and in response to pooling of the blood in the lower extremities. Rest in the side-lying position facilities venous return and enhances kidney function, thus relieving edema of the legs.

Morning edema and edema of the hands and face are not normal and their presence may be suggestive of developing preeclampsia. Rings that become too tight for the woman to wear is one indicator of developing edema.

Urinalysis

The urine is tested at each visit for presence of protein, glucose, and ketones. The significance of these were discussed earlier in this chapter.

Uterine Growth

Recording the fundal height measurement at periodic intervals provides important information about fetal growth. The uterine fundus is palpated halfway between the symphysis and umbilicus at sixteen weeks, rises to just below the level of the umbilicus at twenty weeks, and continues to rise until engagement, which occurs between thirty-eight and forty weeks in primiparas and frequently not prior to the onset of labor in multiparas. Engagement is accompanied by a decrease in fundal height as the presenting part of the fetus descends into the pelvis. Between twenty-four and thirty-six weeks the fundal height (in centimeters) roughly approximates the gestational age of the fetus (see Figure 3-3, Table 3-6, and McDonald's rule, p. 72).

Inconsistencies in fetal growth call for further evaluation. If measurements are either larger or smaller than expected, it may be that the estimate of gestational age is in error and should be carefully reassessed. As discussed, establishing an EDC from the date of the last menstrual period alone is subject to error. Additional parameters, including date of quickening, and date when the fetal heart was first audible with a fetoscope, should be evaluated.

TABLE 3-6 Approximate height of fundus during pregnancy

Gestation (weeks)	Location of the Uterus
1–12	The uterus is a pelvic organ for the first 3 months of pregnancy, palpable on vaginal examination.
12	The uterus fills the pelvic cavity. The fundus is felt level with or just above the upper margin of symphysis pubis. The uterus is the size of a small grapefruit and feels globular and firm.
16	The fundus is halfway between the symphysis and the umbilicus and is ovid in shape.
20	The fundus is about at the umbilicus or 1–2 finger breadths below the umbilicus.
24	The fundus is 1–2 finger breadths above the umbilicus and may rotate to the right. Fundus feels less firm.
28	The fundus is halfway between the umbilicus and the xiphoid, about 3 finger breadths above the umbilicus.
32	The fundus is 3/4 the distance between the umbilicus and the xiphoid, or about 3 finger breadths below the xiphoid.
36	The fundus is at, or just below, the xiphoid.
40	The fundus drops several finger breadths, particularly in primigravidae.

From Antepartum module. Medical University of South Carolina, School of Nursing, Nurse-Midwifery Program, 1975. With permission.
Note: See Figure 3-3 for illustration of these changes.

If the uterus is larger than expected, the possible causes are multiple including multiple pregnancy, hydramnios, hydatidiform mole, or ovarian or uterine tumors. In cases of multiple pregnancy there is often a rapid increase in fundal measurements, particularly during the second trimester. Thus, it is important to review the pattern of uterine growth during the pregnancy as well as the periodic measurement. Hydramnios can also be determined clinically by ballottement or tapping on the woman's abdomen and sensing the rebound fullness on the other side of the abdomen. The conditions contributing to unusually large uterine growth may well be detected by ultrasound. If the fetus is suspected to be large for gestational age (LGA), the mother should be tested for gestational diabetes, since this is often a contributing factor of LGA infants.

If uterine growth is less than expected, the fetus may be small for gestational age, perhaps related to intra-uterine growth retardation from placental insufficiency. This is a high-risk condition for the fetus, and is due to a variety of etiologies including hypertensive disorders, infectious processes, uterine anomalies, and severe malnutrition. Growth retardation is most accurately determined through serial ultrasound examinations, which document inadequate fetal growth over time. Other causes of inadequate uterine growth include fetal structural abnormalities, oligohydramnios (often related to fetal anomalies), or fetal death. In the situation of fetal demise, uterine growth will cease as opposed to the continued but inadequate growth seen in fetal growth retardation.

Whenever intra-uterine growth does not coincide with the gestational age of the pregnancy, the cause must be sought; continued planning for adequate care during pregnancy for mother and fetus hinges on whether or not the intra-uterine growth is normal.

Fetal Assessment

There are other methods for estimating gestational age, evaluating the adequacy of fetal growth, and assessing fetal maturation:

Quickening Initial fetal movements felt by the expectant mother are called *quickening.* These movements have been described as fluttering abdominal movements that gradually increase in intensity. Quickening usually occurs between the sixteenth and twentieth weeks of pregnancy. Perception of fetal movement may be delayed with maternal obesity. Multiparas generally become aware of fetal movement earlier than primigravidas, so quickening may be a less than accurate method of determing the EDC.

Fetal Heart Tones Hearing the fetal heart pulsations provides a positive diagnosis of pregnancy. The heartbeat usually cannot be detected through a fetoscope until the eighteenth to twentieth week. Instruments such as the Doptone, an ultrasonic device, have recently been developed that make it possible to detect the fetal heart toward the end of the first trimester.

With periodic auscultation, it is difficult to detect changes in the fetal heart rate indicative of distress. However, the presence and rate of the fetal heart beat should be evaluated at each visit to assure the prospective mother that her baby is alive and well. If bradycardia (fetal heart rate less than 120) or tachycardia (fetal heart rate greater than 160) is noted, evaluation of fetal well-being by a nonstress test or other methods may be indicated (Jarrell & Sokol, 1979; Paul & Miller, 1978).

Fundal Height Measurements (McDonald's Rule)

During the second and third trimesters, McDonald's rule can be used to estimate gestational age from the fundal height measurement as follows: height of fundus (measured in centimeters from the top of the symphysis pubic) divided by 3.5 equals gestational age in lunar months from the sixth month until term (Gluck, 1978, p. 548).

Not only is the fundus of a typical size for a given gestation, but uterine growth continues throughout pregnancy. The fundal height may not increase after thirty-six weeks; it may even decrease with engagement and descent of the presenting part. Fundal measurements are most accurate when *consistently* obtained by as few examiners as possible. If a minimum of examiners consistently measure a woman's fundal height, they will know how their measurements usually compare and be better able to evaluate fundal growth as her pregnancy progresses.

Ultrasound

Ultrasonic echo sounding (sonar) is a technique that is used to assess gestational age and fetal growth, as well as to diagnose many fetal and maternal problems. The abdomen is scanned using intermittant high frequency sound waves, which are projected onto a screen and converted into a picture. The intensity of the reflection of the waves is dependent on the density of the tissue or fluid penetrated. This technique is considered safer than roentgenograms.

Ultrasound can be used first to determine if a woman *is* pregnant. The gestational sac can be visualized by the fifth week of pregnancy. The gestational age can be extrapolated from uterine or gestational sac size prior to twelve weeks. After twelve weeks of pregnancy, gestational age can be extrapolated from the biparietal diameter, which correlates well with fetal age between sixteen and thirty-two weeks of gestation. The best time for corroborating gestational age with the use of ultrasound is during the second trimester. Serial ultra-sound measurements can be used to document adequacy of fetal growth when intra-uterine growth retardation is a concern. Ultrasound is also useful in establishing a diagnosis of twins, hydatidiform mole, hydramnios, or pelvic tumors or masses. It can also be used to determine the presentation of the fetus and to localize the placenta. Thus, ultrasound is an important aid in many situations. It is particularly useful when uterine growth is inconsistent with gestational age estimates derived from dates of the last menstrual period (Gottesfeld, 1978; Hertz & Zador, 1979).

X-Ray Visualization

Concern about exposure of the mother and fetus to radiation and the availability of other diagnostic aids such as ultrasound have limited the use of x-ray for evaluating fetal growth, but through x-ray visualization of the distal femoral and proximal tibial epiphyses, fetal age can be determined based upon available parameters.

Amniocentesis

Through amniocentesis, the amniotic fluid can be analyzed, providing information for prenatal diagnosis of genetic abnormalities (Simpson, 1981). Late in pregnancy, the technique may be utilized to assess fetal maturity. Some of the most frequent biochemical indicators of fetal maturity are as follows (Gluck, 1978):

• Creatinine levels in the amniotic fluid increase with fetal age, as the fetus achieves renal maturity. When the creatinine value is 2 mg/100 ml, the fetus is assumed to be mature. However, creatinine levels are influenced by maternal renal disease, dehydration, and fetal anomaly, so findings should be viewed with caution.

• Cytologic examination of the amniotic fluid can measure the number of fetal lipid-containing exfoliated cells (stained with Nile blue sulfate). The number of fat cells increases with fetal age, and when twenty percent of the total cells are stained, the fetus is considered to be mature.

• Fetal lung maturity is measured by examining the ratio of surfactants, lecithin and sphingomyelin, in the amniotic fluid. A lecithin/sphingomyelin ratio greater than 2 indicates adequate lung maturity for extra-uterine life. This occurs after thirty-six weeks of gestation.

Fetal Movement

There is growing interest in the mother's subjective evaluation of fetal movement as a measure of fetal well-being. An exact standard for the number of fetal movements indicative of fetal well-being has not been established, but it is generally accepted that a decided reduction in fetal activity may be an indication of deterioration of fetal status. Many women believe the old adage that the baby gets quiet before labor begins. Women need counseling to dispel this misinformation, and it is advocated that all women be taught to note fetal activity as an easy, noninvasive means of monitoring the fetus' well-being. Those who report decreased fetal movement need more extensive evaluation of fetal well-being and may require the care of a high-risk obstetrical team (Coleman, 1981; Fischer et al., 1981; Sadovsky, 1978; Worley, 1980).

Pelvic Examination

A pelvic examination is not usually repeated unless the patient interview reveals symptoms that indicate the need for one. A pelvic examination may be done close to term to assess pelvic measurements and to determine physical changes accompanying the initiation of labor, such as softening of the cervix, effacement, and dilation, and to evaluate the fetal presenting part and its degree of descent into the pelvis.

Continuing Risk Assessment

Throughout pregnancy a woman should continually be reassessed for her risk of developing problems. Her risk status may change during pregnancy as new problems arise or existing problems are resolved. In Table 3-7, Babson et al. (1980) identify risk factors that may develop at different times during pregnancy.

The impact of a diagnosis of a high-risk pregnancy on the woman and her family should be considered. The intensity of care that is required, including the array of diagnostic tests, can add stress to an already difficult experience. The uncertainty of pregnancy outcome for the mother and baby cannot be relieved until delivery. Developing complications may drastically alter the plans and expectations the woman had for her pregnancy experience. For some women, a high-risk pregnancy is a sign of failure and may involve a loss of self-esteem. It is normal for the woman to experience grief over the loss of her expected normal pregnancy, and her plans for her pregnancy should be followed as nearly as possible so that she can find satisfaction in her experience.

Assessment of Parenting

Throughout the prenatal period the development of parenting should be assessed. This includes exploring preparation for parenting, development of attachment, and potential for parenting problems.

Many women have had little previous experience with infants and children and thus find themselves overwhelmed at the idea of being a parent. The nurse can review the woman's previous experience and expectations about parenthood. Referral to prenatal classes or parenting classes that discuss child care and parenting responsibilities may be appropriate. Included in this assessment is the type of support that is available to the woman: Will she have relatives and friends to assist in child care and to serve as role models?

An essential part of parenting is the attachment that develops between parent and child. Attachment begins prior to pregnancy with planning the pregnancy. During the prenatal period confirming the pregnancy by various aspects of pregnancy diagnosis, accepting the pregnancy, feeling the fetus move and hearing the fetal heart, all contribute to the development of attachment. (Klaus & Kennell, 1976) An unplanned or high-risk pregnancy may inhibit the development of attachment. Signs that attachment is occurring include planning room for the new baby, selecting names, fantasizing, and talking about the baby as an individual.

An assessment of parenting includes identification of potential risk for parenting problems. The following factors have been identified as variables that can be identified that influence an individual's potential for abuse (Caulfield et al., 1977).

- *Parent's background:* A lack of adequate parenting role models may interfere with an individual's ability to parent. Abusive parents often were abused as children.
- *Personality:* Low self-concept and lack of self-confidence, lack of empathy, and tendency to use physical punishment are antecedents to abuse.
- *Attachment:* Interference with attachment may lead to later parenting problems.
- *Social network resources:* Abusive parents tend to be social isolates and have difficulty coping with stressors in their environment.
- *Attitudes about childrearing:* Parenting problems often result when parents have unrealistic expectations for their child's behavior. Knowledge of normal growth and development may assist parents in having appropriate expectations.

Health Maintenance During Pregnancy

The expectant mother can be aided in having a healthy and enjoyable pregnancy through activities that will promote and maintain her health and that of her baby. She may have questions or concerns about activities during pregnancy or about the prevention or treatment of common discomforts.

TABLE 3-7   Risk factors associated with different stages of pregnancy

Stage	High-Risk Factors	Moderate-Risk Factors
Early pregnancy	Failure of or disproportionate uterine growth	Unresponsive urinary tract infection
	Exposure to teratogens (radiation, infection, chemicals)	Suspected ectopic pregnancy
		Suspected missed abortion
	Pregnancy complicated by isoimmunization	Severe hyperemesis gravidarum
	Need for antenatal genetic diagnosis	Positive VDRL test
	Severe anemia (9 g or less hemoglobin)	Positive gonorrhea screening
		Anemia not responsive to iron treatment
		Viral illness
		Vaginal bleeding
		Mild anemia (9–10.9 g hemoglobin)
Late pregnancy	Failure of uterine growth or disproportionate uterine growth	Hypertensive states of pregnancy (mild)
	Severe anemia (less than 9 g hemoglobin)	Breech, if Cesarean section is planned
	More than 42 ½ weeks' gestation	Uncertain presentations
	Severe preeclampsia	Need for fetal maturity studies
	Eclampsia	Postdate pregnancy (41–42 ½ weeks' gestation)
	Breech, if vaginal delivery is planned	Premature rupture of the membranes (more than 12 hours without labor if gestation is more than 38 weeks long)
	Moderate to severe isoimmunization (necessitating intra-uterine transfusion or neonatal exchange transfusion)	
	Placenta previa	Induction of labor
	Hydramnios or oligohydramnios	Suspected fetopelvic disproportion at term
	Antepartum fetal death	Floating presentations 2 weeks or less from the EDC
	Thromboembolic disease	
	Premature labor (less than 37 weeks' gestation)	
	Premature rupture of membranes (less than 38 weeks' gestation)	
	Tumor or other obstruction of birth canal	
	Abruptio placenta	
	Chronic or acute pyelonephritis	
	Multiple gestation	
	Abnormal oxytocin challenge test	
	Falling urinary estriols	
	Prolonged rupture of membranes	
	Diabetes	

From Babson, S., Benson, R., Pernoll, M., & Benda, G. (1980). *Management of high-risk pregnancy and intensive care of the neonate* (ed. 4). St. Louis: C. V. Mosby Co., pp. 18–19. With permission.

Exercise and Rest

The pregnant woman can generally participate in any activity during her pregnancy that she engaged in prior to the pregnancy. Physical exercise will not only help to keep her body in good condition for labor and delivery, but also will promote relaxing sleep and increase her feeling of well-being. The woman should recognize that she may tire more easily and be alert to signs of fatigue as a guideline for the amount and type of physical activity that is best for her (Clark, 1978; Corbitt, 1978; Erdelyi, 1962; Jokl, 1956; Sibley et al., 1981; Zaharvieva, 1972).

Strenuous sports or activities should be undertaken with caution. Little is known about the possible dangers of many of the sports in which women are engaging today; e.g., distance running, sky diving, skuba diving, bicycle racing, and mountain sports at high altitudes. These may be dangerous to the fetus because of significant redistribution of blood flow away from the uteroplacental circulation at times of maximum stress, and the development of maternal hyperthermia. More data are needed in this area to adequately advise the pregnant woman (Laurence et al., 1968; Miller et al., 1978; Smith et al., 1978).

The enlarging uterus may disrupt the woman's balance late in pregnancy and interfere with her coordination. During any activity, she should utilize good body mechanics to avoid unnecessary strain to her body. Information about proper body mechanics should be included as part of a prenatal education program.

The pregnant woman has increased needs for rest and sleep, probably due to increased metabolic requirements, yet physical discomfort, fetal movements, and emotional tension may interfere with normal sleep, especially toward the end of pregnancy. The nurse can encourage exercise and help the woman to explore and improve her usual sleep habits and routines and examine her work schedule to find time for rest periods throughout the day. Late in pregnancy, the woman may be most comfortable sleeping with an extra pillow under her head or under her uterus when in a side-lying position. Rest at this time is particularly important so that the woman enters labor in a well-rested state.

Sexual Activity

The expectant mother probably can safely continue sexual activity, including coitus, throughout pregnancy unless she experiences bleeding, premature labor, or rupture of membranes. Sexual activity may be risky in women who have a history of recurrent pregnancy loss or premature birth. There is conflicting evidence as to the effect of coital activity during pregnancy (Naeye, 1979; Wegsteen & Wagner, 1977). Certainly more research and information is warranted.

Changing sexual feelings and interest are common during the prenatal period. Some women experience a decrease in sexual desire in the first trimester when they are easily fatigued and adjusting to pregnancy. In the third trimester the increasing physical size may make usual sexual behaviors awkward or difficult, and the couple may benefit from counseling regarding alternative methods for achieving sexual satisfaction. Many women experience increased sexual responsiveness during pregnancy. Any changes in sexuality that the pregnant woman experiences, and the concerns she or her partner may have, can create strain and should be included in prenatal assessment and counseling. If the woman develops symptoms of pain, bleeding, or unusual vaginal discharge she should seek care as soon as possible so that appropriate treatment can be initiated (Bing & Colman, 1977).

Alcohol, Smoking, and Drugs

There is increasing evidence that smoking, alcohol, and caffeine use during pregnancy are harmful to the developing fetus. The woman's usual habits of use of these substances should be explored as part of the prenatal history, and she should be encouraged to stop her use of these substances ("Cigarette Smoking and Pregnancy," 1979; Clarren & Smith, 1978; Davidson, 1981; Diebel, 1980; Hanson, et al., 1976; Himmelberger et al., 1978; Landesman-Dwyer et al., 1978; Lindor et al., 1980; Little, 1978; Weathersbee et al., 1977).

It is now recognized that the placenta is not an effective barrier to drugs taken by the mother during pregnancy. The greatest risk of drug-related fetal malformations occurs during the first trimester. Before any medication is prescribed for the pregnant woman, the benefits should be carefully weighed against the potential risks. Iron, vitamins, and folic acid supplements are commonly prescribed for the expectant mother. If these are indicated, their use can usually be delayed until after the period of organogenesis. Women should also be cautioned against use of nonprescription and "street" drugs (Alberman, 1978; Blinick et al., 1976; Doering & Stewart, 1978; Fraser, 1976; Hill et al., 1977; O'Brien & McManus, 1978; Rothman, 1977; Schardein, 1976).

Dental Care

Regular dental care should be continued throughout pregnancy It is generally believed that necessary dental repair, under local anesthesia, can be done without danger to the fetus. However, extensive dental work or dental roentgenograms should be undertaken with caution. The expectant mother should inform dental personnel of her pregnancy so that safe care can be planned.

Breast Care

The breasts undergo many changes during pregnancy. Their increased size requires extra support to maintain comfort and prevent poor body alignment and resulting backache. Support can best be provided by a maternity bra that has wide, adjustable (nonelastic) straps and can be adjusted to permit adaptation to increasing breast size. Bra size may change with each trimester and with lactation. Some women find they are most comfortable if they wear the bra during sleep as well as during periods of activity.

Colostrum forms in the breasts about the sixteenth week of pregnancy. Secretion of colostrum may cause crusts to form around the nipple and lead to irritation of the nipple tissue. Use of soap on the nipples should be avoided since it causes dryness and irritation of the nipples.

Preparation of the breasts for later breast-feeding can be started during the prenatal period. Preparation will be discussed in Chapter 17.

Clothing

Clothing worn during pregnancy should be comfortable and functional. An attractive appearance can promote feelings of well-being during pregnancy. Clothing should not be constrictive. Use of hose or stockings with bands that restrict circulation in the lower extremities should especially be avoided. Shoes should be chosen that are comfortable and supportive. Generally, a low-heeled shoe will be most comfortable and safe since a high heel increases spinal lordosis and may disrupt the woman's balance and posture. Milinaire (1974) offers excellent practical suggestions on clothing for pregnancy.

Managing Common Discomforts

Nausea and Vomiting

One of the most common and distressing symptoms of early pregnancy is the nausea and vomiting. The etiology of this symptom has already been discussed. The majority of women are bothered with this in the morning when their stomachs are empty. Thus, one helpful remedy is to keep some food in the stomach by eating small meals frequently throughout the day (i.e., six small meals instead of three large ones). It can also be beneficial to keep dry toast or crackers at the bedside

to eat before arising, or to separate liquid and solid intake by about one-half hour. If these measures are not successful, an antiemetic, such as Bendectin (Dow), can be prescribed *after the eighth week of gestation*. Out of respect for the possibility of a teratogenic effect, all drugs, unless absolutely necessary, should be avoided in the period of organogenesis.

Heartburn (Pyrosis)

Relaxation of the cardiac sphincter to the stomach and relaxation of the lower end of the esophagus contribute to heartburn. Decreased gastrointestinal motility, and pressure from the enlarging uterus cause regurgitation of the stomach contents into the esophagus. If heartburn is a problem, spicy and fatty foods should be decreased. Symptoms can be managed with antacids such as aluminum hydroxide or magnesium hydroxide (one tablespoon, every two to three hours, as necessary), or chewable antacids. Antacids containing sodium (i.e., sodium bicarbonate) should be avoided since they may promote undesired fluid retention. Elevating the head on several pillows at night may prevent some of the regurgitation of gastric acid that contributes to heartburn.

Constipation

Constipation commonly occurs due to decreased transit time of food in the large intestine and resulting absorption of large amounts of water. Iron supplements may also contribute to constipation. The pregnant woman can decrease the problem by increasing her fluid intake to five to seven glasses of water or other fluid per day and adjusting her diet. Foods that increase bulk, such as bran cereals, raw bran, vegetables, and fruits such as prunes and prune juice should be added to the diet. Stool softeners such as dioctyl sodium sulfosuccinate (50–200 mg/day), or the *occasional* use of a laxative such as milk of magnesia may be precribed. Mineral oil should be avoided because it decreases absorption of fat soluble vitamins from the gastrointestinal tract and the resulting lack of vitamin K may lead to hemorrhagic disease in the newborn.

Hemorrhoids and Varicose Veins

Hemorrhoids can cause a great deal of concern and discomfort. Keeping stools soft and preventing constipation can minimize this problem. It is also useful to maintain regular bowel habits and avoid long periods of standing. If hemorrhoids do occur, a warm sitz bath or application of astringents (witch hazel, Epsom salts) or a local anesthetic (Anusol, Warner-

Chilcot; Americaine, Arnar-Stone; Nupercainal, Ciba) may be soothing.

Varicosities of the vulva or lower extremities occur in about twenty percent of pregnant women and seem to have a familial tendency. Avoiding constrictive clothing —especially knee-high stockings and garters—is recommended. Sitting with the legs elevated and uncrossed, lying in a recumbent position, avoiding long periods of standing, elevating the hips, and use of support stockings are also helpful. For some women, prescription elastic stockings (i.e., Jobst) may be indicated.

Backache

Backache and other pelvic discomfort may be the result of softening of supportive ligaments from hormonal influences during pregnancy and changes in body alignment and balance as a result of the enlarging uterus. Poor posture, improper body mechanics, and use of high-heeled shoes also contribute to backache. Exercises and education about body mechanics can prevent some of these discomforts. If backaches are a problem, local applications of heat, gentle massage, and rest are indicated. The pelvic rock is an excellent exercise for prevention and treatment of backache and can easily be taught during prenatal visits.

Leg Cramps

Sudden muscle spasms often occur when stretching with toes pointed or after assuming a recumbent position. There are several theories as to the cause of these cramps. Leg cramps have been attributed to the pressure of the uterus on nerves of the lower extremities. This theory is consistent with the finding that leg cramps occur most frequently between the twenty-fourth and thirty-sixth week of gestation (Abrams & Aponte, 1958; Page & Page, 1953). Another theory is that muscle tetany results from an imbalance in the body's calcium/phosphorus ratio. Calcium and phosphorus exist in a constant ratio in the blood that can be altered by differing the intake of either in foods. If phosphorus is in excess, it will bind calcium in the gastrointestinal tract and reduce the amount of calcium absorbed. Page and Page (1953) suggested that the relative deficiency of calcium resulting from excess phosphorus intake causes muscle irritability. They recommended reducing milk intake because of its high phosphorus content and supplying calcium with oral tablets (i.e., calcium lactate). Leg cramps have also been found to be relieved by taking aluminum hydroxide gel. These gels bind phosphorus in the gastrointestinal tract and prevent it from interfering with calcium

absorption. (Page & Page, 1953; Worthington-Roberts, 1981). Abrams and Aponte (1958) failed to demonstrate a relationship between dairy product ingestion and leg cramps; they also found that calcium lactate was not efficacious in the prevention or alleviation of cramps.

Since milk supplies vital calcium, vitamin D, and other nutrients, limiting the expectant woman's milk intake is not advised. Instead, limiting high phosphorus foods such as processed snacks and soda pop (Worthington-Roberts et al., 1981) may also be beneficial.

Immediate treatment of leg cramps includes flexing the foot and applying local heat. Massaging the contracted muscle should be cautioned against, in case the pain is caused by phlebitis. Often just lying down or getting off one's feet will relieve the cramps by relieving pressure of the uterus on nerves of the lower extremities.

Leukorrhea and Vaginitis

Vaginal and cervical secretions tend to increase during pregnancy and may be very annoying to the woman. Cotton undergarments and frequent bathing may well relieve symptoms. If there is no burning, itching, discoloration, or foul odor to the discharge, no treatment is needed.

If symptoms are present, a vaginal infection is suspected and should be diagnosed through microscopic examination or culture (see "Sexually Transmitted Diseases and Vaginitis," *Women's Health: Ambulatory Care*).

Braxton Hicks Contractions

During the early weeks of pregnancy, irregular and painless contractions of the uterus begin, and recur periodically at intervals of five to twenty minutes throughout the pregnancy. The woman is usually not aware of these contractions early in her pregnancy, but as the pregnancy progresses, she may become aware of periodic tightening and hardness of her abdomen. The primigravida is often not aware that these sensations are contractions, and usually doesn't perceive them until the last six weeks of pregnancy. The multipara may notice Braxton Hicks contractions as early as the sixth month of pregnancy. Braxton Hicks contractions can be palpated on bimanual exam early in pregnancy and later in pregnancy can be palpated abdominally.

While Braxton Hicks contractions are a normal physiological occurrence, they can cause a great deal of concern for the expectant mother. She may worry that she is in premature labor, particularly if the contractions persist, as they often do as term approaches. The contractions can be distinguished from labor contractions by their irregular pattern and because they do not continue to cause progressive effacement and dilation of the cervix.

A long bout of Braxton Hicks contractions may cause the woman to be uncomfortable and may be distracting or prevent rest. Measures such as walking or relaxing in a warm bath often stop the contractions. The woman can also be encouraged to practice relaxation and breathing techniques taught in prenatal classes. The avoidance of stimulating substances such as coffee and nicotine is advised. A massage or the ingestion of warm, relaxing fluids may help the woman to relax and thus rest. Any effort that will promote rest is advised so that the woman may avoid fatigue should labor ensue.

REFERENCES AND ADDITIONAL READINGS

Abrams, J., & Aponte, G. (1958). The leg cramp syndrome during pregnancy: The relationship to calcium and phosphorus metabolism. *American Journal of Obstetrics and Gynecology, 76,* 432–437.

Alberman, E. (1978). Fertility drugs and contraceptive agents. In J.B. Scrimgeour (Ed.), *Towards the prevention of fetal malformation.* Edinburgh: Edinburgh University Press.

Alford, C.A., Stagno, S., & Reynolds, D.W. (1975). Diagnosis of chronic perinatal infections. *American Journal of Diseases of Children, 129,* 455–463.

Andriole, V.T. (1975). Bacteria infections. In G.N. Burrow & T.F. Ferris (Eds.), *Medical complications during pregnancy.* Philadelphia: Saunders.

Babson, S., Benson, R., Pernoll, M., & Benda, G. (1980). *Management of high-risk pregnancy and intensive care of the neonate* (ed. 4). St. Louis: Mosby.

Beers, P. (1979). Update on pregnancy testing. *Lab 79,* April, 17–22.

Bing, E., & Colman, L. (1977). *Making love during pregnancy.* New York: Bantam Books.

Blinick, G., Wallach, R., Jerez, E., & Ackerman, B. (1976). Drug addiction in pregnancy and the neonate. *American Journal of Obstetrics and Gynecology, 125*(2), 135–142.

Bowman, J. (1978). Suppression of Rh isoimmunization. *Obstetrics and Gynecology, 52,* 388–393.

Brandes, J.M. (1967). First trimester nausea and vomiting as related to outcome of pregnancy. *Obstetrics and Gynecology, 30,* 427.

Butler, N.R., Goldstein, H., & Ross, E.M. (1972). Cigarette smoking in pregnancy: Its influence on birth weight and perinatal mortality. *British Medical Journal, 2,* 127–130.

Cabrera, H. (1972). Pregnancy tests. In J.J. Rovinsky, (Ed.), *Davis' gynecology and obstetrics* (vol. 3). Hagerstown: Harper & Row.

Caplan, G. (1957). Psychological aspects of maternity care. *American Journal of Public Health, 47,* 25–31.

Carr, M. (1974). Managing iron deficiency in pregnancy. *Contemporary OB/GYN, 4*(13), 15–19.

Caulfield, C., Disbrow, M., & Smith, M. (1977). Determining indicators of potential for child abuse and neglect: Analytical problems in methodological research. *Committee Nursing Research, 10,* 41–162.

Cigarette smoking and pregnancy. (1979). ACOG Technical Bulletin, no. 53. Chicago: ACOG Publications.

Clark, H.H. (1978). Physical activity during menstruation and pregnancy. *Physical fitness research digest* (series B, no. 3). Washington, D.C.: President's Council on Physical Fitness and Sports.

Clarren, S., & Smith, D.W. (1978). The fetal alcohol syndrome. *New England Journal of Medicine, 298,* 1063–1067.

Coleman, C.A. (1981). Fetal movement counts: An assessment tool. *Journal of Nurse-Midwifery, 26*(1), 15–23.

Committee on Maternal Nutrition, Food and Nutrition Board, National Research Council, National Academy of Sciences. (1980). *Maternal nutrition and the course of pregnancy.* Washington, D.C.

Corbitt, R.W. (1978). Physical activity during menstruation and pregnancy. *Physical fitness research digest* (series B, no. 3). Washington, D.C.: President's Council on Physical Fitness and Sports.

Danforth, D., & Holly, R. (1977). Other disorders due to pregnancy. In D. Danforth (Ed.), *Obstetrics and gynecology* (ed. 3). New York: Harper & Row.

Davidson, S. (1981). Smoking and alcohol consumption: Advice given by health professionals. *Journal of Obstetric, Gynecologic, and Neonatal Nursing, 10*(4), 256–258.

Diebel, P. (1980). Effects of cigarette smoking on maternal nutrition and the fetus. *Journal of Obstetric, Gynecologic, and Neonatal Nursing, 9,* 333–336.

Doering, P.L., & Stewart, R.B. (1978). The extent and character of drug consumption during pregnancy. *Journal of the American Medical Association, 239,* 843–846.

Ellis, D.J. (1980). Sexual needs and concerns of expectant parents. *Journal of Obstetric, Gynecologic, and Neonatal Nursing, 9*(5), 306–308.

Erdelyi, G.J. (1962). Problems and inquiries: Gynecological survey of female athletes. *Journal of Sports Medicine and Physical Fitness, 2,* 174–179.

Erikson, E. (1963). *Childhood and society* (ed. 2). New York: Norton.

Ferreira, A. (1969). *Perinatal environment.* Springfield, Ill.: Charles C Thomas.

Fischer, S., Fullerton, J.T., & Trezie, L. (1981). Fetal movement and fetal outcome in a low-risk population. *Journal of Nurse-Midwifery, 26*(1), 24–30.

Fraser, A.C. (1976). Drug addiction in pregnancy. *Lancet, 2* (7991), 896–899.

Gluck, L. (1978). Evaluating functional fetal maturation. *Clinical Obstetrics and Gynecology, 21*(2), 547–559.

Gottesfeld, K. (1978). Ultrasound in obstetrics. *Clinical Obstetrics and Gynecology, 21*(2), 311–327.

Greenberg, J. (1980). Implications for primary care providers of occupational health hazards on pregnant women and their infants. *Journal of Nurse-Midwifery, 25*(4), 21–30.

Grossman, J. (1977). Congenital syphilis. *Teratology, 16,* 217–224.

Guidelines on pregnancy and work. (1977). Chicago: ACOG Publications.

Hanson, J., Jones, K., & Smith, D. (1976). Fetal alcohol syndrome: Experience with 41 patients. *Journal of the American Medical Association, 235,* 1458–1460.

Harter, C., & Benirschke, K. (1976). Fetal syphilis in the first trimester. *American Journal of Obstetrics and Gynecology, 124,* 705–711.

Hertz, R., & Zador, I. (1979). Ultrasound cephalometry: A clinical discussion. *Clinical Obstetrics and Gynecology, 22*(3), 561–569.

Hill, R.M., Craig, J., Chaney, M., Tennyson, L., & McCulley, L. (1977). Utilization of over-the-counter drugs during pregnancy. *Clinical Obstetrics and Gynecology, 20,* 381–394.

Himmelberger, D., Brown, B., & Cohen, E. (1978). Cigarette smoking during pregnancy and the occurrence of spontaneous abortion and congenital abnormality. *American Journal of Epidemiology, 108,* 470–479.

Hobel, C. (1978). Risk assessment in perinatal medicine. *Clinical Obstetrics and Gynecology, 21,* 287–295.

Holder, W., & Knox, J. (1972). Syphilis in pregnancy. *Medical Clinics of North America, 56,* 1151–1160.

Hook, E.P. (1976). Changes in tobacco smoking and ingestion of alcohol and caffeinated beverages during early pregnancy—Are these consequences, in part, of feto-protective mechanisms diminishing maternal exposure to embryotoxins? In S. Kelly (Ed.), *Birth defects: Risks and consequences.* New York: Academic Press.

Horst, T. (1976). The effects of caffeine: A review of the literature and implications during pregnancy. (Unpublished paper written for Pregnancy and Health Study, Department of P.B.S.).

Hunt, V.R. (1977). *The health of woman at work.* Evanston, Ill.: Northwestern University, Program on Women.

Hytten, F., & Chamberlain, G. (1980). *Clinical physiology in obstetrics.* Oxford: Blackwell Scientific.

Janerich, D.T., Lawrence, C., & Jacobson, H. (1976). Fertility patterns after discontinuation of use of oral contraceptives. *Lancet, 1*(2), 1051–1053.

Jarrell, S., & Sokol, R. (1979). Clinical use of stressed and non-stressed monitoring techniques. *Clinical Obstetrics and Gynecology, 22*(3), 617–632.

Jensen, M., Benson, R., & Bobak, I. (1977). *Maternity care: The nurse and the family.* St. Louis: Mosby.

Jokl, E. (1956). Some clinical data on women's athletics. *Journal of the Association for Physical and Mental Rehabilitation, 10,* 48–49.

Klaus, M., & Kennell, J. (1976). *Maternal–infant bonding.* St. Louis: Mosby.

Knox, E. (1978). How infection damages the fetus. *Contemporary OB/GYN, 12*(1), 96–102.

Landau, B. (1976). *Essential human anatomy and physiology.* Glenview: Scott, Foresman.

Landesman-Dwyer, S., Keller, L.S., & Streissguth, A.P. (1978). Naturalistic observations of newborns: Effects of maternal alcohol intake. *Alcoholism: Clinical and Experimental Research, 2,* 171–177.

Laurence, K.M., Carter, C.O., & David, P.A. (1968). Major central nervous system malformations in South Wales: II pregnancy factors, seasonal variation and social class effects. *British Journal of Preventive Social Medicine, 22,* 212–222.

Ledger, W. (1981). Infectious disease. In S.L. Romney, M.J. Gray, A.B. Little, J. Merrill, E.J. Quilligan, & R. Standler (Eds.), *Gynecology and obstetrics: The health care of women* (ed. 2). New York: McGraw-Hill.

Levin, J., & Algazy, K. (1975). Hematologic disorders. In G.N. Burrow & T.F. Ferris (Eds.)., *Medical complications during pregnancy.* Philadelphia: Saunders.

Lindor, E., McCarthy, A., & McRae, M.G. (1980). Fetal alcohol syndrome: A review and case presentation. *Journal of Obstetric, Gynecologic, and Neonatal Nursing, 9*(4), 222–228.

Little, R. (1977). Moderate alcohol use during pregnancy and decreased infant birth weight. *American Journal of Public Health, 67,* 1154–1156.

Marshall, G.W., & Newman, R.L. (1977). Roll-over test. *American Journal of Obstetrics and Gynecology, 127,* 623–625.

McCammon, C. (1951). A study of 475 pregnancies in American Indian women. *American Journal of Obstetrics and Gynecology, 61,* 1159.

McCauley, C.S. (1976). *Pregnancy After Thirty-Five.* New York: Dutton.

McFee, J. (1973). Anemia in pregnancy—A reappraisal. *Obstetrical and Gynecological Survey, 28*(11), 769–793.

Milinaire, C. (1974). *Birth.* New York: Harmony Books.

Miller, P., Smith, D.W., & Shepard, T.N. (1978). Maternal hyperthermia as a possible cause of anencephaly. *Lancet, 1*(1), 519–521.

Modlin, J.F., Herrmann, K., Brandling-Bennett, A.D., Eddins, D., & Hayden, G. (1976). Risk of congenital abnormality after inadvertent rubella vaccination of pregnant women. *New England Journal of Medicine, 294,* 972–974.

Monif, G.R.G. (1974). *Infectious diseases in obstetrics and gynecology.* Hagerstown: Harper & Row.

Naeye, R.L. (1979). Coitus and associated amniotic fluid infection. *New England Journal of Medicine, 301*(2), 1198–1200.

Nahmais, A.J. (1974). The torch complex. *Hospital Practice, 9*(5), 65–72.

Nesbitt, R. (1977). Coincidental medical disorders complicating pregnancy. In D. Danforth (Ed.), *Obstetrics and gynecology* (ed. 3). New York: Harper & Row.

Nesbitt, P., & Aubry, R. (1969). High risk obstetrics. II. The value of semiobjective grading systems in identifying the vulnerable group. *American Journal of Obstetrics and Gynecology, 103,* 972–985.

Nuckolls, K., Cassel, J., & Kaplan, B. (1972). Psychosocial assets, life crisis and the prognosis of pregnancy. *American Journal Epidemiology, 95,* 431–441.

O'Brien, T.E., & McManus, C.E. (1978). Drugs and the fetus: A consumer's guide by generic and brand name. *Birth and the Family Journal, 5,* 58–86.

Oxorn, H. (1980). *Human labor and birth* (ed. 4). New York: Appleton-Century-Crofts.

Page, E., & Page, E. (1953). Leg cramps in pregnancy: Etiology and treatment. *Obstetrics and Gynecology, 1,* 94.

Paul, R., & Miller, F. (1978). Antepartum fetal heart rate monitoring. *Clinical Obstetrics and Gynecology, 21*(2), 375–384.

Pritchard, J., & MacDonald, P. (1980). *Williams obstetrics* (ed. 16). New York: Appleton-Century-Crofts.

Quilligan, E.J. (1981). Prenatal care. In S. Romney, M.J. Gray, A.B. Little, J. Merrill, E.J. Quilligan, & R. Standler (Eds.), *Gynecology and obstetrics: The health care of women* (ed. 2). New York: McGraw-Hill.

Quilligan, E.J. (1977). Maternal physiology. In D. Danforth (ed.), *Obstetrics and Gynecology.* Hagerstown: Harper and Row.

Rees, D. (1978). Urinary tract infection. *Clinics in Obstetrics and Gynecology, 5*(1), 169–192.

Reid, D.E., Ryan, K.J., & Benirschke, K. (1972). Diagnosis and conduct of pregnancy. *Principles and management of human reproduction.* Philadelphia: Saunders.

Roberts, F. (1977). *Perinatal nursing.* New York: McGraw-Hill.

Rothman, M.J. (1977). Fetal loss, twinning and birth weight after oral contraceptive use. *New England Journal of Medicine, 297,* 486–471.

Rubin, R. (1970). Cognitive style in pregnancy. *American Journal of Nursing, 70,* 502–508.

Sadovsky, E. (1978). What do fetal movements tell about it's well-being. *Contemporary OB/GYN, 12*(6), 59–70.

Schardein, J.L. (1976). *Drugs as teratogens.* Cleveland: CRC Press.

Shneider, K. (1978). *Primary care of the pregnant woman: Laboratory tests.* Series 2, Prenatal Care. White Plains, N.Y.: National Foundation/March of Dimes.

Sever, J.L. (1978). Viral infections in pregnancy. *Clinical Obstetrics and Gynecology, 21,* 477–487.

Sever, J., Larsen, J., & Grossman, J. (1979). *Handbook of perinatal infections.* Boston: Little Brown and Company.

Shaver, J. (1979). Maternal physiologic adaptations to nurture the fetus. In A. Clark & D. Affonso (Eds.), *Childbearing: A nursing perspective.* Philadelphia: Davis.

Sibley, L., Ruhling, R.O., Cameron-Foster, J., Christensen, C., & Bolen, T. (1981). Swimming and physical fitness during pregnancy. *Journal of Nurse-Midwifery, 26*(6), 3–12.

Simpson, J.L. (Ed.). (1981). Symposium: Antenatal diagnosis of genetic disorders. *Clinical Obstetrics and Gynecology, 24*(4), 1005–1168.

Sites, J. (1972). Hyperemesis gravidarum. In J.J. Rovinsky (Ed.), *Davis' gynecology and obstetrics* (Vol. 1). Hagerstown: Harper & Row.

Smith, D.W., Sterling, K.C., & Harvey, M.A.S. (1978). Hyperthermia as a possible teratogenic agent. *Journal of Pediatrics, 92*(6), 878–883.

Sohar, E., Shoenfeld, V., Shapiro, Y., Ohry, A., & Cabili, S. (1976). Effect of exposure to Finnish sauna. *Israel Journal of Medical Science, 12*(11), 1275–1282.

Speert, H., & Guttmacher, A.F. (1954). Frequency and significance of bleeding in early pregnancy. *Journal of the American Medical Association, 155,* 712.

Squier, T.L. (1972). Laboratory examination: Urine, blood chemistry, etc. In J.J. Rovinsky (Ed.), *Davis' gynecology and obstetrics* (Vol. 3). Hagerstown: Harper & Row.

Stetlman, J.M. (1977). *Women's work, women's health.* New York: Pantheon Books.

Streitfeld, P.P. (1978). Congenital malformation: Teratogenic foods and additives. *Birth and the Family Journal, 5,* 7–19.

Varney, H. (1980). *Nurse-Midwifery.* Boston: Blackwell-Scientific.

Waterson, A.P. (1979). Virus infections (other than rubella) during pregnancy. *British Medical Journal, 2,* 564–566.

Weathersbee, P.S., Olsen, L., & Lodge, J.R. (1977). Caffeine and pregnancy: A retrospective survey. *Postgraduate Medicine, 62*(3), 64–68.

Wegsteen, L., & Wagner, N. (1977). Physiological aspects of sexuality during pregnancy. *Fertility and Contraception, 1*(April), 26–30.

Worley, R.J. (1980). What we know and don't know about influences on fetal responses. *Contemporary OB/GYN, 16*(5), 123–135.

Worthington-Roberts, B., Vermeersch, J., & Williams, S.R. (1981). *Nutrition in pregnancy and lactation* (ed. 2). St. Louis: Mosby.

Zaharvieva, E. (1972). Olympic participation by women: Effects on pregnancy and childbirth. *Journal of the American Medical Association, 221,* 992–995.

Zipursky, A. (1981). Isoimmune hemolytic diseases. In D. Nathan & F. Oski (Eds.), *Hematology in infancy and childhood.* Philadelphia: Saunders.

Chapter 4 | Nutrition During Pregnancy

Allison Singleton Parsons

A WOMAN'S NUTRITIONAL NEEDS are determined by her life cycle and lifestyle; her nutritional status is influenced by her social and economic pressures, and her knowledge. Many women today are assuming a more active role in their personal health care and are recognizing nutrition as an essential component. With the additional challenge of pregnancy, nutrition achieves its greatest potential.

Nutrition is a process that continually affects all of our lives; yet for women, it can assume an even greater significance. In 1977 the provisional total for births in the United States numbered 3,313,000 (USHEW, 1978). It has been substantially documented that a woman's nutritional status during pregnancy has a significant impact on the outcome of that pregnancy. She becomes responsible for simultaneously nourishing her own body and that of her unborn child. Every pregnant woman needs nutritional assessment and followup. We cannot assume the heightened consciousness for nutrition that many women develop with pregnancy will be sufficient to ensure the necessary dietary adjustments, nor can we assume that her nutritional course will be a normal one. Many women begin their pregnancies at nutritional risk and others develop nutrition-related complications during their pregnancies. Of the many significant factors contributing to the outcome of pregnancy, nutrition represents the factor most within patient control. Yet, for lack of better information or understanding of their changing needs, many women make serious nutritional errors during the course of their pregnancy. Health care providers must prepare themselves to prevent these nutritional errors.

As an important component of prenatal care, nutrition has never been an issue of controversy. We are, however, now realizing the true impact of nutrition on the mother and fetus, and consequently, on pregnancy outcome. Yet, there is a grave need for improvement in this area.

Nutritionists have specific knowledge of foods' nutritive qualities, and practice nutritional assessment and patient counseling as a responsibility of their patient interaction, but the clinical settings having access to the specialized services of nutritionists or related professionals are in the minority. This dilemma does not justify the exclusion of nutritional services to prenatal patients. Many health professionals are unfamiliar with the basics of nutrition, but the need for an accurate, concise approach to nutrition for use by those professionals providing the majority of prenatal care is recognized.

NUTRITIONAL RISK FACTORS DURING PREGNANCY

Much can be learned about a patient's nutritional health from the basic components of routine prenatal care. The medical and social histories, physical examination, and routine laboratory results will often reflect the client's past nutritional habits and current nutritional status and may indicate her future nutritional intake.

The key is to examine these data for nutritional significance. For example, the demographic data of a specific pregnancy, including age, parity, race, weight, and weeks of gestation, as well as past obstetrical history, and social, economic and environmental influences, should be recognized for their nutritional significance. A familiarity must be developed with those factors that place the pregnant patient in a category of risk. For instance, the obstetrical patient is very likely to be at nutritional risk if, at the onset of pregnancy (ACOG, 1978):

- She is an adolescent, 15 years of age or younger.
- She has had three or more pregnancies within the past two years.
- She has a history of poor obstetric or fetal performance.
- She is economically deprived (an income less than the poverty line or a recipient of local, state, or federal assistance).
- She is a food faddist, ingesting a bizarre or nutritionally restrictive diet.
- She is a heavy smoker, a drug addict, or an alcoholic.
- She has a therapeutic diet for chronic systemic disease.
- Her prepartum weight at her first prenatal visit was less than 85 percent or greater than 120 percent of standard weight.

She is also likely to be at nutritional risk if, during prenatal care (ACOG, 1978):

- She has a low or deficient hemoglobin/hematocrit (low is defined as hemoglobin less than 11.0 g, hematocrit less than 33 percent; deficient, as hemoglobin less than 10.0 g, hematocrit less than 30 percent).
- She has inadequate weight gain (any weight loss during pregnancy or gain less than 2 lb/month).
- She has excessive weight gain during pregnancy (greater than 2 lb/week).
- She is planning to breast-feed her infant.

Adolescence Adolescent pregnancies have been associated with low birth weight, short gestation periods, and perinatal mortality. A pregnant adolescent who conceives within three years of menarche is particularly apt to have such problems. For these patients, pregnancy creates a dual growth demand. She is still growing herself and the pregnancy superimposes additional nutritional needs. Compounding this, adolescent girls traditionally have poor dietary habits or frequently restrict their caloric intakes, resulting in nutritional inadequacies even without the additional burden of a pregnancy. Though biological readiness can obviously be the crucial factor in reproductive performance of the adolescent, emotional, psychological, financial, and educational factors are other important aspects of an adolescent pregnancy.

Frequent Conceptions Any patient who has had three or more pregnancies in a two-year span is prone to depleted nutritional stores. This situation can potentially compromise both maternal and fetal outcome. Therefore, careful monitoring of the woman's nutritional status is warranted.

Poor Reproductive Performance A reproductive past characterized by abortions, pregnancy complications, low-birth-weight infants, or perinatal loss signals a high risk for a current pregnancy. Overlapping nutritional factors may be involved.

Economic Deprivation Economic disadvantage is probably the most readily identifiable nutritional risk category. If the pregnant woman is to be able to provide herself and her unborn child with the necessary calories, protein, minerals, and vitamins during pregnancy and lactation, an adequate dietary increase is necessary. Programs such as the USDA Food Stamps and WIC (Supplemental Food Program for Women, Infants and Children) may be available for assistance. Eligibility for these programs is based upon economic need and a medical referral related to nutritional risk. Local or state health departments provide sources of information for these programs.

Food Faddist The dietary practices of the food faddist, the patient who has unusual dietary requirements, or the one who practices pica (the regular and excessive ingestion of nonnutritive foods) often preclude the ingestion of adequate nutrients for pregnancy.

Many fad diets, of questionable use for most nonpregnant women, are absolutely contraindicated for use by the pregnant patient. Pregnancy is no time to experiment with requirements that can jeopardize the supply of essential nutrients to a developing fetus. Vegetarianism is not what is meant by a *fad* and will be addressed in the section on Nutritional Education.

It is essential to guide each of these patients into good nutritional practices for at least the length of the pregnancy, and the period of lactation. Ethnic or cultural customs may also place dietary restrictions on a patient. When circumstances suggest such, inquire into these factors.

Drug Addiction Addiction to any drug—alcohol, nicotine, prescription drugs, or illegal narcotics—can induce major physiological and nutritional problems as a result of the habit. Malnutrition is often an indirect result, either because of altered metabolism or by failure to purchase or ingest proper food. These patients require particularly close nutritional surveillance.

Chronic Systemic Disease Nutritional health can be compromised by any chronic systemic disorder. Medical or surgical gastrointestinal disorders and medications used in their treatment, for example, may interfere with the ingestion, absorption, and utilization of nutrients. Nutritional counseling for women presenting such complications should combine nutritional guidance for prenatal care with diet therapy for the patient's particular medical condition.

Prepregnant Weight A woman who begins pregnancy with a weight that is below 85 percent or higher than 120 percent of the standard weight for height is at increased risk. (Ideal body weight is explained later in this chapter). Both of these problems may be reflective of life-long nutritional inadequacies with increased risk for deficiencies of specific nutrients. The obese patient must be taught to improve the quality of her diet and to control the quantity. Diminishing risk in pregnancy is not accomplished by weight reduction for this patient; to the contrary, weight reduction during pregnancy has been associated with neuropsychological abnormalities in the infants.

Low prepregnancy weight may result in a low-birth-weight infant. This patient must be taught to improve both the quality and quantity of her intake. Gaining her weight deficit should be accomplished during pregnancy *in addition to* the normal desired weight gain of pregnancy.

ASSESSMENT OF DIETARY INTAKE PATTERNS

Numerous approaches, requiring varying degrees of skill and accuracy, have been used to evaluate the nutritional adequacy of diets. A Typical Day's Intake, a Twenty-Four-Hour Food Recall, and Food Frequency Lifts are among the most common. The success of any assessment depends as much on the collection of data as on the interpretation of those data. Of course, with diet assessments, the more knowledge the interviewer has of foods and their nutritive qualities, the more accurate the data collection and the interpretation are apt to be. Most health care professionals are experienced with interviewing, and efficient diet assessment is possible once an appreciation and understanding of the method of assessment is achieved.

At the Montreal Diet Dispensary in Quebec, Canada, dieticians closely examine their patients' dietary habits. This method simultaneously records meal patterns, total caloric intake, protein supplements, food likes and dislikes, and other factors influencing dietary patterns. Each is essential to assessing maternal nutrition. Additionally, this tool provides the perfect aid for patient education. Necessary diet changes are easily introduced as modifications of current habits. As assessments are regularly repeated, a cumulative view of patient progress is available.

Figure 4-1 shows one intake assessment tool. Modified from the guide used at the Diet Dispensary, this sheet encourages interviewer–patient interaction (Figure 4-2). The interviewer begins with a discussion of the patient's daily activity and food intake—for example:

Interviewer: Ms. Thomas, let's review. You said that before you became pregnant you never took time for breakfast, and your husband only wanted coffee, but now you make an effort to have a morning meal before work. This is usually cold cereal with milk, or toast and juice, and maybe coffee. You are away from home at lunchtime but there is a snackbar in your office building and lunch is either soup and salad with crackers, or a sandwich with chips and always milk. Since you only work until 3 o'clock you said usually you don't have snacks at the office but will have fruit and sometimes cheese when you get home. Now, tell me about your evening meals. Do you do the shopping and meal preparation? Can you identify a pattern to what you buy and prepare?

Patient: Oh yes, that's simple. My husband and I enjoy our big meal of the day in the evening. We always

Name: _____   Date: _____

Meal Pattern

Morning:

Noon:

Evening:

Snacks:

Weekend differences:

					Initial Intake			Modifications		
	Food Items	Serv	Cal	Prot g	Amt	Cal	Prot g	Amt	Cal	Prot g
PROTEIN	Beef/chicken/fish	4 oz	200–300	25						
	Protein sandwich fill.	11/2 oz	120	7						
	Peanut butter / nuts	2 Tbs	150	7						
	Eggs	1	70	7						
	Cheese, cheddar	1 oz	120	8						
	Cheese, cottage	4 oz	120	16						
	Yogurt	8 oz	200	8						
	Milk, whole	8 oz	160	8						
	Milk, 2% / skim	8 oz	125/80	8						
ENERGY	Breads	1 slice	70	2						
	Cereals, breakfast	1/2 cup	70	2						
	Rice / pasta	1/2 cup	70	2						
	Legumes	1/2 cup	100	7						
	Potatoes	1 sm	70	2						
	French fries	10	150	2						
	Soup	1 cup	100	2						
	Vegetables	1/2 cup	25	2						
	Citrus fruits / juice	4 oz	40	1						
	Other fruits / juice	4 oz	60	1						
	Margarine / butter	1 Tbs	135	–						
	Oils / salad dressings	1 Tbs	100	–						
	Milk desserts	1/2 cup	150	4						
	Cookies / pastry / cakes	2 oz	200	2						
	Sugar	1 Tbs	45	–						
	Soft drinks	12 oz	150	–						
	Beer / wine / liquor	1 oz	12/25/75	–						
	Popcorn / chips	1 cup	100	1						
	Other:									

Calories / Protein   Actual: _____   Recomd: _____

Comments:

RECORD

Vit/Min Supplement: ____ Yes ____ No ____ Amt

Cigarettes: ____ Yes ____ No ____ Amt

Height/Ideal Weight ____ / ____

Weight/Weight Gain ____ / ____

Age/Activity ____ / ____

Week of Gestation ____

Calorie	Guide
5–7 x wk =	1 serving
3–4 x wk =	1/2 serving
1–2 x wk =	1/3 serving

FIGURE 4-1   Intake assessment sheet.

Name: Thomas, A.   Date: Jan. 30, 1979

Meal Pattern

Morning:
Cereal c̄ milk
or
Toast / Juice / coffee

Noon:
Soup / Salad / Crackers
or
Sandwich c̄ chips
Milk (always)

Evening:
meat
Vegetables
Potatoes (sometimes bread)
fruit
milk + coffee

Snacks:
afternoon –
fruit / cheese

Weekend differences:
2 meals / day?
Desserts = pie or cake

Calorie	Guide
5–7 x wk =	1 serving
3–4 x wk =	1/2 serving
1–2 x wk =	1/3 serving

	Food Items	Serv	Cal	Prot g	Initial Intake Amt	Initial Intake Cal	Initial Intake Prot g	Modifications Amt	Modifications Cal	Modifications Prot g
PROTEIN	(Beef) / chicken / fish	4 oz	200–300	25	4 oz	300	25			
PROTEIN	Protein sandwich fill.	11/2 oz	120 (3x wk)	7	(1/3 serv)	40	2			
PROTEIN	Peanut butter / nuts	2 Tbs	150	7						
PROTEIN	Eggs	1	70	7	1	70	7			
	Cheese, cheddar	1 oz	120	8	2	240	16			
	Cheese, cottage	4 oz	120	16						
	Yogurt	8 oz	200	8						
	Milk, whole	8 oz	160	8	24 oz	480	24	+8 oz.	160	8
	Milk, 2% / skim	8 oz	125/80	8						
	Breads	1 slice	70	2	2	140	4	+2 serv	140	4
	Cerals, breakfast	1/2 cup	70	2	1/2 serv	35	1			
	Rice / pasta	1/2 cup	70	2						
	Legumes	1/2 cup	100	7						
	Potatoes	1 sm	70	2	1	70	2			
	French fries	10	150	2						
	Soup	1 cup	100	2	1	100	2			
	Vegetables	1/2 cup	25	2	1c	50	4			
ENERGY	Citrus fruits / juice	4 oz	40	1	4 oz	40	1			
ENERGY	~~Other fruits~~ / juice	4 oz	60	1	1	60	1			
ENERGY	(Margarine) / butter	1 Tbs	135	–	1	135	–			
ENERGY	Oils / salad dressings	1 Tbs	100	–	1	100	–			
ENERGY	Milk desserts	1/2 cup	150	4						
	Cookies / pastry / cakes	2 oz	200 wkends	2	(1/3 serv)	70	–			
	Sugar	1 Tbs	45	–	1 tsp.	15	–			
	Soft drinks	12 oz	150	–						
	Beer / ~~wine / liquor~~	1 oz	12/25/75	–						
	Popcorn / (chips)	1 cup	100	1	(1/2 serv)	50	–			
	Other:									
	Calories / Protein				Actual: 1995 / 89			Recomd: 2320 / 75		

RECORD

Vit/Min Supplement: ✓ Yes __ No
Cigarettes: ✓ Yes __ No __ Amt
Height/Ideal Weight 5′6″ / 128
Weight/Weight Gain 138 / 10 lbs
Age/Activity 24 / Sed.
Week of Gestation 21

Comments:
– Diet is great
– Routinely recommend 32 oz. milk
– Encourage increasing bread intake for additional calories to spare protein.

FIGURE 4-2 Example of a completed intake assessment sheet.

TABLE 4-1 Nutrition in pregnancy

Nutrient	Pregnancy Need	Reasons for Increased Nutrient Need in Pregnancy	Food Sources
PROTEIN	76–100 g	Rapid fetal tissue growth; amniotic fluid; placental growth and development; maternal tissue growth: uterus and breasts; increased maternal circulating blood volume: increased hemoglobin and plasma protein; maternal storage reserves for labor, delivery, and lactation	Milk; cheese; yogurt; eggs; poultry; seafood; meat; grains and flours; nuts and seeds; nutbutter; legumes (i.e., soy beans, lentils, limas, split peas, kidney beans, pinto beans)
CALORIES	2400	Increased basal metabolic rate: increased energy needs; protein sparing	Carbohydrates; fats; proteins
MINERALS			
Calcium	1200 mg	Fetal skeleton formation; fetal tooth bud formation (development of enamel-forming cells in gum tissue) increased maternal calcium metabolism	Milk; cheese; whole grains; leafy vegetables; egg yolk
Phosphorus	1200 mg	Fetal skeletal formation; fetal tooth bud formation; increased maternal phosphorus metabolism	Milk; cheese; lean meats
Iron	18+ mg (plus 30–60 mg supplement)	Increased maternal circulating blood volume: increased hemoglobin; fetal liver iron storage; high iron cost of pregnancy	Liver; meats; eggs; whole or enriched grain; leafy vegetables; nuts; legumes; dried fruits
Iodine	125 μg	Increased basal metabolic rate: increased increased thyroxine production	Iodized salt
Magnesium	450 mg	Coenzyme in energy and protein metabolism; enzyme activator; tissue growth and cell metabolism; muscle action	Nuts; soyeans; cocoa; seafood; whole grains; dried beans and peas

have a meat, vegetable, potato, bread (although I don't always have bread) and fruit for dessert, plus milk and coffee. This is usually rather late, 8 o'clock or so, so we seldom have any late-night snacks.

Interviewer: Are most of your weekdays similar to this pattern, Ms. Thomas, and are weekend meals any different for you?

Patient: I'd say with working, my weekdays are pretty routine. Weekends, though, can be a bit different. Sometimes we may only have two meals, a late breakfast and an earlier evening meal. And too, our desserts may be pie or cake instead of fruit.

After this information is obtained, the patient's habits become much clearer. It is easy to see that food habits are influenced by other family members, work routines, and weekend schedules. Additionally, this gives an indication of those foods the patient includes routinely and those she may seldom have, but a closer look is helpful.

To accommodate the tremendous growth demands of pregnancy, caloric, protein, and specific vitamin and mineral needs increase significantly (Table 4-1). Certainly, the interviewer must emphasize high-quality protein and energy foods with the patient. Table 4-2 provides a comparison of food energy and protein content of some common protein foods. Only by examining the patient's actual intake and comparing it to her specific needs can the interviewer show the patient both where and how to improve her diet.

Referring back to Figure 4-1, food groups are shown with caloric and protein values for average portions. Foods common to most diets can be categorized within these groups. Each food group should be discussed with the patient in an attempt to estimate the sources of her daily calories and proteins. The guide in the lower left corner of the assessment sheet of Figure 4-1 can be useful in determining how calories should be counted when a food is eaten less than daily. The list is divided into those foods that supply protein energy, nonprotein

Nutrient	Pregnancy Need	Reasons for Increased Nutrient Need in Pregnancy	Food Sources
VITAMINS			
A	5000 IU	Essential for cell development, hence tissue growth; fetal tooth bud formation; fetal bone growth	Butter; cream; fortified margarine; green and yellow vegetables
D	400 IU	Absorption of calcium and phosphorus; mineralization of bone tissue; tooth bud formation	Fortified milk; fortified margarine
E	15 IU	Tissue growth; cell membrane integrity; red blood cell integrity	Vegetable oils; leafy vegetables; cereals; meat; egg; milk
C	60 mg	Tissue formation and integrity; cement substance in connective and vascular tissues; increases iron absorption	Citrus fruits; berries; melons; tomatoes; chili peppers; green peppers; leafy vegetables; broccoli; potatoes
Folic acid	800 μg (plus 200–400 μg supplement	Increased metabolic demand in pregnancy; prevention of megaloblastic anemia in high-risk patients; increased heme production for hemoglobin; production of cell nucleus material	Liver; leafy vegetables
Niacin	15 mg	Coenzyme in energy and protein metabolism	Meats; peanuts; beans and peas; enriched grains
Riboflavin	1.5 mg	Coenzyme in energy and protein metabolism	Milk; liver; enriched grains
Thiamine	1.3 mg	Coenzyme for energy metabolism	Pork; beef; liver; whole or enriched grains; legumes
B_6 (pyridoxine)	2.5 mg	Coenzyme in protein metabolism	Wheat; corn; liver; meat
B_{12}	4.0 μg	Coenzyme in protein metabolism, especially vital cell proteins such as nucleic acid; formation of red blood cells	Milk; eggs; meat; liver; cheese

Adapted from Williams, 1976.

energy, or both, making it easier to identify the patient's specific needs and where additional calories may need to be added.

The next step of the interview involves reviewing a list of common foods with the patient to find out which ones she eats and how often. This guide is used to assess both quality and quantity of the patient's intake. Any food that she has less than once a week cannot be counted as a significant contributor of calories or protein. It is important that the interviewer find out what kinds of protein the patient eats most often. If she has fish and chicken more often than beef or pork, the value for the lower range of meat calories should be used in the calculations. If she frequents fast-food restaurants, or has frankfurters and luncheon meats often, the higher caloric values should be used because the fat content is greater.

The interviewer needs to ask specific questions to estimate the patient's average portion sizes, such as,

"When you have chicken, Ms. Thomas, which pieces do you usually have?" "If you have pork chops for dinner, do you have one or more?" "How much meat do you use in your casseroles and what is your serving from the dish?" If 4 or 5 ounces is estimated as the patient's usual portion size each day, and if she is having beef more often than other protein sources, then 4 ounces, 300 calories (Cal)* and 25 g of protein are recorded for her meat intake (see Figure 4-2).

As shown in Figure 4-2, Ms. Thomas reported eating sandwiches at work. The type of sandwich filling and frequency eaten need to be determined. If she has a sandwich twice a week, then the interviewer records one-third of the total 120 Cal and 7 g of protein (from the guide on the assessment sheet) that the patient

---

*In this chapter, all caloric values are for *large calories,* which are abbreviated either Cal or kcal.

TABLE 4-2 Protein and caloric content of some common protein foods

Food Group	Portion Size	Calories	Protein (g)
Cereals			
All-Bran	1/3 cup	70	3.0
Cheerios	1 cup	102	3.4
Cream of Wheat, cooked	1 cup	130	4.4
Oatmeal, cooked	1 cup	148	5.4
Quaker 100% natural	1/3 cup	186	5.3
Special K	1 cup	60	3.2
Sugar Crisp	1 cup	126	2.3
Wheat germ	1/4 cup	103	7.5
Dairy Products and Eggs			
Eggs, large	1 egg	88	7.0
Cottage cheese	1/2 cup	120	15.3
Natural cheddar cheese	1 oz	115	7.2
Natural Swiss cheese	1 oz	106	7.7
Processed American cheese	1 oz	107	6.5
Milk, whole, fresh	1 cup	162	8.6
Nonfat dry milk solids	1 cup	215	21.4
Ice cream	1/6 qt	186	3.6
Yogurt, from skim milk	1 cup	122	8.3
Flours			
Soy, low-fat	1 cup	356	43.4
White, all-purpose	1 cup	400	11.6
Whole wheat	1 cup	400	16.0
Grains and Pasta			
Barley, pearled, dry	1/4 cup	196	4.6
Cornmeal, dry	1/4 cup	135	2.9
Rice, white, dry	1/4 cup	178	3.3
Brown rice, dry	1/4 cup	176	3.7
Egg noodles, dry	1/4 cup	70	2.3
Macaroni, dry	1/4 cup	101	3.4
Spaghetti, dry	1/4 cup	140	4.8
Legumes			
Kidney beans, dry	1/2 cup	343	22.5
Lentils, dry	1/2 cup	340	24.7
Limas, dry	1/2 cup	345	20.4
Navy beans, dry	1/2 cup	340	22.3
Pinto beans, dry	1/2 cup	349	22.9
Split peas, dry	1/2 cup	348	24.2
Peanut butter	1 tbs	86	3.9
Peanuts, shelled	1 tbs	86	4.0
Soybeans, dry	1/2 cup	403	34.1
Meats and Fish			
Beef			
Ground beef	1/4 lb raw	304	20.3
Ground beef, lean	1/4 lb raw	203	23.4
Chuck roast, good grade	1/4 lb raw	288	16.7
Sirloin steak, choice grade	1/4 lb raw	229	17.8
Round steak, choice grade	1/4 lb raw	216	22.1
Liver	1/4 lb raw	159	22.6

Food Group	Portion Size	Calories	Protein (g)
Chicken			
Whole, ready-to-cook	1/2 lb raw	191	28.7
Breasts	1/2 lb raw	197	37.3
Drumsticks	1/2 lb raw	157	25.6
Thighs	1/2 lb raw	218	30.8
Fish			
Cod, flesh only	1/4 lb raw	86	20.0
Flounder, flesh only	1/4 lb raw	90	19.0
Haddock, flesh only	1/4 lb raw	89	20.8
Perch, flesh only	1/4 lb raw	108	21.6
Salmon, canned	1/4 lb	160	27.0
Tuna, canned in water	1/4 lb	144	32.0
Pork			
Bacon	1/4 lb raw	667	9.3
Ham, picnic	1/4 lb raw	265	15.6
Ham, canned boneless	1/4 lb	189	20.9
Loin chops	1/4 lb raw	266	15.3
Miscellaneous			
Bologna	1/4 lb	345	13.7
Frankfurters, all-meat	1/4 lb	361	14.9
Luncheon meat, canned	1/4 lb	334	17.0
Salami	1/4 lb	352	19.9

Adapted from Williams, 1976.

would have consumed had she eaten a sandwich filling every day.

The number of eggs in the patient's diet are also discussed. The patient is helped to investigate her diet using the meal patterns obtained earlier. If she averages one egg every day, she would receive 70 Cal and 7 g of protein with it; if less, the frequency guide is used to estimate calories.

The interviewer continues through the list of foods, discussing each question and answer with the patient. If there appears to be a contradiction, the interviewer cross-checks by asking the same question with another approach or discussing the inconsistency with the patient. For example, if Ms. Thomas says she drinks three 8-ounce glasses of two-percent (fat content) milk each day, but the interviewer can only find two in her meal pattern (Figure 4-2), this is discussed. When confronted, Ms. Thomas may respond by noting that she has a large glass of milk with her morning cereal four times a week. Therefore, her milk intake would be near the reported 24 ounces.

Breads can be difficult to estimate if the patient varies her meal pattern from day to day. The interviewer may find it easier to total the estimated number of bread servings for a week and divide by seven to get the daily average. This number should then be multiplied by the caloric and protein values for one serving of bread as listed on the assessment tool (Figure 4-1).

The interviewer must remember that if the patient is not having a particular food category every day, calories and protein must be adjusted accordingly. It may be better to underestimate than to overestimate the patient's intake.

When discussing fruits and vegetables included in the patient's diet, the interviewer must check for a source of vitamin C, which is present only in certain foods and may be missing in some diets. Citrus fruits and juices, strawberries, broccoli, tomatoes, and whole potatoes are among the best sources available. Ascorbic acid is a water soluble vitamin C and should be included daily. Vitamin A is also a frequently lacking nutrient, particularly when liver or specific vegetables are not included. Yellow vegetables such as carrots and sweet potatoes are excellent sources. If these two nutrients are not included regularly in the patient's diet, their importance and their food sources should be stressed (see Table 4-1).

Iron is another nutrient of particular concern during pregnancy (Table 4-1), as it is difficult to meet requirement from food sources alone. An iron supplement is, therefore, routinely recommended for most prenatal patients, usually in conjunction with prenatal vitamins. It is necessary to check for both of these supplements in the patient's routine.

Diet assessment skills can be sharpened with practice. The interviewer learns to evaluate the diet during the interview, questioning the intake of specific nutrients and making mental notes to direct attention to diet weaknesses during patient counseling. It is important that judgmental remarks or expressions are not made: the aim is collecting the most accurate information possible, and any indication of disapproval may alter a patient's response.

As the data collection is completed, interpretation becomes the focus of the assessment. The interviewer is familiar with the patient's dietary patterns and has recorded the sources of her total calories and protein. Comparing these with the patient's calculated requirements reveals the need for diet modification and patient education. Additionally, physical and clinical parameters can be examined for further indication of the patient's nutritional status. Table 4-3 can serve as a useful guide. Laboratory tests should not be overlooked. For the status of certain nutrients, specific tests are invaluable. The National Academy of Sciences' 1977 report, *Laboratory Indices of Nutritional Status in Pregnancy,* summarizes this pertinent assessment information.

ENERGY AND PROTEIN NEEDS

There is much to be understood about the relationship between energy and protein. During periods of rapid growth, such as pregnancy, requirements for both are elevated. Yet the demand for energy, not growth, takes first priority. Carbohydrates, fats, and protein are the energy-producing nutrients. In the absence of sufficient amounts of carbohydrates and fats, amino acids will be catabolized as a source of energy and will not be available for synthesis of body proteins. Protein utilization is, therefore, dependent on caloric intake. Increased energy intake alone has been found to be an effective supplement to diets that are marginal in protein (Lechtig et al., 1975). This means that calories

TABLE 4-3 Clinical signs of nutritional status

Body Area	Signs of Good Nutrition
General appearance	Alert, responsive
General vitality	Endurance, energetic, vigorous, sleeps well
Weight	Normal for height, age, body build
Posture	Erect, arms and legs straight
Hair	Shiny, lustrous, firm, not easily plucked, healthy scalp
Skin (general)	Smooth, slightly moist, good color
Face and neck	Skin color uniform, smooth, pink, not swollen
Eyes	Bright, clear, shiny, no sores at corner of eyelids, membranes moist and pink color, no prominent blood vessels or mound of tissue on sclera, no fatigue circles beneath
Lips	Smooth, good color, moist, not chapped or swollen
Mouth, oral membranes	Reddish pink mucous membranes in oral cavity, no swelling or bleeding
Tongue	Good pink color (or deep reddish), not swollen, surface papillae present, no lesion
Nails	Firm, pink
Legs, feet	No tenderness, no weakness, no swelling, good color
Muscles	Well developed, firm, good tone, some fat under skin
Nervous control	Normal reflexes, good attention span (not irritable or restless) psychological stability
Gastrointestinal function	Good appetite and digestion, normal regular elimination, no palpable organs or masses
Cardiovascular function	Normal heart rate and rhythm, no murmurs, normal blood pressure
Skeleton	No malformations

Adapted from National Academy of Sciences, 1977.

from nonprotein sources, such as carbohydrates and fats have a sparing effect on protein calories. A desirable distribution of caloric intake from the energy-producing nutrients is as follows: 46 percent of total calories as carbohydrates (complex starches contain other nutrients and are preferable to sugars), eleven to twelve percent protein calories, (animal or vegetable origin), and the remaining forty-two percent from fat sources (decreasing total saturated fat intake) (Worthington et al., 1977).

In the United States one standard recognized with credence for diet evaluation are the recommended dietary allowances (RDAs). These allowances represent the best estimates available from the evidence of metabolic balance studies and theoretically based calculations of requirements. Published by the Food and Nutrition Board of the National Research Council–National Academy of Sciences, these allowances are periodically reviewed and updated, most recently in 1980 (Table 4-4). The National Research Council has projected the gross energy cost for a nine months' pregnancy as 80,000 kcal. Represented as a daily allowance, an extra 300 kcal/day throughout the pregnancy is considered sufficient for most women.

Flexibility in this recommendation should be realized for nutritionally deficient or active women, who may have greater energy requirements. To accommodate for differences in body size, individual needs can be calculated by allowing 40 kcal/kg ideal prepregnant body weight (Table 4-5) or approximately 18 kcal/lb (Worthington et al., 1977). The energy intake required for adequate utilization of protein during pregnancy in normal, healthy women is 36 kcal/kg; in no case should the daily allowance for energy during pregnancy drop below this figure (NAS, 1980).

Ideal body weight (kb) × 40 kcal =
Caloric intake for pregnancy

The National Research Council allows 44 g/day of protein for the nonpregnant woman, with an additional 30 g/day estimated to allow for maternal protein storage and fetal gain (Table 4-4) (National Academy of Sciences, 1980). On a weight basis, the daily allowance would be 1.3 g protein/kg ideal pregnant body weight or 0.6 g/lb. To adjust protein intake to body size, the following guidelines are suggested (Barness & Pitkin, 1975):

• Mature woman: 1.3 g protein/kg pregnant weight
• Adolescent girls (15–18): 1.5 g protein/kg pregnant weight
• Younger girls: 1.7 g protein/kg pregnant weight

In establishing these protein allowances, the National

Research Council has taken into consideration protein utilization in mixed diets consumed by most pregnant women, including the assumption that energy needs have been met.

Studies show that if caloric and protein intake are within an acceptable range, other nutrients are apt to be also (Jeans et al., 1955). The exceptions are those nutrients whose increments for pregnancy are such that dietary sources must be complemented with supplements for adequate supply of them.

The Higgins Method of Dietary Intervention

Nutritional rehabilitation during pregnancy of underweight and undernourished mothers may be necessary to ensure normal growth and development of the fetus. Agnes C. Higgins, dedicated to this concept-philosophy, began work in 1948 at the Montreal Diet Dispensary providing nutritional counseling to malnourished pregnant women. Over a fifteen-year period Mrs. Higgins gradually developed a nutrition rehabilitation method (1975).

In 1963, in collaboration with the Royal Victoria Hospital, the Diet Dispensary began to test and improve this method. The success of this approach for diet improvement and rehabilitation was validated: a direct relationship was found between maternal weight gains and birth weights and length of time the women received Diet Dispensary service. Today, study continues as the long-term benefits of this prenatal diet enhancement are investigated.

The following is a description of the Higgins Method of corrective allowance for undernutrition, underweight, and special high-risk conditions (perhaps indicative of nutritional stress):

• *Undernutrition* is determined if a protein deficit exists between actual dietary intake and requirements. Calculation of protein requirements is based on the Dietary Standard for Canada (1948) prepared by the Canadian Council on Nutrition. For all expectant mothers over twenty weeks' gestation, 500 Cal and 25 g of protein are added as recommended in the Canadian Standard. *Undernutrition correction* is equal to the protein deficit plus an allowance of 10 Cal for each gram of protein deficiency.

• *Underweight* status is determined when a mother's pregravid weight is five percent or more under the desirable weight for height (see Table 4-5). *Underweight correction* should provide sufficient additional calories and protein to ensure the mother gains this weight deficit during pregnancy. An allowance of 500 Cal and 20 g of protein are provided to permit a gain of 1

TABLE 4-4 Recommended daily dietary allowances*

	Age (years)	Weight (kg)	Weight (lb)	Height (cm)	Height (in)	Energy Needs† (with range) (kcal)	Protein (g)	Fat-Soluble Vitamins — Vitamin A (μg) RE‡	Vitamin D (μg)§	Vitamin E (mgα-TE)¶
Females	11–14	46	101	157	62	2200 (1500–3000)	46	800	10	8
	15–18	55	120	163	64	2100 (1200–3000)	46	800	10	8
	19–22	55	120	163	64	2100 (1700–2500)	44	800	7.5	8
	23–50	55	120	163	64	2000 (1600–2400)	44	800	5	8
	51 +	55	120	163	64	1800 (1400–2200)	44	800	5	8
Pregnant						+ 300	+30	+200	+5	+2
Lactating						+ 500	+20	+400	+5	+3

Reproduced from *Recommended dietary allowances,* ninth edition (1980), with the permission of the National Academy of Sciences, Washington, D.C.
*The allowances are intended to provide for individual variations among most normal persons as they live in the United States under usual environmental stresses. Diets should be based on a variety of common foods in order to provide other nutrients for which human requirements have been less well defined.
†The energy allowances for the young adults are for women doing light work. The allowances for the older age group represent mean energy needs over this age span, allowing for a 2% decrease in basal (resting) metabolic rate per decade and a reduction in activity of 200 kcal/day for women between 51 and 75 years, and 400 kcal for women over 75. The customary range of daily energy output is shown in parentheses, and is based on a variation in energy needs of ±400 kcal at any one age, emphasizing the wide range of energy intakes appropriate for any group of people.
‡Retinol equivalents. 1 retinol equivalent = 1 μg retinol or 6μg β-carotene.
§As cholecalciferol. 10 μg cholecalciferol = 400 IU of vitamin D.
¶α-Tocopherol equivalents. 1 mg *d-α* tocopherol = 1 α-TE.

lb/week. The maximum addition for underweight is 1000 Cal and 40 g of protein (or 2 lb/week).

• *Nutritional stress* is determined if any one of the following maternal conditions exist: pernicious vomiting, pregnancies spaced less than one year apart, previous poor obstetrical history, failure to gain 10 pounds by the twentieth week, or serious emotional problems. *Nutritional stress correction* provides an additional 20 g of protein and 200 Cal for each stress condition.

To augment these specific nutrient recommendations, regular visits are established for those clients with repeat histories; weight checks, encouragement, and support are provided to each patient. Pregnant women whose incomes are below the poverty level are given a food supplement of milk, eggs, and oranges to correct the nutritional deficits. Additionally, all expectant mothers receive a vitamin and mineral supplement.

At the Montreal Diet Dispensary it is difficult, if not impossible, to separate the benefits of the food supplements and specific nutrient recommendations from the counseling expertise. Yet, what is apparent is the value of superior nutritional guidance during prenatal care (Worthington et al., 1977).

NUTRITIONAL EDUCATION

Women who are well informed about pregnancy and childbirth, and who have a positive attitude about their pregnancy, generally have fewer physical and emotional problems (Martin, 1978). In many instances patients may take the initiative in becoming better informed; yet meeting the patient's educational needs remains a major responsibility of the prenatal care providers. Key areas of information should be outlined for short educational sessions throughout the prenatal months. Habits that could affect the fetus should be discussed early in these sessions. Nutrition is a real priority.

All pregnant women can benefit from early nutrition counseling; minimally each should be provided with current guidelines and recommendations. The method of detailed nutritional assessment outlined in this chapter allows a much more individualized approach to be taken.

Referring to the intake assessment sheet (Figure 4-1), note the columns labeled "Modifications." When discrepancies exist between present and recommended intake, correcting the deficits becomes a goal of patient

Water-Soluble Vitamins							Minerals					
Vitamin C (mg)	Thia-min (mg)	Ribo-flavin (mg)	Niacin (mg NE)**	Vitamin B_6 (mg)	Folacin†† (µg)	Vitamin B_{12}(µg)	Calcium (mg)	Phos-phorus (mg)	Mag-nesium (mg)	Iron (mg)	Zinc (mg)	Iodine (µg)
50	1.1	1.3	15	1.8	400	3.0	1200	1200	300	18	15	150
60	1.1	1.3	14	2.0	400	3.0	1200	1200	300	18	15	150
60	1.1	1.3	14	2.0	400	3.0	800	800	300	18	15	150
60	1.0	1.2	13	2.0	400	3.0	800	800	300	18	15	150
60	1.0	1.2	13	2.0	400	3.0	800	800	300	10	15	150
+20	+0.4	+0.3	+2	+0.6	+400	+1.0	+400	+400	+150	‡‡	+5	+25
+40	+0.5	+0.5	+5	+0.5	+100	+1.0	+400	+400	+150	‡‡	+10	+50

**One NE (niacin equivalent) is equal to 1 mg of niacin or 60 mg of dietary tryptophan.

††The folacin allowances refer to dietary sources as determined by *Lactobacillus casei* assay after treatment with enzymes (conjugases) to make polyglutamyl forms of the vitamin available to the test organism.

‡‡The increased requirement during pregnancy cannot be met by the iron content of habitual American diets nor by the existing iron stores of many women; therefore the use of 30–60 mg of supplemental iron is recommended. Iron needs during lactation are not substantially different from those of nonpregnant women, but continued supplementation of the mother for two to three months after parturition is advisable in order to replenish stores depleted by pregnancy.

TABLE 4-5   Desirable weights for women

Height (with 2-inch heels)	Small Frame	Medium Frame	Large Frame
4 ft 10 in	92–98	96–107	104–119
4 ft 11 in	94–101	98–110	106–122
5 ft 0 in	96–104	101–113	109–125
5 ft 1 in	99–107	104–116	112–128
5 ft 2 in	102–110	107–119	115–131
5 ft 3 in	105–113	110–122	118–134
5 ft 4 in	108–116	113–126	121–138
5 ft 5 in	111–119	116–130	125–142
5 ft 6 in	114–123	120–135	129–146
5 ft 7 in	118–127	124–139	133–150
5 ft 8 in	122–131	128–143	137–154
5 ft 9 in	126–135	132–147	141–158
5 ft 10 in	130–140	136–151	145–163
5 ft 11 in	134–144	140–155	149–168
6 ft 0 in	138–148	144–159	153–173

From Metropolitan Life Insurance Co. (October, 1977). *Statistical bulletin.* (Based on data from the *Build and blood pressure study,* 1959), published by the Society of Actuaries.) With permission.

Note: For women aged 18–25, subtract 1 pound for each year under 25.

TABLE 4-6 Modified basic four food guide

Food Group	No. of Servings
Milk and milk products	2
Protein	
Animal sources (3 oz/serving)	2
Legumes and/or nuts	2
Fruits and vegetables (3/4 cup/serving)	
Vitamin-C rich	1
Dark green	1
Other	2
Whole-grain cereals and breads	4
Fats and oils (1 tbsp/serving)	1

From King, J., Cohenour, S., Corrucchini, C., & Schnerman, P. (1978). Evaluation and modification of the Basic Four Food Guide. *Journal of Nutrition Education, 10*, 27–29. With permission.
Note: This guide does not make allowances for the increased nutrient needs of pregnancy. I suggest four servings of milk for its calcium and extra protein, and more servings of whole-grain cereals and breads, fruits and vegetables, and fats for additional calories.

education. Specific changes can easily be outlined with this assessment sheet. For example, if it was determined that a patient's needs included a daily increase of 20 g protein, the counselor can consult the protein-value section of the guide and help the patient plan how the protein increase can be incorporated. Food likes and dislikes, as well as availability, will influence food selection.

Changing eating habits can be traumatic, so only necessary changes should be made. In many instances increasing milk intake is the perfect way to make up for deficiencies in both calories and protein. Dietitions at the Montreal Diet Dispensary have found mothers much more willing to increase their milk intake when told that they are drinking the milk not for themselves but for the baby (Higgins, 1975).

It is important for the counselor to establish a good personal relationship with the patient; as the success of counseling depends largely on the counselor's ability to motivate patient compliance.

In addition to specific dietary habits that may be discussed, it is necessary to provide the prenatal patient with a daily food guide to be used as an on-going form of education and as an aid in food selection. A tool currently in use is the *Basic Four Food Guide*, published by the USDA in 1956 and based on the 1953 Recommended Daily Allowances.

King et al. (1978) evaluated and modified this guide based on the 1974 RDAs for adults. Their Modified Basic Four Food Guide provides a sound foundation for making food choices for a nutritionally adequate diet (Table 4-6).

Using their modified guide, King et al. also computed several alternative diets for individual food preferences: one with no meat, one with no dairy products, and another with no legumes. A guide was also developed that used low-cost foods (Table 4-7).

When milk was excluded, more dark green, leafy vegetables were included for calcium contribution. With no meat, protein sources such as dairy products, legumes, and nuts were increased. With no legumes, animal protein and vitamin-C-rich foods were in-

TABLE 4-7 Modified basic four food guide for special preferences

	No. of Servings			
Food Group	No Meat	No Milk	No Legumes	Low Cost*
Milk and milk products	4	0	1½	1½
Protein foods				
Animal sources	0	4	4	1
Legumes	2	2	0	2
Nuts	1	0	0	0
Fruits and vegetables				
Vitamin-C rich	3	3	2½	0
Dark green	1½	3	2	1½
Other	3	0	0	0
Whole-grain cereals and breads	6	3	4	9
Fats and oils	0	0	0	1

From King, J., Cohenour, S., Corrucchini, C., & Schnerman, P. (1978). Evaluation and modification of the Basic Four Food Guide. *Journal of Nutrition Education, 10*, 27–29. With permission.
*For pregnant women, the low-cost diet could benefit from additional servings of milk and a rich source of vitamin C.

TABLE 4-8 Low-cost versus high-cost protein foods

Sources of Protein	Cost of Protein (100 g)
Expensive	
Bologna	2.00
Leg of lamb	2.05
Round steak	2.14
Frozen pizza	2.20
Soybean-based breakfast sausage	2.58
Salmon, canned	2.68
Sugar Crisp cereal	2.69
Boiled ham	2.88
Lamb chops	3.04
Bacon	3.39
Economical	
Soybeans, purchased dry	0.22
Navy beans, purchased dry	0.35
Lentils, purchased dry	0.38
Kidney beans, purchased dry	0.54
Mackerel, canned	0.55
Peanut butter	0.60
Beef liver	0.64
Powdered milk	0.66
Whole chicken	0.82
Cottage cheese	0.89

From King, J. Cohenour, S., Corrucchini, C., & Schnerman, P. (1978). Evaluation and modification of the Basic Four Food Guide. *Journal of Nutrition Education, 10,* 27–29. With permission.

creased. When cost was minimized, grains were used as the major caloric source. Table 4-8 provides an excellent comparison of the costs of various protein foods.

Vegetarian diets represent a special preference in food selection and with their increase in prevalence in our society, more detailed attention is warranted.

VEGETARIANISM

To many people a vegetarian diet is one that does not contain meat, poultry, or fish. Yet vegetarian diets differ among themselves in the foods allowed; some are more restrictive than others. Foods basic to most vegetarian diets include vegetables, fruits, enriched- or whole-grain flours, breads and cereals, legumes (dried beans and peas), nuts, nut-butters, and seeds. Foods in addition to these may be included:

- A *pure vegetarian,* or *vegan,* diet excludes all foods of animal origin.
- An *ovolacto-vegetarian* diet includes eggs and dairy products but excludes meat, poultry, and fish.

- A *lacto-vegetarian* diet excludes meat, poultry, fish, and eggs, but includes dairy products.

Vegetarianism has been advocated for religious, philosophical, moral, economic, and health reasons, and perhaps in some cultures out of necessity when meat was unattainable. In modern society the most justifiable support for vegetarian tendencies arises from the following attributes:

- The emphasis on the dietary importance of fruits and vegetables
- The emphasis on vegetable foods as an increasingly important protein source, both for economic and nutritional reasons
- The contribution to the selection of foods that lower serum cholesterol

In 1974 the Food and Nutrition Board of the National Research Council-National Academy of Science issued a statement on vegetarian diets, which said, in part, that young adults today have increasingly altered their eating habits from the traditional Western food patterns toward a vegetarian food pattern, and that this

---

EXHIBIT 4-1   Vegetarian food guide

- Follow Modified Basic Food Guide as outlined in this chapter.
- Eat a wide variety of foods, including milk and milk products and eggs.
- If no milk is allowed, use a supplement of 4 g of vitamin B_{12} daily. If goat and soymilk are used, partial supplementation may be needed.
- If no milk is taken, also use supplements of 12 mg of calcium and 400 IU of vitamin D daily. Partial supplementation will be necessary if less than four servings of milk and milk products are consumed.
- Select a variety of plant foods (especially grains, legumes, nuts, and seeds) to obtain "complete" proteins by complementary combinations, as indicated in the table below.
- Use iodized salt

Food	Amino Acids Deficient	Complementary Protein Food Combinations
Grains	Isoleucine, lysine	Rice + legumes
		Corn + legumes
		Wheat + legumes
		Wheat + peanut + milk
		Wheat + sesame + soybean
		Rice + Brewer's yeast
Legumes	Tryptophan, methionine	Legumes + rice
		Beans + wheat
		Beans + corn
		Soybeans + rice + wheat
		Soybeans + corn + milk
		Soybeans + wheat + sesame
		Soybeans + peanuts + sesame
		Soybeans + peanuts + wheat + rice
		Soybeans + sesame + wheat
Nuts and seeds	Isoleucine, lysine	Peanuts + sesame + soybeans
		Sesame + beans
		Sesame + soybeans + wheat
		Peanuts + sunflower seeds
Vegetables	Isoleucine, methionine	Lima beans
		Green beans
		Brussel sprouts, cauliflower, or broccoli + sesame, brazil nuts, or mushrooms
		Green + millet or rice

From California Department of Public Health, MCH Unit. (1975). *Nutrition during pregnancy and lactation.* Sacramento, Ca. With permission.

---

trend raises serious concerns regarding the nutritional quality of the dietary intake. Vegetarian diets may be comprised of plant food sources alone; plant foods and dairy products; or a combination of plant foods, dairy products, and eggs. It is evident that as nutrient sources become less restrictive, there is a greater likelihood that the nutrient requirements will be met. Further, as milk and/or eggs are added to the diet, the risk of inadequate nutrient sources is reduced. Clearly, diets with a wide range of variation are less likely to omit an essential nutrient. If a restrictive diet is adopted, it therefore becomes essential that the nutritional limits of the food sources utilized be carefully considered, so that health is not endangered (Seelig, 1977).

It has been demonstrated that diets of properly selected plant foods can be nutritionally adequate. However, during pregnancy and other periods with increased nutritional needs for growth, particular care must be taken that diets adequately supply all of the essential nutrients. Obtaining an adequate supply of protein and certain minerals and vitamins can be more problematic for vegetarians than for nonvegetarians.

At least eight amino acids known to be essential for the synthesis of body proteins are not manufactured by the human body and must therefore be supplied through our daily diets. Protein from animal sources is known to contain all of these essential amino acids in amounts necessary for the synthesis of body proteins, while plant proteins are known to be incomplete or lacking in one or more of the essential amino acids. Because of this inadequacy, plants are identified as lower-quality protein foods (California Department of Public Health, 1975).

To compensate for these insufficiencies, plant foods can be selected and eaten together so that the combination of their amino acids yields complete proteins, or proteins that are comparable to the high-quality animal proteins (see Exhibit 4-1).

The significance of these protein quality differences partially explains the emphasis placed on careful selection of the vegetarian diet in meeting nutrient needs. Other nutrients likely to be marginal in all-plant diets, particularly with the increases needed for pregnancy, are vitamin B_{12}, iron, calcium, riboflavin and, in areas with insufficient exposure to sunlight, vitamin D (California Department of Public Health, 1975).

Vegetarian diets containing milk and eggs can be altered much more easily to accommodate the increased needs for pregnancy than those that do not. For example, plant foods do not contain vitamin B_{12}. Pure vegetarians should consume fortified soybean milk or a vitamin B_{12} supplement to prevent B_{12} deficiency anemia. Ovolacto-vegetarians will get a satisfactory supply of vitamin B₁₂ from milk and eggs.

A daily intake of 4 cups of milk will generously meet the markedly increased needs for calcium in pregnancy (Table 4-1). Without milk as a daily ingredient of the diet, meeting calcium needs must be a conscious effort (Exhibit 4-1); bioavailability of calcium from plant sources is questionable. Fortified milk is a good source of riboflavin in a diet that contains no meat, as well as being the best dietary source of vitamin D.

Recommended daily allowance for iron during pregnancy, as indicated previously, is difficult to attain from food sources alone. For vegetarians this is even more difficult to achieve. Exhibit 4-1 provides guidelines to help safeguard vegetarian diets from nutrient deficiencies.

MATERNAL NUTRITION AND PREGNANCY OUTCOME

The relationship between maternal nutrition and birth weight of the offspring is becoming more definitive. Both pregravid weight and weight gain during pregnancy are influenced by nutrition. Numerous studies have reported a high correlation between weight gained during pregnancy, maternal pregravid weight, and birth weight of the infant (Butler & Alberman, 1969; National Academy of Sciences, 1970; Singer et al., 1968). The risks for preterm and growth-retarded infants are so well documented that low birth weight itself is considered an unfavorable outcome of pregnancy (Bergner & Susser, 1970; National Academy of Sciences, 1970; Shah & Abbey, 1971; Worthington et al., 1977).

Weight Gain

Normal pregnancy is a time of progressive maternal weight gain and this positive attitude should be conveyed early to the pregnant woman (ACOG, 1978). In the past, much emphasis has been placed on total pounds gained rather than an appreciation for the components and rate of weight gain. Total weight gain may vary among individual women, but a gain of between 26 and 30 pounds in normal pregnancy is shown to produce the most favorable outcome (ACOG, 1978; Barness & Pitkin, 1975; National Academy of Sciences, 1970; Worthington et al., 1977).

The fetus, placenta, amniotic fluid; and increases in uterus, breasts, and blood volume account for approximately 16 pounds. The additional pounds varying from patient to patient are primarily dependent on the extent of extracellular water accumulation and temporary fat stores (Table 4-9). During the first three months, weight gain should be minimal (2–4 pounds total); thereafter a gain of 3–4 pounds each month should be expected. Clinically, it is important to document the progress of weight change during pregnancy to observe patterns of inadequacy or excess (ACOG, 1978; National Academy of Sciences, 1970) (Figure 4-3).

Weight gain alone discloses nothing about the components of the gain. Most of the weight gain with pregnancy should be lean body tissue. A gain from too much fluid or too much fat is not desirable.

A sudden accumulation of weight (greater than 2 lb/week) is indicative of fluid retention, and the patient should be observed for the presence of, or development of other signs of preeclampsia (ACOG, 1978). Over-

TABLE 4-9 Components of the average weight gained in normal pregnancy

Component	Amount (g) Gained at:			
	10 weeks	20 weeks	30 weeks	40 weeks
Total gain of body weight	650	4,000	8,500	12,500
Fetus	5	300	1,500	3,300
Placenta	20	170	430	650
Amniotic Fluid	30	250	600	800
Increase of				
Uterus	135	585	819	900
Mammary gland	34	180	360	405
Maternal blood	100	600	1,300	1,250
Total (rounded)	320	2,100	5,000	7,300
Weight not accounted for (total gain – total [rounded])	330	1,900	3,500	5,200

From National Academy of Sciences, Committee on Maternal Nutrition. (1970). *Maternal nutrition and the course of pregnancy*. Washington, D.C. With permission.

PRENATAL WEIGHT GAIN GRID

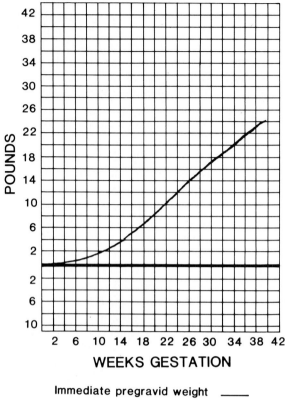

Immediate pregravid weight   _____

Height in inches
without shoes
Plus one inch   _____

Standard weight   _____

(Record weight with shoes)

FIGURE 4-3 Average prenatal weight gain grid for normal pregnancies. (Redrawn from National Academy of Sciences, Committee on Maternal Nutrition. (1970). *Maternal nutrition and the course of pregnancy.* Washington, D.C. With permission.)

whelming evidence indicates that the nutritional status and the quality of weight gained are of vital importance in the maternal patient's defense against the hypertensive diseases of pregnancy.

Excessive weight gain due to an accumulation of fat cell deposition is much less dramatic in terms of time of its accumulation.

When such situations exist the nutritional value of the diet must be investigated for calorically rich components and their elimination.

Weight Loss

Weight reduction is never a safe alternative during pregnancy or lactation (even for the obese patient) because of potential adverse effects on the nutrition, growth, and development of the fetus.

Inadequate weight gain (less than 2 lb/month in the second and third trimesters) is a sign of maternal and fetal malnutrition, and is associated with lowered birth weight, intra-uterine growth retardation, and fetal jeopardy (ACOG, 1978). As with excessive weight gain, nutritional inadequacy of the patient's diet must be evaluated and corrected.

To ensure the desired pattern of weight gain, the pregnant woman must be encouraged to ingest adequate calories and nutrients from the onset of pregnancy to the cessation of lactation (ACOG, 1978).

For the patient who is underweight at the time of conception, a planned weight gain for her pregnancy should include correcting this weight deficit in addition to the average weight gain for normal pregnancy (Barness & Pitkin, 1975). Weight gain is another of the issues of pregnancy requiring individualized management. Guidance toward a planned weight goal is valuable to the most favorable outcome for both mother and baby.

Sodium Intake

Restricting sodium intake during pregnancy is now regarded as potentially hazardous. The great expansion of maternal tissues, in addition to the fetal needs, increase the requirement for sodium during pregnancy. In the past, restricting sodium and the use of diuretics was commonly recommended to combat edema and/or to prevent toxemia. Research has discredited this practice. Pike and Smiciklas (1964) cite studies in which the condition of pregnant women with toxemia improved with additional salt.

In practice, reducing sodium intake often jeopardizes the nutritive quality of diets. Foods such as milk, cheese, peanut butter, canned meats, and fish are valuable to maternal diets but are also high in sodium. Low sodium diets are less palatable and adherence to such regimens may result in decreased food intake.

Additionally, iodized salt is the main source of valuable iodine for most Americans (Clausen et al., 1977). Iodized salt should be used freely during pregnancy.

Supplementation

All pregnant women should receive 30–60 mg of elemental iron daily to meet recommended pregnancy requirements and to protect maternal iron stores (Barness & Pitkin, 1975; National Academy of Sciences, 1980). Requirements for this nutrient are greatly elevated with pregnancy and food sources alone are inadequate to meet this need.

Most anemias in pregnancy are iron deficiency produced; however, megaloblastic anemia, resulting from insufficient folic acid is also a potential problem during pregnancy (ACOG, 1978). Folic acid requirements are greatly increased at this time and daily supplements of 400–800 μg should be prescribed for all pregnant women (Barness & Pitkin, 1975; National Academy of Sciences, 1980).

Food sources for both of these nutrients should be emphasized in addition to supplemental sources (Table 4-1).

Multivitamin supplementation is an extra precaution when dietary intake of these nutrients is questionable or when pregnancies have short interconceptional intervals. Carefully selected vitamin supplements are most valuable if specific deficiencies are proven or suspected. Care should be taken, however, to avoid both misuse of dietary supplements, and the creation of a false sense of security.

LACTATION

Breast-feeding represents the preferred source of nutrition for full-term newborns (see Chapter 17). Care must be taken to ensure this milk supply and its optimal nutrient content for meeting infant needs. Following are current lactation nutrition guidelines:

- The maternal diet should continue to meet the nutrient requirements of the mother and the infant.
- Energy requirements are even higher than those for pregnancy.
- Iron supplements recommended during pregnancy should be continued to replenish maternal iron stores depleted by the pregnancy.
- Vegetarians must include a vitamin B_{12} source if breast milk is their infants' solitary nutrient source (Higginbottom et al., 1978).
- Oral contraceptives may interfere with the amount of milk produced.
- Drugs of any kind should be used judiciously.

CONCLUSIONS

As research continues to provide scientific basis for change, unfounded, often erroneous practices of the past are being replaced. Unfortulately, current philosophies are slow to be accepted and conflicting information does exist. Objectives of prenatal nutrition education should be to ensure that every pregnancy patient has an understanding of the following:

- The significance of maternal nutrition to pregnancy outcome
- A daily food guide that incorporates the necessary increases for energy, protein, minerals, and vitamins
- The jeopardy of weight loss and inadequate weight gain with pregnancy
- The hazards of sodium restriction, use of diuretics, and other drugs during pregnancy (Hanson et al., 1976; USDHEW, 1971)
- The uses of mineral and vitamin supplements for pregnancy
- The special nutritional guidelines for lactation.

REFERENCES AND ADDITIONAL READINGS

American College of Obstetrics and Gynecology (ACOG) (1978). *Assessment of maternal nutrition.* Chicago, Il.: ACOG.

Barness, L., & Pitkin, R. (1975). Symposium on nutrition. In L. Barness & R. Pitkin (Eds.), *Clinics in perinatology.* Philadelphia: Saunders.

Bergner, L., & Susser, M. (1970). Low birth weight and perinatal nutrition: An interpretative review. *Pediatrics, 46,* 946–966.

Butler, N., & Alberman, E.D. (1969). Maternal factors affecting duration of pregnancy, birth weight and fetal growth. In N. Butler & E.D. Alberman (Eds.), *Perinatal Problems.* Edinburgh: Livingstone.

California Department of Public Health, MCH Unit. (1975). *Nutrition during pregnancy and lactation.* Sacramento, Ca.

Clausen, J.P., Flook, M.H., & Ford, B. (1977). *Maternity nursing today.* New York: McGraw-Hill.

Hanson, J., Jones, K., & Smith, D. (1976). Fetal alcohol syndrome. Experience with 41 patients. *Journal of the American Medical Association, 235,* 1458–1460.

Higginbottom, M., Sweetman, L., & Nyhan, W. (1978). A syndrome of methylmalonic aciduria, homocystinuria, megaloblastic anemia and neurologic abnormalities in a vitamin B_{12} deficient breast fed infant of a strict vegetarian. *New England Journal of Medicine, 229,* 317–323.

Higgins, A. (1975). Nutritional status and the outcome of pregnancy. Paper read before the annual meeting of the Canadian Dietetic Association, Moncton, New Brunswick, June 19, 1975.

Jeans, P., Smith, M., & Stearns, G. (1955). Incidence of prematurity in relation to maternal nutrition. *Journal of the American Dietetic Association, 3,* 576–581.

King, J., Cohenour, S., Corruccini, C., & Schnerman, P. (1978). Evaluation and modification of the Basic Four Food Guide. *Journal of Nutrition Education, 10,* 27–29.

Lechtig, A., Habict, J., Delgado, H., Klein, R., Yarbrough, C., & Martorell, R. (1975). Effect of food supplementation during pregnancy on birth weight. *Pediatrics, 56,* 508–520.

Martin, L. (1978). *Health care of women.* Philadelphia: Lippincott.

National Academy of Sciences, Committee on Maternal Nutrition. (1970). *Maternal nutrition and the course of pregnancy.* Washington, D.C.

National Academy of Sciences (1977). *Laboratory indices of nutritional status in pregnancy,* publication F-427.

National Academy of Sciences–National Research Council, Food and Nutrition Board. (1980). *Recommended Dietary Allowances* (ed. 9). Washington, D.C.

Pike, R. (1974). Sodium intake during pregnancy. *Journal of the American Dietetic Association, 44,* 176–181.

Seelig, M. (1977). *Nutritional imbalances in infant and adult diseases. Proceedings of the 1975 Meeting of the American College of Nutrition.* New York: Spectrum.

Seelig, R.A. (1974). Vegetarianism—A review. Washington, D.C.: United Fresh Fruit and Vegetable Association.

Shah, F.K., & Abbey, H. (1971). Effects of some factors on neonatal and post-neonatal mortality. *Milbank Memorial Fund Quarterly, 49,* 35–57.

Singer, J.E., Westphal, M., & Niswander, K. (1968). Relationship of weight gain during pregnancy to birth weight and infant growth and development in the first year of life. *Obstetrics and Gynecology, 31,* 417–423.

United States Department of Health, Education and Welfare (1971). *Health consequences of smoking; A report of the surgeon general: Smoking and pregnancy,* Public Health Service.

United States Department of Health, Education and Welfare (1978). *Monthly vital statistics report, provisional statistics annual summary for the United States, 1977,* publication 79-1120, no. 13. Public Health Service.

Williams, S. (1976). *Handbook of maternal and infant nutrition.* Berkeley, Ca.: S.R.W. Productions, pp. 76–78.

Worthington, B., Vermeersch, J., Williams, S. (1977). *Nutrition in pregnancy and lactation.* St. Louis: Mosby.

Chapter 5 | Childbirth Preparation

Rosemary Cogan

I N THE MID-NINETEENTH CENTURY, two developments took place that profoundly changed the experience of giving birth. In 1837, hypnosis was used to provide three hours of hynotic sleep to a woman who had been in labor for 48 hours. Ten years later, James Simpson gave ether to a woman in labor to ease the pain she was experiencing, thus beginning a long line of developments in the use of pharmacological relief of pain in childbirth.

The history of approaches to pain reduction in childbirth has been reviewed by Chertok (1959) and provides an excellent perspective for understanding current childbirth education. Hypnosis or hypnosuggestive methods came into some general use during the end of the nineteenth century in France, Germany, Austria, and particularly the Soviet Union, where, during the 1940s, attempts were made to use hypnosuggestive methods during childbirth without any preliminary preparation. Investigations showed that prenatal preparation facilitated analgesia during childbirth, particularly if expectant fathers were included in the preparation.

Psychoprophylaxis was developed from hypnosuggestive methods by a team of workers comprising two psychiatrists, Velvovsky and Platonov, and two obstetricians, Plotitcher and Chougom, who reported on the method in 1949. In 1951, the French obstetrician Lamaze observed the labor of women who had received psychoprophylactic preparation for childbirth. Lamaze returned to Paris, an enthusiastic convert to the method. Lamaze and his associate Vellay adapted psychoprophylaxis for their own patients, and described the approach in conferences around the world. The *Lamaze method* is a common approach to childbirth preparation used in the United States at the present time. It is based on relaxation and breathing patterns, which are practiced before birth and used throughout labor contractions. Information about labor and birth is taught to women before they begin labor, and support from a labor coach is stressed as facilitating use of the method during labor. The theoretical basis for the method is thought to be Pavlovian conditioning.

Also in use in the United States at present is the *Read method*, which is usually referred to as "natural childbirth." Grantly Dick-Read developed natural childbirth out of an experience he had in 1914 when a woman whose birth he attended refused his offer of chloroform, saying after the birth, "It didn't hurt. It wasn't meant to, was it, Doctor?" The story of Dick-Read's subsequent work, described in a biography by Thomas (1957), is both interesting and thought provoking. He pointed out that during labor, fear, tension, and pain can easily form a spiral that can be reduced or eliminated by practicing relaxation to be used during labor contractions to reduce tension and fear. The Read method also includes the use of slow, rhythmic, abdominal breathing during labor.

Positive results of childbirth preparation have been repeatedly shown in research studies (Cogan, 1980). Women with childbirth preparation experience less pain, are observed by others to appear less tense and to complain less during labor, and receive less medication during childbirth. Their experience of birth, and their later feelings about the birth are more positive than women who give birth without psychological preparation. Fathers who are involved in prepared childbirth report feeling positively about themselves as helpers during childbirth. Babies whose mothers have childbirth preparation have a more stable heartbeat during labor than other babies. With this multitude of benefits, perhaps it is understandable that there are some differences of opinion as to what the essential elements of childbirth preparation are.

There has been considerable controversy over the definition of natural childbirth, and whether it means that the woman delivers without medication. In the early days of prepared childbirth, women who wanted to use natural childbirth were frequently denied any kind of medication even if they needed it late in their labor and delivery. If the concept of "no medication no matter what" is instilled in the minds of consumers or professionals, the results can be devastating. Flexibility in the use of medication allows the mother who cannot go through her entire labor completely without medication (especially primigravidas) to still feel that she has accomplished something. She should not have to feel as though she has failed because of the need for medication. This more flexible approach, which is being adopted by professionals and childbirth educators, promotes a sense of success in childbearing regardless of the tools used to achieve the goal.

Chertok (1969) has been a particularly thoughtful and articulate contributor to literature on prepared childbirth. Chertok sees the primary purpose of childbirth preparation as psychological analgesia. The central question about preparation programs is whether a program accepts a minimum goal of helping the laboring women, or insists upon a maximum goal of making childbirth painless. Chertok recognizes that psychological analgesia is an ambitious and difficult goal and also that many other psychological values may result from prepared childbirth.

> Painless childbirth leads to new standards for childbirth; a good confinement implies activity, directed by means of a technique, resulting in behavioral control more or less pain free and allowing cooperation with the obstetrician; an emotional participation in the birth; and a positive emotional relation to the child, in the joy of achievement.... Childbirth is an aim in itself, to be experienced as a positive moment in the woman's life.*

One additional psychological value of childbirth preparation that has been a particularly American addition, is the involvement of the father as the labor coach during childbirth. Preliminary research suggests that the involvement of the father in childbirth may have far-reaching implications for his increased involvement in care of the child.

MECHANISMS OF CHILDBIRTH PREPARATION

Chertok has explored the mechanisms by which childbirth preparation accomplishes analgesia during childbirth, and has suggested roles of information, psychophysical techniques, and psychotherapeutic or social-emotional components of preparation.

Information

Virtually all childbirth preparation classes provide students with information about labor and birth. Information has been shown to be associated with reduced pain and medication, and a more favorable attitude toward childbirth, but information about labor and birth seems to have a fairly rapid ceiling effect, and is only one part of a complete program of childbirth preparation. The husband-coach also needs preparation for the work and noise of second-stage labor, or he or she may interpret these as indicating pain when they are not indicative of pain for the woman. Among the books available illustrating the informational content of classes are Beals (1977), Cogan et al. (1979), and Ewy and Ewy (1976).

---

*From Chertok, L. (1959). *Psychosomatic methods in painless childbirth: History, theory and practice.* Elmsford, N.Y.: Pergamon Press. With permission.

Psychophysical Techniques

Breathing Techniques

Breathing skills are components of almost all approaches to childbirth preparation. In Read's Natural Childbirth, slow rhythmic breathing is focused in the abdominal area, while in Lamaze childbirth preparation, the breathing is focused in the chest area. While the focus of breathing has never been shown to be related to the effectiveness of childbirth preparation, it is probably important to have many details of psychophysical techniques fixed, in order to maintain unified and complete programs of preparation.

As it was developed in the Soviet Union, psychoprophylaxis originally included deep, rhythmical breathing at a rate of sixteen to eighteen exchanges per minute. The rhythmical breathing involved inspiration through the nostrils and exhalation through the mouth. As the intensity of contractions increased, women were directed to add a light stroking or effleurage of the abdomen and the depth of the breathing became somewhat deeper. A third technique for pain control utilized pressure on pain-reducing points.

The breathing component of psychoprophylaxis was elaborated by Lamaze, and in most instances includes chest breathing, done at a slow rate and a faster, shallower rate; panting, done at a slow rate and a faster, shallower rate; and pant-blowing, using a moderately forceful blow through pursed lips to help delay pushing. Women learn to combine breathing levels by beginning with a slow rate or level, gradually accelerating to a faster rate or level as a contraction builds to a peak, and then decelerating as the contraction reduces in intensity. All breathing is adapted as needed during labor, although in general chest breathing is used during the latent phase of labor, panting during the active phase, and panting-blowing during transition. Women probably need encouragement both in classes and during labor to stay with slower breathing, since there is a natural tendency for women to hurry into faster breathing as if to hurry labor itself along.

During the 1970s, several modifications of Lamaze's late-labor breathing patterns were proposed in the United States. The modifications were stimulated by the concern that the rapid breathing might be producing hyperventilation during labor. This concern probably reflected a series of articles in medical literature during the late 1960s, in which the relationship between prolonged maternal hyperventilation and fetal well-being was explored with mixed results. Research has since shown that a certain amount of hyperventilation is an essentially universal feature of pregnancy and childbirth, and no differences in the frequency or extent of feelings associated with hyperventilation have been found as a function of late-labor breathing in prepared childbirth. At the same time, students taught slow panting, and those taught *he* breathing (in which a low or moderate pant is combined with a mouth position that leads to a *he* sound during late-labor breathing) experienced more pain during labor than women taught fast panting for use in late labor.

Practice of breathing techniques for a minimum of ten minutes a day during the six to eight weeks of childbirth preparation has been found to be associated with pain reduction during the active phase of labor. More extensive practice times did not evidently lead to further pain reduction during labor or birth.

Relaxation Training

Approaches to relaxation training vary in different childbirth preparation programs, reflecting interests of teachers and students. Approaches all include a chance to focus on muscle tension, release of the tension, and awareness of the feelings of relaxation. Jacobson's (1939) work on relaxation has been adapted for many classes. Vellay's (1959) writing has focused somewhat more on repeated cycles of contracting and releasing; this active approach is widely used. Imagery, part of the relaxation training of Read's program, is being added to relaxation in many imaginative ways and a good variety of approaches to relaxation are developing that can be adapted to students' interests and developing skills at relaxation techniques. Practice of relaxation or release from five to about thirty minutes every day has been found to be the maximum practice time that facilitates pain reduction in prepared childbirth. Either breathing or relaxation techniques used alone are less effective in pain relief than when used in combination. Books illustrating the psychophysical techniques of Lamaze classes include Vellay (1959), Ewy and Ewy (1976), and Cogan et al. (1979). The techniques of Read's classes are described in Fitzhugh (1976).

Psychotherapeutic Components

Many features of classes do serve to reduce anxiety. Information itself is probably an anxiety-reduction aspect of classes, as is gaining confidence in technical skills to be used during labor and birth. Psychotherapeutic or social-emotional components of childbirth preparation are probably the most widely varying aspects of classes. Birth is an event in which the feelings and activities of significant others take on great importance. The importance of an understanding and supportive medical staff has been stressed consistently in Soviet and French literature on childbirth preparation, and has been reaffirmed in research.

American literature has stressed the importance of an individual labor coach who has no technical responsibilities, for every woman in labor. The coach can be any significant person who will gain an understanding of her childbirth preparation, will practice with the woman, and will be available to give her complete, individual, personal help and attention during her labor. While it is helpful to the childbirth education teacher to act as labor coach occasionally, taking on the coach role involves a commitment of many continuous hours of help during labor; most teachers cannot realistically do this often. Helping women find helpers more involved with their own lives probably also has benefits in giving them the direct opportunity to learn about getting help from family and friends. The labor coach can be the husband or father of the baby, or another person significant to the woman such as a friend, sister, mother, or woman in the community who has experienced prepared childbirth and is willing to assume the coaching role. In most instances, the father's participation as labor coach has special urgency for the pregnant woman; his involvement is particularly helpful and important since he will generally be involved in the subsequent care of the family. The presence and support of the father–coach during childbirth has been found to be associated with reduction of pain and medication requirements among women *with* prepared childbirth.

Social-emotional aspects of childbirth preparation are particularly emphasized in the Bradley approach to prepared childbirth, sometimes called Husband Coached Natural Childbirth. The Bradley approach lessens emphasis on breathing techniques, sometimes teaching only slow chest-breathing in classes, and elaborates on the interaction patterns between the husband and wife (Bradley, 1974; Hartman, 1975). Kitzinger's psychosexual approach focuses upon the psychological dynamics of pregnancy and birth (Kitzinger, 1977). Approaches to childbirth based on Yoga also emphasize social-emotional factors, and focus on birth as a spiritual experience with considerable focus on the woman's "becoming one" with her contractions and fully experiencing all the positive physical and emotional sensations of labor and birth.

There is no reason why childbirth preparation cannot be adopted to the interests, temperament, and belief systems of groups with strong orienting viewpoints that differ from those of the community at large. Lamaze childbirth preparation has been adapted readily, for instance, to a transactional analysis point of view and to a Christian point of view. These modifications tend to adjust the specific psychotherapeutic aspects of childbirth preparation to the viewpoint shared by students and teacher, while still teaching information about labor and birth, and relaxation and breathing techniques to be practiced and used in labor and birth. Two exceptionally helpful books are available in which the psychotherapeutic aspects of childbirth preparation are explored. These books are Kitzinger (1977) and Edwards (1976). Helpful and thought-provoking examples of the effects of social-emotional factors on the birth experience may be found in Gaskin's (1978) collection of midwife-attended birth reports from The Farm.

CLASSES

It seems that, in order to be effective, classes must be small enough so that interaction between class members is practical, and so that the needs of each individual can be recognized by the teacher. It seems likely that six to eight couples is the most effective class size to accomplish this. Childbirth preparation is typically taught in a series of six to eight classes during the last weeks of pregnancy. Childbirth preparation can be taught in fewer classes, but since it is not possible to predict which class members will give birth before their expected due dates, teachers and students are reluctant to begin classes much closer than six weeks before the expected due date.

There is an alternative format for providing childbirth education classes that is being adopted by many groups of childbirth educators and various hospitals providing prenatal education. This new format consists of three classes offered at about sixteen to twenty weeks' gestation. These classes include discussions of the physiology of pregnancy, nutrition, and fetal development. Another three to five classes are offered late in pregnancy and discuss labor and delivery and the immediate postpartum period. The last group of two to four classes focus on early parenting and start two to four weeks postpartum. The rationale for arranging the classes in this manner is that it keeps the group together longer and meets emotional and educational needs of parents at times more acceptable to them.

Because the childbirth educator acts as a role model for couples it is most effective if these educators have had positive prepared childbirth experiences. It is evidently extremely difficult for women who have not themselves experienced prepared childbirth to fully realize that childbirth preparation *can* produce analgesia, and that the feelings of labor and birth are often extremely positive.

COMMUNITY NEEDS

In program planning, it is important to evaluate the needs of a community with respect to childbirth preparation. The health care worker who is interested should attend several class meetings of existing childbirth preparation groups. It is important not to base ideas about classes on secondhand, often distorted information. The worker should observe several women in labor who have had classes from existing programs, and/or should talk with several women who have recently given birth and have had classes from existing classes. In talking with women about their experiences with prepared childbirth, it is particularly important to pay attention to what their *expectations* had been for their birth experience, as well as their feelings about their actual experience. It is possible for classes to suggest such minimal goals that students may be content but, in fact, may have had birth experiences characterized by extensive medication or pain. Finally, it can be helpful to formally survey women who have had babies by sampling from birth announcements in public records and actually doing a study. Such a study can be done by mail and can shed a great deal of light on the situation and needs of a community.

If classes are effective, women with classes usually report experiencing less pain during each phase of labor in comparison to women without classes. Women with childbirth preparation frequently require and receive less medication, and should feel positively about their experiences. No effective method of evaluating the extent of the ecstatic nature of the experience has yet been reported in the literature. This is clearly an outcome measure that would be of great interest, and several investigators are working on ways of looking at positive feelings towards the birth experience. Community evaluations should be repeated every few years, since classes and situations do change.

The results of two such surveys are summarized in Figures 5-1 and 5-2, in which the primary purpose of prepared childbirth is explored in two different communities.

If effective classes already exist in the community, the nurse or social worker can go on to look at other areas of need. In most communities, the women who take childbirth preparation classes tend to be a selected part of the childbearing population. They tend to be well

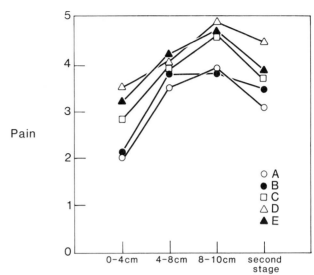

Experiences of Women	Childbirth Education Classes				
	A	B	C	D	E
Some hyperventilation during labor	32%	44%	28%	33%	34%
Some backache during labor	55%	66%	83%	67%	76%
Some medication before second stage	32%	33%	76%	93%	61%
Husband present during birth	91%	100%	90%	64%	27%
Women conscious during birth	100%	100%	97%	87%	88%
Breast-feeding initiated	97%	100%	72%	64%	50%

FIGURE 5-1 Childbirth experiences of women electing different childbirth preparation classes in city A. Group E is a comparison group of women who did not attend such classes.

educated, well adjusted, have a more extensive work history, and a higher family income than women who do not take classes. They more often plan to and do breast-feed their babies. Women in less fortunate circumstances have urgent needs for childbirth preparation. This work will require skills and ideas that childbirth educators, generally accustomed to working with the families who currently tend to select classes, may not have gained. Materials from the International Childbirth Education Association are available to help in the development of outreach childbirth education classes, or childbirth educators in the community may be interested in collaborating on development of an outreach program.

Most communities have a good many needs associated with childbearing that have not yet been met. A preconception meeting scheduled regularly can help families prevent birth defects and maximize their readiness for pregnancy and parenthood. Classes for women expecting Cesarean births can be extremely helpful. A chance to explore feelings and answer questions can be very helpful to the couple who experiences an unexpected Cesarean birth. Hospitals may vary in the extent to which education is provided during the hospital stay.

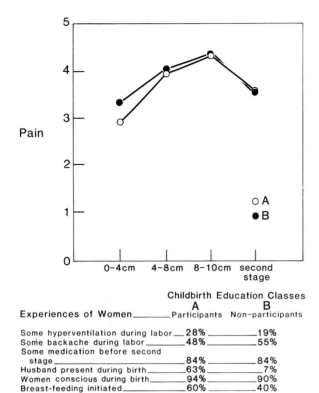

Experiences of Women	Childbirth Education Classes	
	A Participants	B Non-participants
Some hyperventilation during labor	28%	19%
Some backache during labor	48%	55%
Some medication before second stage	84%	84%
Husband present during birth	63%	7%
Women conscious during birth	94%	90%
Breast-feeding initiated	60%	40%

FIGURE 5-2 Childbirth experiences of women electing or not electing childbirth preparation in city B. Group A consisted of women who did attend childbirth preparation classes; those in Group B did not.

Literature suggests that help with family planning, infant care, breast-feeding, normal behavior and development of the newborn, and parenting can be extremely helpful to new parents. Hospital rules need to be reviewed, and perhaps revised; the health care worker can be an extremely effective agent for producing change in this area. What is essential is for each of us to review our community situations and our own skills, and then direct our energies where they are most likely to be helpful.

REFERENCES

Beals, P. (Ed.) (1977). *I.C.E.A. parent's guide to the childbearing year.* Milwaukee, Wi.: I.C.E.A.

Bradley, R. (1974). *Husband-coached childbirth.* New York: Harper & Row.

Chertok, L. (1959). *Psychosomatic methods in painless childbirth: History, theory and practice.* New York: Pergamon.

Chertok, L. (1969). *Motherhood and personality: Psychosomatic aspects of childbirth.* Philadelphia, Pa.: Lippincott.

Cogan, R. (1980). Effects of childbirth preparation. *Clinical Obstetrics and Gynecology, 23,* 1–13.

Cogan, R., Logan, S., & Tipton, L. (1979). *Joyful beginnings with Lamaze preparation for childbirth* (ed. 2). Lubbock, Tx.: Parent Education Programs.

Edwards, E. (1976). *Communications: Dimensions in childbirth education.* Seattle: Catalyst Publications

Ewy, D., & Ewy, R. (1976). *Preparation for childbirth.* New York: Signet.

Fitzhugh, M.L. (1974). *Preparation for childbirth.* San Rafael, Ca.: Associates Printing.

Gaskin, I.M. (1978). *Spiritual midwifery,* (revised). Summertown, Tn.: Book Publ. Coop.

Hartman, R. (1975). *Exercises for true natural birth.* New York: Harper & Row.

Jacobsen, E. (1939). *Professional measures for relaxation.* Chicago: University of Chicago Press.

Kitzinger, S. (1977). *Education and counseling for childbirth.* London: Cassel & Collier Macmillan.

Thomas, N.A. (1957). *Doctor courageous: The story of Dr. Grantly Dick-Read.* New York: Harper.

Vellay, P. (1959). *Childbirth without pain.* New York: Dutton.

Part 3

Family Health Care Through Labor and Birth

HUMAN LABOR AND BIRTH have experienced a myriad of changing trends throughout history. With the development of new technologies allowing evaluation of the woman and fetus during labor and birth came a distrust of nature and her forces. A birthing woman was viewed as a hospitalized patient and was stripped of her rights, choices, and decision-making power. In response, during the 1960s and 1970s steps were taken to return the labor and birth process to the woman and her loved ones. Professionals and other concerned people became involved in philosophical, political, and technical aspects of birth, so that today birth has assumed the status of a social issue.

The woman, her loved ones, and the unborn child have the right to a safe and satisfying childbirth experience. Further, they must assume the responsibility for this themselves. The delicate nature of the unborn child's physiological balance must be acknowledged. Labor and birth are highly critical periods for the fetus with only a very narrow margin for error. Birth attendants and other involved professionals should have a thorough knowledge of the physiological responses of the woman and the fetus in labor and birth; should use their knowledge, technology, and skill appropriately; and should try to meet the physical, psychological, and social needs of the woman, her loved ones, and the newborn child.

Nurses have an unparalleled opportunity to influence people's lives as they experience birth. Roles for nurses in the care of women and their families during labor and birth are numerous and varied. The potential for personal satisfaction in providing professional services is great: the advent of family-centered care reinforced the role of the nurse as educator, counselor, and facilitator of parent–infant bonding and successful parenting. In addition to participating in birth as a family event, the nurse is needed as an educator before and during the event of labor and throughout the postpartum period.

The first chapter in this section is devoted to labor and the essentials of care during the intrapartum period. Elaboration upon maternal–fetal physiology during labor is extensive, and specific aspects of care are discussed in terms of their physiological, scientific basis. With a thorough understanding of the normal, healthy response to labor, the nurse can provide highly individualized, safe care to women and their families as they give birth.

The chapter on birth describes how the nurse cares for, supports, and guides the woman and her family successfully through the birth process. Because we are still in an era where women often seek choices in birth that are not obtainable in all health care facilities, the nurse has a responsibility to be an agent of change.

The nurse also has the responsibility of knowing how to safely perform an emergency delivery. The focus of the chapter on emergency delivery assumes an inevitable birth, acknowledges the danger of any measures that forcibly impede birth, and provides explicit information on how to provide safe care for mother and baby at birth.

Even though this volume is devoted to women with low-risk pregnancies, nature sometimes deals the unexpected. In spite of the most careful surveillance, babies are born who unexpectedly need resuscitation.

For the benefit of all who are around newborn infants, the essential components of resuscitation are presented.

After the birth, the nurse has a great responsibility to evaluate and to assure the baby's and mother's physical adaptations. In the first few hours after birth both mother and baby are in their most physiological labile states. Soon after birth, important psychosocial processes begin for the newborn and family. The chapter on the immediate postdelivery period is concerned with the nurse's role in observing and facilitating physiological stability and psychosocial interaction for the newborn, mother, and family.

In keeping with the perspective that labor and birth are currently the focus of great social concern, the last chapter in this section deals with birth alternatives. Traditional birth systems are explored, as are other alternatives.

Chapter 6

Labor and Intrapartum Care

Joan E. Hoffmaster

I N OUR CHANGING SOCIETY, nurses are called on to respond to the changing needs and desires of parents involved with childbirth. The actual birth event is being recognized as a significant time for human relationships as well as biophysiological occurrences.

As traditional practices, responsibilities, rights, areas of decision making, and other factors related to childbirth and parenting are questioned and examined, the basic concept of the nurse's role is also questioned, and thus, ethical considerations of practices must be examined continually.

The evolving concepts of self-care and self-responsibility for the state of health, consign to the nurse increasing responsibility for educating and informing the childbearing families. Nurse involvement in normal labor and birth has become less one of managing labor, and more one of facilitating the environment and the family integrity, although this does not preclude the consistent surveillance of mother and baby.

Ethical questions of human values are being raised with an urgency probably unequaled since pregnancy and childbirth entered the "sickness model" or "medical model." For this reason a brief look at some of the ethical components of childbirth is called for.

RESPONSIBILITY IN INTRAPARTUM CARE

The terms *responsibility, accountability, informed decision making,* and *contract* are in frequent usage relating to health care and nursing practice and appear commonly in discussions of childbearing, pregnancy, and parenting.

Responsibility includes the ability to deliberate rationally, to understand and make decisions concerning rules of conduct (or agreements), and to conform to the decisions made (or carry through with expressed intent); and the capacity to avoid neglect and to accept the consequences of actions. These elements are interrelated and interdependent. For example, if an agent is held responsible for the outcome of her or his actions, then it is assumed the agent has the capacity of reason and foresight to avoid harmful outcome (Donagan, 1977; Hinshaw, 1977; Twiss, 1977).

In the traditional concept of moral responsibility, the assessment of accountability for actions on the part of the responsible agent (e.g., the nurse) assumes a limitation of the time span, or a short-range causal connection between actions and their consequences. Twiss (1977) points out that advanced technology in health care has effected an extension of this concept, with the introduction of new and variable elements of moral significance. There is, for example, an expansion of time as a result of the increasing predictability of long-term or irreversible consequences. This implies an ethic of long-range responsibility, which includes the moral responsibility of acquiring predictive knowledge of the possible long-range outcomes prior to implementing newer therapies, technologies, drugs, and so on. The responsibility to exercise caution and restraint when a lack of such information exists follows. This raises a spectrum of implications for nurses and others involved in the labor and birth process (Twiss, 1977).

In view of the normal outcomes of over ninety percent of births, questions concerning childbirth practices and policies were considered at the 1977 Hastings Center Conference on Values Underlying the New Childbirth Technology. This multidisciplinary gathering of philosophers, midwives, pediatricians, historians, obstetricians, policy makers, and others expressed a diversity of values, based upon whether childbirth and pregnancy were viewed primarily as social and psychological events sometimes requiring medical assistance, or primarily as medical events. An outcome of this conference was the identification of three issues considered to need further scrutiny:

> First, when dedicated clinicians control much of the information and inevitably use it to advocate their favored policy, how can policy makers or parents make responsible decisions about pregnancy and childbirth? ...Second, should parents adhere strictly to what the dominant medical opinion declares is the safest method of childbirth, or is there, in fact, a range of options within which parental choice should not only be allowed but facilitated? ...Third, in assessing alternative approaches, how much support should policy makers give to the view that the health care system ought to promote active parental involvement in decision making, childbirth, and newborn care?*

These questions reflect the changing social relationships between health care providers and recipients, in which the recipients are providing new social definitions relative to certain aspects of health care (e.g., birth, health and sickness, options, responsibilities, and rights). A partner relationship is emerging between health care providers and recipients, in which all participants are mutually obligated to share information, to become knowledgeable and informed, and to act responsively and responsibly.

---

*From Steinfels, M.O. (1978). New childbirth technology: A clash of values. *The Hastings Center Report, 8*(1), 9–12. Reprinted with permission of the Hastings Center.

Such a contract may include the expectant mother's choices about such things as who will participate in the birth event, the kind of help that is desired from the birth attendants, her wishes regarding use or nonuse of drugs, the means of surveillance for well-being of mother and baby, areas of further informational needs or special concern, and self-help needs.

The contract can be an effective vehicle in the process of informing the parents, since expectations, options, risks, limitations, and other information that the parents need in order to make judgments are appropriately discussed in the face-to-face, ongoing planning and revision that enters into the contract. Contracts, when developed in good faith and honored by all those involved, are the essence and the body of the processes of assessment, planning, and intervention in health care.

ETIOLOGY OF LABOR ONSET

Human pregnancy is considered to be about 280 days when calculated from the first day of the last menstrual period. Hammes and Treloar (1970) reported a study of vital records showing that fifty percent of women begin labor by 280 days, seventy-seven percent by 287 days, ninety-six percent by 301 days, and about ninety-nine percent by 315 days.

The precise cause of labor onset is unknown, but a number of theories exist. There is a recognized increase in the activity of the myometrium toward the latter part of pregnancy, but there is, as yet, no proven cause for the transition from Braxton Hicks contractions of pregnancy to the contractions that result in the cervical dilation of labor. The mechanisms involved appear to encompass a complexity of interrelated factors.

Labor onset is not adequately explained by the occurrence of uterine contractions, since the uterus in the nonpregnant state, as well as throughout pregnancy, contracts. Contractions occur with greater regularity and higher intensity during both menstruation and labor (Hendricks, 1964). It has been postulated that molecular changes occur in the myometrium during pregnancy; the changes are believed to be exaggerations of similar processes of the menstrual cycle (Theobald, 1968) and are considered to be prerequisites to the generally coordinated activity of the myometrium that is seen during menstruation or labor. Such myometrial organization is accompanied in pregnancy by physiochemical changes in the collagen of the cervix, leading to increased cervical compliance at term (Bryant et al., 1968).

The precise mechanisms by which this kind of molecular process is induced are not understood, but some of the factors that have been implicated include the prostaglandins, oxytocin, the fetus, uterine distention, and estrogen and progesterone.

Fetal Endocrine System

There are indications that the endocrine system of the fetus plays a role in the initiation of labor by way of the fetal pituitary–adrenal pathway. It is known that in normal pregnancy the cortisol levels rise in the fetal circulation and in the amniotic fluid before birth (Silman et al., 1977).

Evidence of fetal endocrine involvement in the initiation of labor has been derived from observations of prolonged pregnancies associated with fetal adrenal and pituitary abnormalities in human and other species. Human pregnancies associated with anencephaly, in the absence of hydramnios, have been the longest pregnancies reported. Gestations of forty-three to fifty-three weeks in five of fifteen incidents of anencephaly without hydramnios were recorded by Comerford (1965). From about the twentieth week of pregnancy, the fetal zone of the adrenal gland in anencephalics undergoes atrophy, resulting in an adrenal gland that is smaller than normal (Benirschke, 1956).

Such observations suggest that the normally functioning fetal adrenal gland has some role in the initiation of labor. However, since labor usually begins soon after intra-uterine fetal death rather than at forty weeks' gestation, adrenal insufficiency alone does not explain prolongation of pregnancy. Rather, the fetal endocrine system may be interrelated with the roles played by estrogen and progesterone (Silman et al., 1977).

Estrogen and Progesterone

For the necessary uterine response of stretching to take place, it is postulated that there must be an optimal relationship of estrogen to progesterone. Estrogen influence is important to the orderly progression of contraction waves from one part of the uterus to the next; progesterone prevents such progression. It has been proposed that the withdrawal of this progesterone block allows stimulation factors to take over, and labor to begin. These stimulation factors include the increased influence of estrogen with concomitant myometrial activity, and the increased release of prostaglandins by the myometrium (Danforth & Hendricks, 1977; Pritchard & MacDonald, 1976).

From studies of the properties of myometrial cells, it appears that a number of pacemakers are contained in a sheet of uterine muscle. Cellular membrane potential is increased by estrogens, thereby decreasing the contraction frequency while increasing the amplitude. Presumably, individual myofibrils contract "all or none," but contraction of the total organ requires that the contraction wave spread to involve other myofibrils. With stimulation of the estrogen-dominated myometrium at any point, there is a spread of the excitation evoked, whereas the myometrium under progesterone domination contracts only at the point stimulated. Hence, during pregnancy the myometrial tendency to conduct an impulse over its surface disappears, apparently due to progesterone effect. At the end of pregnancy, when the progesterone block is withdrawn, the tendency to conduct impulses is regained (Csapo & Jung, 1963; Woodbury et al., 1963).

Production of estrogen during pregnancy is influenced by the fetal adrenal system. Cortisol and precursors produced by the fetal adrenal gland are converted to estrogen in the placenta. Maternal plasma levels of 17 β-estradiol rise from 2 ng/ml in early pregnancy to 12 ng/ml at term (Munson et al., 1970).

Progesterone production, on the other hand, does not require an intact fetal–placental unit. It is synthesized by the human placenta from the precursor, cholesterol, which is derived from maternal plasma (Hellig et al., 1970). Levels of plasma progesterone gradually increase during pregnancy until a plateau is reached at about thirty-two weeks' gestation (Johansson, 1969).

Oxytocin Stimulation

Around the twentieth week of pregnancy, or shortly thereafter, a physiological increase in spontaneous uterine activity occurs, and is followed by a progressive responsiveness to oxytocin as pregnancy progresses. Because of the increased sensitivity of the uterus to stimulation by parenterally administered oxytocin, there have been postulations that endogenous oxytocin plays a role in the start of labor, but this has not been proved (Silman et al., 1977).

Attempts have been made to delineate the physiological role of oxytocin by observing the course of labor in women who had experienced hypophysectomy and in women with diabetes insipidus. However, reports of these labor observations have not been consistent; some of the women required exogenous oxytocin while others had normal labors. It appeared that some women with diabetes insipidus, who did not secrete vasopressin, retained the ability to secrete oxytocin. Thus, oxytocin may be released directly from the hypothalamus in instances of ablation of the neurohypophysis (Caldeyro-Barcia et al., 1971).

There is evidence of increased maternal pituitary secretion of oxytocin during the latter part of labor. There is also an associated secretion of oxytocin by the fetal neurohypophysis, with the greatest amount at the time of birth, lesser amounts in early labor, and the least in the absence of labor. It has been hypothesized that fetal oxytocin may act directly on the myometrium, either as a result of fetal urinary excretion of oxytocin into the amniotic fluid, or by passage through the umbilical artery. There may be an indirect effect via the pituitary adrenal axis. It has also been suggested that the levels of maternal endogenous oxytocin remain unchanged during pregnancy while the uterine responsiveness to the unchanged levels becomes greater as pregnancy progresses (Silman et al., 1977).

Fetal Membrane Prostaglandins

Recently, there has been interest in the possible role of prostaglandins in the onset of uterine contractions. Higher levels of prostaglandins or their metabolites appear in the blood of women immediately before and during labor and in the amniotic fluid of laboring women. Arachidonic acid, essential to the synthesis of prostaglandins, has been shown to be present in concentrations of eightfold increase in the amniotic fluid of women in labor, and appears to be stored preferentially in the fetal membranes (McDonald et al., 1974).

In addition to the presence in amniotic fluid and decidua; prostaglandins have been demonstrated in menstrual fluid, umbilical cord, endometrium, and human seminal fluid. Although the physiological role of the prostaglandins is unidentified, their possible involvement in the initiation of labor is suggested by an oxytocinlike effect. In a study of blood samples from pregnant women, Karim (1968) found prostaglandins in the blood of women during labor, but not at any other time during pregnancy.

Uterine Distension and Stretch

The stimulus of stretch is provided by the rapidly growing fetus in late pregnancy. The effects of uterine distention and stretch on the beginning of labor are unclear, although distention is considered to be a direct stimulus to uterine activity, along with an associated increase in electrical activity. It has been shown that progesterone depresses, and estrogen enhances, this activity (Danforth & Hendricks, 1977).

PHYSIOLOGY OF LABOR

Uterine Contractions

Physiological Basis

Whatever the influence triggering the onset of labor it eventually acts on the contractile elements of the uterine myometrium. Free calcium is believed to induce contraction of uterine smooth muscle as it does in striated muscle; evidence suggests the existence of bound calcium in smooth muscle. Released to the myofibril of the uterine muscle from a binding-storage site in the surrounding sarcoplasmic reticulum, calcium may induce a muscle contraction by interacting with myofibril proteins, and then returning to the storage system. The process leading to an increased intracellular concentration of liberated calcium may be the inhibitory action of prostaglandin E_2 and prostaglandin $F_{2\alpha}$: by preventing the binding of calcium to the sarcoplasmic reticulum, uterine contractions may be initiated (Carsten, 1968; Pritchard & MacDonald, 1976).

Measurement

In attempts to learn more about uterine contractility, numerous methods have been used to measure uterine activity, ranging from electrical or mechanical instrumentation to clinical assessment by palpation. Variations in results may be due to differences of systems, site of recording instruments, or to the differences in uterine activity of individual women in labor. Direct or indirect instrumentation methods may be employed; instrumental measurement of any kind of uterine contractility is generally known as *tocometry*. These may be external by pressure recording from the abdominal wall, or internal by means of intra-uterine pressure transducers, balloons, and catheters.

Standards for quantitative assessment of uterine activity also vary. In one situation, intensity of a contraction has been defined as the rise in amniotic fluid pressure produced by contractions; tonus may be defined as the lowest or resting pressure between contractions. More exact measures or units of activity, such as the Montevideo unit, express the product of the frequency and intensity of contractions (Serr, 1977).

The measurement of electrical waves to study uterine activity has resulted in the description of two kinds of electrical wave groups—low frequency and high frequency. Low frequency electrical activity has been compared to the resting pressure between contractions, and high frequency to the tetanic contraction. A correlation has been shown between a contraction frequency wave and the clinically palpable uterine firmness; an increased activity has also been recorded in response to emotion, mechanical stimulation of the uterus, and sexual excitement. The changes in electrical activity recorded from the lower uterine segment during labor, prior to and after cervical dilation of 5 cm, indicates the uterus functioning in a unified fashion after 5 cm of dilation with these contractions. Cervical dilation has also been observed to occur more rapidly (Serr).

Characteristics

Overall variability of the involuntary uterine contraction has long been recognized; the degree of individual variability of laboring women has also been demonstrated. However, general characteristics and patterns of activity can be identified.

In the description of contradictions, frequency may be used to refer to the time period from the onset of one contraction to the onset of the next, or to the number of contractions in a ten-minute period. The interval of uterine relaxation between contractions is necessary for adequate uteroplacental blood flow. During the later part of labor this interval may be as short as one to two minutes (Pritchard & MacDonald, 1976).

Intensity of contractions is the *height,* or the rise in intra-uterine pressure as measured in millimeters of mercury (mm Hg). During normal, spontaneous labor this pressure may vary from 25 to 55 mg Hg during the active phase. Duration of contractions during active dilation varies from thirty to ninety seconds, with an average of sixty seconds (Schulman & Romney, 1970).

In most visceral smooth muscle, cephalad or fundal dominance is present. This fundal dominance, rather than the theory of specific site pacemakers that initiate and control rhythmic uterine contractions, may explain contractile waves. With every uterine muscle cell having equal potential as a pacemaker, activation of contractility may begin in a variety of sites and spread according to the receptivity of neighboring cells. The variable duration, as well as intensity of each succeeding contraction, is due to varying activating points. Regularity of intensity and duration tends to increase around the end of the first stage.

Measurements of intensity and duration differential of activity during normal labor in the upper and lower segments of the uterus have shown a gradient of decreasing physiological activity from the fundus to the cervix. Intensity of contractions is greater in the fundal zone than in the midzone, and greater in the midzone than below. Similarly, the duration of contractions

decreases from the fundal zone to the midzone and from the midzone to the area below. Dilation and progress of labor are related to this synchronization of contractions with fundal dominance, or decreasing gradient of activity; in the absence of this gradient or dominance, equalization of intensity and duration of contractions in all zones may occur, with resulting failure of cervical dilation (Pritchard & MacDonald, 1976).

During labor the upper and lower segments of the uterus exhibit distinctly different anatomical and physiological characteristics: the upper segment, due to successive contraction and shortening (retraction) of the muscle fibers with each contraction, becomes thickened, smaller, and maintains sustained contact with the contents in an effort to diminish its size; in response, the lower segment fibers stretch and remain fixed at the greater length attained with each contraction of the upper segment, resulting in a thinning of the lower segment.

The boundary between the uterine segments is known as the *physiologic retraction ring.* This ridge on the inner uterine surface may become prominent in obstructed labor, due to extreme thinning of the lower segment, forming a pathological retraction ring.

Cervical Changes

If the membranes remain intact, the force of uterine contractions exerts hydrostatic pressure through the membranes and against the lower uterine segment and cervix; if membranes have ruptured, the presenting part exerts this downward pressure. The hydrostatic pressure in the amniotic cavity rises to about 60 mm Hg at the peak of a normal contraction, while as much as 200 mm Hg pressure may be exerted against the largest diameter of the fetal head in contact with the lower segment.

With this downward pressure the membranes are pouched into the cervical canal; the combined factors help in the development of the lower uterine segment and the thinning of the cervix effacement. The combination of the hydrostatic action of the amniotic sac and uterine contractions produces a wedgelike pressure on the cervix and helps to effect dilation. Normally, there is a loosening of the attachment of the fetal membranes in the lower segment during early labor to facilitate dilation. When the cervix is completely effaced or "drawn up" into the lower segment, only the external os remains. When complete dilation of the cervix is achieved it often rises out of reach, and with the descent of the fetal head there is a retraction of the cervix, possibly as high as the pelvic inlet plane. The uterine supports (fascia and ligaments) are then involved in providing the resistance against which the uterus works to propel the baby through the birth canal.

Rupture of the Membranes

The fetus is enclosed in a sac known as *the membranes,* or *bag of waters,* which comprises the inner amnion and outer chorion layers; a portion of the sac is uncovered by the dilating cervix and may pouch into the cervical opening. With the progression of cervical dilation, the intact membranes may bulge through the os. However, if there is a snug fit between the fetal head and the lower segment and adherent membranes, there may be no protrusion. Usually, intact membranes become tense under the increasing pressure and protrude or bulge through the os during, and relax between, contractions.

Frequently, the spontaneous rupture of membranes occurs during the course of labor, although they may rupture before the beginning of contractions or ongoing cervical dilation. If they remain unruptured throughout the birth, the infant is said to be born in the "caul," which must be removed from the head immediately at birth to allow breathing.

Often the spontaneous rupture occurs at the height of a contraction and is accompanied by a gush of water of variable quantity that is normally clear, colorless, or mildly rubid in appearance. In advanced labor the spontaneous rupture of membranes may be accompanied by descent of the fetus lower into the pelvis.

Pelvic Floor and Vagina

The passage of the fetus through the birth canal is resisted during the first stage of normal labor by the soft, lower portions of the uterus and during the second stage by the vagina and pelvic floor. This resistance offered by soft tissues is to a large extent dependent on the size of the presenting part.

The functional closure and support of the birth canal is performed by several layers of tissue forming the pelvic floor. One of the more important of these is the levator ani muscle, because of its function in closing the vagina. The levator ani muscle begins to stretch when the fetal head passes through the cervix and rests on the pelvic floor; the muscle bundles separate, and along with the vaginal mucosa and perineal skin, allow the vaginal canal to stretch to an adequate circumference to permit the passage of the fetal head.

Acid–Base Metabolism

Hyperventilation, with an associated decrease in carbon dioxide tension and increase in oxygen tension, is a maternal response to uterine contraction that frequently results in a moderate hypocapnia. Characteristically, a small decrease of pH is found at the end of normal labor as a result of metabolic acidosis, which is associated with a parallel increase of lactate concentration (Low, 1977).

The blood lactate concentration has been shown to increase during labor up to the time of birth, with mean values increased to 24 mg% from the initial, normal resting level of 12–13 mg%. The rise continues to about 34 mg% in the first half-hour postpartum, and then decreases again. The blood lactate concentration during muscular work may be considered an index of anaerobic metabolism in the active musculature. In some instances, a moderate to considerable increase of the concentration of blood lactate has been reported to occur in close proximity to the time of birth, possibly indicating the high degree of activation of the relatively small mass of muscles utilized in the second stage of labor (Gemzell et al., 1957).

It has been noted that the body reacts to intermittent muscular work with a marked increase in blood lactate concentration, a decreased mechanical efficiency of muscular work performance, and a corresponding increase in the mean rate of oxygen uptake. The subjective feelings of fatigue and muscular pain in labor may be associated with the intermittent pattern of intense activity (Gemzell et al., 1957). Examination of umbilical vein and artery blood at birth has demonstrated that the response of the normal fetus to normal labor is a slight decrease of pH due to metabolic acidosis, as shown by an increase of base deficit (Low, 1977).

Marx and associates (1969) found that the maternal labor response to apprehension and pain may result in development of abnormal blood gas tensions, possibly as a result of very rapid breathing or with low tidal volumes. Pain relief reportedly reverses this process and improves oxygenation.

In another study of the correlation between painful contractions and hyperventilation, Bonica (1973) noted that in primigravidas with no prenatal psychological preparation and no analgesia or sedation during the first stage of labor, ventilation increased significantly (100 to 350 percent above prelabor ventilation), causing a large but transient reduction of arterial carbon dioxide.

Clinical implications indicate the need for reduction of pain and anxiety of labor through psychological preparation and the elimination or reduction of anxiety- and stress-producing procedures and practices.

The Maternal Cardiovascular System

Throughout pregnancy, the total blood volume is augmented about forty-five percent, with consistent red cell and plasma volume increases. The early increase of cardiac output rises to approximately thirty to fifty percent above nonpregnant levels by twenty-eight weeks' gestation, then decreases in the direction of nonpregnant levels again near term (Hansen & Ueland, 1973).

During labor and birth, cardiovascular changes vary according to the position of the mother, the manner of birth (i.e., vaginal or Cesarean section), the amount of work necessary to give birth, fluid intake of the mother, and the effect of drugs, including anesthetics that may be used (Hansen & Ueland, 1973).

The cardiovascular changes of labor are largely related to maternal apprehension, according to Burch (1977); associated with uterine contractions is a rise in mean heart rate, arterial blood pressure, cardiac output, systemic venous pressure, and right ventricular pressure. Also in connection with uterine contractions is an increase of heart rate ranging in the first stage from 6 to 29 beats/min and in the second stage from 10 to 52 beats/min (Winner & Romney, 1966).

Following birth, maternal heart rate consistently slows by about 5 to 7 beats/min. This bradycardia may continue for about two weeks postpartum (Hollman, 1977).

Frequently associated with first-stage contractions is an elevated blood pressure of 15–37 mm Hg systolic and 5–22 mm Hg diastolic. Increased changes of the second stage and bearing down may raise the systolic pressure by as much as 75 mm Hg (Winner & Romney, 1966).

Hansen and Ueland (1973) reported an average increase in blood pressure of 20 mm Hg systolic and 10 mm Hg diastolic during contractions (maternal supine position), with an increased pulse pressure. They have described the physiological effect of bearing down (Valsalva maneuver) with contractions, noting raised intrathoracic pressure and the drawing of blood from the lungs into the left heart, with an increase of both diastolic and systolic blood pressure. With the continued holding of the breath and the impeded return of blood to the chest, there is a steady drop in the blood pressure with a narrowing of pulse pressure. At the time of release of the breath, the pulmonary vascular beds fill, accompanied by a rapid fall in blood pressure, the degree of which seems to depend on the length of time of breath-holding. This decrease of pressure due to breath-holding release occurs at the end of the contraction and simultaneously with the decreased uterine perfusion with blood, thus compounding the lowered oxygenation of the fetus at that time. There is an evident cumulative effect on the degree of blood pressure elevation, with subsequent efforts of breath-holding and bearing down, but no greater increase of intrathoracic pressure.

Cardiac output undergoes considerable change during labor. Recent studies have shown that with each uterine contraction there is an increase in cardiac output, accumulative to a maximum of eighty percent after vaginal birth with local anesthesia. The cardiac output has been found to decline only slightly at one hour postpartum, even in the face of estimated blood loss of 500–600 ml in vaginal birth (Hansen & Ueland, 1973). Immediately postpartum, however, there is a significant rise in cardiac output due primarily to increased venous return to the heart as a result of removal of uterine pressure on the inferior vena cava and the marked decrease in volume of the uteroplacental vascular bed. An increased cardiac effort and left ventricular work continues for at least four days postpartum (Rovinsky, 1977).

Hansen indicates that while maternal posture markedly influences the hemodynamic effect of contractions, pain relief has no significant influence (Hansen & Ueland, 1973). It has also been reported that less prominent variations in cardiac output were found when the squatting position was assumed for labor and the Sims' or left lateral position for the birth (Hansen & Ueland, 1966).

Immediately after birth, rapid changes occur in plasma volume. On the basis of hematocrit changes, Duhring (1962) proposes that there is an immediate postpartum transfer of a volume of plasma to the extravascular from the intravascular compartment (over and above actual loss of blood), and that on the second or subsequent postpartum days there is a return of this plasma to the intravascular compartment. A moderate decrease of red cell volume at time of birth is attributed solely to blood loss (Rovinsky, 1977).

Losses of total blood volume following normal vaginal birth have variously been reported as ranging from 400 to 800 ml, but there is general agreement that restoration of the nonpregnant blood volume occurs by four to six weeks postpartum (Rovinsky, 1977).

Supine Position and Occlusion of the Inferior Vena Cava

When the pregnant woman assumes the supine position during late pregnancy or in labor, she may experience a reaction to occlusion of the inferior vena (the *supine hypotensive syndrome*) characterized by a sudden drop in heart rate, arterial blood pressure, and peripheral resistance. Pallor, complaints of dizziness or faintness, or "not feeling well" frequently accompany this; nausea and vomiting may occur. Scott (1973) considers this to be a vasovagal attack caused by a large drop in cardiac output *(low-flow state)* with a sharp drop in peripheral resistance, heart rate, and arterial blood pressure. Symptoms disappear quickly when the woman is turned on her side, increasing the cardiac output. As vasovagal reflexes are transient in nature, the event is self-limiting (Scott, 1973).

For some pregnant women, inferior vena cava occlusion in late pregnancy may occur without symptoms and without hemodynamic changes, as a result of collateral circulation through the azygos system that permits venous return to continue at a normal level (Scott, 1973).

Changes in the Blood Coagulation Mechanism During Pregnancy

Several of the factors involved in the blood coagulation mechanism are increased during pregnancy, including the procoagulants factor VIII and fibrinogen. One of the most important is the plasma fibrinogen (factor I) content, which averages 300–350 mg/100 ml of blood in nonpregnant women and increases by approximately fifty percent in normal pregnancy to about 450–500 mg/100 ml (Scott, 1978). Such a marked increase in the concentration of fibrinogen contributes to an increased sedimentation· rate in normal pregnancy, a phenomenon that adds to the error-proneness of some laboratory tests performed on the blood during pregnancy, as in the employment of the sedimentation rate for the assessment of the activity of rheumatic heart disease in pregnancy. Also, the prothrombin time as measured by the Quick method is shortened, as is the partial thromboplastin time.

Factors VII, VIII, IX, and X are also found to be increased consistently in normal pregnancy, factors XI and XIII are decreased, and platelets do not seem to change in function or concentration. Even though a number of coagulation factors are increased in pregnancy, no hypercoagulable state has been detected (Scott, 1978). The exertion and stress of labor may contribute to a further increase in the level of factor VIII.

Voiding

Urine will not ordinarily pass into the urethra from the bladder unless the force of expulsion of the bladder musculature equals or exceeds the opposing resistance to urine flow that occurs at the neck of the bladder and in the urethra. Voluntary contractions of the detrusor muscle of the bladder occur as a result of impulses from the stretch receptors in the bladder muscle when the tension in its walls rises above a threshold value; this is known as the *micturition reflex* (Brobeck, 1973; Reid et al., 1972).

The functions of the bladder are to hold and to periodically expel urine under voluntary control. The internal urethral orifice at the neck of the bladder is normally closed due to collagen and elastic tissues in that area; the extension of these tissues down the urethra helps to produce resistance to flow. In the presence of straining, as in the bearing down efforts of labor, the increased intra-abdominal pressure is transmitted equally to the bladder. The high pressure within the bladder may not permit sufficient resistance to flow by the elastic tissues of the urethra to maintain closure. The result is that the bearing down actions are frequently accompanied by small spurts of urine.

Since urine is normally confined to the bladder, leaving the proximal urethra empty, the external urethral sphincter is involved mainly with interruption and termination of the urine flow, and not particularly with the normal state of continence (Brobeck, 1973; Guyton, 1977; Reid et al., 1972). In contrast to the smooth muscle of the bladder, the external sphincter (comprised of the urogenital diaphragm through which the urethra passes at a few centimeters beyond the bladder) is a voluntary skeletal muscle that normally remains tonically contracted by impulses received via the pudendal nerves, but can be voluntarily or reflexly relaxed at the time of voiding. The external sphincter is controlled by the pudic nerve, which originates in the first two sacral segments of the spinal cord. The physiological elements of the bladder, and of voiding, are influenced by altered anatomical relationships during labor (Brubeck, 1973; Ganong, 1975; Guyton, 1977).

The location of the bladder at various stages of labor and the possible effects of the same on the course of labor were investigated by Kantor et al. (1949). They found that the location of the bladder was dependent upon the degree to which the presenting part filled the pelvis.

As determined by cystographic study, the bladder position varies with individual pelvic capacity and the descent of the presenting part, but is unrelated to cervical dilation. In early labor, a large portion of the bladder remains in the pelvis, and until the presenting part is well below the ischial spines, the distended bladder can impede descent; usually, however, it is not obstructive after the presenting part is on or near the pelvic floor, even though a portion of the bladder still remains in the pelvis.

Kantor et al. (1949) also noted that moderate bladder distention did not interfere with delivery of the shoulders or the body of the fetus, and that routine catheterization prior to vaginal delivery (spontaneous or outlet forceps) was unnecessary. They further concluded that emptying of the bladder is essential in early labor to prevent obstruction, but that the presence of some abdominally palpable urine in the bladder just prior to delivery may be physiological and therefore not an indication for catheterization unless hyperdistention is present, since catheterization at this time is technically difficult, is an additional source of pain to the woman, may be traumatizing, and may introduce the potential for bladder infection (Kantor et al., 1949).

The micturition reflex, mediated in the voluntary center for micturition in the cerebral cortex, causes either urination or a conscious desire to void. Generally, the first feeling of a desire to void is experienced as a vague feeling in the perineum when the bladder filling has reached about 150–250 ml. As filling continues and the desire to void intensifies through the feelings of fullness, discomfort, and finally pain, continence is maintained and the spinal reflex center for micturition is inhibited by impulses via the cortico-regulatory tracts preventing efferent impulses from leaving the spinal center. When there is an opportunity to void, this voluntary restraint upon the spinal micturition center is removed and urination occurs automatically. The micturition reflex occurs as a complete single cycle of bladder contraction leading to a rapid and progressive increase in pressure, a period of sustained pressure, and then a cessation of the reflex and rapid lessening of the bladder contraction and a return to basal tonic pressure of the bladder. The bladder normally is completely empty at the end of micturition (Brobeck, 1973; Reid et al., 1972).

If the micturition reflex has occurred but has not succeeded in emptying the bladder, the reflex nervous elements usually remain in an inhibited state for a period of a few minutes to an hour or more before another reflex occurs. Although the reflex is a completely automatic cord reflex, it can be facilitated or inhibited by higher brain centers, which normally exert final control (Guyton, 1977).

The bladder position during labor, and the characteristics of the micturition reflex have clinical care (see section on Bladder Function, under Assessment of Continuing Needs). Clinical applications include the following:

- Prevention of delay or failure to urinate that may be caused by interference with the micturition reflex through inappropriate timing of any necessary activities (e.g., auscultations of fetal heart sounds)
- Facilitation of an atmosphere and environment of normalcy in which fear and anxiety are prevented, and anesthesia and analgesia needs minimized
- Anticipation and attention to the physical and psychological needs and comfort of the woman, including her ability to go to the bathroom and void in the normal manner
- Observation of the bladder status frequently, with reminders to void, and with use of measures to encourage voiding if the administration of a regional anesthesia has obtunded bladder sensations and impaired bladder emptying
- Consideration of the stage of labor and the position of the presenting part when assessing the status of the bladder, prior to the use of interventive measures to empty the bladder—possibly unnecessarily (e.g., when catheterization is being considered during the latter part of second-stage labor when there is only moderate bladder distention and labor progress is consistent)

Gastric Motility and Emptying

Emptying of the stomach is partially controlled by the degree of filling of the stomach and the activity of stomach peristalsis. Probably more important are feedback signals from the duodenum, including the enterogastric reflex and hormonal feedback. In general, stimulation of the parasympathetic nerves produces increased muscle activity, while stimulation of the sympathetic nerves usually results in decreased, or inhibited, activity.

The rate at which food leaves the stomach is determined by a combination of factors, including the total volume, consistency, pH, osmolar concentration, and chemical composition of the gastric contents (Brobeck, 1973).

It has been found that, for any type of meal, and for any individual, amount of evacuation in a particular unit of time depends on the volume; i.e., the greater the volume of material in the stomach at any particular time, the greater the rate of gastric emptying. This relationship between gastric volume and rate of emptying is due to stimulation of mechanoreceptors in the stomach wall in proportion to the degree of distention, with brain-mediated impulses resulting in vagal stimulation of gastric contraction (Brobeck, 1973; Guyton, 1977).

A comparison of liquids with solids reflects the effect of consistency on the rate of emptying. Inert liquids, which do not stimulate either osmotically or chemically, leave the stomach rapidly. For example, water begins to leave the stomach almost as soon as it enters, while solids are not normally evacuated until they are reduced to a semifluid or fluid state (Brobeck, 1973; Ganong, 1975).

It is known that strong acid solutions leave the stomach slowly, and that neutralization of the acid accelerates the rate of emptying. In like manner, osmolar concentrations can affect emptying time, as has been demonstrated by the slow emptying of gastric contents made hypotonic or hypertonic with respect to the blood. The type of food eaten also affects the emptying rate: food rich in carbohydrate leaves the stomach in a few hours; protein-rich food leaves more slowly, and fat empties most slowly (Guyton, 1977; Mountcastle, 1974; Selkurt, 1976).

Various factors (e.g., fats, hydrogen ions) exert an inhibitory effect by acting through a reflex involving the vagus nerves (the enterogastric reflex) or through a hormone (enterogastrone), or both. Stressful stimuli have been shown to have variable effects on gastric secretion. Epinephrine and norepinephrine, secreted in large amounts during some stresses, inhibit gastric secretion. Fear and anxiety have been associated with slowing of gastric emptying (Ganong, 1975; Mountcastle, 1974; Selkurt, 1976).

During pregnancy the enlarging uterus causes some changes in the position of the stomach and intestines. The stomach is rotated to the right and displaced upward in a somewhat horizontal position, along with upward movement of the large intestine. Gastric motility has been considered to be decreased during pregnancy and labor. There also tends to be a lowered gastric acidity level during pregnancy, possibly due to acidic neutralization by the duodenal contents rather than to an actual decrease in secretion of hydrochloric acid. Gastric emptying time has been reported to be slowed during active labor, and to be further prolonged by narcotic analgesics (Davision et al., 1970; Reid et al., 1972) (see section on Nutritional and Fluid Needs).

USUAL MECHANISM OF LABOR

The *mechanism of labor* is the term applied to the movements that the fetus undergoes in accommodating itself to the irregularly shaped birth canal under the influences of the forces of labor and of gravity. Since not all diameters of the mature fetal head are capable of passing through all diameters of the pelvis, a process of accommodation of certain diameters of the head to particular portions of the pelvic cavity is necessary. In negotiating the birth canal, there is initial movement downward and backward to the level of the ischial spines; at this location of bony attachment of the muscles of the pelvic floor, the direction changes and movement of the presenting part proceeds downward and forward. The passage of the fetus through the pelvis is due to the downward push of each uterine contraction, which causes the passive descent against the resistance of the bony pelvis and soft tissues.

The main movements involved in the normal labor mechanism for the head to traverse the pelvis in the occiput positions are *descent, flexion, internal rotation, extension,* and *external restitution* (Figure 6-1). These constitute a combination of movements taking place at the same time.

Since there are many variations of pelvic shape and size, the mechanism is not exactly the same for each pelvis. Other variables that influence the passage of the head through the pelvis are (1) the anterior curvature of the birth canal; (2) the degree of disproportion between size of the pelvis and fetal head size; some relative disproportion can be overcome by extremely efficient uterine forces and molding of the head; and (3) the degree of flexion of the head.

These mechanisms rest on the assumptions of an average-sized female pelvis, efficient uterine contractions, adequate flexion of the head, average amount of molding, occiput presentation, and a baby large enough to utilize the available pelvic space, but not too large. The characteristics of the major pelvic shapes (gynecoid, android, platypelloid, and anthropoid) also influence the labor mechanism to a great extent, since the inlet shape largely determines the position of engagement when available space is utilized, as in the occurrence of occiput transverse positions in the flat or platypelloid type of pelvis.

Two significant principles in determining changes of the fetal head position in its movement through the birth canal are (1) the occiput tends to rotate to that portion of the pelvis that has the greatest space at any given level, and (2) the narrowest presenting diameter (biparietal) of the head must go through the narrowest pelvic diameter at any given level.

LABOR POSITIONS

Positions, or postures, for labor and birth are debated as to their relative cultural significance, safety, benefits, convenience, labor effectiveness, comfort, and evolutionary aspects. Some studies raise questions about

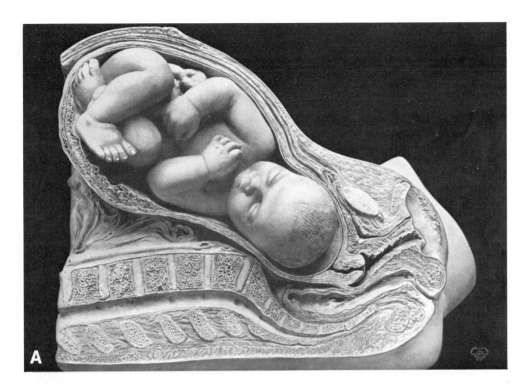

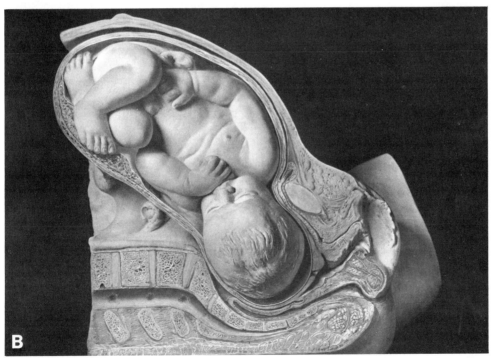

FIGURE 6-1 Usual mechanism of labor with average-sized female pelvis and vertex presentation. (A) The head approaches engagement in the occiput transverse position. (B) *Flexion* increases, along with *descent* into the midpelvis, permitting the relatively small suboccipitobregmatic diameter of the head to present. (C) *Internal rotation* to the occiput anterior position begins. (D) With further descent, the head negotiates the pelvic curve by *extension*, and the occiput passes through the outlet. (E) By further extension, the sinciput sweeps along the posterior (sacral) portion of the birth canal so that the bregma, forehead, nose, mouth, and chin in sequence are born over the perineum. (F) The head undergoes *restitution* back to resume its former relationship with the shoulders, which traversed the pelvis in oblique diameter without rotating. As the shoulders rotate to the anteroposterior diameter of the pelvis, the head further *rotates externally* to continue the normal relationship with the shoulders and assume its former occiput transverse position. (From the Maternity Center Association (1968). *Usual mechanisms of labor.* New York: Birth Atlas. With permission.) *(Continued on pp. 120–121.)*

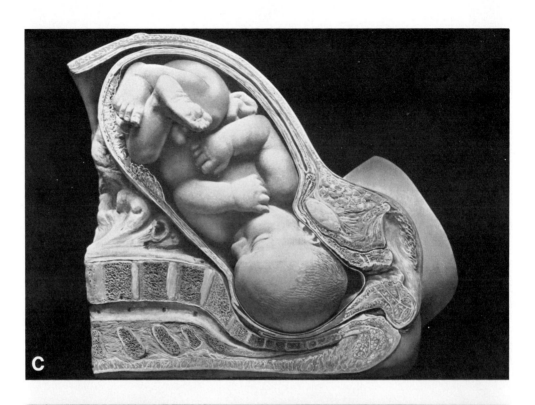

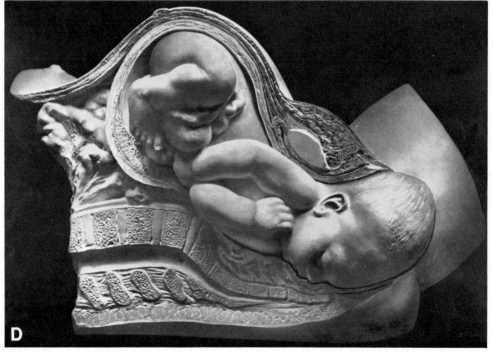

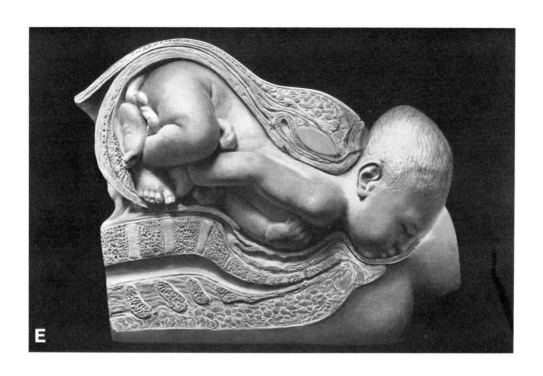

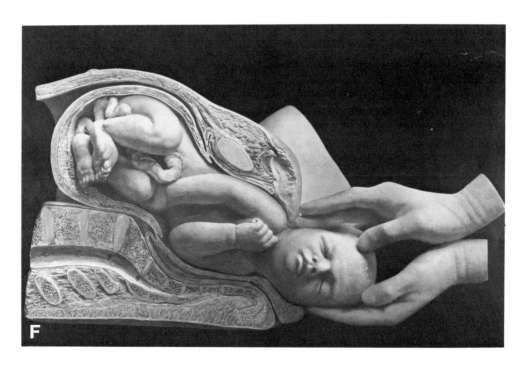

what have become "traditional" positions for labor and birth in this country.

As a basis for the following discussion, the types of positions are divided into two broad categories: *vertical* and *horizontal*. Vertical positions include (1) standing, (2) squatting, (3) kneeling, and (4) sitting. Horizontal positions include (1) supine (dorsal, recumbent), (2) knee-chest or knee-elbow, (3) semirecumbent, (4) prone, and (5) lateral. Variations of the horizontal positions include (1) head-down (Trendelenburg), (2) lithotomy or exaggerated lithotomy, (3) lateral prone, and (4) hanging-leg (Atwood, 1976; Dunn, 1976, 1978; Irwin, 1978; McManus & Calder, 1978; Smyth, 1974). Historically, the evolution of many of the variant positions follows the evolution of practices of the early accoucheurs (man–midwives) and later science of Western obstetrics.

The field of Western obstetrics is considered by some to be a culture by virtue of its learned behavior patterns that have become accepted practice that is universally used and passed on to succeeding generations. The behavior patterns that have become associated with childbirth, and positions for birth are a part of the culture to which the laboring woman does not belong. This then becomes a matter of an outsider accepting the cultural behaviors expected within the cultural environment in which she seeks help with childbirth (Atwood, 1976; Dunn, 1976; Smyth, 1974).

From an anthropological viewpoint, a review of the evolution of positions related to birth, with comparisons of cultural similarities, differences, and changes over a period of time does not permit inferences to be drawn, but does suggest the following instructive impressions:

- The selected posture of the mother for birth is determined by culturally resultant behaviors, not by physiological processes.
- The adaptability of the human female permits a variety of birth positions.
- There is no single "correct" position for birth.
- The negative and positive aspects of each position should be weighed with respect to its effects on the individual and as an integral part of cultural influences.
- Most of the parturitional positions developed by obstetricians are related to obstetrical complications.
- Data suggest that prior to contact with Western medicine the majority of primitive cultures used a vertical (upright) position for birth.
- A comprehensive consideration of birth positions requires that both the cultural and physiological aspects of childbirth be acknowledged.

- There is a generally recognized paucity of knowledge with respect to labor and birth postures.
- If the structure of the health care community and obstetrical culture does not accept mutual and informed decision making and the woman's options for alternatives, she may opt increasingly for birth settings and birth attendants that are not part of the obstetrical culture (Atwood, 1976; Haire, 1972; Rothman, 1977).

Fetal–Maternal Safety

Supine position during labor and birth has been associated with decreased contraction intensity and less efficient uterine contractility, lowered cord blood pH, increased duration of cervical dilation, and maternal hypotension with reduced cardiac output known as the *inferior vena cava occlusion syndrome* (Caldeyro-Barcia, 1976; Haire, 1972; Irwin, 1978; Wood, 1976). The problems of supine hypotension are discussed in detail elsewhere and are not repeated here; this same syndrome is found in relation to the lithotomy position (Atwood, 1976; Caldeyro-Barcia et al., 1960). Further, the lithotomy position has been implicated in prolonged stirrup and strap pressures on the popliteal area of the legs, which may lead to thrombosis in leg veins or nerve damage, particularly of the peroneal nerve. Continued pressure on the lateral aspect of the knee from the weight of the leg itself on the stirrup or knee crutch has been enough in some instances to produce peroneal nerve injuries. Additional leaning on the leg by an attendant adds to the possible injury (Hunter et al., 1954).

Back, hip, and leg pain following the use of stirrups has been found to be a result of arching of the lumbosacral area in association with abduction and outward rotation of the thighs. Arching is produced by stretching of the abductors of the thigh (attached to the pubic rami) and the stretching of the iliopsoas (attached to the lesser trochanteric area of the femur) and capsule of the hip joint. Resulting strains and pulls cause disability and discomfort that is not radiographically demonstrable (Hunter et al., 1954).

The position of the mother has been linked to significant cord blood pH differences as reported by Wood (1976). Comparing dorsal and tilted positions, a definite fall in cord pH was associated with mothers who were in the dorsal position during second-stage labor; this was not found in those instances in which the mothers were in a tilted position.

Following labor and birth in a thirty-degree upright position compared with recumbent posture, no significant difference was noted by Liu (1974) in one-minute Apgar scores of the experimental and control groups of newborn infants. Irwin (1978) reported that Apgar scores at one and five minutes of life for 102 infants born vaginally with the mother in the left lateral position suggested no fetal compromise traceable to the position or method of delivery.

Requirement of forceps delivery has been found to be less frequent among women who labor in an upright position than with women laboring in a recumbent position (Caldeyro-Barcia, 1976).

Efficiency of Labor

Uterine efficiency has been found to be higher in the laboring woman when she is vertical (standing up) when compared to horizontal (lying in bed) (Caldeyro-Barcia, 1976). When comparing lateral and supine positions for labor, it is reported that uterine contractions have a greater intensity and a lower frequency when the woman lies on her side than when she lies on her back. Contractions also appear to be better coordinated and uterine tonus lower in the lateral position. The decreased tonus may be due to the diminished frequency of contractions, which allows more time for uterine relaxation. This observation has useful clinical application in reducing excessive uterine contractility and tonus by placing the woman in the lateral position. While the mechanisms by which position changes affect uterine contractility are unknown, Caldeyro-Barcia et al. (1976) note that "the characteristics of the contractions suggest that those produced when the patient lies on her side should be more efficient for the progress of labor than those produced when the patient lies on her back."

In comparison of standing and supine positions, Mendez and co-workers (1975) found the intensity of contractions to be significantly higher, and the frequency to be diminished in women laboring in the standing position. They also found the mean duration of labor was shorter for normal nulliparas than the reported standard clinical experience and the published data showed. No clear arguments were found against the use of the standing position for labor.

A higher intensity and greater regularity of frequency, with no significant difference in duration of uterine contractions, was found among women laboring and giving birth in a thirty-degree upright position than among women in a flat, recumbent position. Shorter first and second stages of labor were also reported in the upright position (Liu, 1974).

Utilization of the gravitational force is not well documented, but has been considered to be sufficient to supply much of the force required for descent of the baby through the birth canal when the mother is in an upright position (Dunn, 1978). Some have contended that the horizontal positions (supine, lithotomy) tend to negate the natural forces of gravity and the pelvic axis in aiding passage of the baby through the birth canal, and to increase the need for the use of forceps, episiotomy, and fundal pressure, particularly in the presence of regional anesthetics (Dunn, 1976; Haire, 1972; Smyth, 1974).

Comfort

The left lateral Sims' position for childbirth has been cited as having the particular advantage of comfort. It represents a natural sleep position, eliminates restriction of movements associated with the use of stirrups, avoids hypotension, and efforts to bear down are not inhibited. Greater relaxation of the perineal muscles and skin result from extension of the leg on one side, decreasing the need for episiotomy. Generally, the laboring women can remain in this position for relatively long periods of time with physiological safety and comfort (Irwin, 1978).

There are reports of greater overall comfort and less pain with contractions in both standing and sitting positions, rather than recumbent (Dunn, 1978; Mendez-Bauer et al., 1975). Leg cramping is common when the mother is placed in the lithotomy position with leg stirrups.

Another effect of the lithotomy position is the psychological vulnerability involved; the dimensions and effect of this are immeasurable and have been largely neglected. This position also causes concern (not unfounded) to the mother about the possibility of her baby being dropped when her buttocks are projecting over the edge of the delivery table.

Convenience to the Birth Attendant

It has been postulated that the customary use of the supine position for childbirth originated with the beginning use of forceps, and has continued as an obstetrical convenience. The possible need for forceps or other intervention at the time of birth is still given as a reason to continue the traditional lithotomy position.

Other reasons cited in support of the lithotomy position include (1) feces contamination of the area can be prevented more easily; (2) maintenance of asepsis is made easier; (3) the fetal heart can be auscultated without difficulty; (4) anesthetic management is better facilitated; (5) management and control of the second and third stages are easier; (6) episiotomy and repair can be accomplished more readily; and (7) physicians are not trained to work with the mother in other positions.

The appropriate position for labor and birth, barring a threat to the well-being of the mother or baby, is the position that each woman indicates "feels right" for her. Nursing care should be based on the woman's choices as labor progresses, and should accommodate her needs and choices by altering or facilitating the labor environment, while continuing with nonintrusive clinical surveillance of both mother and baby.

The mother may decide that a squatting position feels better at certain times during labor than does being in bed. Or, she may find that walking to a kitchen or refreshment area and having some nourishment provides for greater relaxation and calm. Women who are experiencing intense low-back pain associated with posterior presentation of the baby often experience relief when encouraged to try nontraditional positions, such as standing and leaning forward on a comfortable prop. She may choose to spend her entire labor out of bed. On the other hand, she may choose to be in bed.

The nurse can assess labor changes and progress, or lack of it, by observation of psychological responses, facial reactions, physical responses associated with transition, the beginning urge to bear down, and so on, rather than totally depending on vaginal examinations, which require that the woman lie down. By working with, not against, the mother's choice of activities and positions for labor, the nurse facilitates her ability to work with the forces of labor rather than against them.

NORMAL PROGRESS OF LABOR

Prelabor Course

Cervical Dilation

The prelabor period, or last four weeks of pregnancy, constitutes a time when physiological preparation for labor is beginning for many women. Cervical changes take place; the lower uterine segment is being prepared for labor, with progressive cervical effacement and dilation resulting from the intermittent, irregular uterine contractions commonly experienced. Prelabor dilation, along with the initial rate of dilation, may actually be predictive of the outcome of labor.

Rather than beginning labor at 0 cm dilation of the cervix, it has been documented that during the last three days prior to the onset of labor the average cervical dilation for nulliparas is found to be 1.8 cm and for multiparas is 2.2 cm. At the time of the first examination during labor, cervical dilation averages 2.5 cm for the nullipara and 3.5 cm for the multipara. As a rule, the nulliparous cervix is found to efface more rapidly but dilate less rapidly than the multiparous cervix over the three-day prelabor period.

Lightening

Lightening, or the settling of the fetal presenting part into the upper pelvis, may occur several weeks before the onset of labor, particularly among Caucasion primigravidas. Descent of the presenting part occurs in conjunction with the development and elongation of the lower uterine segment and cervical effacement.

The mother may feel the baby "drop" and may note a change of abdominal shape, and the ability to breath easier due to lessened pressure on the diaphragm. At the same time she often experiences greater frequency of urination and more pelvic region discomfort as the presenting part presses on the pelvic structures.

False Labor

In *false (prodromal) labor* the contractions are usually irregular and of short duration, possibly with discomfort that is confined to the lower abdomen and groin areas; these may occur with some regular contractions of two- to three-minute intervals followed by scattered, less intense contractions at ten-minute or longer intervals. Often the discomfort is lessened by walking. This irregular contraction pattern and the obviously more regular contractions of the latent phase of early labor, are not accompanied by the progressive cervical dilation that occurs during active labor.

By contrast, *true labor* manifests by cervical dilation, the fundamental clinical phenomenon of the first stage of labor. Contractions of true labor usually begin in the fundal region of the uterus and radiate over the uterus and to the lower back. The pattern of contractions is regular, with a progressive increase of duration and frequency.

In the event of false labor, or even mistaken evidence of ruptured membranes, the woman's (and companions') long awaited start of labor and its attached anxieties, relief, and expectations suddenly become crushed and subdued. The feelings of letdown and disappointment require that the woman and her companions be reassured that seeking advice was the right thing to do. She needs to be given an opportunity to vent her disappointment, frustration, or anger. She also needs to know that it is often equally difficult for those providing care to differentiate between false and true labor. She should be encouraged to seek advice again under similar circumstances and at any time she feels the need, and to utilize comfort measures to relax tense muscles, such as a warm bath and backrub. (See Friedman (1978) for further discussion of differences between primiparous and multiparous labors.)

Labor Course

Labor can be defined as the complex integration of physiological, biomechanical, and psychological work, with synchronized efforts directed toward the bearing of an infant through the birth canal. There are four stages:

- *First stage* (dilation of the cervix): the onset of a regular pattern of contractions (five- to ten-minute frequency) accompanied by progressive dilation of the cervix, ending with complete cervical dilation
- *Second stage* (birth): complete dilation of the cervix, ending with the completed birth of the baby
- *Third stage* (placenta): complete birth of the baby, ending when the placenta and membranes are expelled
- *Fourth stage* (immediate postdelivery period) (see Chapter 10)

Labor Length

First and Second Stages

The cervix is usually dilated 1–3 cm when labor begins. It is relatively common for first labors to be completed (active phase with progressive dilation) within eight hours and subsequent labors within three to six hours. However, there may be a latent period of one to eight hours or more in which contractions of variable patterns of intensities may occur without dilating the cervix.

The relationships between the presenting part and its size, the amount of resistance to be overcome, and the quality of uterine contractions determine the duration of second-stage labor. In the nullipara, or the multipara with a large baby, a considerably longer period of bearing down may be necessary than in the instance of the multipara with a small baby. A second-stage duration of more than one to two hours can be considered to be prolonged. Duration of the second stage can be quite variable, but the median time for nulliparas is fifty minutes and for multiparas twenty minutes.

It should be stressed that parameters are established only to serve as guidelines for assessment of progress and of potential problems (see Figure 6-3). Fetal and maternal response to the labor process is the primary significant factor in determining what variations of time periods and processes are normal for the individual labor. One baby may tolerate a two-hour second stage with no difficulties, while another may have problems with thirty minutes or one hour of second-stage labor. The same applies to other stages. Progress of labor and care of the laboring woman must be clinically monitored and determined by data presented by the individual mother and baby and not by averages and charts.

INTRAPARTUM CARE

Initial Contact

The first contact that the laboring woman and her labor partner has with the nurse or other attendants sets the tone and foundation for the subsequent working relationship throughout the duration of labor, birth, and the period thereafter. The first minutes can affect not only their response to the entire childbirth experience, but their reponse to the newborn as well.

Once labor has begun, and the initial status of the labor is found to be normal or low risk, there are four principal areas of nursing involvement: (1) *care and comfort* of the mother and her partner or others she chooses to be with; (2) *safety of mother and baby* through consistent clinical surveillance of the status of both; (3) *facilitation of the environment* to make it conducive to the support of all relationships involved in the labor (mother, father, baby, or others); and, possibly assuming the role of labor partner and primary support person in those instances when family or others do not assume this role; and (4) *appropriate nonintervention,* or knowing when to do nothing, except be available.

It is emphasized that these are priority bases of care of the normal mother in labor, and all subsequent discussion of helping and caring for the laboring woman will rest on these. The surveillance of the well-being of the mother and baby during normal labor emphasized here is the utilization of sharpened clinical assessment skills (eyes, ears, and hands) in the evaluation of labor to determine deviations from the expected or normal range of events, and then to guide the need for, and judicious use of, technological surveillance and measures of intervention when indications exist.

Initial screening (physical and psychosocial) of the normal laboring woman and baby should proceed in an unrushed, nonobtrusive, and noninterfering manner to reduce anxiety and facilitate the woman's undisturbed continuation of control over herself, her labor, her environment, and the general atmosphere of the labor (see case studies in later sections). The nurse's introduction of herself and her *role* is a good place to begin. The woman and her labor partner should be told the name by which the nurse prefers to be called, and the nurse should find out how these individuals wish to be addressed. This name identification of the laboring woman is of even greater significance when support and companionship during labor is solely the responsibility of the nurse. If this is clarified early on, it may benefit verbal communications and her responsiveness later in labor.

An introduction of the woman and her companion to the physical environment, and their understanding that it is to be adapted by them to their needs (rather than the needs of attendants or the health care facility) facilitates their developing a comfortable, individualized "territory" of their own for their birth experience. Judgments about priorities can be accomplished jointly without pressuring or rushing the woman. Most women will give birth without problems regardless of perineal shaving, enema, "putting to bed," or other routine procedures. These can be eliminated in deference to the true priorities of assessing and facilitating the physical and emotional well-being of mother and baby.

Prenatal Record and Labor

Either before or upon arrival of the woman and her labor partner the nurse, nurse–midwife, or other labor and birth attendants can be quickly reviewing the prenatal record, which should always be easily accessible at the onset of labor.

Immediate prenatal information of note includes gravidity, parity, age, expected date of confinement (EDC), last normal menstrual period (LNMP), present week of pregnancy, past labors and births (including size of baby, duration of labor, problems of mother or baby), and any risk factors or indicators of the kind of labor that may be anticipated. This record could also contain the plan of care or contract with attendants for labor and birth care, plus such information as the preference for feeding the baby, plans for keeping or giving up the baby, past health history (including surgery), indications of specific needs for support or reassurances during labor, allergies, status concerning blood transfusions, and laboratory findings.

Prenatal laboratory findings provide indices of the woman's general health status at the outset of labor and a baseline for comparison of any studies that may be necessary to repeat during labor (see Chapter 3).

Of these tests, the relationship of several to the intrapartum period should be noted:
- *Hemoglobin* The usual level is 11.0 g/100 ml or higher (higher at higher altitudes) near term of healthy pregnant women.
- *Hematocrit* The usual level is thirty-three percent or higher (higher at higher altitudes) in the latter weeks of pregnancy. Reassessment at the onset of labor,

or during the course of labor is sometimes done to detect hidden bleeding, a drop due to iron malabsorption or failure to take iron. Maternal anemia, if severe, may result in lowered fetal iron stores. In acute anemia of recent onset there is greater potential for fetal distress during labor, while with chronic anemia the baby tends to tolerate labor.
- *White Blood Cell Count* A white blood cell rise to 12,000 before labor and to 25,000 or more during labor and immediately after birth may be normal. The cause of this markedly increased leukocyte count in labor is unknown but resembles the leukocyte increase accompanying strenuous exercise.
- *Urine Examination for Glucose, Albumin, and Acetone* When done at the initial assessment in labor, and at intervals during labor, it provides early warning of developing problems. Findings during labor should also be compared with those of the prenatal course. Presence of albumin of +1 or more may be due to such factors as preeclampsia, vaginal contamination of the specimen, abnormal kidney function, or urinary tract infection. When albumin is present, the cause should be sought, including careful attention to blood pressure, edema, and central nervous system responses (tendon reflexes) during labor if evidence of preeclampsia is developing. Glycosuria may be present, particularly if intravenous dextrose solutions are used. Ketonuria or acetonuria may reflect a starvation state and indicate a need for administration of oral or intravenous glucose solutions.
- *Blood Group and Rh* Determination of Rh and blood type allows for identification of potential candidates for Rh-immune globulin after childbirth and for ABO incompatibility. The prenatal screening for atypical antibodies may also alert the nurse during labor to the presence of certain antibodies creating the possibility of great difficulty in the cross-matching of blood in the event that it should be needed.
- *Serology* This is done to detect and allow for treatment of syphilis before it affects the fetus.

Current History

After assessment of the prenatal course it is necessary to gather further information by history and by examination in order to establish normalcy of labor at the present time. The current history is primarily concerned with the beginning of labor and the period of time since the last prenatal assessment.

History of the onset of labor is determined by the mother's account of when the contractions became regular and stronger, usually with about five- to ten-minute frequency. Other factors for assessing labor are listed in Exhibit 6-1.

EXHIBIT 6-1 History of labor onset: Assessment factors

Contractions
- Frequency.
- Duration.
- Time when contractions developed regular patterns.
- Perceived intensity: Are they bothersome? Beyond distractibility?
- Where contractions are felt: Lower abdomen only? As a radiating to the back region? Only in back?

Other signs or symptoms
- "Show" of blood-streaked mucus discharge vaginally.
- When she last slept and ate.
- Loss of fluid from vagina (either as sudden gush or as sensation of continuous leaking), indicating rupture of membranes; if so, when?
- Loose stools associated with beginning signs and symptoms of labor is relatively common.
- Anything that has bothered her in the past days or weeks, and possibly since her last prenatal examination.

Any recent problems
- Vaginal bleeding.
- Unusual pain.
- Unusual edema.
- Recent need to take any drugs.

Overall physical assessment
- Height and weight (from prenatal record).
- Blood pressure.
- Temperature.
- Pulse and respirations.
- Weight: a decrease often indicates onset of labor; an increase may be a sign of toxemia.
- Observe for edema and a blood pressure elevation.
- Abdominal examination for:
    Height of uterine fundus; lie, presentation, and position of fetus by palpation; estimate of size of baby in relation to amount of amniotic fluid; palpations done gently *between* contractions.
    Presence of palpable contractions; relaxation of uterus between contractions.

Presence of auscultated fetal heart sounds (FHS) between 120–160 beats/min; where maximal FHS is located.
- Inspection of extremities for:
    Edema.
    Presence of varices.
    Neurological response (signs of hyperreflexia).
- Vaginal examination for:
    Status of cervix: dilation, effacement, position, consistency.
    Presenting part and position.
    Station.
    Palpability of protruding or bulging membranes through cervical os.
- Detection of ruptured membranes: If there is a question of possible rupture of membranes, there are several means of attempting detection. First, observe for leakage of amniotic fluid from the vaginal orifice. Second, observe the escape of amniotic fluid from the cervical os with speculum examination. Third, test the acidity or alkalinity of the vaginal fluid by nitrazene test. The normal pH of vaginal secretions ranges from 4.5 to 5.5, while that of the amniotic fluid is more alkaline, about 7.0 to 7.5. This can be checked by inserting a sterile cotton-tipped applicator into the vagina, touching it to a piece of nitrazene paper, and comparing with a color chart to determine whether it has changed to the blue-green to deep blue colors of the alkaline range, indicating probable rupture of membranes. This test may also be done by placing nitrazene paper against the upper vaginal mucosa, preferably in the posterior fornix, through a speculum, and observing color of the paper. A false reading is likely in the presence of intact membranes but a large amount of bloody show, since blood, like amniotic fluid, is alkaline. Fourth, look for "ferning" in vaginal material that is placed on a slide, allowed to dry, and viewed under the microscope. The presence of ferns, or a frondlike crystalline pattern, is caused by the sodium chloride present in the amniotic fluid and suggests ruptured membranes; blood will interfere with the ferning.

Psychosocial Assessment

The significance to labor of psychosocial elements of the woman's life pertains primarily to the presence or absence of self-strengths and the supportive strengths provided by others whom she chooses to be with her in labor; and the manner in which the nurse can best complement these strengths or intervene in their absence. Some of the factors that warrant consideration are shown in Exhibit 6-2.

Unspoken needs require sensitive nursing assessment and interventive actions in order to prevent growing anxiety, and to establish feedback from the mother to guide the nurse and labor partner in their efforts to help. The need for information is frequently greatest when information is not requested. Even for those who have prepared themselves for the childbirth experience, the stresses of normal labor tend to strain the usual communicative abilities, behavioral response patterns, and means of relating to others.

The importance of self-control, not only by the mother but by those in attendance to her, was noted by Grantly Dick-Read (1946). The persons surrounding the laboring woman have the potential to help prevent, or to cause, disruptive effects on her mental state, and

EXHIBIT 6-2 *Psychosocial assessment factors*

- What is the initial impression of her manner of dealing with the present situation of labor?
- Does she seem to be able to communicate concerns or needs to either the nurse or her labor partner?
- Is there information available from the prenatal record concerning any psychological or social situations that might have bearing on intrapartum events? For example: major changes in the living situation, relationships and lifestyle, work or financial situations, child care problems, indications of feelings about the pregnancy and parenthood, special concerns about labor or the baby.
- What comments or other clues does she give concerning her outlook on this time and event in her life?
- Is there a helping person or labor partner (father of the baby, family member, friend) who will be with her during labor?
- What is the planned involvement or participation of the woman and her labor partner in this labor? What are the desires and expectations for this labor and birth experience, and afterwards?
- Has there been any means of preparation (e.g., psychoprophylaxis) for labor and birth? Did she choose not to? Were preparations made concerning the feeding and care of the baby?
- Does she indicate an understanding of the labor process, what to expect, and how to work with the forces of labor?
- Is she using her energies in a manner appropriate to the status or progress of her labor?
- What kind of help does she want? From whom?
- What were her prior experiences with labor and childbirth, if any?
- What information needs are evident or expressed at this time?

thus, on the course of labor. For instance, doubts are created in the woman's mind when information concerning findings of observations and examinations are withheld, and by simply not giving her reinforcement and encouragement that what she is doing is right and that labor is progressing.

The woman's self-assurance or confidence is one of the primary strengths that carries her through the stresses of labor. This strength may be exhibited by aggressive and independent behavior that needs the acceptance and support of the nurse. However, the same woman may experience the need for a degree of dependence on others at some time during labor. Nursing care appropriately provides the support that is needed to get through a temporary period of dependence, but fosters independence and self-confidence whenever possible. Whatever the woman's choices and

preferences during labor, there is a need to respect them and to take care not to impose unnecessary provider-made decisions on her.

Clinical Evaluations

Most of the information needed to assess the ongoing progress of labor, to update the risk assessment during the remainder of labor, and to make judgments about the well-being of mother and baby can be obtained by consistent, careful clinical observations and examinations. The information accumulated throughout labor by auscultation, palpation, and visualization can be determinants of whether there are developing problems that require technological surveillance of baby and mother. These parameters require experience both in their use and in their interpretation. Clinical surveillance of the laboring woman does not have to interrupt her work, the activities or positions she may choose, or her working relationship with her labor partner; it is safe, requires touch and consistent contact with the woman; and it assures her of the presence of the care provider, and can lay the groundwork for better communication. It provides a medium through which the hands and words of the care provider can convey gentleness, comfort, and caring to alleviate anxiety and stress, and can possibly decrease the need for analgesics or anesthetics.

These skills are learned at the side of the laboring woman, both from her and through the guidance of an experienced mentor. During all clinical assessments, the parents need to be included and informed of progress, to listen to the baby's heartbeat, to feel the baby's position abdominally, to know what to anticipate next, and to be aware of problems if they develop. This is part of the planning and intervention processes that facilitate parental decision making.

General Physical Assessment

Vital Signs

Blood pressure, pulse, and temperature may be checked every two hours unless otherwise indicated in early labor. Blood pressure and pulse are checked more frequently as labor progresses to active phase, late first- and second-stage labor; the normal rise in arterial pressure during contractions should be kept in mind (see section on The Maternal Cardiovascular System).

Characteristics of the contractions and the fetal heart sounds that are normal for each woman and baby can be established by periodic palpation and auscultation.

The interrelationship of the contractions and the fetal heart rate can be monitored clinically, thus obtaining information that might otherwise be sought through electronic monitoring.

Fetal Heart Auscultation

In early labor, fetal heart auscultation should be done at approximately half-hour intervals, increasing to fifteen-minute intervals as the active phase of first stage progresses, and to every five minutes in second-stage labor. Auscultation is necessary at the time rupture of membranes occurs to detect changes in fetal heart sound that could indicate cord compression or prolapse; vaginal examination may also be done for the latter reason immediately after rupture of membranes. Additionally, any beginning signs of deviant fetal heart sounds or labor patterns are indications for more frequent or constant clinical monitoring by auscultation. The woman in labor should be assisted in listening to her baby's heartbeat whenever she wishes; this frequent reassurance can have a positive influence on her labor.

Auscultation of the fetal heart during labor may reveal changes of rate or rhythm, such as bradycardia, tachycardia, and decelerations or accelerations occurring before, during, or after uterine contractions. The area of maximum intensity of fetal heart sounds is also noted at each auscultation as one index of change of fetal position and descent.

Since auscultation is periodic rather than constant, however, it should be performed in a manner that permits these types of deviations to be picked up early and consistently. One means of doing this is by listening through, and for at least forty seconds after, contractions, as well as during uterine rest periods. As contractions become quite close during late labor, particularly during the more rapid fetal descent of second stage, the fetal heart sounds should be auscultated through several sequential contractions and the rest intervals between, covering several minutes (preferably using a Doppler instrument for the woman's comfort and convenience in whatever posture she is laboring). In second stage, during each contraction there is commonly a decrease in rate of 10 or more beats below the baseline rate. As the uterus relaxes the rate returns to the original level. This bradycardia concurrent with the contraction may be due to pressure on the fetal head and vagus nerve stimulation during a contraction.

A second means of improving the method of evaluation by auscultation is by recording fetal heart rates in graphic form to improve the collection of baseline information and the identification of notable changes (Figure 6-2).

As with any series of observations or assessments, the reliability is increased when the assessments are consistently made by the same person.

Normal range of the fetal heart rate is from 120 to 160 beats/min. The rhythm is usually regular, although occasional skipped beats are not uncommon. Any gross changes in rhythm, rate, or both, particularly if exaggerated during or after uterine contractions, are considered signals of fetal distress (hypoxia). Maternal pulse rate should be checked concurrently with the fetal heart rate periodically to differentiate the two and to rule out the possibility of maternal tachycardia being misinterpreted as a normal fetal heart rate.

Fetal *bradycardia* is a heart rate of less than 120 beats/min that persists for at least five minutes or through two complete contractions. Moderate bradycardia consists of 100–120 beats/min; marked, 70–100; and severe, below 70. Fetal *tachycardia* is a heart rate of more than 160 beats/min that persists for at least five minutes or through two complete contractions. It is moderate at 160–180 beats/min and severe above 180.

Moderate fetal bradycardia may be a physiological response to fetal skull compression during second stage and in instances of relative cephalopelvic disproportion, or in an unfavorable vertex presentation such as occiput transverse or posterior; upon spontaneous rotation to a more favorable position the fetal heart sounds may be expected to return to normal. The heart rate in this instance is usually not affected by maternal position change or by administration of oxygen. Thus, such a finding is not a sign of gross fetal distress, but signals a need for further evaluation of the cause, including vaginal examination to determine position of the vertex and indications of possible disproportion.

Bradycardia recognized by auscultation is considered to correlate with poor fetal condition, especially if the episode extends beyond the end of the contraction. This definition, however, does not exclude the possibility of late decelerations indicative of poor fetal status (p. 137). Tachycardia, although considered more innocuous, sometimes precedes the development of bradycardia.

If signs of fetal distress are detected by clinical assessment during labor, and are not quickly alleviated by appropriate corrective measures (see section on Fetal Distress: Intervention), continuous electronic monitoring of fetal heart and maternal contractions can be utilized if available. If electronic surveillance is used, individuals with the expertise to interpret the recorded patterns, and the ability to make action judgments based on total assessment data must be present, and

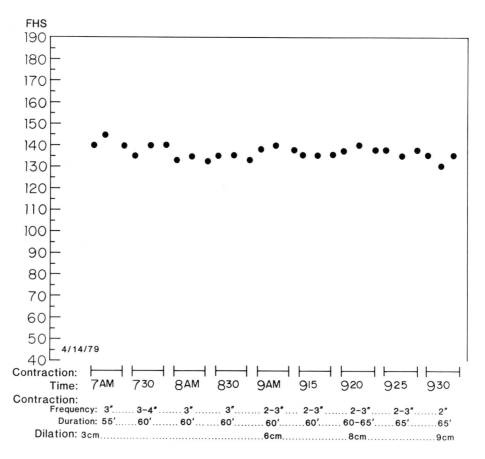

FIGURE 6-2 Contraction graph of fetal heart sounds (FHS).

periodic auscultation of fetal heart sounds and evaluation of maternal pulse concurrent with electronic monitoring to discover any machine malfunction or artifact.

Uterine Contractions: Perception by Palpation

Palpation of the abdomen in the fundal area of the uterus during contractions with the flat of the fingers in gentle motion (not with stabbing movements of fingertips) will elicit information about the frequency, duration, and quality (indentability and mobility) of the uterine contractions. Evaluation should also be made in the relaxation period (uterine indentability) between contractions. Contraction quality as assessed by palpation can be compared with amniotic fluid pressure (related to myometrial tension) that could be obtained by intra-uterine pressure measurement. The duration of a contraction as estimated clinically is shorter than the actual duration (as might be ascertained by intrauterine pressure measurement) since the very beginning

and end are not perceptible by palpation. With the fingers kept lightly in place, resting on the fundal area of the uterus through several contractions, uterine relaxation between contractions can be evaluated as well as the pattern of activity for quality, frequency, and duration of contractions.

Contractions are perceived as a hardening and slight rising of the abdomen, especially over the uterine fundus area. They become palpable after the amniotic pressure has risen above the normal uterine resting pressure (tonus) by 10 mm Hg. The experience of the examiner, thickness of the abdominal wall, and intensity of the contraction itself influence the threshold of perception by palpation. Mild contractions of less than 20–30 mm Hg are easily indentable. This would be typical of latent or early active labor when contractions may be occurring with a frequency of six to fifteen minutes, and a thirty- to forty-second duration (probable 1–3 cm dilation of the cervix). As active labor and progressive dilation take place (possible dilation of 4 cm or more) contractions usually increase in frequency to about three to five minutes, with a duration of forty-five to sixty seconds. When the corresponding intra-uterine pressure (intensity) reaches 30–40 mm Hg (moderate contraction), the uterine wall can be indented with the fingers by exerting moderate counterpressure. When intensity reaches about 40–60 mm Hg or more (strong contraction), the uterine wall resists indentation; this may be expected in advanced or late labor (near the end of the first stage or into the second stage) when contraction frequency has increased to as often as one contraction every two to three minutes, with a sixty- to eighty-second duration.

Some individual contractions of late labor may intensify to a peak of 80–100 mm Hg; this is felt as an intensely rigid, unindentable uterus. Although the resting pressure may also rise slightly in late labor (from a usual range of 5–10 mm Hg, to 12–14 mm Hg between contractions), the uterus continues to be palpable as distinctly relaxed, softened, and again easily indentable as each contraction is completed.

With abnormal uterine activity, the uterine tonus may become elevated above the normal range, rendering it impossible to perceive the changes of uterine intensity during contractions; this usually occurs when the uterine tonus has become elevated beyond 30 mm Hg. Lack of palpable uterine relaxation between contractions is an indication of dysfunctional uterine contractility and potential fetal distress due to the prolonged decrease in uterine blood flow (see section on Fetal Distress: Intervention).

Mobility (side to side) of the uterus and baby is relatively easy in early labor, but decreases by the time 3–7 cm of cervical dilation is reached. Approaching the second stage of labor the uterus becomes relatively fixed as the supporting ligaments become taut and exert their pull on the uterine corpus in a forward direction, thus contributing to fetal descent and to the parallel alignment of the uterine axis with the pelvic inlet.

Contractions should be assessed about every thirty minutes to an hour in early labor, every fifteen minutes in the latter half of first-stage labor, and at least every five minutes and in conjunction with auscultation of fetal heart sounds in second-stage labor. The woman and her labor companion can assess contractions if they have been taught and wish to do so.

Vaginal Examination

Both for the comfort of the woman and to prevent infection, vaginal examinations during labor should be kept to a minimum. Usually, in a slowly progressive first labor, examinations every three hours are adequate to show labor progress. Evidence of unusually slow or rapid progress is an indication for examination.

In order that few examinations need be done, all possible information should be obtained at each examination and should include the following:

- *Cervix:* degree of dilation and effacement; consistency; and position in relation to the presenting part
- *Presenting part:* positive determination of the part presenting and position if possible
- *Status of membranes:* protrusion of membranes; palpable through the cervical os
- *Station:* degree of descent of presenting part into the birth canal in relation to the ischial spines
- *Pelvic structures:* relative adequacy (available space) of the pelvis in regard to sacrum, ischial spines, diagonal conjugate, and pelvic sidewalls
- *Vagina and perineum:* distensibility

Vaginal examinations should be done gently, with slow movements of the hand, and with as gentle pressure of the fingers as is possible. The labia are separated prior to introducing the gloved examining fingers into the vagina in order to avoid any contamination of the sterile glove.

Urine Examination

Urine can be examined for the presence of protein by dipping an indicator strip in the urine. The woman can be taught to do this herself; in fact, she may have been doing the test during the prenatal period, and thus, may be familiar with its significance. This aspect of her reliance on her own skills should be continued into labor just until she wants to turn the responsibility over to her attendants.

Normally, proteinuria does not occur during pregnancy except for occasional slight amounts during or shortly after vigorous work or exercise. Its presence during the course of labor in greater than trace amounts, in the absence of any previous proteinuria, hypertension, or other signs of problems, may indicate the possible emergence of problems (e.g., preeclampsia) during labor and thus a need for more intense and frequent surveillance of blood pressure, urine, and urine output pattern to detect developing problems early.

Initial Assessment of Clinical Findings and Establishment of Baseline

The initial examination provides a baseline for comparison with the normally expected findings of early labor, as well as with subsequent changes as labor progresses.

TABLE 6-1 Expected clinical findings during labor

Contraction				Cervix		Presenting Part
Frequency (contractions per min)	Duration (sec)	Quality*	Uterine Pressure (mm Hg)†	Dilation (cm)	Effacement (percentage)	Station
>5‡	15–30	Mild‡	20–30	0–3	25–50	0 to −2
3–4	30–45	Moderate	<40	3–7	50–75	0 to ±1‡
2–3	60	Strong	>40	7–10	75–100‡	≥ +1

Courtesy of B.D. Reeves, M.D.
*Assessed in terms of uterine indentability and mobility during contraction. *Mild:* uterus is indentable and mobile; *moderate:* uterus is indentable but not mobile; *severe:* uterus is neither indentable nor mobile.
†Comparison of intra-uterine pressure with equivalent findings by abdominal palpation.
‡Represents eighty-five percent of Caucasian primigravidas at time of labor onset.

The characteristic clinical findings when at term or in early labor, and the expected pattern of change in these findings as labor progresses, are shown in Table 6-1. Not all women will present findings within these characteristic ranges when at term, or as labor begins and progresses, but if findings are markedly different, a reason for, and the potential impact of, these deviations should be assessed.

Since labor that does not progress in an expected manner may lead to adverse effects on both the baby and the laboring woman, it is important to discriminate between the usual and the deviant courses of labor. Progressive changes, as shown in Table 6-1, can provide some direction to the overall assessment of this ongoing process and can be correlated with the labor curve as defined by Friedman (Figure 6-3).

Graphic Labor Record

Measureable results of labor are found in the determination of cervical dilation, descent of the presenting part, and to a lesser extent, effacement of the cervix. The work of Friedman and others has resulted in practical guides for the assessment of the progress of individual labors through the graphic plottings of ongoing clinical findings.

By observing the rates of change of the relationships between progressive cervical dilation and elapsed time in labor, and between progressive descent of the presenting part and elapsed time in labor, potentially abnormal labor can be identified relatively early.

Labor progress and the phases of labor up to delivery have been defined in functional terms by Friedman (1978), who developed a graphic means of following the

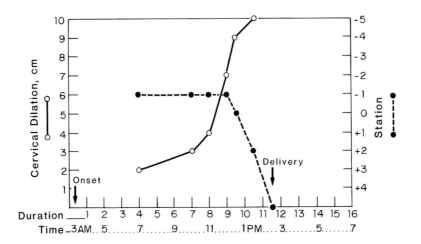

FIGURE 6-3 A graphic labor record. (Redrawn from Friedman, E.A. (1978). Diagnosis of abnormal labor. *The Female Patient*, 3(5), 71–74. With permission.)

TABLE 6-2 The patterns of abnormal labor

Pattern	Diagnostic Criterion
Prolonged latent phase	
Nulliparas	Duration of 20 hr or more
Multiparas	Duration of 14 hr or more
Protracted active-phase dilation	
Nulliparas	Maximum slope of dilation of 1.2 cm/hr or less
Multiparas	Maximum slope of dilation of 1.5 cm/hr or less
Protracted descent	
Nulliparas	Maximum slope of descent of 1.0 cm/hr or less
Multiparas	Maximum slope of descent of 2.0 cm/hr or less
Prolonged deceleration phase	
Nulliparas	Duration of 3 hr or more
Multiparas	Duration of 1 hr or more
Secondary arrest of dilation	Cessation for 2 hr or more
Arrest of descent	Cessation for 1 hr or more
Failure of descent	Lack of expected descent during deceleration phase and second stage
Precipitate dilation	
Nulliparas	Maximum slope of dilation of 5 cm/hr or more
Multiparas	Maximum slope of dilation of 10 cm/hr or more
Precipitate descent	
Nulliparas	Maximum slope of descent of 5 cm/hr or more
Multiparas	Maximum slope of descent of 10 cm/hr or more

From Friedman, E.A. (1978). *Labor: Clinical evaluation and management* (ed. 2). New York: Appleton-Century-Crofts. With permission.

progress of labor through a comparison of cervical dilation in centimeters, descent of the fetus, and the duration in hours. In normal labor, an S-shaped (sigmoid) curve develops as periodic estimates of cervical dilation for the laboring woman are plotted against time on a graph; descent of the presenting part is also plotted. With knowledge of the outer limits of normal range of dilation and descent over specific time periods, deviations from the normal can be recognized quickly (Figure 6-3). Both dilation and descent are expected to continue without interruption once they have begun. This analysis of labor defines the first stage as a *latent phase* in which there is little cervical change. This stage normally lasts less than twenty hours in the nullipara and less than fourteen hours in the multipara. About ten percent of the time, contractions will eventually stop, and labor will subsequently be determined to have been false.

The second phase of labor is termed the *active dilation phase* in which both dilation and descent take place. This phase is characterized by a maximum of dilation, expected to progress approximately 1.2 cm/hour for nulliparas and 1.5 cm/hour for multiparas. Two possible problems of this phase are protraction of either dilation or descent. While the causes are frequently unknown, with continued emotional and physiological support, vaginal delivery usually ensues.

The third phase, called the *deceleration* or *pelvic phase* involves the period when many of the mechanisms of labor, such as rotation, occur. This phase normally lasts about three hours in nulliparous women and about one hour in multiparas. A prolongation of this part of the active phase is frequently associated with cephalopelvic disproportion.

Normally, descent during the deceleration phase is expected to proceed at about one station (1 cm) per hour in nulliparas and two stations per hour in multiparas. Cessation or failure of dilation progress for two hours (termed *secondary arrest of dilation*) or a failure of fetal descent for one hour or more indicates a deviation from normal. These problems may also be related to cephalopelvic disproportion.

These various parameters of normal progress in labor are useful for early detection, proper identification (see Table 6-2), and appropriate actions associated with various deviations.

Again, it is emphasized that parameters and averages serve as guidelines of normal variations as well as of possible abnormal deviations. Cohen (1977) presents data challenging current obstetrical concepts maintaining that labor should be terminated if duration of the second stage exceeds two hours. Labor data from 4403 nulliparous women were analyzed to determine whether the length of the second stage of labor influenced

TABLE 6-3 Maternal and fetal risk factors

Finding	Possible Significance
Maternal	
Fever < 100.4°F (38°C)	Dehydration; infection
> 100.4°F	Extra- or intra-uterine infection (amnionitis)
Rising blood pressure	Preeclampsia
Falling blood pressure	Supine hypotension; sign of shock; analgesic or anesthetic drug reaction
Maternal tachycardia	Fever; impending shock; pain response; bleeding
Vaginal discharge (purulent or foul)	Amnionitis (potential fetal sepsis)
Vaginal bleeding (clots or liquid form)	Traumatized maternal soft tissues; placental abruption; placenta previa; marginal separation of placenta
Complaint of excessive pain	Undetected uterine abnormality; individual level of reaction to pain; reaction to drug
Cyanosis	Cardiac problem; maternal hypoxia; reaction to drug (anesthetic)
Pallor, air hunger, and cool skin	Sign of shock; bleeding
Unconsciousness	Reaction to drug; shock; seizure (eclampsia; previous disorder; unknown cause)
Labor Process and Progress	
Failure of dilation progress	Prolonged or arrested labor; potential for fetal distress
Abnormal abdominal tenderness or pain (hypersensitivity to touch; rigidity)	Placental abruption; uterine rupture (associated with abrupt cessation of contractions)
Decreased contraction frequency, duration, regularity, quality (intensity)	False labor; abnormal uterine contractility; excessive medication
Uterine tetany (failure of uterus to relax between contractions)	Placental abruption with intra-uterine bleeding; oxytocic drugs
Failure of descent of presenting part after complete dilation	Malposition; disproportion; error in cervical dilation estimate
Fetal	
Amniotic fluid with port-wine color	Placental abruption or ruptured vasa previa
Prolapsed cord	Potential fetal death
Abnormally slow, rapid, or irregular fetal heart sounds	Fetal distress/hypoxia; reaction to anesthesia
Meconium-stained amniotic fluid (from heavy, dark green, and tenacious to light and yellow or greenish); passage of stained fluid after clear fluid previously	Fetal distress (potential for meconium aspiration)

maternal puerperal morbidity or perinatal outcome. Findings of this study showed no significant increase in the frequency of perinatal mortality, neonatal mortality, or low five-minute Apgar scores with long second stages of more than two hours' duration. An increase in puerperal hemorrhage after more than three hours of second-stage labor was related to the use of midforceps procedures; no such increase was found in vaginal deliveries, even after a second-stage duration exceeding three hours, when midforceps operations were excluded from analysis. I feel that the elective termination of labor simply because an arbitrary period of time has elapsed in the second stage is unwarranted. At the same time a long second stage should not be ignored; while the data of Cohen's study indicate no immediate deleterious effects on the fetus after long second stages, there is a need for well-controlled prospective data concerning long-term neurological follow-up of such infants.

Ongoing Assessment of Risk

Having determined a normal, low-risk labor at its onset or first evaluation, the continuing assessment of risk is a matter of familiarity with the ranges of normal labor and recognition of deviations that may adversely affect the well-being of mother and baby. These deviations may be reflected in the labor process and progress (as shown in Table 6-1) in maternal systemic changes or fetal response to maternal changes, in placental factors, or in intrinsic factors. The risk factors may also be reflected in the mother's psychological forces, her strengths or weaknesses, or her expressed or evidenced needs for dealing with the work at hand.

Risk factors that develop during ongoing labor may appear either insidiously or abruptly. Examples are given in Table 6-3.

Among the intrapartum risk factors determined by Hobel and co-workers (1976) to be significantly related to poor neonatal outcome are the following: toxemia, meconium staining of amniotic fluid, hydramnios, prolonged latent phase, amnionitis, premature rupture of membranes, abruptio placentae, abnormal presentation, excessive magnesium sulfate, fetal tachycardia, pitocin augmentation, outlet forceps, shoulder dystocia, precipitous labor of less than three hours, and second stage labor of more than two and a half hours. Hobel et al. noted additional factors, which include fetal bradycardia (first and second stage), high forceps, and prolapsed cord.

Risks of Teenage Labor

The risks associated with adolescent pregnancy seem to be related primarily to care received in pregnancy and childbirth rather than to age per se. Those teenagers who have been assessed as having low-risk pregnancies can and should be prepared and guided through the same options of low-risk care during labor that are provided for other age groups. This is an aid in reducing anxieties and the need for intervention, and thereby helping the adolescent to continue the normalcy she has achieved up to the time of labor onset. The developmental "unfinished business" of moving from adolescence to adulthood should guide the helping efforts on behalf of the young woman in labor; her future and her child's future can be influenced by the

care provided now—especially as it affects her willingness to maintain an ongoing, close contact with care providers that is essential to future preventive health maintenance and education.

Social change, earlier menarche (12.3 years), and earlier sexual activity have contributed to a marked increase in the number of teenage pregnancies. For those adolescents who obtain prenatal care, many of the risk factors will have been identified and possibly diminished by the time of labor onset.

The actual incidence of high-risk factors among pregnant teenagers is variously reported. Recent reports seem to indicate that the findings of health problems among pregnant teenagers may have been biased in that some of the risks that were attributed to being pregnant at a young age (e.g., toxemia, low-birth-weight infants, syphilis, pyelonephritis, anemia) may have been due largely to inadequate prenatal care received by teenagers. Several of the pregnancy-related problems previously reported to occur more frequently in first pregnancy at a young age are shown to occur with increased incidence in nonwhite, low socioeconomic groups of any age. Some of the differences in pregnancy complications and risk factors between the teenage and older populations have been minimized in studies utilizing pair-matched control groups; prematurity by weight may be one of those factors that is an effect of socioeconomic elements rather than of young age (Abbott, 1978; Duenhoelter et al., 1975; Youngs et al., 1977).

Labor outcomes have been reported by Youngs et al. (1977) for teenagers aged 17 and under showing that, with consistent prenatal care, a large percentage (eighty-three percent) deliver within twelve hours of the rupture of membranes (with about an eight percent occurrence of premature rupture of membranes). Evrard and Gold (1977) found only about three percent of the labors to be prolonged beyond twenty-four hours, while about twelve percent had labors of less than three hours. Their study results dispute earlier claims that fetopelvic disproportion is more common in the young. Complications were largely hypertensive disorders associated with pregnancy.

Cesarean section rates have been reported to range from 0.8 to twelve percent, and include indications of fetal distress, breech presentation, fetopelvic disproportion, malpresentation, and abruptio placentae (Evrard & Gold, 1977). Semmens' (1965) study found the Cesarean delivery rate to be 1.4 percent and the rate of prolonged labor eight percent.

These factors are of particular importance in evaluating the manner in which appropriate and effective care can be provided so that teenagers who arrive in labor without major problems and who are basically low-risk, achieve a good pregnancy outcome. The principles of care during normal labor and birth are appropriate for gravidas of all ages.

Electronic and Biochemical Surveillance

Clinical surveillance of the normal labor, both in terms of initial assessment and the progression of labor, has been discussed. If other means are deemed necessary, electronic monitoring of fetal heart rate and uterine contractions and fetal blood sampling may be utilized.

The concepts and criteria for utilization of these means of surveillance vary from selective use in specific instances of indicated need or suspected increased risk to suggestions for use during every labor without qualification. Studies concerning the benefits, costs, and risks of these methods vary markedly in their findings, as do opinions and views based on experience with their use.

The following questions are being raised by health care providers as well as by parents:

- To what extent have these specific methods of surveillance contributed to decreased perinatal mortality in the United States or in the world?
- Can the effect of this surveillance method be isolated from other factors possibly contributing to decreased perinatal mortality, such as improved neonatal care, improved nutrition, lower maternal parity and age, expanded knowledge of perinatology, contraceptive availability, and liberalized sterilization and abortion laws?
- What are the potential benefits in comparison to overall expenses and to direct consumer cost?
- Is there an increased incidence of infection (fetal or maternal) that can be attributed to invasive intrapartum monitoring techniques? If so, is this related to the duration of monitoring?
- Is there a relationship between monitored labors and an increased number of Cesarean sections, and if so, what is the significance of this?
- Does the woman with a normal (low-risk) labor at onset and a normal prenatal course need these methods of surveillance? And, under such circumstances, do these methods interfere with the woman's ability to work with the forces of labor without unnecessary anxiety or analgesia? Can their use introduce problems in an otherwise normal (low-risk) labor?
- Does a restriction of activities and positions during labor affect the labor process in any way?

- Is there a potential morbidity due to trauma (e.g., maternal, as in uterine perforation during insertion of catheters to measure intra-uterine pressure; or fetal, as in hemorrhage or scalp infection due to incision of the fetal scalp to measure the blood pH)?
- Does use of these surveillance methods lead to an increased frequency of vaginal examinations, other intravaginal manipulations, or early amniotomy? If so, is there any significant relationship between these factors and maternal–infant outcomes, or on the labor process itself?

A slowing effect on the progress of active labor has been reported to result from intravaginal manipulations (as in amniotomy or intravaginal fetal monitoring) as well as from malposition or disproportion, as shown in a study with continuous ultrasonic recording of cervical dilation. In the same study, Sokol et al. (1976) suggested that active labor, especially with intravaginal manipulation, sometimes proceeds with nonlinear progression rather than linear as has generally been reported.

In low-risk pregnancies and labors the use of some modes of anesthesia and of elective acceleration of labor, with their respective possibilities for risk of hypotension and uterine hyperstimulation, may be associated with a determined need for surveillance by electronic uterofetal monitoring. However, Haverkamp and associates (1976) demonstrated equally satisfactory fetal outcomes when mother and fetus are closely monitored by appropriately trained attendants using auscultation.

Uterofetal Electronic Monitoring

There has long been knowledge of the reflection of fetal hypoxia in the fetal heart rate changes. The work of Hon et al. (1975) and others has demonstrated specific patterns of fetal heart rate response to uterine contractions, and specific alterations in the heart rate recordings related to fetal distress.

Normally, pressure within the placental intervillous space during uterine contractions is lower than the capillary pressure in the placental villi. This is maintained by fetal blood pressure changes, thus preventing collapse of the villi and impeded blood flow through fetal vessels, and allowing the exchange of materials between maternal and fetal circulations even during contractions. There is, however, a temporary reduction in flow of maternal oxygenated blood through the placental intracotyledonary spaces during each uterine contraction, which creates a source of stress on the fetus during labor. This may be compounded by other sources of fetal stress such as cord compression, maternal hypotension, drugs administered for anesthesia or analgesia, placental disease, maternal disease, and inherent fetal disease. In order to detect fetal distress during labor, it has been urged by Hon et al. (1975) and others that continuous fetal heart rate beat-to-beat recording be carried out in concomitance with pressure changes resulting from uterine contractions. Detection and monitoring equipment is available for monitoring uterine contractions and the fetal heart rate.

Two methods of uterine contraction–fetal heart rate monitoring are available; *internal* and *external.* Internal methods may be used only after membranes have ruptured and the cervix is dilated adequately to allow application of a fetal scalp electrode to directly record the fetal heart rate in correlation with changes in intrauterine pressure. Uterine contractions are measured directly by a catheter threaded through the cervix and into the uterus. This direct method of recording provides more precise and accurate fetal heart rate data than indirect recording.

External methods, while less exact than internal, have the advantage of use when conditions do not permit use of internal monitoring (intact membranes or insufficient cervical dilation). In external monitoring, the fetal heart rate recording is by ultrasonocardiography, abdominal fetal electrocardiography or phonocardiography. Uterine activity is commonly evaluated by a pressure-sensing tocodynamometer. Both instruments are held in place on the abdomen of the mother with belts, and simultaneous recordings are made of contractions and fetal heart rate.

Some of the indicated conditions for continuous monitoring include meconium-stained amniotic fluid with vertex presentation of the fetus, abnormal fetal heart rate on auscultation, previously determined high-risk status, poor progress of labor, premature labor, preeclampsia or other medical or obstetrical complications, and use of oxytocin.

The normal controlling mechanisms affecting the fetal heart rate, an interplay of stimuli from the autonomic nervous system, may be lost due to hypoxia or central nervous system damage. This is reflected in the recorded fetal heart rate pattern. Of the various patterns that may be demonstrated in combination or alone, attention has focused especially on the early, late, and variable deceleration patterns and on loss of beat-to-beat variability.

Hon et al. (1975) have described the heart rate patterns of babies with impaired oxygen supply during labor (Figure 6-4). The *early deceleration* pattern coincides with the onset of the uterine contraction and returns to baseline when the contraction subsides. These are believed to be related to heat compression during the contraction and to be innocuous.

Variable deceleration is associated with umbilical cord compression, and is variable in onset with regard to uterine contractions, is variable in shape, and is usually sporadic and variable in degree. Typically there is a precipitous drop from normal rate to 50–60 beats or less per minute followed by a variable interval of bradycardia ending with an abrupt return to the baseline rate. This pattern is sometimes ablated by a change of maternal position, possibly relieving pressure on the cord due to compression between the maternal pelvis and the fetal head. Generally, no major therapeutic steps are taken if there is an abrupt and prompt return of the fetal heart rate to the baseline level and if there is no significant smoothness of the baseline heart rate, or associated tachycardia.

Late deceleration pattern is considered to be ominous and is frequently associated with hypoxia in conjunction with metabolic derangement due to uteroplacental insufficiency. This repetitive deceleration usually begins around the time of the peak of the uterine contraction or at some time after the start of the contraction, and reaches maximum bradycardia and returns to baseline after the contraction has subsided.

Usually in late pregnancy there is a beat-to-beat variation in the fetal heart rate. Although demonstrated by internal monitoring, this may not be apparent from external recordings. This beat-to-beat variability is evidently due to the continuous interplay of decelerator and accelerator cardiovascular reflexes, and its absence in late pregnancy has been associated with fetal compromise; lack of variability has also been attributed to meperidine, diazepam, and magnesium sulfate effects.

Baseline tachycardia, a persistent acceleration of rate (considered severe in excess of 170 beats/min) in the absence of decelerations could be caused by a response to fetal hypoxia or a maternal febrile state. *Baseline bradycardia* is a persistent deceleration of the heart rate which, in the absence of either accelerations or decelerations, is not necessarily due to fetal distress. It can be associated with congenital heart lesions. Also, fetal death may appear to be fetal bradycardia, with the maternal heart rate recorded by the electronic monitor.

It should be noted that the absence of an ominous fetal heart rate pattern as recorded by electronic monitor is not absolutely predictive of good fetal outcome. Hayashi and Fox (1975) reported a fetal cardiac arrest and subsequent death that was not preceded by an ominous fetal heart rate pattern during the course of labor induction.

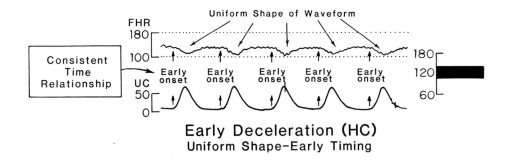

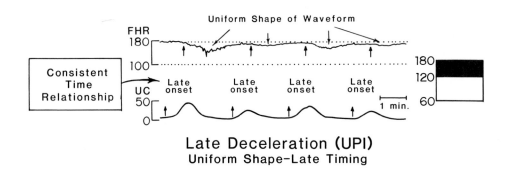

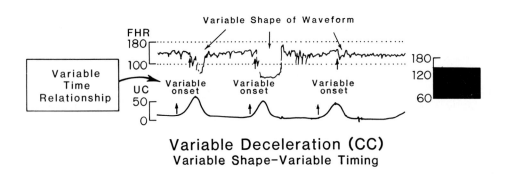

FIGURE 6-4   Fetal heart rate (FHR) patterns.

Fetal Blood Sampling

Another method of diagnosing fetal hypoxia is by measuring pH (and possibly P_{O_2} and P_{CO_2}) of blood obtained during labor by incising the fetal scalp. The fetus normally develops a combined metabolic and respiratory acidosis with a drop in pH, a base deficit, and a rise in P_{CO_2} in the latter part of the active phase of labor. If hypoxia develops, these changes are exaggerated. In the event of clinical evidence of hypoxia (e.g., meconium in the amniotic fluid in vertex presentation, ominous fetal heart rate pattern), repeated scalp blood sampling is performed. A pH of 7.20 or less is considered evidence of acidosis or serious fetal distress.

Fetal Distress: Intervention

When signs of fetal distress are signaled by an abnormal fetal heart rate pattern, steps need to be taken to relieve the distress. While the cause of distress may be evident, more often intervention is based on potential causes and fetal response to the immediate interventive actions. Basic intervention measures include the following:

• The woman's position should be changed to a lateral position in order to decrease pressure on the inferior vena cava and aorta by the uterus and baby. The position change may also relieve pressure on the umbilical cord and may change uterine activity, sometimes increasing the interval or rest period between contractions and thereby increasing uteroplacental perfusion and fetal blood supply.

• Oxygen should be administered to the mother in order to increase oxygen content of her blood above normal and to increase the content in fetal circulation. This is useful when blood flow to the baby is decreased, even if the mother is not hypoxic.

• Fluids should be administered intravenously to the woman in the presence of hypovolemia or hypotension.

• If oxytocin is being administered (in which case the labor is no longer considered to be normal or low-risk), it should be discontinued immediately to decrease uterine tone, to increase the rest interval between contractions, and to reduce mechanical interference with perfusion of the intervillous space. The excessive uterine activity caused by administration of oxytocin is one of the common causes of inadequate uteroplacental perfusion.

• If severe fetal distress continues in the face of corrective measures and with confirmation of fetal distress by those means available, including *auscultation* by several persons, preparations should begin for the birth to be accomplished by the most expeditious and safe route with respect to both the woman and her baby.

The occurrence of a persistent abnormal fetal heart rate pattern places a compelling responsibility on the nurse to initiate these interventive measures with extreme calm and with precise, honest explanation to the woman and her labor companion of what may be occurring, why these measures are being used, and the possible results. The total inclusion of both the woman and her labor partner, as well as their continued involvement in whatever measures are undertaken, is of vital importance to the woman's continued control and ability to assist in bringing about improvement of her baby's status. Maintaining a low level of anxiety in the woman at this time may have as much effect on fetal recovery (and uteroplacental sufficiency) as other combined measures.

Planning and Providing for Continuing Needs

Nutritional and Fluid Needs

Increased energy requirement during any kind of vigorous work or exercise is met by rapid metabolism of glycogen, which results in liberation of lactate. Likewise, carbohydrates are broken down to meet the energy requirements of labor, accompanied by an increase in maternal arterial lactate. It is not uncommon for maternal metabolic acidosis to exist during labor in

direct relationship to the beginning of intense uterine contractions. This should not be associated with fetal acidosis under normal circumstances. In abnormal situations of severe maternal acidosis there may be an accompanying fetal acidosis. The over-all energy expenditure of the woman in labor does indicate a need for carbohydrate intake orally, or glucose intravenously, depending on individual needs and circumstances (e.g., labors lasting for long periods).

Generally, the woman will be able to, and will want to, continue her oral fluid intake during most or all of labor. In normal labor there should not be a fluid or electrolyte imbalance in spite of increased fluid loss through lungs and skin, salt losses are negligible except with vomiting.

Concerns about drinking liquids or light eating during labor are based on the use of general anesthesia and its associated risk of aspiration of gastric contents. Pritchard and MacDonald (1976) noted that, while aspiration of undigested food may cause airway obstruction, the highly acidic gastric juice that follows a period of fasting is probably more dangerous and more commonly aspirated than are gastric contents. For these reasons, in the event of need for general anesthesia, specific prophylactic precautions have been recommended, including the emptying of the stomach by nasogastric tube or other means and the ingesting of antacids to neutralize gastric acidity.

There is little information available with regard to nourishment during labor, to the motility, emptying, and absorptive actions of the gastrointestinal tract, and possibly more importantly, to factors which affect these aspects of labor; such factors may include the individual perception and response to pain, complications, length of labor or intensity of muscle activity involved, analgesia or anesthesia, fear and anxiety, and others.

A study was done by Hendrie (1975) utilizing a high-calorie, high-protein, low-fat content liquid diet (dried milk product) during labor to provide nutrition and hydration. In preliminary studies to assess the emptying time of 230 ml of the test meal it was found that sixty-five to seventy percent of the meal had left the stomach in half an hour. This liquid meal was associated with an increase of the gastric pH (above the critical level of 2.5) and a decreased incidence of urinary ketosis during labor.

In order to reduce the risk of acid aspiration during Cesarean section, Roberts and Shirley (1974) studied preventive measures in 100 women undergoing this surgery. The administration of oral antacid within four hours of inducing anesthesia was found to significantly raise the gastric pH. This resulted in a tenfold reduction of the number of women at risk for developing pneumonitis due to acid aspiration (defined as those having at least 25 ml of gastric juice with pH below 2.5 in the stomach at delivery).

It would seem reasonable to use such preventive measures with the relatively small number of women who may require them rather than to have women who are experiencing normal labor restrict their oral intake in order to be prepared for the possible need for a general anesthetic.

Overall this remains an area where more data are needed to conclusively identify the risks and benefits of oral intake by women in labor.

Ambulation

There is generally no contraindication to ambulation during labor. Ambulation, along with various positions to increase comfort and to aid the work of labor, should be the choice of the mother. Ambulation and upright positions are facilitative of gravitational effect and of the freedom and control of self and surroundings that is exercised by the laboring woman.

Enemas

In a study by Toppozada and co-workers (1967), enemas were shown to have no significant effect on overall uterine activity. If, at the time of vaginal examination, there is a large amount of stool in the rectum that may obstruct the descent of the baby, an enema may be needed but enemas have not been shown to stimulate labor. Fecal contamination is not necessarily a greater problem without the enema, and may be less of a problem since any stool is less likely to be of liquid consistency. Further, enemas may be a source of discomfort to the woman in labor. The best solution may be to offer the woman a choice.

Voiding

A woman in early labor usually has no difficulty voiding, but in the latter part of the active phase urination may become difficult. Inability to void may be due to pressure of the fetal presenting part against the urethra and trigone, pain, position (maternal and fetal), inability to relax muscles, tension due to surroundings and circumstances—particularly in conjunction with attempts to use the bedpan; and in some instances, sedation. Distention of the bladder can cause interference with uterine action, delay of labor progress, increased pain in the bladder region, and later hypotonia of the bladder accompanied by urinary retention, or the possible predisposition to cystitis. Results of a study reported by Toppozada and associates (1967) showed notable effect on uterine activity following evacuation of the distended bladder, with marked increase of the amplitude of contractions, and a less marked increase in the frequency.

As the lower segment lengthens and the cervix is retracted, and as the fetal head becomes engaged, the bladder is pulled upward and becomes located entirely abdominally. It can usually be seen and palpated above the symphysis as a soft, fluctuant mass. Both palpation and percussion are useful in outlining a distended bladder.

During the active phase of labor the woman may not experience the urge to void, and should be encouraged to empty the bladder at regular intervals. Voiding is generally facilitated by the upright sitting position, ambulation, privacy, and the ability or sufficient time to relax muscles between contractions. Suggestion, with the use of running water or pouring of warm water over the perineal area, is sometimes helpful. If a bedpan must be used, a sitting position is preferable, either in a chair or on the edge of the bed with the legs over the side and feet on the floor.

If all attempts to facilitate voiding fail and the woman has not urinated for several hours, and there is visible and palpable distention, or if there is a failure of labor progress over several hours along with these conditions, catheterization is indicated. Since catheterization is accompanied by the increased risk of urinary tract infection, however, the need for catheterization should be weighed against the degree and present effects of any distention.

Prevention is the keynote of nursing planning and intervention. Keeping the bladder empty by consistent encouragement and reminding of the woman in labor is preferable to recognizing a distended bladder and having to intervene at that point.

Perineal Shave

The routine procedure of shaving the perineum during labor continues even in the face of evidence that this is unnecessary. Bases for the shaving of perineal hair have included the need for improved asepsis, better visualization to perform and repair the episiotomy, and greater ease of postpartum care.

The improvement of asepsis, or a lowered incidence of infection, through the use of this procedure has been contradicted by study findings. In a study of postpartum complications based on the incidence of endometritis, fever, or readmission among 7600 women not receiving perineal shaves, Burchell (1964) reported the omission of the shave to be favorable in terms of complications. Kantor et al. (1965) investigated seventy-five women for whom four contrasting methods of preoperative perineal preparation were utilized (shaving and nonshaving in conjunction with either pHisohex [Winthrop] or providone-iodine), found the differences in shaving and nonshaving to be insignificant with respect to the number and types of bacteria left on the perineum after the four methods of preparation. In another study, Seropian and Reynolds (1971) compared shaving with the use of depilatory creams and with the use of no preparation. They reported a postoperative wound infection rate of 5.6 percent after shaving compared with rates of 0.6 percent after the use of both depilatory cream and no method of preparation (155 of the total 406 people in the study received no preparation). It was further concluded that preparation by shaving contributed to risk of surgical wound infection rather than reducing it. Even earlier observations by Johnston and Sidall (1922) supported the omission of this procedure as it relates to infection incidence.

Rupture of the Membranes

Caution is advised relative to amniotomy in early labor (Caldeyro-Barcia, 1976; Caldeyro-Barcia et al., 1972; Martell et al., 1976; Schwarcz et al., 1973). Routine amniotomy early in the first stage of labor for the purpose of employing interval monitoring or to shorten an otherwise normal labor may cause cord prolapse or compression, infection, early deceleration patterns, and disalignment of the parietal bone (Charles, 1976; Caldeyro-Barcia et al., 1972; Schwarcz et al., 1973). Lower pH values in newborns have been associated with early amniotomy, as reported by Martell et al. (1976). It has also been found that artificial rupture of membranes in early or midlabor causes changes in the fetal heart rate patterns that must be taken into consideration in evaluating fetal status (Caldeyro-Barcia, 1976).

Early deceleration patterns often associated with early artificial rupture of membranes, although thought to be innocuous, are not proved to be so (Caldeyro-Barcia, 1976). These decelerations are related to fetal vagal stimulation that may be caused by umbilica occlusion or by uneven compression of the fetal head (Schwarcz et al., 1973). Fedrick and Butler (1971) reported an increased incidence of cerebral birth trauma (subdural hemorrhage) associated with length of time between rupture of membranes and delivery.

The effect of amniotomy on the progress of labor is a highly controversial topic. According to Friedman and Sachtleben (1963), the progress of labor is not significantly influenced by the timing of amniotomy during labor. Other researchers have not confirmed the frequently held view that early amniotomy significantly shortens the duration of labor (Caldeyro-Barcia et al., 1972; Schwarcz et al., 1973). For that matter, evidence is lacking to support that a shorter labor is necessarily beneficial to the mother or to the baby. Early amniotomy may intensify her feelings of pelvic pressure or of the contractions, making it difficult to be in control of what she feels and what is happening to her. An inability to "work with" the situation created may lead to an increased need for analgesia.

Amniotomy remains a frequently employed intervention in the management of labor in this country. Hendricks (1977) described amniotomy as the single most effective maneuver for facilitating the progress of labor. I feel that the data do not support the use of amniotomy in normal labor. (The use of amniotomy in labor that deviates from normal is a separate issue and will be discussed further in *Women's Health: Illness and Crisis in Childbearing*.)

When rupture of the membranes occurs, the fetal heart should be listened to. A sterile vaginal examination can be done to check for possible prolapse of the umbilical cord (see section on Fetal Heart Auscultation).

The Perineum and Pelvic Support Structures

Concern for the perineum during childbirth extends to ancient times when Aristotle advocated salves and other emolients to soften and relax the perineum and so reduce perineal resistance (Laufe & Leslie, 1972). Midwives were instructed by Soranus, in first- and second-century Rome, in a technique of providing artificial support to the perineum with a linen pad while the head advanced (Graham, 1960).

Another technique used to protect the perineum involved restraining the head from rapid descent during second stage. Along with this, Harvie, in the early eighteenth century, advised vaginal lubrication with hog's lard in a technique for ironing out the perineum and reducing perineal resistance (Graham, 1960).

In 1855, Ritgen recommended, in addition to surgical incisions, other methods of protecting the perineum:

(1) Prevention, if at all possible, of the supplementation of labor in painful deliveries; (2) letting the head or breech, which ever presents, pass through without obstruction, if the lower vaginal area is sufficiently prepared, without any pressure on the perineum; (3) holding back the presenting head until the lower vaginal area is sufficiently prepared, provided the intensity of the contractions does not render dangerous the continued holding back of the head; (4) pushing the presenting head through between pains; (5) letting through, or guiding through, the presenting head in

the usual way, and not by means of forceps if they have been applied and three-fourths or two-thirds of the circumference of the head has been delivered; (6) guiding through the shoulder girdle, and delivering the shoulder at the public arch, before the shoulder at the perineum; (7) softening inunctions of grease in the vagina and perineum; (8) softening injections into the vagina; (9) softening poultices on the outer vaginal orifice; (10) steam baths at the vaginal orifice; (11) softening douches; and (12) otherwise required local or general active treatment.*

Ritgen also advocated laboring in the left lateral position, or the right lateral position if preferred by the woman. He noted that the woman would usually choose to lie on whichever side the baby's back was directed toward, with the bed thus providing support for the baby. Since the back of the head would most frequently be coming from the left side of the mother's pelvis to begin moving under the public arch, it was reasoned that the left lateral position would usually be chosen by the woman. These measures were considered an alternative to surgical incision or episiotomy.

Episiotomy is often referred to as a simple, routine procedure that is now, as in the past, frequently debated in obstetrical publications mainly in terms of where the incision should be made (Bekhit, 1976; Beynon, 1974; Ould, 1742; Walker, 1974). First advocated by Sir Fielding Ould in 1742, the operation of episiotomy was defined and described in the *Treatise of Midwifery*. The procedure was further popularized by Pomeroy in 1918 and suggested as a routine procedure for primiparous women to reduce pressure on the baby's head. It was first advocated for prophylactic use by De Lee in 1920.

The incidence of episiotomy in the United States has been reported as having ranged between one and approximately 43 percent in different hospitals in 1930 (Tritsch, 1930), to a range of seventy (Jacobs & Adams, 1960) to ninety-five percent by the mid-1960s (O'Leary & O'Leary, 1965). Klopfer et al. reported in 1975 an episiotomy frequency of eighty-eight percent among women who had participated in childbirth education classes.

In other countries there seems to be a lower frequency of episiotomy. In Australia, for example, Beischer (1967) reported an episiotomy rate of thirty percent for a large number of women, while Vellay (1975) described a rate of five percent for multiparas and thirty-three

percent for primiparas in France. The rate in the Netherlands has been reported as eight percent (Stewart & Stewart, 1976).

Evidence to support the routine use of episiotomy is lacking in the literature. Several reasons, however, have been advanced.

Shortening of Second-Stage Labor In order to reduce pressure to the fetal head, and thereby neurological impairment in instances where there is no sign of fetal distress, episiotomy may be performed. A seven-year follow-up of 17,000 children born in Great Britain indicated that, for full-term, average-for-gestational-age infants who show no signs of fetal distress, the incidence of neurological impairment is not increased by a second stage of labor lasting as long as two and a half hours (Laufe & Leslie, 1972).

Although Laufe and Leslie (1972) did show a decrease in the peak force required to accomplish birth after an episiotomy takes place, the significance of this decrease on normal labor outcome is unclear. A long-term investigation of perinatal hazards reported by Butler and Alberman (1960) revealed no relationship between length of time or force for birth during normal labor, and the subsequent neurological development of the child.

Reduction of Trauma or Damage to Pelvic Floor Few data exist concerning the condition of the pelvic floor after birth, except those associated with the use of forceps or episiotomy; in the studies that are available, controls are frequently lacking. In one study, published by O'Leary and Erez (1965), pelvic support at six weeks postpartum was reported for two groups of women having an equal frequency of forceps' use (forty-four percent). One-half of the 100 women were administered hyaluronidase during vaginal term births. The rate of episiotomies was sixty-eight percent in the group who did not receive the drug and thirty-six percent in the group that received it. At the six-week postpartum assessment of pelvic support, equally good results were reported for both groups.

Kaltreider and Dixon (1948) reported on a study of 43,503 deliveries to determine the immediate incidence and resulting complications of third-degree lacerations (involving the sphincter or a portion of the rectum, but excluding lacerations of the rectum with intact sphincter). Among the women with episiotomies, the majority being midline, a 4.49 percent incidence of third-degree lacerations was reported; among women without episiotomies the incidence was 0.25 percent. Thirteen percent of the women with lacerations experienced later

---

*Ritgen, G. (1855). (R.M. Wynn, trans.). Concerning his method for protection of the perineum. *Monatschrift für Geburtskande, 6,* 21. (*American Journal of Obstetrics and Gynecology,* 1965, *93*(3), 421–433.) With permission.

complications including vaginoperineal sinus and incision breakdown. Rectovaginal fistula occurred in an additional 2.25 percent of the women. Lacerations were due primarily to use of forceps, occiput transverse and occiput posterior positions, primigravidity, and experience of the attendant.

Walker (1974) advocated routine midline episiotomy with rectal or sphincter incision when necessary, and in his study of the use of episioprectotomy (episirectomy) in 262 consecutive deliveries, reports good-to-excellent results based upon perineal anatomical results and subjective impressions of pain at examinations four and eight weeks postpartum.

Some attempts have been made to study variables related to perineal lacerations. In a retrospective study of 210 women, Fischer (1979) analyzed the relationship of major and minor perineal lacerations to thirty separate factors. First- and second-degree lacerations were found to be associated with multiparity, prepregnant obesity, short second stage, low weight gain, large infant weight, and absence of forceps, anesthesia, and episiotomies. Third- and fourth-degree lacerations were found to be strongly related to use of forceps, young age, low parity, and episiotomies.

Danielson (1957), in writing about the clinical aspects of prolapse of the uterus and vagina, and associated pelvic connective tissue supports, reported on a review of 600 cases from Stockholm. Several theories, based on numerous investigations, are provided concerning the principal support of the genital organs, and the possible cause and prevention of problems related to support of the pelvic structures. Among these are the following:

- The pelvic floor provides support for the genital organs; however, it has been found that trauma, such as laceration of the levator muscles, is not necessarily followed by prolapse.
- Although both the pelvic floor muscles and the pelvic ligaments interact as a functional unit, the ligaments—particularly the cardinal ligaments—are of primary importance in support.
- Trauma of childbirth (especially related to repeated births at short intervals, large infants, high forceps deliveries) is the commonest cause of injury to the supportive structures. Stretching and laceration of the pelvic connective tissues—notably the cardinal ligaments—cannot be avoided even in a normal birth. Additionally, it is probable that this stretching of tissues has already begun in pregnancy, therefore not even Cesarean section will fully eliminate this danger.

- Median episiotomy is considered by several American authors to help bring the levator muscles together again in the midline; "however, the value of episiotomy from the preventive standpoint has not yet been demonstrated statistically. It is undoubtedly best to allow childbirth to proceed quite spontaneously wherever possible" (Danielson, 1957, p. 115).
- Adequate rest and diet during the puerperium are essential to prevention.
- Avoidance of urinary bladder distension is important, especially during the puerperium, since this may be conducive to retroflexion and subsequent relaxation of supportive structures.
- Preventive levator-muscle exercises designed to strengthen the pelvic floor should be taught routinely to every woman.
- Hormonal deficiency contributes to loss of elasticity and weakening of supporting tissues of genital organs.
- Metabolic endocrine, or systemic, disorders have been suggested to be contributory causes.
- Congenital weakness of supporting tissues may be a contributing factor in some women, causing these tissues to be incapable of resisting intra-abdominal pressure (as in bearing down during childbirth, as in ascites caused by pathological disorders, or as in frequent straining down at defecation).

This review shows a multiplicity of potential contributing factors involving either congenital or acquired weakness of supporting tissues. Muscles of the pelvic floor are associated with the uterine support systems—notably the cardinal ligaments—so that the presence of cystocele, rectocele, and other weaknesses of vaginal tissues contribute to the total pelvic connective tissue structural support system.

Maintaining Sexual Response The overriding question in this rationale is whether female or male sexual satisfaction is more likely to be associated with the perineum that has undergone incision and repair of episiotomy or with the perineum that has undergone preventive or restorative levator-muscle exercises. While the use of the episiotomy is advocated by some including Shute (1959) who suggests that overstretching of the vulvar elastic connective tissues can be prevented by a well-timed episiotomy, which ensures both anatomical and "conjugal normalcy" restoration, data do not exist to support this position. Haire (1972) cites interviews with obstetrician-gynecologists of various countries indicating agreement that "a superficial, first-degree tear is less traumatic to the perineal tissue than an incision which requires several sutures for reconstruction."*

Women need to be aware that lack of tone and support in pelvic floor–perineal muscles is associated with nutritional status, general preventive health self-care, standing for long periods, bearing down strenuous for bowel movements, general tissue condition, hormonal influences, failure to exercise these muscles appropriately, and other factors that require attention in nonpregnancy as well as in pregnancy. Regardless of cause, intervention for many of these muscle support problems exists in the form of specific exercises.

Levator-muscle exercises have a place in women's health care with or without the involvement of childbirth, but are specifically indicated for both preventive and restorative purposes following pregnancy and birth. This type of exercise and muscle reeducation has been, and is being, successfully used in dealing with some sexual problems, specific sphincter control, relaxed vaginal walls, and other pelvic support problems.

When a pregnant woman is taught this exercise, a verbal description might be that she try to contract her urinary and vaginal openings as though trying to prevent urinating, with a "sucking-in" and "closing" movement of the vagina and rectum. Assessment of the vaginal wall support and muscle tone and demonstration of the "squeezing down" actions of the sphincter and pubococcygeal muscle can be accomplished by having the woman squeeze down on the examiner's fingers. However, a woman can more effectively determine how to contract these muscles, and the strength of her contraction, by inserting her own fingers into the vagina and contracting the vaginal muscles. This may be done in any comfortable position, such as squatting or lying on the back with knees flexed. Use of her own fingers also helps the woman to develop familiarity and awareness of her own body.

It may be difficult for the postpartum woman to effectively contract the right muscles. If she is asked to stop the urine flow in midstream a few times at each voiding, she usually has no difficulty finding the muscle group and contracting it with effectiveness. Also, the woman may find the voluntary contraction of these muscles during coitus to be desirable and pleasing for herself and her partner. Once learned, the exercise can be done daily at any time without interrupting

---

*From Haire, D. (1972). *The cultural warping of childbirth.* Milwaukee: International Childbirth Education Association. With permission.

routines. The exercise consists of contracting the pelvic floor muscles as tightly as possible, holding the contraction for ten seconds, releasing and relaxing completely, and then contracting again in a series of twenty to thirty contractions three to four times a day, or more according to individual need and endurance levels. The woman should be encouraged to continue performing the exercises intensely for several months after childbirth in order to restore muscle tone; but their ongoing, lifelong benefit to pelvic support, bladder and bowel tone, and sexual awareness should be stressed.

Psychological Responses to Labor

The woman is usually pleased and excited with the realization that "this is it" and the long wait is finally coming to an end. Early in labor she is talkative and in a light, cheerful mood, with a degree of anxious anticipation. At this time she can be rather easily distracted from the contractions and can occupy herself with the completion of last minute preparations and arrangements, usual activities around home, reading, and so on.

From the beginning, the presence of the baby's father, or other labor partner whom she chooses to be with during labor, is important to her ease of mind and physical relaxation. There is no need for their separation at any time unless by their choice. She is especially open to learning at this point, and so it is a good time to discuss any questions she may have about labor or birth.

She should be guided to conserve her mental and physical energies through distraction and relaxation; having the same attendants with her throughout the intrapartum period is very helpful. One of the best combatants of fear is the constant presence of consistent, caring people—both her labor companion and the attendants. The helping, sustaining relationship of her labor partner can have a positive influence on the total labor and birth experience. It may also affect future relationships between parents and baby and between the parents themselves.

As labor progresses, the woman will need increasingly more reassurance that everything is proceeding normally; the father or others need to be supported in the same manner. The laboring woman will be more concerned about her ability to get through labor as the contractions increase in strength and duration. She will also require more intense guidance and direction with breathing techniques through each contraction, with measures of distraction, and with relaxation. As she becomes totally focused on working with the contractions, she will need to be reminded of the need to void frequently, to try various comfort measures and postural changes, and to let her attendants know what she is feeling.

Toward the latter part of the first stage (transition) the laboring woman often becomes somewhat irritable, easily agitated, restless, impatient, demanding, and discouraged; this may be expressed verbally, facially, or with actions. The transition period is a time of great testing and requires encouragement that she can do it. She may feel that she "can't stand anymore of this" and may stop trying to work with her labor forces. Calm, firm, and confident reassurance by all those around her, along with frequent reminding of her progress and use of physical comfort measures, will help her in progressing to the second stage of labor.

Usually there is relief, both physical and emotional, with the bearing down efforts of the second stage. There is increased active work and energy expenditure with each contraction and an equally increased need to be helped to relax and rest between contractions. There is frequently a natural desire to sleep between contractions at this time if relaxation can be achieved. Some women need and desire medication during the active phase of labor. Regardless of her preferences and individual circumstances, she needs to be reassured that she can accomplish the job that is required of her.

Pharmacology and Labor Pain

Ideally, any relief measures during labor will have the following characteristics: (1) perceived relief of pain by the woman in labor, (2) clarity of the woman's mental state, (3) ability of the woman to maintain control of decision-making capacities and of the work involved in labor, (4) lack of deleterious effect on the fetus (immediate or future), and (5) lack of undesired effect on the course of labor (e.g., uterine contractility and the voluntary expulsive forces).

Increased study and scrutiny are being applied to the possible long-term effects on the baby of pain relief measures. Experience with intervention measures to alleviate pain has included such things as psychological and pharmacological methods such as hypnosis and acupuncture.

The pain associated with the physiological uterine contractions of labor has not been clearly explained. Some of the suggested causes of pain during the first and second stages of labor include: hypoxia of the myometrium when contracted; stretching of the cervix and lower uterine segment; compression of cervical and lower uterine nerve ganglia by interlocking muscle bundles during myometrial contraction; stretching of the supportive ligaments and overlying peritoneum; and stretching of the vagina, vulva, and perineum in the second stage.

The hypothesis that first-stage labor pain is due to compression of nerve ganglia of the cervix and lower uterus, and to the stretching of these structures during uterine contractions, is supported by the finding that the pain of subsequent contractions is generally diminished appreciably following paracervical infiltration with a local anesthetic. The pain of contractions is also reduced during caudal anesthesia, which blocks the nerves coursing through the cervix but not those innervating the upper uterine segment. These first-stage pain impulses travel by way of sensory pathways, accompanying the sympathetic nerves and entering the spinal cord via the posterior roots of the eleventh and twelfth thoracic nerves.

The pain impulses of the second stage (associated with stretching of the vagina, vulva, and perineum) are carried by sensory pathways that are constituents of the pudendal nerves, with fibers entering the spinal cord by way of the posterior roots of the second, third, and fourth sacral nerves.

These two routes involved with pain transmission during labor may be interrupted pharmacologically at specific sites. The techniques include paracervical, caudal, and pudendal blocks.

Some of the specific effects of these techniques, along with those of particular pharmacological analgesic agents, are shown in Table 6-4. It may be noted that some of these procedures (e.g., paracervical and uterosacral blocks) involve motor as well as sensory nerves to the uterus, so their use in early labor can cause uterine contractility to stop. The procedures of caudal epidural, pudendal, and saddle blocks eliminate the involuntary reflex urge to bear down that is initiated by the stretching of the perineum by the baby's head, and the consequent stimulation of sensory nerve receptors. However, with the use of low concentrations of local anesthetic, motor blockage may not necessarily be involved, and thus the woman will retain the ability to use her muscles to bear down when she is instructed of the presence of contractions.

Anesthetic Side Effects Maternal hypotension is a common side effect of epidural, caudal, and spinal blocks. In severe cases, it may be related to a concomitant compression of the inferior vena cava or a systemic toxic reaction. Persistent hypotension is followed by lessened uteroplacental blood flow, with fetal effects such as bradycardia and depression of the neonate.

It is well established that paracervical block is frequently accompanied by fetal bradycardia. There is also a relationship between the fetal blood level and the amount of local anesthetic; high fetal blood levels associated with fetal acidosis have been found in

TABLE 6-4 Anesthetic techniques and agents for labor and their effects

Agent or Technique	Optimal Dose or Concentration	Therapeutic	Cardiovascular	Respiratory
Bilateral pudendal block	10 ml	Analgesia in perineum; useful during delivery	None	None
Bilateral lumbar sympathetic block	10 ml at L-2 bilaterally	Block of uterine pain; analgesia during labor	No direct effect; mild hypotension in 5%–10%	None usually; mild depression with hypotension

Inhalation analgesia
  Nitrous oxide
  Trichloroethylene
  Cyclopropane
  Methoxyflurane
	
	40%–50%
	0.4%–0.6%
	3%–5%
	0.3%–0.6%
		Complete or partial analgesia in 75%–90% of the parturients without loss of consciousness	None	Little or no depression

Psychological analgesia
  Hypnosis
  Natural childbirth
  Psychophylaxis
	Intense preparation during pregnancy and reinforcement during labor	Analgesia in 20%; decrease in pain in 50%; modification of mood and behavior; amnesia in 20%–50%	Not studied in gravida; deleterious effects are probably seen only when technique fails	

Inhalation anesthesia
  Cyclopropane
 	
  Diethyl ether
 	
  Halothane
 	
  Methoxyflurane
	
	5%–12%
	
	2%–5%
	
	0.5%–1%
	
	0.4%–0.8%
		Used for maintenance of *light* anesthesia; higher concentration needed for induction	Mild increased cardiac output; arrhythmia
			Increased cardiac output; tachycardia
			Mild to moderate hypotension
			Bradycardia; slight decrease in cardiac output; hypotension
				Depression → hypoventilation
				Hyperventilation
				
				Depression → hypoventilation
				Depression → hypoventilation

Balanced anesthesia
  Thiopental or thiamalyl for induction → succinylcholine or *d*-tubocurarine → tracheal intubation → maintenance with N₂O₂-O₂ relaxant
    or
  Cyclopropane-O₂ relaxant
	Barbiturate, 100–150 mg IV; succinylcholine, 40–60 mg IV, *d*-tubocurarine, 9–12 mg IV; N₂O₂ 70%; O₂ 30%
	
	Cyclopropane 5%–10%; oxygen 90%–95%
		Barbiturates; rapid smooth induction; succinylcholine and *d*-tubocurarine; muscle relaxation; others: maintenance of *light* anesthesia	Little or no depression	Depression and respiratory muscle paralysis require controlled ventilation

Hepatorenal	Other	Labor	Fetal	Remarks
Not studied; probably none	Relaxation of perineum; convulsions with systemic reactions	Loss of bearing-down reflex	None except with complications	Paracervical–pudendal block combination provides complete analgesia with less alterations than other regional techniques
Not studied; probably none	None	Same as paracervical	Same as extradural	Excellent analgesia during labor; helps to correct incoordinate uterine activity
Little or no depression	None, except occasional nausea	None	None	Better analgesia than with narcotics
Not studied in gravida; deleterious effects are probably seen only when technique fails	None when properly used; psychiatric disturbances in patients with underlying emotional disorders	None	None; conditions of fetus better than with other methods of analgesia and anesthesia	Of benefit to all patients but must be complemented with other analgesics in most parturients
Mild transient depression Greater than cyclopropane Same as diethyl ether Same as diethyl ether	Emetic symptoms in 25%–40% Emetic symptoms in 40%–60% Little or no emetic symptoms Same as halothane	None with OD*; mild depression with deep anesthesia	Mild depression with OD; moderate to severe depression with deep or prolonged anesthesia	Best all around inhalation anesthetic Good, but conducive to overdosage; best agent for uterine relaxation
Little or no depression	None	None	Mild depression	Best anesthetic in patients with hypovolemia, anemia, hypotension, or other disorders contraindicating regional anesthesia; excellent for Cesarean section *(continued)*

TABLE 6-4 *(continued)*

Agent or Technique	Optimal Dose or Concentration	Therapeutic	Cardiovascular	Respiratory
Sedatives				
Barbiturates	100 mg IM 50 mg IV	Sedation and sleep	None with OD; mild depression with overdose	None with OD; depression with overdose
Ataractics	Dose varies with drug	Sedation and tranquility; antiemetic; potentiation of narcotics	None except hypotension with some (phenothiazine)	None with OD; hyperventilation with restlessness with overdose of promethazine (Phenergan)
Scopolamine	0.3 mg IM	Amnesia and sedation	None (minimal vagolytic effect)	None alone; depression when combined with barbiturate
Narcotics				
Morphine	8–10 mg IM; 2–5 mg IV	Analgesia, sedation, sleep, euphoria, decrease of anxiety, apprehension, and fear	With OD, none, except orthostatic hypotension; depression of all parameters with overdose	With OD, mild depression antagonized by pain; severe depression with overdose
Meperidine (Demerol)	75–100 mg IM; 25–35 mg IV slowly			
Other potent narcotics	Equianalgesic doses			
Regional techniques				

Continuous extradural block
  Lumbar epidural
  Caudal
	Analgesia to T-10 for labor and vaginal delivery	Greater degree of pain relief than with any other method	No direct effects; mild mild (10–15 mm Hg) hypotension (30 mm Hg or more) in 5% of patients due to vasomotor block and supine syndrome	No direct effects; mild depression with severe hypotension

Subarachnoid block ("saddle" block)	Same levels as in extradural techniques	Analgesia for labor and delivery	No direct effects; mild hypotension frequent; severe hypotension in 5%–10%; hypotension more rapid on onset than with extradural route	Same as extradural block
Bilateral paracervical block	10 ml bilaterally	Block of uterine pain; analgesia during labor	None	None

From Barber, H.R.K., & Graber, E.A. (1974). *Surgical disease in pregnancy.* Philadelphia: W B Saunders. With permission.
*OD = optimal dose.

Hepatorenal	Other	Labor	Fetal	Remarks
None	Gastric emptying retarded	None with OD	None with OD; depression with overdose	Useful during early (latent) phases of labor
None	Some produce neurological complications	None	None	Useful in combinations with narcotics
None	Restlessness; disorientation; marked dryness of mouth	None	May produce minimal depression	Should not be used in cardiac patients
None with OD except decreased kidney function	Gastric emptying retarded; emetic symptoms; dizziness	None if properly used (OD during active phase); retarded if given too early	Mild depression with OD; severe depression with overdose	Effective analgesics for moderate to severe pain in 75%–90% of parturients
None, except minimal decrease in renal blood flow and glomerular filtration → oliguria → prompt return to normal	None	None, unless started too early → prolongation of latent phase; loss of bearing-down reflex during second stage	None unless severe and sustained hypotension occurs → depression	Best all around analgesia for labor and vaginal delivery
Same as extradural block	Headache in 3%–30% (depending on size of needle); neurological sequelae rare	Same as extradural block	Same as extradural block	Excellent analgesia-anesthesia for pregnant cardiac patients except in those with hypovolemia, hypotension, anemia, CNS disease, etc.
Not studied; probably none	None; convulsions with improper technique	Same as extradural but bearing-down reflex not lost	Bradycardia in 15%–25% with complications → depression	Excellent analgesia during labor but does not prevent perineal pain; must be combined with pudendal or other technique

association with rapid transarterial diffusion of mepivacaine, as reported by Steffenson et al. (1970).

Local anesthetics administered to induce pudendal nerve, paracervical, epidural, or local infiltration anesthesia are absorbed rapidly from the injection site, cross the placental barrier, and appear in the blood of the fetus. The significance of this placental crossing depends on the resulting fetal blood level and the presence of preexisting fetal compromise from any cause. In most cases where fetal blood levels are low, there are no ill effects in the newborn.

The need for pain relief measures during labor is highly individualized and depends on many factors such as different fetal presentations and positions, rate of progress, or size of the baby. Each woman also brings her personal psychological make-up to the labor experience. This aspect includes such variables as her efforts to become psychologically and physically prepared; her sense of fear, anxiety, and apprehension; her feelings about pregnancy and becoming a mother; the stability of the parent-to-parent relationship; and her normal, individual perception and tolerance of pain.

Related to these factors is the labor environment. A soothing physical environment combined with the support of a labor partner, and backed up by the care providers can make a major impact on the kind and extent of relief measures required. Since no single measure is suitable for all women, a great deal of flexibility must be exercised in meeting the individual desires and needs for pain relief.

The work of pain may be viewed as an inherent part of the work of labor. The dimensions, or tasks, of pain work as analyzed by Strauss et al. (1974) include the expression of pain, the diagnosis of the meaning of pain, the minimizing or prevention of pain, and the endurance of pain. According to their observations, nurses have to deal with their own reactions to the expressions of the person experiencing pain. The management of pain was found to be equated with relief of pain, possibly due to advanced drug technology. The endurance of pain, which is linked with the expression of pain, may be a source of misunderstanding between the woman in labor and those providing care; the two may have different expectations about what constitutes the appropriate expression of pain, the appropriate endurance of pain, and when medication is appropriate.

Caring for the woman who is working with the pain of labor places the responsibility on the care takers of recognizing that each woman approaches these tasks of pain work differently, that pain is what the woman experiencing it says it is, and that the appropriate expression, endurance, or intervention of pain is what she deems it to be.

The pain of labor is unlike that of any other life situation: it has both temporal and spatial elements that are directly related to the physiological and biomechanical occurrences of the labor process; it is associated with the beginning of life rather than with illness or injury; and it has universal identification with labor contractions, in that labor is to each woman what she "feels."

In the context of childbirth and the laboring woman, pain can be conceptualized as a force of labor, along with the other physiological, psychological, and biomechanical forces and energies involved in labor. Pain, in this sense, has a potential positive involvement in the work that culminates in birth: it is part of the complex of labor forces with a pattern of energies and responses having a purpose—that of childbirth (Figure 6-5).

The pain of labor is interpreted by many women as a welcome signal for the beginning of the work of labor. It then continues to serve her as a guide to what is occurring physiologically, and how she can best use available time and activities during labor. As a positive force of labor, pain can be harnessed for optimal use in conserving energies and accomplishing the purpose of labor, rather than being accepted as negative, opposing force. The positive force of pain is enhanced by muscle relaxation, psychological calm, self-confidence, and a sense of control over what is occurring. The positive force of pain then works in unison with the other forces (uterine muscle contractions, cervical dilation, gravitational force, abdominal muscle force, and psychological forces) rather than in opposition.

In contrast, unharnessed pain becomes a negative force, operating not in conjunction with the other labor forces, but in opposition to them. Anxiety, fear, and tension enhance the negativity of pain, as described by Grantly Dick-Read (1959).

Negative response to the force of pain may take the form of avoidance, or reaction, or a combination of these. *Avoidance* is a passive response that includes the individual's capacity for tolerance. *Reaction* is an active response, in degree and in kind, to pain that is unavoidable. The harnessing of pain, and the manner of harnessing, is dependent on the individual.

Harnessing efforts may encompass both avoidance and reaction responses, and are influenced by such variables as the meaning of pain for the individual woman; her beliefs and culture; her relationships; her knowledge of the labor process; her general state of mind as well as the overall atmosphere for laboring. Her psychological preparation for the work of labor

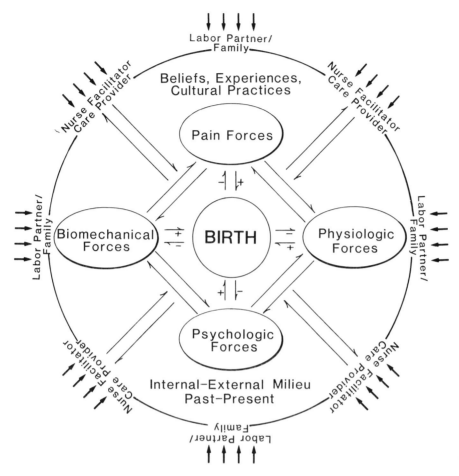

FIGURE 6-5 The complex of labor forces.

and her ability to cope with unexpected deviations will also greatly contribute to her capability of using the positive forces of pain.

Psychological Intervention There are many forms of psychological intervention in the pain process, some of which are practiced in psychoprophylactic methods of preparing for childbirth. In order to decrease anxiety and give direction to childbirth efforts, various distraction or coping techniques can be learned and used during labor.

Fear of the unknown can be removed with education, and pain can be influenced with techniques of intervention such as (1) diversion, dissociation, or distraction activities including breathing or physical actions (e.g., stroking or rubbing the abdomen or back, or exerting pressure on the lower back); (2) focusing methods like visual concentration, use of control words, interaction with another person; and (3) specific meditation techniques such as Zen Buddhism and

Yoga, or Transcendental Meditation; others may rely on prayer as a positive help. Thus, through the use of competing sensory stimuli and cognitive processes, the pain experience is altered for women during labor.

Effects of Psychological Analgesia Psychological techniques of analgesia do alter pain. Studies of the effects of these techniques have reported reduction of fear and anxiety levels (Klusman, 1975), lower levels of pain, higher levels of enjoyment during childbirth (Charles et al., 1978), lower levels of anesthesia and analgesia requirements (Zax et al., 1975), less frequent use of narcotics, less frequent use of conduction anesthesia, and a higher frequency of spontaneous vaginal deliveries following psychoprophylactic preparation (Scott & Rose, 1976).

There is a need for constant and refined evaluation of the long-range effects on the mother and baby of all methods of relief of maternal discomfort. Adamsons and Fox (1975) point out that it is no longer adequate to

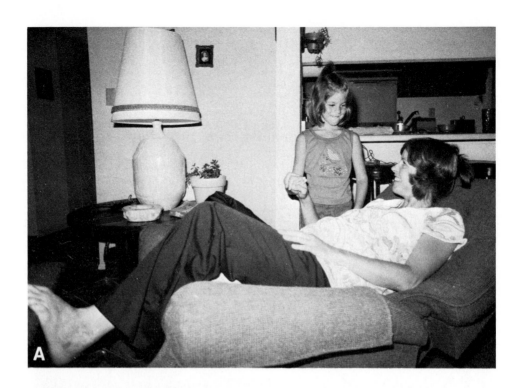

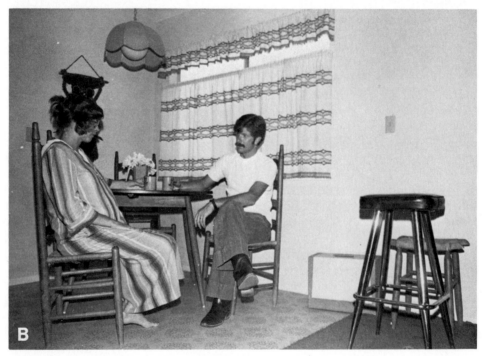

FIGURE 6-6 Labor-birth environment for normal, low-risk pregnancy. (A) In early labor, the woman and one of her children spend time in lounge-kitchen area of birth setting, relaxing with each other before the woman changes clothes. (B) The woman and her partner eat in the kitchen area. (C) The labor partner checks a contraction as a child shares this time with them (the children also shared in the preparation and practice for labor and birth). (D) As active labor progresses, more comfortable dress and surroundings—including a bed—are sought for periodic rest and position changes. Intensity of a contraction is checked by the laboring woman. (E) Resting. (F) Trying an alternative position for back discomfort, surrounded by helpers. (G) Finding relief by standing and leaning forward. (H) Concentrating on total relaxation. (I) Helper applies back pressure during transition. (J) Teamwork continues during second-stage bearing-down efforts. (Photographs courtesy of Jim Testa, El Paso, Texas.) *(Continued on pp. 153–156.)*

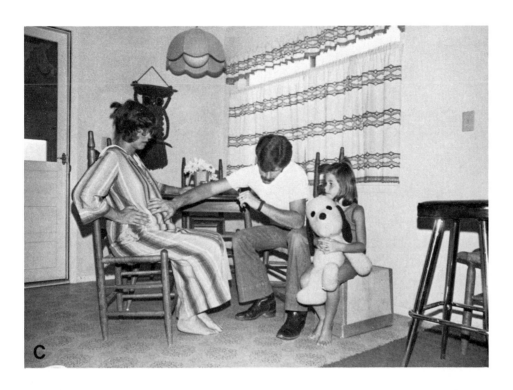

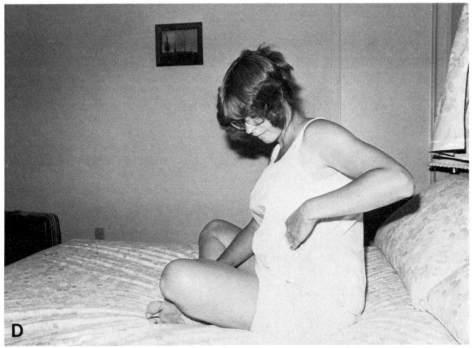

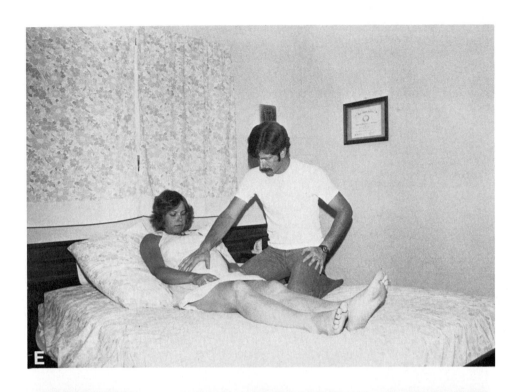

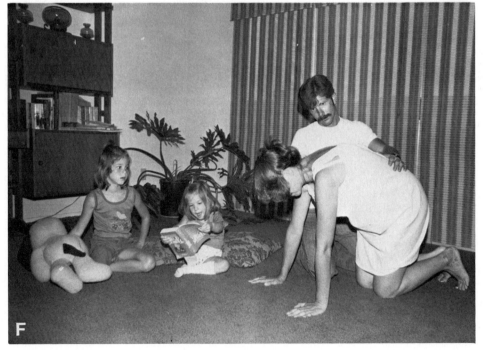

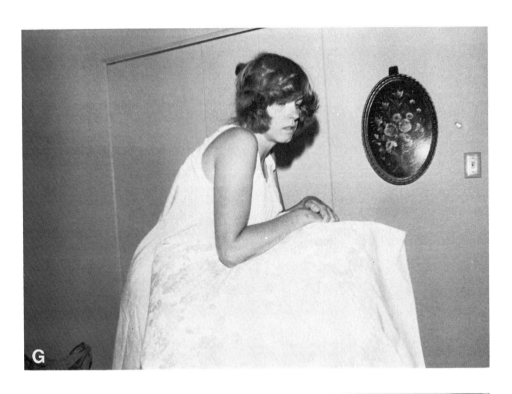

G

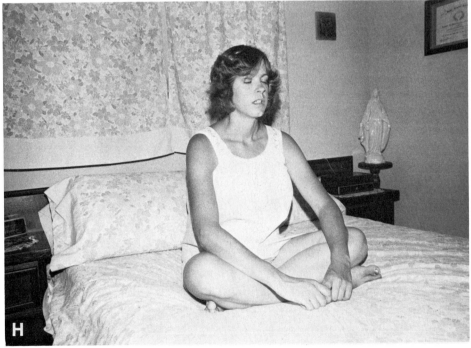

H

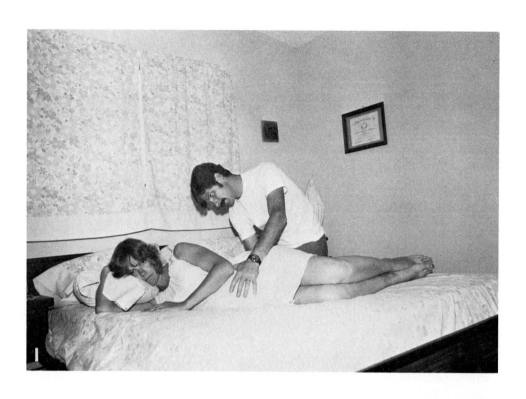

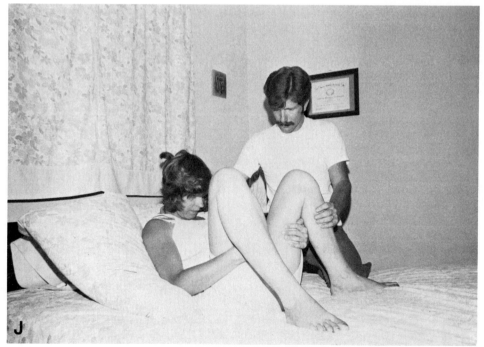

EXHIBIT 6-3 Helping the laboring woman and her companion apply learned childbirth techniques

To assist the couple in using the techniques of a prepared childbirth method, the nurse should do the following:

- Learn the techniques as they are learned and practiced prenatally by the woman and her companion. Be familiar with the exercises, postures, comfort measures, controlled relaxation, and breathing, and know what each is intended to accomplish.
- Become familiar with the helping role of the laboring woman's companion and how this person can most effectively be supported, backed up, and augmented.
- Whenever possible, work through the companion in offering suggestions or help.
- Avoid interference with the couple or the techniques being used when the two are working together; try not to undermine their efforts.
- Avoid stereotyped or rigid expectations with respect to "results" the woman should experience with any particular technique at any point in labor.
- Assist the labor companion in recognizing changes of the woman's responses (to labor and to the techniques being used). Supply encouragement to the woman, and carry out comfort measures such as back pressure, back rub, changes of position, effleurage or stroking of the body or limbs for relaxation, mouth rinses, nourishment, wiping face with cool cloth, keeping lips moistened, and others.

- Offer reassurance that their efforts are appropriate and productive.
- Assist the companion in recognizing the beginning of each contraction by palpation and in coordinating the breathing pattern with the contractions, and with changes in the contractions and overall labor.
- Interpret variations of normal labor (e.g., the "back labor" associated with posterior presentation), offer modifications of techniques if appropriate, and reassure the woman and her companion of the progress in labor, the effects of their efforts, and the fitness of the baby and the mother.
- Help them assess the need and desire for analgesia or anesthesia.
- Be particularly aware of changes and behaviors of the transition phase of labor, and be available to help interpret these, to carry both the woman and her companion through this difficult period, to help maintain or regain control, and to remind them of the more rapid progress and "shorter distance to go" from this time to the birth.
- Offer to relieve the companion or companions periodically, or "stand in" for them at intervals if this is desired; labor companions also need nourishment and time to "recharge" in order to continue dealing with the stress that is being shared and to give strength and encouragement.
- Remain constantly available during the bearing-down efforts to provide guidance, to dispel fears associated with the feelings of immense rectal pressure, burning, or tearing, and to relieve the fear of being unattended when the baby is born.

use the absence of a narcotized, limp, apneic infant, or even the presence of a high Apgar score as outcome criteria for maternal analgesia. Thermoregulation of the newborn, maternal attachment behaviors, and behaviors of the child as he or she develops are examples of measures to be given serious attention.

Childbirth Preparation

Assistance with Prepared Techniques

Nurses can help individuals to use any of the prepared childbirth methods. Providing such help requires that the nurse maintain an attitude of support of the techniques being used and the persons involved, including possibly relinquishing some traditional "nursing tasks" to the labor companion (Figure 6-6). The nurse also should learn the specific principles and techniques involved in the various methods.

Exhibit 6-3 lists broad areas and means for providing this help.

Preparation During Labor

The woman who, for whatever reason, has not undertaken a recognized method of preparing for childbirth prior to the onset of labor, with or without a labor companion, can be "talked" and "walked" through the preparation as a part of her care. The nurse should begin with whatever is appropriate to her stage of labor at the time, and proceed on a contraction-by-contraction basis.

If the nurse's first contact with the woman occurs in early labor (2–4 cm dilation) she will probably still be amenable to a beginning assessment of her labor status, and her informational and other needs, in a relatively social atmosphere. On the other hand, the woman who is in advanced active labor (6 or more cm dilation) at first meeting may be better served by the simple act of having the nurse constantly with her, explaining only the necessities and what is to be expected immediately ahead; her ability to take in external or auditory stimuli at this time is becoming quite limited. Responsiveness of the woman at this stage is usually much greater to the physical presence or nearness of another caring person (this may be a husband-partner, sister, friend, nurse, or other), and to comfort measures and verbal guidance in quiet, slow, deliberate tones. The atmosphere or pace that is set by the attendant is frequently picked up by the laboring woman, and reflected in her responses: Slow speaking and demonstration of breathing usually elicits a slowing, and calming of her breathing and responses to the contractions and other sensations of labor. In contrast to this, a rushed effort to get her "properly attired" in a gown, or to shave the perineal area will set the tone for excitable responses.

The constant presence of the same companion, combined with simplicity of words and actions, provides a good foundation for support of the laboring woman's own physical and emotional strengths. Same level, eye-to-eye contact as well as touch can help to strengthen nonverbal or verbal communication, although it should be recognized that some persons do not wish to be touched and respond negatively to physical contact. Initially, it is important to determine what concerns or bothers her most at the time and to give attention to helping her with that, whether it is pain, concern about the unborn baby, how her other children are managing, fear about how she will do when the labor becomes stronger, or something else.

Once it is established that the woman and her baby are well, and that a normal, low-risk labor is in progress, there are few reasons to rush any aspect of care. The woman may be more comfortable walking, and should wear whatever clothes are comfortable at her time in labor. Alternating activities and positions of sitting, walking, taking nourishment, lying down if desired, visiting with her family, or whatever she prefers, are beneficial to mental diversion and relaxation, and tend to promote descent of the presenting part. It is important that she be encouraged to try different positions and activities and to choose what is right for her.

Her stage of labor or response to labor may be such that it is first necessary to focus her attention in order to help her. Some clues to this may include her withdrawal and inability to respond to verbal or touch stimuli, pulling away from any attempted communication; thrashing about in bed; eyes closed—or opened wide, with an unfocused stare of fear; responding with screams of continuous, disorganized, uncontrolled terror, as opposed to the moaning or organized noise making associated with contractions and the work of labor. Usually a slow, quiet, gentle, but firm approach will reach her first during the period *between* contrac-

tions. During the contractions, her sensory perceptions (auditory, visual, tactile, and so on) will probably be somewhat blocked by her perception of pain and other labor forces.

A beginning step in getting her attention may be eye-to-eye contact initiated by the nurse's efforts and by the nurse's own postural change as needed to be in the most effective position to work with the woman in whatever position she has chosen. Sometimes simply sitting with her, placing a hand on her arm, and waiting will get results; or, finding out where it hurts and beginning to apply pressure, massage, or whatever seems helpful. Other times she may be helped by a change of positions to alleviate discomfort and allow for back pressure or massage, to facilitate relaxation. Any response, even an initial negative response such as telling the nurse to "leave her alone" is an opening to communications and an outlet for her feelings. Acceptance of any kind of response goes a long way toward a helping relationship.

Magee (1976), in writing of her own experience both as a laboring woman and as an obstetrician, emphasized the need to let the person who is hurting know that it is all right to make noise, to cry, to say what is on her mind, or to respond in whatever manner gives her relief.

After getting her attention or response, an attempt can be made (between contractions) to help the woman identify and understand the characteristics of her contractions, by describing to her how the present one is ending; how the next one will begin and come to a peak, then gradually ease; that there is a time between contractions when she needs to "loosen up" to help her uterus, and her entire body and mind to rest until the next one. The term "relax" frequently does not have meaning during intense labor and stress, and often elicits a response of anger. If she can identify the contractions, what they are accomplishing, and how she can help by "untightening" her body to work with them, she can more easily begin to follow a breathing pattern as it is demonstrated by the nurse, so the two of them can do this together with the next contraction. She is asked to "follow me and breathe with me." A simple, easily adapted technique of breathing for women who have not been exposed to any form of preparation for labor is that of slow breaths, exhaled or "blown out," through pursed lips.

If she is nearing or in transition, and the stress of the labor necessitates it, the breathing is changed to a more rapid, shallow, puffing (as if blowing out a match or candle). Continued eye contact is important to her "following" and changing speeds or rhythms as needed to work with each contraction. Some women respond well to repetitive movement of the hand or fingers with a rhythmic, pendulum motion to provide a sense of timing for breathing; or, to rhythmic touch or stroking of the arm. Touching may bother others at this time. Tactile communication assumes major importance if verbal communication is limited for any reason. Such limitation may be due only to the effects or stage of labor, but may also include language differences, difficulties with speech, hearing, and other problems affecting verbal–auditory communications.

The nurse and labor companion are guided by palpating the onset, peak, and end of contractions, having the woman initiate her breathing at the first palpable tensing and "rising" of the uterus, and adjusting the breathing rhythm with the contraction itself and according to the woman's response to what she feels: facial expressions, body tensing, gripping the hands of other people, losing the breathing pattern, and so on. She should be told frequently that she is doing a good job.

Between contractions, a continuing explanation should be given of what will be happening next, how it may feel, and how she can help. She should also be reassured that the nurse will be staying there to help. She needs to be constantly reminded of the progress *she is making* and encouraged to continue the good work. Also, it is essential that she be assured that both she and the baby are doing well, and that she be allowed to listen to the baby's heartbeat as she desires.

While working together with her, other means of providing comfort include the occasional change to fresh dry clothes if she is perspiring; wiping her face with a cool cloth; keeping her lips lubricated and moist, offering ice chips, hard candy, or some means of keeping her mouth and throat moistened for easier breathing.

If signs of hyperventilation occur, such as dizziness, tingling, a feeling of stiffness around the mouth, or contraction and stiffness of the fingers, the woman should be assisted to breathe into a paper bag placed over her nose and mouth, or into cupped hands (her's or another person's), in order to increase the carbon dioxide level and help relieve the hyperventilation. At the same time, attempts should be made to equalize and slow her rate of inhaling and exhaling.

Generalized shivering, or uncontrollable shaking of the legs may occur around the time of transition. This may be relieved by asking her to "let them go" while they are supported by the nurse or labor companion and the inner thighs are massaged or stroked from knees to near the perineum.

If severe back pain is present, a change of position may provide relief. Any position that she finds helpful is appropriate.

Massage, light stroking, or firm counter-pressure at specified points of the sacrolumbar region are often helpful; the pressure may be applied constantly in one location, or with a firm movement of the heel of the hand, moving the skin over the underlying bones with circular or rocking motions. Either warm or cold compresses may be applied to this region as well.

During the first or second stage of labor, usually near transition (about 7–10 cm dilation) when there is increased descent of the baby, the woman may experience a feeling that the pelvic bones or "hips" are being spread apart. This is sometimes described as a feeling of extreme pressure, to which she frequently responds by exerting counter-pressure over one hip with her hand; or she requests that this be done for her. As the head descends further, the back pain moves lower, with feelings of massive distention at the base of the spine (soft tissue area below the coccyx). Descent of the head past the bladder into the vagina is accomplished by stretching of the vagina and labia with sensations of "splitting" or tearing; there may also be feelings of warmth and "burning." The cause of these feelings must be interpreted for the woman, and emphasized as "progress," and being "good" in bringing the baby nearer to birth. It must be stressed to her that while the tissues *are* being stretched and pulled, she is not actually tearing, and need not be afraid to bear down when the cervix is completely dilated, letting the buttocks drop down and the heavy, bulging feeling in the vagina drop downward as well; the sensation of how to release the pelvic floor muscles and let the perineal muscles relax or "go loose" can often be better understood by having her contract and tighten them with the buttocks lifted, followed by a dropping and releasing of the entire area. Some women find the use of a mirror helpful with this, but others find it distracting.

The bearing-down reflex may begin as a sense of pressure in the rectum at the peak of contractions, and then become an ever increasing bulge and heaviness, causing a feeling of urge to defecate. It is emphasized to her that her bearing down is *through the vagina.*

She is best guided in her breathing and her position for bearing down by her urge to do so, rather than by a preplanned pattern of, or position for pushing. Not all contractions will be equally accompanied by the same degree of bearing-down urge or for the same number of times. Some contractions may not be accompanied by any bearing-down sensation, and she may not want or need to bear down with those. There may be unusual circumstances, due to position of presenting part, or lack of descent of the presenting part to the pelvic floor for initiation of the bearing down reflex. In these unusual instances, if other measures to facilitate descent (e.g., position or postural changes to maximize gravitational effect) are not successful, the woman may need guidance in her efforts to bear down with contractions of good quality. Complete cervical dilation, however, is not necessarily an indication in itself to begin bearing down immediately.

By having her work *with* what she is feeling, and by waiting for the bearing-down urge to develop spontaneously as the head descends and stimulates neuroendocrine receptors, it is usually possible for her to exhale or "blow away" during the bearing-down exertion, thereby avoiding the holding of her breath. Extreme physical exertion to bear down while holding the breath (Valsalva maneuver) may have negative effects by contributing to: (1) increased blood pressure elevation with a cumulative effect in subsequent breath-holding efforts, followed by a sudden drop to a low level at the moment of release of breath-holding. This, along with the usual decreased uteroplacental circulation during the contraction, may further decrease the oxygen supply to the baby at that time (see section on The Maternal Cardiovascular System); (2) over-utilization of energy reserves by forced exertion of uterine and abdominal muscles, and of arms when used to pull back on legs; (3) increased stress on pelvic floor and perineum due due to involuntary contraction of the sphincter muscles. Breathing out allows for relaxation of these muscles and for stretching of tissues; and (4) taking away from the woman her sense of control and timing that she needs in order to go along with the way she feels her body is guiding her.

As the time of birth approaches, the position best suited for bearing down and for birth continue to be the choice of the laboring woman. Interference with her work of bearing down, or insistence that she "not push" in order to delay the birth until the arrival or readiness of the birth attendant is not justifiable. The manner of bearing down is important both to the efficient use of energy and to protection of the perineum.

Case 1

A young primigravid woman, recently arrived in the United States from Asia, came to the hospital's labor area in early active labor. A labor and birth attendant (nurse-midwife) was called to be with the woman. The woman, who had not previously met the people who would be providing care, was at that time turning from side-to-side in bed and showing facial expressions of pain with each contraction. A language barrier prevented verbal communication between the non-English-speaking woman and her attendant; however, while awaiting the arrival of her husband, some universal sign language served to establish that her back was hurting and that she needed to void. After going to the bathroom, the woman removed the hospital gown and assumed a squatting position on the floor. It was indicated to her (and to all other persons involved in her care) that this was a good position for labor; she, in turn, indicated relief of the pain in her back.

Her husband arrived shortly thereafter and seemed somewhat surprised at the laboring position his wife had chosen. They had participated in a childbirth preparation program and had practiced laboring positions and breathing and relaxation techniques in the traditional American manner, and in accordance with Western and American cultures.

This woman clearly understood what was happening to her in labor, was well in control of the labor, and was doing what was normal labor behavior for her. Her husband showed some discomfort with the situation in the beginning and asked if she should be in bed. He was assured that her squatting position was a good position for labor, that it seemed to be providing greater comfort for her, and that it presented no difficulties in her care. He talked with her about this, and then stated that she wished to continue in that position; he remained present during the entire labor, helping his wife and the attendant communicate more readily, with care being given by the attendant, as desired by the woman.

All labor assessments were done with the woman in the squatting position. Contractions were palpated with no difficulty, and the fetal heart tones were assessed by use of a Doppler instrument on an intermittent basis. The attendant sat on a stool on the same level with the woman, which made assessment of contractions, fetal heart tones, and labor changes quite easy, and allowed eye-to-eye contact.

Progress of labor was assessed by the woman's actions, facial expressions, statements, gestures, and physical signs of changing status. Vaginal examinations were not performed after the initial nursing assessment (membranes had ruptured spontaneously two hours after the onset of contractions and prior to coming to the hospital). Amniotic fluid was seen to be clear, and continued to be lost from the vagina throughout labor, for which easily changed linen protectors were placed on the floor beneath her to absorb the leaking fluid. She walked to the bathroom frequently to void and then return to the same position.

During the course of early labor and into the active phase, uterine contractions by palpation progressively increased in intensity (decreased indentability of the uterus) and in frequency and duration; as labor continued, progressive descent of the baby could be gauged by abdominal palpation and by the descending location of the point of maximal sound of the fetal heart tones lower in the abdomen.

Within three hours, signs of transition appeared, including beads of perspiration on the upper lip and face; flushing on the face; belching and occasional hiccuping; widening of the eyes during some contractions with an expression of distress and a signaling of some feelings of losing control; and, an occasional involuntary catching of the breath in the throat and holding it with some contractions, indicating the beginning signs of the reflex urge to bear down with descent of the presenting part. Within the next hour she was experiencing involuntary bearing down as the baby's head reached the pelvic floor (with no evidence of any reason to discourage this; i.e., no unusually increased vaginal bleeding to suggest early bearing down against an incompletely dilated cervix, or laceration of the cervical tissues, and no unusual fetal heart tone pattern).

Progress of descent during her bearing down was assessed first by observing, and placing the palm of the hand over the soft, hollow area of the back located between the coccyx and the rectum. Distention or bulging of this area can be seen and palpated as the baby's head descends past the coccyx and onto the pelvic floor; with further stretching of the soft pelvic-floor structures, the head begins to distend first the rectal and then the vaginal openings until the head is directly visible.

At this point, the woman indicated that she wished to go to the bed; she was told that she could, but that if she preferred, she did not need to. She chose a semisquatting, semisitting position on the bed, with back support provided by another attendant. The vulva and perineal area was washed with a warm cleansing solution while she remained in that position with hips elevated slightly by a wedge.

Her 7-lb girl was born without need for an episiotomy. The cervix, vagina, vulva, and perineum were examined after the birth and no lacerations were found. No attempt had been made to perform an episiotomy, or to interfere in any manner with the woman and her labor, her position, or her ability to maintain control at the crucial time just prior to the birth of the baby's head.

In talking about the experience afterwards, the husband emphasized that his wife was quite happy (a feeling she conveyed to her attendants without the use of words) to have labored in the manner that she had learned by being with her own mother during the labors and births of four younger siblings at home. She seemed to be satisfied with her own accomplishment and the work she had done to achieve it.

Protection of the Perineum

Bearing-down efforts during second-stage labor can be performed slowly over a sufficient period of time to facilitate gradual stretching of the vaginal outlet and perineum and to avoid the need for episiotomy. The woman is encouraged to bear down according to her "feeling of need," rather than in accordance with a predetermined schedule. This contributes to more gradual stretching of vaginal and perineal tissues, optimum utilization of total energy, and prevention of overworking of the uterine muscle and of her total energies, all of which can lead to decreased effectiveness of uterine contractions and to extreme fatigue as she nears the end of the second stage. Both of these

sometimes result in intervention with such measures as oxytocin augmentation or forceps assistance. The pacing of bearing-down efforts in harmony with the reflex urge is an effective guide to the woman's efficiently performing the work of second-stage labor, and maintaining control of her labor.

Protection of the vagina, perineum, and external genitalia (including the periurethral area) is accomplished through patience by the birth attendant, and the continuation of the slow, gradual stretching of tissues by the presenting part. This, too, requires the woman's control of breathing and bearing down, with assistance and encouragement from the birth attendant and the labor companion, so that minute-by-minute guidance is given to "blow out" and "breathe the head out" slowly during contractions, rather than pushing forcefully by holding the breath.

Some women find their bearing-down efforts are helped when they are able to watch the progressive descent (bulging and crowning) of the baby's head in a mirror.

Stress on the perineal area and associated lacerations can be lessened and prevented by a position in which the thighs are not widely separated or abducted, and which allows for relaxed, nonstressed perineal tissues (sitting or semisitting, lateral, or squatting positions, for example). In addition to this benefit, the woman may experience a change in her urge to bear down in relation to certain positions, so that the position may influence either a decrease or an increase in that reflex and in her ability to respond to it. The nurse's encouragement to try different positions may reveal to the woman her best position for the maximum urge to bear down and for greatest comfort in doing so.

SEXUALITY OF LABOR

In discussing the female reproductive triad of coitus, birth, and lactation, Newton (1973) noted that there is a tendency in this society to emphasize the first, and ignore sexual aspects of the other two. Deutsch (1945) described childbirth and coitus as somewhat analogous in biological terms with respect to the double task of the female reproductive organs and the rhythm of retention and expulsion that dominates both. It is emphasized by Kitzinger (1972) that labor constitutes but one part of a woman's psychosexual life, with the whole of her life rhythm comprising puberty and menarche, ovulation and menstruation, love-play and intercourse, pregnancy and labor, involution and breast-feeding, and menopause. The psychosocial elements of all of these are seen as interrelated, so that a characteristic of one may carry over into other psychosexual life situations. For example, what the woman learns about herself in labor may contribute to her sexual relations in the future: "sensations of which she becomes aware, rhythms to which she is able to surrender herself, whether in reaching orgasm or in the remarkably similar urge to bear down in the second stage of labour, for instance, are interconnected" (Kitzinger, 1972, p. 147).

The marked similarities of the three reproductive acts just discussed require their having a place in any consideration of women's sexuality. Newton (1973) suggests that, while the neurohormonal involvement in parturition, coitus, and lactation is not completely understood, there is experimental evidence of some similarity among these physiological processes, including the involvement of oxytocic substances.

The sexual aspects of labor, when related consciously or unconsciously to other psychosexual experiences may bring into focus for the woman her feelings about her own sexuality, about labor, about the baby's father, and in some instances, about the baby. This can be a problem of great significance to any woman, but especially to the teenager.

Special Considerations for the Teenager

The teenager is in the midst of physical, biological, social, and emotional changes. The passage from childhood to adulthood involves the striving for independence (with a source of security), maturity (with approval for periodic return to childhood fantasies), identity (with resolution of conflicts and synthesis of a personal belief system), and sexuality. Keats and Bjorksten (1978) defined the various stages of adolescent sexual development to include (1) *sexual awakening*, the stage believed to occur between the ages of 13 and 15, with the development of secondary sex characteristics and confrontation with peer comparisons; (2) *practicing*, the stage occurring between ages 14 and 17 and involving practice of social skills needed to form intimate relationships; (3) *acceptance of sexual role*, the stage extending from age 16 to 19, with more intense sexual relationships, greater comfort with the role that is chosen, and a growing isolation from peers and family; and (4) *choice of permanent relationships*, the stage commonly occurring between ages 18 to 25 and beyond.

When pregnancy is added to the normal developmental tasks and stages of adolescence prior to their resolution, the pregnant teenager often becomes even more isolated from her usual sources of peer or family support and reassurance. Depending on her stage of sexual development and her relationship with the father of the baby, the teenager who is pregnant may have great difficulty coping with her isolation, as well as the uncertainties of her own sexual feelings and expressions, and intimate relationships. These factors often present the teenager with anxiety and fear that is intensified as labor approaches and begins, and in turn intensifies her perception of pain.

It is extremely important that the teenager not be left alone during labor. Open communication by a consistent, gentle care provider can help the laboring teenager to get more in touch with her body, her feelings about herself and her sexuality, her baby, and the forces of labor. Helping her to feel good about herself and the way she deals with her labor can have a significant impact on how she feels about her baby initially.

FEARS, FANTASIES, AND EXPECTATIONS

Some women approach and begin labor with an overall sense of harmony, control, inner strength, and of being generally pleased with themselves, while having some doubts and anxieties. Other women begin labor with a dominating sense of self-doubt, fear, anxiety, conflict, inadequacy, and hostility. For some, the reality does not match the expectation that childbirth should be a time of harmony and fulfillment, with freedom from feelings of disappointment, conflict, stress, hostility, or even emptiness.

In certain instances the woman may, for reasons possibly linked to her relationship with her partner, or to origins in her own childhood, attempt to retreat from the reality of a labor and birth experience that is for her overwhelming. She may wish for a labor in which she does not experience any sensations—physical or emotional. This could be expressed as resisting, fighting, or blocking out her body sensations and others around her. In the desire "not to feel anything," deep analgesia-anesthesia may be requested before labor begins.

The woman's feelings about her body and about childbirth exert an effect on the process and progress of labor. Kitzinger (1972, p. 149) comments on the effects of the woman's attitude in normal labor:

In a normal straightforward labour a woman's attitude of mind, her approach to the task that awaits her, and her preconceptions concerning the nature of the work that her body has to do, are more important than any sort of physical preparation she can make in advance. Whatever athletic exercises she may essay, however controlled her breathing, however complete her muscular relaxation, in the last resort the thing that matters most is, essentially, the kind of woman she is, and the sort of personality she has....Controlled muscular activity can assist her in making of her labour something she creates, rather than something she passively suffers, but her capacity for achieving this physical coordination is dependent upon her mind—upon her fearlessness and sense of security, her intelligence, her joy in the baby's coming, her courage, her self-confidence, and the understanding she has of herself.*

Common Fears

The final weeks of pregnancy and the beginning of labor superimpose different conditions of emotional crises on the individual woman; these frequently consist of doubts and fears concerning both herself and the baby. In a study of the fears of primigravid British women, MacDonald (1969) reported that a majority of primigravidas had fears about pain during labor; the next most common fears and anxieties, in order, were the following:

1. Congenital abnormality of the infant
2. Inability of the woman to meet the demands of infant care during the first few days of life (fear of feeding problems, of letting the baby fall, and of injuring the baby while bathing it)
3. Inability to identify the onset of labor
4. Being left alone during labor
5. General apprehension about the unknowns of a new experience
6. Loss of sympathy, or alienation, by attendants in labor due to "cowardly" behavior or through making too much noise
7. Inability of the father to love and accept the child
8. The possibility of stillbirth
9. Damage to external genitalia through tearing in second stage

Only two percent of this group expressed fears induced by "old wive's tales"; seventy-two percent of the women believed that the presence of their husband or partner could have greatly dispelled the anxieties they experienced in the first stage of labor.

Case 2

During the labor of a young primigravid nurse, who for the past several years had been involved in the cares of newborns with problems or abnormalities requiring intensive care,

---

*From *The Experience of Childbirth* by Sheila Kitzinger (Taplinger Publishing Co., Inc., 1972). © 1962, 1967, 1972 by Sheila Kitzinger. Reprinted by permission.

progress slowed and subsequently stopped with cervical dilation of 6 cm, descent of the presenting part at −1 station, and strong (by index of indentability) contractions of sixty-second duration occurring regularly at two-and-a-half- to three-minute intervals; membranes had ruptured spontaneously one hour prior to the onset of contractions.

During the early phase of active labor the woman had experienced persistent low-back pain and pressure, which intensified through the labor; abdominal and vaginal examination confirmed the baby to be in occiput posterior position. Various positional changes were used to relieve this, with some relief obtained in the vertical position, standing and leaning forward on a raised table padded with pillows, which allowed her to rest her folded arms and head on the pillows when desired while hand pressure was applied to her lower back by her labor companion. Both the nurse-midwife and others in attendance were well known to the couple through involvement with them during prenatal visits and classes to prepare for childbirth; open and direct exchanges of information took place before and during labor. Explanations were given of changes occurring in labor and of what to expect next, with no assumptions being made about informational needs or lack of needs because she was a nurse.

With the growing effects of fatigue and lack of progress in labor over a period of hours, she began to ask repeatedly "Is the baby really in posterior position?" "Why isn't the position changing?" Reassurance was given of the position and that some change was occurring; however, the position became right occiput transverse and remained so. Evidence of lack of progress of labor and signs of distress for the baby began developing. The fetal heart tones had been monitored while she labored in the standing position by using a Doppler instrument to listen through each contraction and for at least thirty seconds or more into the interval between contractions. Both the woman and her companion listened to the baby frequently and were informed of changes, including the need to alter the original plans for labor and birth to now include measures to improve the status of the baby.

Significant late decelerations of the fetal heart tones had begun to occur in the range of 100–110/min, with a duration of twenty-five to forty seconds past the end of palpable contractions, representing a deviation from the previous range of 128–144/min with no decelerations. Placing herself in the lateral positions and breathing oxygen did not lead to improvement of the fetal signs of distress; instead, a persistent bradycardia (fetal heart rate of 90/min) developed. These findings were confirmed on auscultation by two attendants. Intravenous infusion of fluids had been started and the changing status of the baby explained. The possible need for birth of the baby by Cesarean section had been introduced to the couple by this time and the situation further evaluated by the obstetrician.

Throughout all the earlier measures—position changes, application of pressure to the back, and changes of breathing pattern to accommodate her intense need to bear down when cervical dilation was 6 cm—the woman's questioning persisted: "Are you sure the baby is in that position?" Reassurance of this, as well as the progress that had occurred, was repeated. On several occasions she was also assured that the attendants were not aware of any situation or information that she did not know about; however, her reluctance to be able to accept this explanation continued and she freely verbalized this.

After the couple's final preparation, including plans for the labor companion to be present and remain with her during surgery, a Cesarean section was performed. At the time of birth, the woman immediately asked her companion if there was something wrong with the baby "other than having been in that position." His reassurance, and her seeing her new son immediately, was the first evident relief of her anxieties. Several hours later, while verbally reconstructing her labor, she expressed to the nurse-midwife the fear that she had been unable to express earlier—that the baby was hydrocephalic and that this was the cause of all the problems during labor; she associated this fear and anxiety, which had begun during the third trimester, to her experiences with infants for whom she had provided nursing care in the intensive care nursery. The very real possibility of her baby being hydrocephalic had become her unshared burden for several months and throughout an agonizing labor.

Retrospectively, it was recognized that this person, because of her previous close relationship and caring for infants with severe physical and nervous system deviations, had a need for someone to ask about the feelings and concerns that she had in order that she might have been able to acknowledge, to express this fear, and to share it with someone, possibly alleviating her anxiety much earlier.

ROLE FULFILLMENT–REVERSAL AND LOSS-SEPARATION

Among the multiple sources of anxiety during pregnancy and birth are the woman's concerns about her ability to give birth to a normal baby, and her capacity to fulfill societal expectations of the maternal role and to accept responsibility for the completely dependent newborn, particularly with the first birth. Gordon (1978, p. 204) observes that many women "cannot spontaneously 'switch on' maternal feelings the moment they are presented with their babies, and it is immensely helpful to them to know that their uncertain, initial responses do not necessarily indicate the lack of a maternal instinct."

A woman may not have experienced a satisfying relationship with her own mother and may as a result look to her baby to provide the protection, love, and gratification for which she has longed in the past. In so doing, a role reversal takes place with the woman

seeking a parent in the infant who is incapable of fulfilling this role, resulting in mutual frustration, anxiety, withdrawal, or more extreme acting out of feelings of hate. Other unresolved conflicts may include earlier sibling rivalries causing maternal perception of the newborn as a previously hated brother or sister, or the childhood experience of death of a sibling or parent, which can cause distorted responses to her baby at this time due to unresolved blame or guilt association.

Past, unresolved experiences of the mother may make it impossible for her to respond appropriately to her own infant. Relatively early signs of maternal and infant distress or disharmony may be communicated by the manner in which the mother holds, looks at, feeds, touches, or talks to her infant, and how she responds to the baby's cries or other signs of distress. Early indications of a failure of mother–baby communications and disturbed relationships require further exploration and assessment of the mother's need for help in relating to her baby. Likewise, the father's relationship and interactions with the baby, as well as his ability to provide emotional support for the mother, are dependent on his own childhood relationships and experiences.

Feelings of loss during labor can be related directly to loss of control of bodily functions. Fear of loss-separation may be attached to feelings of involuntary regression to earlier, infantile bodily functionsd as labor progresses. Although intellectually anticipated, the escape of amniotic fluid from the vagina, sensations of pressure or involuntary pushing—possibly accompanied by loss of urine or feces—can be a source of extreme anxiety as loss of control of body functions is experienced.

FAMILY MEMBERS PRESENT DURING LABOR AND BIRTH

Children

Separation of the mother from her other children at the time of labor and birth has been compared with the trauma of death, in terms of the dehumanization of family members that may result from institutionalization for either of these events (Enkin, 1975; Kubler-Ross, 1976; Mauksch, 1975; Mehl et al., 1977). One answer to the separation of families, and the associated dehumanization of the birth process, has been the home birth movement (Arms, 1975; Hazell, 1969; Sousa, 1976; Ward & Ward, 1976). Other responses have included alternative birth settings with hospital affiliations.

The inclusion of children in the labor and birth experience at an alternative birth room was reported by

Goodman (1976) to have no untoward effects on children. However, there has been objection by some to the involvement of children on the basis that birth is not a part of the activities of childhood (Brazelton, 1977). Still others consider the age of the child, especially between 1½ and 5 years, and the possible pressuring of the child to see the birth, as potentially leading to adverse effects. It has been cautioned that the facial reactions of the mother in labor, as well as the sight of blood, may be associated with physical injury in the prior experiences of a child (Sousa, 1976). In many cultures the presence of children at birth is an acceptable part of the life experience, since the outcome of birth affects every member of the family (Sousa, 1976).

Separation of families, and the exclusion of other children in the family during the time of labor and birth, may not only be traumatic for the woman, but may mark the beginnings of more intense sibling rivalry and jealousy (Ginott, 1965; Hazell, 1969; Sousa, 1976; U.S. Government Report, 1970). Ginott (1965, p. 146) proposes that "in contrast to their parents, children do not question the existence of jealousy in the family.... Regardless of how thoroughly they were prepared, the arrival of a new baby brought jealousy and hurt." In particular, the birth of the second baby presents a crisis in the life of the young child, and a change in his or her spatial boundaries.

As pregnancy progresses, the young child notices that the mother is beginning to be less available, more tired, and has less room on the lap for sitting—that space being occupied by "the intruder." Ginott suggests that preparations begin during pregnancy to try to understand and deal with the child's unasked questions and unexpressed worries, including that of being replaced, and of the hurt that is involved in sharing the mother. The child can be introduced to the coming baby by being able to feel and hear the baby inside of the mother, by an honest approach (being told the good *and* the bad to be expected in living with the new baby), and by not being forgotten or shut out as the family sphere widens.

A child's greatest fear is that of being abandoned and unloved. The stress of separation at childbirth intensifies the fantasy of being left alone in the world (Ginott, 1965). Older children can be included in talking about, and planning for, the new baby; and in small doses, the older child can learn that there is room for another and that he or she will not be shut out or forgotten. The child under 3 years may need to be "babied" again and may return to earlier habits during this adjustment period (U.S. Government Report, 1970).

Mehl et al. (1977) studied the beliefs and sexual attitudes of twenty children between the ages of 2 and 14 years, who had been present at the labor and delivery of siblings, and compared them to an equal number of children who had not been present at delivery. The children and their fifteen families were interviewed. The children in both groups were also observed at play, to study and interpret activities related to their sharing of this experience. It was found that parents of children present at delivery held attitudes that birth was a positive, normal family event that should involve the other children of the family. Children of these families tended to have accurate notions about "where babies come from," and to view birth as a happy, positive event. This was contrasted with the puzzling, inaccurate concept of birth expressed by children not present at birth. The results of the study are interpreted to suggest that the presence of children at birth allows for the development of an attitude of birth as a normal process in families having this ideology.

The Father

The father's presence and involvement in the labor and birth has, in this country, been influenced greatly by hospitalization and association of illness with childbirth, just as the woman's labor behaviors have been altered to fit this model.

The changing role of the father, of the family, and of styles of living seem to allow for integration of the concepts of tenderness, affection, and caring in male as well as female roles (English, 1965). Gentleness, empathy, tenderness, and emotional response are being recognized as human rather than male or female traits. Josselyn (1956) identifies the meanings the child has for the father, and the expression of tenderness and gentleness in a man toward his baby—the binding forces—as human characteristics and as fatherliness.

Early contact with the newborn seems to have an effect on the father as well as the mother. The father who attends the birth, holds the newborn, and sees him or her in the first hours of life, tends to remain more closely tied to the child and to experience an increased feeling of self-esteem (Greenberg & Morris, 1974; Hersch & Levin, 1978). The father's inclination toward early contact and interaction with the newborn is affected by preparation for this and by having his emotional needs met during pregnancy; this is further facilitated by his receiving needed support during labor and childbirth.

According to Tanzer and Block (1972), the father, through involvement in childbirth, sees himself as important, competent, and performing valuable emotional and physical functions. Benedek (1970) considers empathy as the vehicle of communication within the psychological field of the family; the man is preparing himself for parenthood by supporting and empathizing with his mate during pregnancy and birth and by becoming a part of the family triad, thus strengthening the bonding between mates. The nurturing responses and behaviors of the father are brought about by the gratification received from his responsive and receptive infant (Hersch & Levin, 1978).

The role of the father during labor is primarily that of comforter, supporter, and at times, interpreter of the woman's actions, responses, needs, and wishes. As such, he needs to know that he has a place and an important part to play during labor, and to know also, that there is someone available at all times to help him, and to "stand in" for him if he needs to leave at any time.

If the man seems reticent to go ahead with offering the woman comfort measures, assisting with relaxation and breathing techniques, and other aides to the laboring woman that they were taught (or that the two of them have worked out together), the labor attendant may help him to get started by demonstrating help through a few contractions and by providing some comfort measures jointly with his help at first. At other times his support is best elicited by backing away and allowing the two of them to work out how they can most effectively work with the labor, unless they indicate a desire for suggestions or help, or there is evidence of a developing problem for which all parties need to begin working toward a correction.

Some women may reject the man's presence during labor. This may be due to an insecure relationship, lack of trust, his noninvolvement in the entire pregnancy, or her feeling threatened by his involvement with the newborn, a function she may consider her own; her reasons may be of a cultural or religious nature; or, there may be other bases for the woman's decision about who will be with her during labor and birth. Regardless of the origin of the decision, it must be respected.

Case 3

A 22-year-old woman and her husband came to the hospital with their second pregnancy. She had had five hours of labor with her first baby, and had been awakened from sleep two hours ago with mild contractions that were now becoming regular and stronger, radiating from her lower back. The couple was from Saudi Arabia and had moved to this country only recently and temporarily. Since the woman did not speak English, her husband provided information concerning her health, the previous and current pregnancies and the onset of this labor. He indicated that he and his wife were Muslim, what his involvement would be in the labor and birth, and

what the plan was for them as a family after the baby was born (a short hospital stay was requested in order that the father, mother, 2-year-old child, and newborn could be together at home soon). He would be there with his wife during labor to help her and to facilitate communications with her, but he would not be present for the actual birth. The couple had requested a female birth attendant, and a nurse-midwife (female) met them at the time of their arrival.

Since this was the first meeting between the attendant and the couple, the woman was asked about her first labor and birth, and how she wanted this birth. She stated that most of her first labor had been spent driving for several hours to reach the hospital, she had received a local perineal anesthetic, did not require any "stitches," and had given birth to the baby in the bed in which she had labored. She wished to have this baby in the same manner, and was told that every effort would be made to help her to do so.

At this time contractions were occurring every four minutes, with a duration of one minute, and examination revealed cervical dilation of 5 cm. Within two hours, during which her husband was at her side, talking with her and stroking her forehead, her labor had progressed to 7–8 cm dilation, with contractions becoming more intense and occurring every three minutes. Her husband, remembering that he needed to make arrangements to be relieved at his work as a pilot, informed his wife and the attendant that he would need to leave for a short time and would then return.

Up until that time the woman had been sitting on the side of the bed, responding to each contraction by opening her eyes to look at her husband, while breathing more rapidly and moaning at times. When her husband left she seemed to become very drowsy; she lay down on her side, and slept soundly (without medication) while palpable contractions continued for the next thirty minutes. About twenty minutes after her husband's return she went to the bathroom and voided, then returned to the bed in a semisitting position and resumed her earlier response to the contractions, which were now quite intense and occurring every two minutes. Within a short time the membranes ruptured spontaneously, she began feeling a need to bear down with contractions, and the loss of amniotic fluid from the vagina was accompanied by a small amount of blood. Her husband stepped out of the room; her perineum was washed and a sterile towel was placed under the perineal area for the baby's arrival. She remained in the same position with legs outstretched and knees slightly flexed.

With the next contraction the head was born. Communication at that point (in the husband's absence) was dependent on touch, and hand and face gestures, to which she responded knowingly and from experience. The baby boy was placed skin-to-skin on the mother's abdomen and both were covered with warmed blankets. There was no episiotomy and no lacerations. After a few minutes (and after dry, warm linens were placed under her) she began breast-feeding, with her husband there to help. Their 2-year-old child came to see that her mother was all right, and, after a period of observation of mother and baby, an early discharge was arranged.

REFERENCES

Abbott, M.I. (1978). Teens having babies. *Pediatric Nursing, 4*(3), 23–26.

Abe, T. (1940). The detection of the rupture of fetal membranes with the nitrazene indicator. *American Journal of Obstetrics and Gynecology, 39,* 400–404.

Adams, C.J. (1977). Intrapartum risk factors and neonatal mortality. *Journal of Nurse-Midwifery, 22*(1), 35–40.

Adamsons, K., & Fox, H.A. (Eds.). (1975). *Preventability of perinatal injury.* New York: Liss.

Ademowore, A.S., & Myers, E. (1977). Use of the problem-oriented medical record by nurses caring for high risk antepartum patients. *JOGN Nursing, 6*(1), 17–22.

Aiken, L.H. (1977). Primary care: The challenge for nursing, *American Journal of Nursing, 11,* 1828–1832.

Ammon, L.I., & Rich, O.J. (1973). Expressions of hostility in early labor. *Maternal–Child Nursing Journal, 2,* 215–220.

Anderson, C. (1976). Operational definition of "support." *Journal of Obstetric, Gynecologic, and Neonatal Nursing, 5*(1), 17–18.

Anderson, S.F. (1977). Childbirth as a pathological process: An American perspective. *MCN: The American Journal of Maternal Child Nursing, 2*(4), 240–244.

Angelini, D.J. (1978). Nonverbal communication in labor. *American Journal of Nursing, 78*(7), 1221–1222.

Arms, S. (1975). *Immaculate deception.* Boston: Houghton Mifflin.

Atwood, R.J. (1976). Parturitional posture and related birth behavior. *Acta Obstetricia et Gynecologica Scandinavica, 57* (Suppl.), 5–25.

Aubry, T.H., & Pennington, J.C. (1973). Identification and evaluation of high-risk pregnancy: The perinatal concept. *Clinical Obstetrics and Gynecology, 16*(1), 3–27.

Baer, E.D., McGowan, M.N., & McGivern, D.O. (1977). How to take a health history. *American Journal of Nursing, 77*(7), 1190–1193.

Barber, B. (1976). Compassion in medicine: Toward new definitions and new institutions. *New England Journal of Medicine, 295*(17), 939–943.

Bayer, M., & Brandner, P. (1977). Nurse/patient peer practice. *American Journal of Nursing, 77*(1), 86–90.

Bean, M. (1975). Birth is a family affair. *American Journal of Nursing, 75*(10), 1689–1692.

Beard, R.W. (1974). The detection of fetal asphyxia in labor. *Pediatrics, 53*(2), 157–159.

Beazley, J.M. (1975). The active management of labor. *American Journal of Obstetrics and Gynecology, 122*(2), 161–168.

Beischer, N.A. (1967). The anatomical and functional results of mediolateral episiotomy. *Medical Journal of Australia, 2,* 189–192.

Beischer, N.A., & Mackay, E.V. (1967). *Obstetrics and the newborn.* Sydney: Saunders.

Bekhit, M. (1976). The use of episiotomy. *Nursing Times, 72,* 1231–1233.

Benedek, T. (1970). The family as psychologic field. In E.J. Anthony & T. Benedek (Eds.), *Parenthood, its psychology and psychopathology.* Boston: Little, Brown.

Benirschke, K. (1956). Adrenals in anencephaly and hydrocephaly. *Obstetrics and Gynecology, 8,* 412–413.

Beynon, C.L. (1974). Midline episiotomy as a routine procedure. *Journal of Obstetrics and Gynaecology of the British Commonwealth, 81,* 126–130.

Bonica, J.J. (1967). *Principles and practice of obstetric analgesia anesthesia.* Philadelphia: Davis.

Bonica, J.J. (1972). *Obstetric analgesia and anesthesia.* Heidelberg: Springer-Verlag.

Bonica, J.J. (1973). Maternal respiratory changes during pregnancy and parturition. *Clinical Anesthesia, 10*(2), 4–19.

Bonica, J.J. (1978). Pathophysiology of pain. In *Hospital practice. Proceedings: Current concepts in postoperative pain. A symposium.* New York: American Society of Anesthesiologists, pp. 4–14.

Brazelton, T.B. (1977). Cited in Children at birth: Effects and implications. *Journal of Sex and Marital Therapy, 3*(4), 275–277.

Brobeck, J.R. (Ed.). (1973). *Best and Taylor's physiological basis of medical practice* (ed. 9, sec. 2). Baltimore: Williams & Wilkins.

Bryant, W.M., Greenwell, J.E., & Weeks, P.M. (1968). Alterations in collagen organization during dilatation of the cervix uteri. *Surgery, Gynecology and Obstetrics, 126,* 27–31.

Burch, G.E. (1977). Heart disease and pregnancy. *Obstetrical and Gynecological Survey, 32*(8), 516–519.

Burchell, R.C. (1964). Predelivery removal of pubic hair. *Obstetrics and Gynecology, 24,* 272–273.

Butler, N.R., & Alberman, E.D. (Eds.). (1960). *Perinatal problems.* London: Livingstone.

Buxton, C.L. (1962). *A study of the psychoprophylactic methods of the relief of childbirth pain.* Philadelphia: Saunders.

Caldeyro-Barcia, R. (1976). Return to squatting position for delivery advised. *Obstetrical Gynecological News, 11*(22), 1, 43.

Caldeyro-Barcia, R. (1978). The influence of maternal bearing-down efforts during second stage on fetal well-being. In T. Simkin & C. Reinke (Eds.), *Kaleidoscope of childbearing.* Seattle: Penny Press.

Caldeyro-Barcia, R., Alvarez, H., & Reynolds, S.R.M. (1950). A better understanding of uterine contractility through simultaneous recording with an internal and a seven channel external method. *Surgery, Gynecology and Obstetrics, 91,* 641–644.

Caldeyro-Barcia, R., Melander, S., & Coch, J.A. (1971). Neurohypophyseal hormones. In F. Fuchs & A. Klopper (Eds.), *Endocrinology of pregnancy.* New York: Harper & Row.

Caldeyro-Barcia, R., Noreiga-Guerra, L., Cibils, L.A., Alvarez, H., Posiero, J.J., Pose, S.V., Sica-Blanco, Y., Mendez-Bauer, C., Fielitz, C., & Gonzalez-Panizza, V.H. (1960). Effect of position changes on labor. *American Journal of Obstetrics and Gynecology, 80*(2), 284–290.

Caldeyro-Barcia, R. Schwarcz, R.L., & Althabe, O. (1972). Effects of rupture of membranes on fetal heart rate pattern. *International Journal of Gynaecology and Obstetrics, 10*(5), 169–172.

Caldeyro-Barcia, R., Schwarcz, R.L., Belizan, J.M., Martell, M., Nieto, F., Sabatino, H., & Tenzer, S.M. (1974). Adverse perinatal effects on early amniotomy during labor. In L. Gluck (Ed.), *Modern perinatal medicine.* Chicago: Year Book.

Caplan, G. (1954). The mental hygiene role of the nurse in maternal and child care. *Nursing Outlook, 2*(1), 14–19.

Caplan, R.M., & Sweeney, W.J. (1978). *Advances in obstetrics and gynecology.* Baltimore: Williams & Wilkins.

Carsten, M.E. (1968). Regulation of myometrial composition, growth, and activity. In N.S. Assali (Ed.), *Biology of gestation, the maternal organism* (Vol. 1). New York: Academic Press.

Chapman, C.R. (1978). Psychological aspects of pain. In *Hospital practice. Proceedings: Current concepts in postoperative pain. A symposium.* New York: American Society of Anesthesiologists, pp. 15–19.

Charles, A.G., Norr, K.L., Block, C.R., Meyering, S., & Meyers, E. (1978). Obstetric and psychological effects of psychoprophylactic preparation for childbirth. *American Journal of Obstetrics and Gynecology, 131*(1), 44-52.

Charles, D. (1976). Sepsis is still a major cause of maternal death. *Obstetrical Gynecological News, 11*(22), 3.

Chinn, P.L. (1979). Issues in lowering infant mortality: A call for ethical action. *Advances in Nursing Science, 1*(3), 63-78.

Chiota, B.J., Goolkasian, P., & Ladewig, P. (1976). Effects of separation from spouse on pregnancy, labor and delivery and the postpartum period. *JOGN Nursing, 5*(1), 21-23.

Clark, R.B. (1973). Analgesia during labor: Effect on the fetus and neonate. *Clinical Anesthesia, 10*(2), 140-155.

Clark, R.B. (1978). Regional versus general anesthesia for obstetrics. *Perinatology/Neonatology, 2*(2), 18-21.

Cohen, W.R. (1977). Influence of the duration of second stage labor on perinatal outcome and puerperal morbidity. *Obstetrics and Gynecology, 49*(3), 266-269.

Collaborative Perinatal Study of the National Institute of Neurological Diseases and Stroke. (1972). *The women and their pregnancies,* (NIH)73-379. U.S. Department of Health, Education and Welfare, National Institutes of Health.

Colman, A., & Colman, L. (1971). *Pregnancy: The psychological experience.* New York: Herder & Herder.

Comerford, J.B. (1965). Pregnancy with anencephaly. *Lancet, 1,* 679-680.

Copp, L.A. (1974). The spectrum of suffering. *American Journal of Nursing, 74*(3), 491-495.

Crawford, M.I. (1968). Physiological and behavioral cues to disturbances in childbirth. *Bulleton of the Sloane Hospital for Women, 14,* 132-142.

Csapo, W., & Jung, H. (1963). Effects of progesterone on uterine contractility. In J.M. Marshall & W.M. Burnett (Eds.), *Initiation of labor: Proceedings of Interdisciplinary Conference on the Initiation of Labor,* no. 1390. U.S. Department of Health, Education and Welfare, Public Health Service.

Curtin, L.L. (1979). The nurse as advocate: a philosophical foundation for nursing. *Advances in Nursing Science, 1*(3), 1-10.

Danforth, D.N., & Hendricks, C.H. (1977). Physiology of uterine action. In D.N. Danforth (Eds.), *Obstetrics and gynecology* (ed. 3). New York: Harper & Row.

Danielson, C.O. (1957). Prolapse of the uterus and vagina, clinical and therapeutic aspects: Review of 600 cases. *Acta Obstetricia et Gynecologica Scandinavica, 36*(Suppl. 1), 9-16, 114-115.

Davis, J.W., Hoffmaster, C.B., & Shorten, S. (Eds.). (1978). *Biomedical ethics.* New York: Humana Press.

Davison, J.S., Davison, M.C., & Hay, D.M. (1970). Gastric emptying time in late pregnancy and labour. *Journal of Obstetrics and Gynaecology of the British Commonwealth, 77,* 37-41.

De Lee, J.B. (1920). The prophylactic forceps operation. *American Journal of Obstetrics and Gynecology, 1,* 34-35.

Dershimer, F.W. (1936). The influence of mental attitudes in childbearing. *American Journal of Obstetrics and Gynecology, 31,* 444-454.

Deutsch, H. (1945). *The psychology of women. Volume II: Motherhood.* New York: Grune & Stratton.

Donagan, A. (1977). Informed consent in therapy and experimentation. *The Journal of Medicine and Philosophy, 2*(4), 307-329.

Duenhoelter, J.H., Jimenez, J.M., & Baumann, G. (1975). Pregnancy performance of patients under fifteen years of age. *Obstetrics and Gynecology, 46*(1), 49-52.

Duhring, J.L. (1962). Blood volume in pregnancy. *American Journal of Medical Science, 243,* 808-810.

Dunn, H.L. (1961). *High-level wellness,* Richmond, Va.: R W Beatty.

Dunn, P.M. (1976). Obstetric delivery today—for better or for worse? *Lancet, 1*(7962), 790-793.

Dunn, P.M. (1978). Posture in labour. *Lancet, 1*(8062), 496-497.

Eastman, N.J., & Hellman, L.M. (1961). *Williams obstetrics* (ed. 13). New York: Appleton-Century-Crofts.

English, O.S. (1965). The psychological role of the father in the family. In R.S. Cavan (Ed.), *Marriage and family in the modern world,* (ed. 2). New York: Cromwell.

Enkin, M. (1975). The family in labour. *Birth and the Family Journal, 2,* 133-136.

Ernst, E.K.M., & Forde, M.P. (1975). Maternity care: An attempt at an alternative. *Nursing Clinics of North America, 10*(2), 241-249.

Evrard, J.R., & Gold, E.M. (1977). Adolescent pregnancy. *Perinatal Care,* 8-12.

Fedrick, J., & Butler, N.R. (1971). Certain causes of neonatal death. Cerebral birth trauma. *Biology of the Neonate, 18,* 321-324.

Fischer, S.R. (1979). Factors associated with the occurrence of perineal lacerations. *Journal of Nurse-Midwifery, 24*(1), 18-26.

Fitzgerald, D., Herman, E., Ventre, F., & Long, T. (1976). *Home oriented maternity experience.* Washington, D.C.: H.O.M.E., Inc.

Friedman, E.A. (1978). *Labor: Clinical evaluation and management* (ed. 2). New York: Appleton-Century-Crofts. (a)

Friedman, E.A. (1978). Diagnosis of abnormal labor. *The Female Patient, 3*(5), 71-74. (b)

Friedman, E.A., & Sachtleben, M.R. (1963). Amniotomy and the course of labor. *Obstetrics and Gynecology, 22,* 755-770.

Ganong, W.F. (1975). *Review of Medical Physiology* (ed. 7). Los Altos, California: Lange.

Gassner, C.B., & Ledger, W.J. (1976). The relationship of hospital-acquired maternal infection to invasive intrapartum monitoring techniques. *American Journal of Obstetrics and Gynecology, 126*(1), 33-37.

Gemzell, C.A., Robbe, H., Stern, B., & Strom, G. (1957). Observations on circulatory changes and muscular work in normal labour. *Acta Obstetricia et Gynecologica Scandinavica, 36,* 75-92.

Ginott, H.G. (1965). *Between parent and child.* New York: MacMillan.

Goldstein, A. (1978). The endorphins—their discovery and significance. In *Hospital practice. Proceedings: Current concepts in postoperative pain. A symposium.* New York: American Society of Anesthesiologists.

Goodlin, R.C., & Lowe, E.W. (1974). Multiphasic fetal monitoring: A preliminary evaluation. *American Journal of Obstetrics and Gynecology, 119*(3), 341-357.

Goodman, M. (1976). Experiences with a labor/delivery room. *Birth and the Family Journal, 3,* 123-125.

Gordon, B. (1978). The vulnerable mother and her child. In S. Kitzinger & J.A. Davis, (Eds.). *The place of birth.* Oxford: Oxford University Press.

Graham, H. (1960). *Eternal eve.* London: Hutchinson.

Greenberg, M., & Morris, N. (1974). Engrossment: The newborn's impact upon the father. *American Journal of Orthopsychiatry, 44*(4), 520-531.

Greenhill, J.P. (1965). *Obstetrics* (ed. 13). Philadelphia: Saunders.

Greenhill, J.P., & Friedman, E.A. (1974). *Biological principles and modern practice of obstetrics.* Philadelphia: Saunders.

Gruenberg, S.M. (1970). *The wonderful story of how you were born.* Garden City, N.Y.: Doubleday.

Guyton, A.C. (1977). *Basic Human Physiology: Normal Function and Mechanisms of Disease* (ed. 2). Philadelphia: Saunders.

Haire, D. (1972). *The cultural warping of childbirth.* Milwaukee: International Childbirth Education Association.

Haire, D. (1980). *The pregnant patient's bill of rights.* Minneapolis, Mn.: International Childbirth Education Association. (a)

Haire, D. (1980). *The pregnant patient's responsibilities.* Minneapolis, Mn.: International Childbirth Association. (b)

Hammes, L.M., & Treloar, A.E. (1970). Gestational interval from vital records. *American Journal of Public Health, 60,* 1496-1505.

Hansen, J.M., & Ueland, K. (1966). The influence of caudal analgesia on cardiovascular dynamics during labor and delivery. *Acta Anaesthesiologica Scandinavica* (Suppl.), *23,* 449-454.

Hansen, J.M., & Ueland, K. (1973). Maternal cardiovascular dynamics during pregnancy and parturition. *Clinical Anesthesia, 10*(2), 22-35.

Haverkamp, A.D., Thompson, H.E., McFee, J.G., & Cetrulo, C. (1976). The evaluation of continuous fetal heart rate monitoring in high-risk pregnancy. *American Journal Obstetrics and Gynecology, 125*(3), 310-320.

Hayashi, R.H., & Fox, M.E. (1975). Unforeseen sudden intrapartum fetal death in a monitored labor. *American Journal of Obstetrics and Gynecology, 122,* 786-788.

Hazell, L.D. (1969). *Commonsense childbirth.* New York: Tower.

Hellig, H., Gattereau, D., Lefebure, Y., & Balte, E. (1970). Steroid production from plasma cholesterol. I. Conversion of plasma cholesterol to placental propesterone in human. *Journal of Clinical Endocrinology, 30,* 624-631.

Hendricks, C.H. (1964). The use of isoxsuprine for the arrest of premature labor. *Clinical Obstetrics and Gynecology, 7,* 687-692.

Hendricks, C.H. (1977). Distocia due to abnormal uterine action. In D.N. Danforth (Ed.), *Obstetrics and gynecology* (ed. 3). New York: Harper & Row.

Hendricks, C.H., Brenner, W.E., & Kraus, G. (1970). Normal cervical dilatation pattern in late pregnancy and labor. *American Journal of Obstetrics and Gynecology, 106*(7), 1065-1082.

Hendrie, M.J.M. (1975). Liquid food for obstetric patients. *Nursing Times, 71*(2): 60-62.

Hersh, S.P., & Levin, K. (1978). How love begins between parent and child. *Children Today, 7*(2), 2-6, 47.

Heymans, H., & Winter, S.T. (1975). Fears during pregnancy: Interview study of 200 postpartum women. *Israel Journal of Medical Sciences, 11,* 1102-1105.

Highly, B.L., & Mercer, R.T. (1978). Safeguarding the laboring woman's sense of control. *MCN, 3*(1), 39-41.

Hines, J.D. (1971). The forgotten man. *Nursing Forum, 10*(2), 177-200.

Hinshaw, A.L. (1977). Preventive aspects of liability in obstetrics and gynecology. *Clinical Obstetrics and Gynecology, 20*(1), 19-24.

Hobel, C.J. (1976). Recognition of the high-risk pregnant woman. In W.N. Spellacy (Ed.), *Management of the high risk pregnancy.* Baltimore: University Park Press. (a)

Hobel, C.J. (1976). Problem-oriented risk assessment during labor. *Contemporary Obstetrics and Gynecology, 8*(1), 120-124. (b)

Hollman, A. (1977). Cardiac function. In E.E. Philipp, J. Barnes, & M. Newton (Eds.), *Scientific foundations of obstetrics and gynaecology.* Chicago: Year Book.

Hon, E.H., Zannini, D., & Quilligan, E.J. (1975). The neonatal value of fetal monitoring. *American Journal of Obstetrics and Gynecology, 122*(4), 508-519.

Hott, J.R. (1976). The crisis of expectant fatherhood. *American Journal of Nursing, 76*(9), 1436-1440.

Hunt, J.N., & Murray, F.A. (1958). Gastric function in pregnancy. *Journal of Obstetrics and Gynaecology of the British Empire, 65,* 78-83.

Hunter, R.G., Henry, G.W., & Larsen, I.J. (1954). Stirrups and postoperative backache. *Obstetrics and Gynecology, 4*(3), 344-347.

Huprich, P.A. (1977). Assisting the couple through a Lamaze labor and delivery. *MCN: The American Journal of Maternal Child Nursing, 2*(4), 245-253.

Illich, I. (1976). *Medical nemesis: The expropriation of health.* New York: Pantheon.

Irwin, H.W. (1978). Practical considerations for the routine application of left lateral Sims' position for vaginal delivery. *American Journal of Obstetrics and Gynecology, 131*(2), 129-133.

Jacobs, W.M., & Adams, B.O. (1960). Midline episiotomy and extension through the rectal sphincter. *Surgery, Gynecology and Obstetrics, 111,* 245-246.

Jeffcoate, W.J., Rees, L.H., McLoughlin, L., Ratter, S.J., Hope, J., Lowry, P.J., & Bessner, G.M. (1978). Beta-endorphin in human cerebrospinal fluid. *Lancet, 2*(8081), 119-121.

Johansson, E. (1969). Plasma levels of progesterone in pregnancy measured by a rapid competitive protein binding technique. *Acta Endocrinologica, 61,* 607-611.

Johnston, R.A., & Sidall, R.S. (1922). Is the usual method of preparing patients for delivery beneficial or necessary? *American Journal of Obstetrics and Gynecology, 4,* 645-650.

Jonas, H. (1974). *Philosophical Essays.* Englewood Cliffs, N.J.: Prentice-Hall.

Jonas, H. (1979). Toward a philosophy of technology. *The Hastings Center Report, 9*(1), 34-43.

Josselyn, I.M. (1956). Cultural forces, motherliness, and fatherliness. *American Journal of Orthopsychiatry, 26,* 267, 269.

Kaltreider, D.F., & Dixon, D.M. (1948). A study of 710 complete lacerations following central episiotomy. *Southern Medical Journal, 41*(9), 814-820.

Kantor, H.I., Miller, J.E., & Dunlap, J.C. (1949). The urinary bladder during labor. *American Journal of Obstetrics and Gynecology, 58*(2), 354-364.

Kantor, H.I., Rember, R., Tabio, P., & Buchanon, R. (1965). Value of shaving the pudendal–perineal area in delivery preparation. *Obstetrics and Gynecology, 25,* 509-512.

Karim, S.M.M. (1968). Appearance of prostaglandin $F_{2\alpha}$ in human blood during pregnancy and labour. *British Medical Journal, 4,* 618-620.

Keats, C.M., & Bjorksten, O.J.W. (1978). Adolescent sexuality. In A.K.K. Kreutner & D.R. Hollingsworth (Eds.), *Adolescent obstetrics and gynecology.* Chicago: Year Book.

Kinlein, M.L. (1977). The self-care concept. *American Journal of Nursing, 77*(4), 598-601.

Kitzinger, S. (1972). *The experience of childbirth.* New York: Taplinger.

Kitzinger, S. (1977). Giving support in labor. *Nursing Mirror, 144,* 20-22.

Kline, N.S., Li, C.H., Lehmann, H.E., Lajtha, A., Laski, E., & Cooper, T. (1977). β-Endorphin-induced changes in schizophrenic and depressed patients. *Archives of General Psychiatry, 34:*1111-1113.

Klopfer, F.J., Cogan, R., & Henneborn, W.J. (1975). Second stage medical intervention and pain during childbirth. *Journal of Psychosomatic Research, 19,* 289-293.

Klusman, L.E. (1975). Reduction of pain in childbirth by the alleviation of anxiety during pregnancy. *Journal of Consulting and Clinical Psychology, 43*(2), 162-165.

Kowalski, K., Gottschalk, J., Greer, B., & Bowes, W.A., Jr. (1977).

Team nursing coverage of prenatal–intrapartum patients at a university hospital. *Obstetrics and Gynecology, 50*(1), 116–119.

Kramer, M., & Schmalenberg, C.E. (1978). Conflict: The cutting edge of growth. *Nursing Digest, 5*(4), 59–65.

Krieger, D. (1975). Therapeutic touch: The imprimatur of nursing. *American Journal of Nursing, 75*(5), 784–787.

Kubler-Ross, E. (1976). *Death: The final stage of growth.* New York: Harper & Row.

Lamaze, F. (1972). *Painless childbirth: The Lamaze method.* New York: Simon & Schuster.

Lamaze, F., & Velay, P. (1957). *Psychologic analgesia in obstetrics.* New York: Pergamon.

Laufe, L.E., & Leslie, D.C. (1972). The timing of episiotomy. *American Journal of Obstetrics and Gynecology, 114*(6), 773–774.

Lesinski, J. (1975). High risk pregnancy. *Obstetrics and Gynecology, 46*(5), 599–603.

Lesser, M.S., & Keane, V.R. (1956). *Nurse–patient relationships in a hospital maternity service.* St. Louis: Mosby.

Levine, C. (1979). Ethics and health cost containment. *The Hastings Center Report, 9*(1), 10–13.

Levine, N.H. (1976). A conceptual model for obstetric nursing. *Journal of Obstetric, Gynecologic, and Neonatal Nursing, 5*(2), 9–15.

Levine, J.D., Gordon, N.C., & Fields, H.I. (1978). The mechanism of placebo analgesia. *Lancet, 2*(8091), 654–657.

Levison, G., & Shnider, S.M. (1973). Placental transfer of local anesthetics: Clinical implication. *Clinical Anesthesia, 10*(2), 174–185.

Levy, D.M. (1966). *Maternal overprotection.* New York: Norton.

Lewin, K. (1935). On the structure of the mind. In K. Lewis (Ed.), *A dynamic theory of personality.* New York: McGraw-Hill.

Liebeskind, J.C. (1976). Pain modulation by central nervous system stimulation. In J.J. Bonica & D. Albe-Fessard (Eds.), *Advances in pain research and therapy* (Vol. 1). New York: Raven Press.

Lindgren, L. (1973). The influence of uterine motility upon cervical dilatation in labor. *American Journal of Obstetrics and Gynecology, 117*(4), 530–536.

Liu, Y.C. (1974). Effects of an upright position during labor. *American Journal of Nursing, 74*(12), 2202–2205.

Long, A.E. (1967). Unshaved perineum at parturition. *American Journal of Obstetrics and Gynecology, 99,* 333–336.

Low, J.A. (1977). Maternal and fetal blood gas and acid-base metabolism. In E.E. Philipp, J. Barnes, & M. Newton, (Eds.), *Scientific foundations of obstetrics and gynaecology.* Chicago: Year Book.

Lubic, R.W. (1975). Developing maternity services women will trust. *American Journal of Nursing, 75*(10), 1685–1688.

MacDonald, E.A. (1969). Major fears of primigravid patients. *Journal of Obstetrics and Gynaecology of the British Commonwealth, 76,* 71–72.

MacDonald, P.C., Schultz, F.M., Duenhoelter, J.H., Gant, N.F., Jimenez, J.M., Pritchard, J.A., Porter, J.C., & Johnston, J.M. (1974). Initiation of human parturition: I. Mechanics of action of arachidonic acid. *Obstetrics and Gynecology, 44,* 629–636.

Magee, J. (1976). Labor: What the doctor learns as a patient. *The Female Patient, 1*(11), 27–29.

Maltbie, A.A., Cavenar, J.O. Hammett, E.B., & Sullivan, J.L. (1978). A diagnositc approach to pain. *Psychosomatics, 19*(6), 359–366.

Martell, M., Belizan, J.M., Nieto, F., & Schwarcz, R. (1976). Blood acid–base balance at birth in neonates from labors with early and late rupture of membranes. *Journal of Pediatrics, 89*(6), 963–967.

Martin, J.E., & Pauerstein, C.J. (1973). The initiation of labor. *Clinical Anesthesia, 10*(2), 52–69.

Marx, G.F., Macatangay, A.S., Cohen, A.V., & Schulman, H. (1969). Effect of pain relief on arterial blood gas values during labor. *New York State Journal of Medicine, 69,* 819–822.

Masters, W.H., & Johnson, V.E. (1966). *Human sexual response.* Boston: Little, Brown.

Matadial, L., & Cibils, L.A. (1976). The effect of epidural anesthesia on uterine activity and blood pressure. *American Journal of Obstetrics and Gynecology, 125*(6), 846–854.

Matousek, I. (1968). Fetal nursing during labor. *Nursing Clinics of North America, 3*(2), 307–314.

Mauksch, H.O. (1975). The organizational context of dying. In E. Kubler-Ross (Ed.), *Death: The final stage of growth.* Englewood-Cliffs, N.J.: Prentice Hall.

Mayer, D.J., & Price, D.T. (1976). Central nervous system mechanisms of analgesia. *Pain, 2,* 379–382.

Mayle, P. (1973). *Where did I come from?* Secaucus, N.J.: Lyle Stuart.

McDonald, J.S. (1977). Preanesthetic and intrapartal medications. *Clinical Obstetrics and Gynecology, 20*(2), 447–459.

McLachlan, E. (1974). Recognizing pain. *American Journal of Nursing, 74*(3), 496–497.

McManus, T.J., & Calder, A.A. (1978). Upright posture and the efficiency of labour. *Lancet, 1*(8055), 72–74.

Mehl, L.E., Brendsel, C., & Peterson, G.H. (1977). Children at birth: Effects and implications. *Journal of Sex and Marital Therapy, 3*(4), 274–279. (a)

Mehl, L.E., Brendsel, C., & Peterson, G.H. (1977). Psychophysiological aspects of childbirth. I. Childbirth as psychotherapy. Paper presented at the 130th Annual Meeting of the American Psychiatric Association, Toronto, Ontario, Canada, May 5. (b)

Melmed, H., & Evans, M.I. (1976). Predictive value of cervical dilatation rates. *Obstetrics and Gynecology, 47*(5), 511–514.

Melzack, R., & Wall, P.D. (1965). Pain mechanisms: A new theory, *Science, 150,* 971–979.

Mendelson, C.L. (1946). The aspiration of stomach contents into the lungs during obstetric anesthesia. *American Journal of Obstetrics and Gynecology, 52,* 191–193.

Mendez-Bauer, C., Arroyo, J., Garcia, R.C., Menendez, A., Lavilla, M., Izquierdo, F., Villa, E.I., & Zamarriego, J. (1975). Effects of standing position on spontaneous uterine contractility and other aspects of labor. *Journal of Perinatal Medicine, 3,* 89–99.

Messing, R.B., & Lytle, L.D. (1977). Serotonin—containing neurons: Their possible role in analgesia. *Pain, 3,* 1–4.

Montagu, A. (1971). *Touching: The human significance of the skin.* New York: Harper & Row.

Morrison, J.C., Whybrew, W.D., Rosser, S.I., Bucovaz, E.T., Wiser, W.L., & Fish, S.A. (1976). Metabolites of meperidine in the fetal and maternal serum. *American Journal of Obstetrics and Gynecology, 126*(8), 997–1002.

Mountcastle, V.B. (Ed.) (1974). *Medical Physiology* (Vol. 2). St. Louis: Mosby.

Munson, A.K., Mueller, J.R., & Yannone, M.E (1970). Free plasma 17β-estradiol in normal pregnancy, labor and the puerperium. *American Journal of Obstetrics and Gynecology, 108,* 340–344.

Newton, N. (1970). Childbirth and culture. *Psychology Today, 4*(6), 75.

Newton, N. (1973). Interrelationships between sexual responsiveness, birth, and breast feeding. In J. Zubin & J. Money (Eds.), *Contemporary sexual behavior: Critical issues in the 1970s.* Baltimore: Johns Hopkins University Press.

Newton, N. (1976). Childbirth and self-esteem. Paper presented at The annual conference of the American Foundation for Maternal and Child Health, New York.

Newton, N., & Newton, M. (1972). Childbirth in crosscultural perspective. In J.G. Howells (Ed.), *Modern perspectives in psychoobstetrics.* New York: Brunner/Mazel.

Nimmo, W.S., Wilson, J., & Prescott, L.F. (1975). Narcotic analgesics and delayed gastric emptying during labor. *Lancet, 1,* 890–893.

Okada, D.M., Chow, A.W., & Bruce, V.T. (1977). Neonatal scalp abscess and fetal monitoring: Factors associated with infection. *American Journal of Obstetrics and Gynecology, 129*(2), 185–189.

O'Leary, J.A., & Erez, S. (1965). Hyaluronidase as an adjuvant to episiotomy. *Obstetrics and Gynecology, 26,* 66–69.

O'Leary, J.L., & O'Leary, J.A. (1965). The complete episiotomy; analysis of 1224 complete lacerations, sphincterotomies, episi-proctotomies. *Obstetrics and Gynecology, 25,* 235–240.

Ould, F. (1742). *A treatise of midwifery.* Dublin: Milton & Head.

Packer, J., & Cooke, C.W. (1976). The interdependent team approach in caring for the pregnant adolescent. *Journal of Obstetric, Gynecologic, and Neonatal 5*(4), 18–25.

Pellegrino, E.D. (1978). Ethics and the moment of clinical truth (editorial). *Journal of the American Medical Association, 239*(10), 960–961.

Perl, E.R. (1976). Sensitization of nociceptors and its relation to sensation. In J.J. Bonica & D. Albe-Fessard (Eds.), *Advances in pain research and therapy* (Vol. 1), proceedings of The First World Congress on Pain. New York: Raven Press.

Peterson, G.H., Mehl, L.E., & Leiderman, P.H. (1977). Effects of childbirth upon women's self esteem. Paper presented at the 130th Annual Meeting, American Psychiatric Association, Toronto, Ontario, Canada, May 5.

Philipp, E.E., Barnes, J., & Newton, M. (Eds.) (1977). *Scientific foundations of obstetrics and gynaecology* (ed. 2). Chicago: Year Book.

Phillips, J.C., Hochberg, C.J., Petrakis, J.K., & Van Winkle, J.D. (1977). Epidural analgesia and its effects on the "normal" progress of labor. *American Journal of Obstetrics and Gynecology, 129*(3), 316–323.

Pies, H.E. (1976). The right of a father to be present in the delivery room. *American Journal of Public Health, 66*(7), 599–689.

Pomeroy, R.H. (1918) Shall we cut and reconstruct the perineum in every primipara? *American Journal of Obstetrics, 78,* 211–212.

Post, J.A. (1972). Expectations and reality in the expected day of confinement of a primigravida. *Maternal-Child Nursing Journal, 1,* 87–100.

Pritchard, J.A., & MacDonald, P.C. (1976). Physiology of labor. In *Williams obstetrics* (ed. 15). New York: Appleton-Century-Crofts.

Ralston, D.H., & Shnider, S.M. (1978). The fetal and neonatal effects of regional anesthesia in obstetrics. *Anesthesiology, 48*(1), 34–64.

Randolph, B.M. (1977). Birth and its effects on human behavior. *Perspectives in Psychiatric Care, 15,* 20–26.

Read, G.D. (1946). Correlation of physical and emotional phenomena of natural labour. *Journal of Obstetrics and Gynaecology of the British Empire, 53,* 55–61.

Read, G.D. (1959). *Childbirth without fear* (ed. 2). New York: Harper & Row.

Reid, D.E., Ryan, K.J., & Benirschke, K. (1972). *Principles and management of human reproduction.* Philadelphia: Saunders.

Reynolds, D.V. (1969). Surgery in the rat during electrical analgesia induced by focal brain stimulation. *Science, 164,* 444–445.

Reynolds, S.R.M., Hellman, L.M., & Bruns, P. (1948). Patterns of uterine contractility in women during pregnancy. *Obstetrics and Gynecological Survey, 3,* 629–632.

Richman, J., & Goldthorp. W.O. (1978). Fatherhood: The social construction of pregnancy and birth. In S. Kitzinger & J.A. Davis (Eds.), *The place of birth.* Oxford: Oxford University Press.

Rising, S.S. (1975). A consumer-oriented nurse–midwifery service. *Nursing Clinics of North America, 10*(2), 251–262.

Ritgen, G. (1855). (R.M. Wynn, trans.). Concerning his method for protection of the perineum. *Monatschrift für Geburtskunde, 6,* 21. (*American Journal of Obstetrics and Gynecology,* 1965, *93*(3), 421–433.)

Roberts, R.B., & Shirley, M.A. (1974). Reducing risk of acid aspiration during cesarean section. *Anesthesia and Analgesia: Current Researches, 53,* 859–868.

Roehner, J. (1976). Fatherhood: In pregnancy and birth. *Journal of Nurse-Midwifery, 21*(1), 13–16.

Rothman, B.K. (1977). The social construction of birth. *Journal of Nurse-Midwifery, 22*(2), 9–13.

Rovinsky, J.J. (1977). Blood volume and the hemodynamics of pregnancy. In E.E. Philipp, J. Barnes, & M. Newton (Eds.), *Scientific foundations of obstetrics and gynaecology.* Chicago: Year Book.

Rubin, R. (1976). Maternal tasks in pregnancy. *Journal of Advanced Nursing, 1,* 367–376.

Ryden, M.B. (1977). Energy: A crucial consideration in the nursing process. *Nursing Forum, 16*(1), 71–82.

Sasmor, J.L., Castor, C.R., & Hassid, P. (1973). The childbirth team during labor. *American Journal of Nursing, 73*(3), 444–447.

Scanlon, J.W., Brown, W.V., & Alper, M.H. (1971). Neurobehavioral responses of newborn infants after maternal epidural anesthesia. In proceedings of the Annual Meeting of the American Society of Anesthesiologists (abstract).

Schmitt, M. (1977). The nature of pain. *Nursing Clinics of North America, 12*(4), 621–629.

Schulman, H., & Romney, S.L. (1970). Variability of uterine contractions in normal human parturition. *Obstetrics and Gynecology, 36*(2), 215–221.

Schwarcz, R., Althabe, O., Belitzky, R., Lanchares, J.L., Alvarez, R., Berdaguer, P., Capurro, H., Belizan, J.M., Sabatino, J.H., Abusleme, C., & Caldeyro-Barcia, R. (1973). Fetal heart rate patterns in labors with intact and with ruptured membranes. *Journal of Perinatal Medicine, 1,* 153–165.

Scott, D.B. (1973). Inferior vena caval occlusion in late pregnancy. *Clinical Anesthesia, 10*(2), 38–50.

Scott, D. (1978). Hemodynamic changes of pregnancy. In What's new and important in ob-gyn: A postgraduate symposium in obstetrics and gynecology. Dallas: Texas Technical University, Department of Obstetrics and Gynecology, pp. 89–91.

Scott, J.R., & Rose, N.B. (1976). Effect of psychoprophylaxis (Lamaze preparation) on labor and delivery in primiparas. *New England Journal of Medicine, 294*(22), 1205–1207.

Sears, R.R., Macoby, E.C., & Levin, H. (1957). *Patterns of child rearing.* New York: Harper & Row.

Seiden, A.M. (1976). The maternal sense of mastery in primary care obstetrics. *Primary Care, 3*(4), 717-726.

Selkurt, E.E. (Ed.). (1976). *Physiology* (ed. 4). Boston: Little, Brown.

Semmens, J.P. (1965). Implications of teen-age pregnancy. *Obstetrics and Gynecology, 26*(1), 77-85.

Seropian, R., & Reynolds, B.M. (1971). Wound infections after preoperative depilatory versus razor preparation. *American Journal of Surgery, 121,* 251-254.

Serr, D.M. (1977). The uterus and cervix. In E.E. Philipp, J. Barnes, & M. Newton (Eds.), *Scientific foundations of obstetrics and gynaecology.* Chicago: Year Book.

Shainess, N. (1963). The psychologic experience of labor. *New York State Journal of Medicine, 10*:2923-2932.

Shnider, S.M., Asling, J.H., Holl, J.N., & Margolis, A.J. (1970). Paracervical block anesthesia in obstetrics. I. Fetal complications and neonatal morbidity. *American Journal of Obstetrics and Gynecology, 107,* 619-624.

Shute, W.B. (1959). A physiologic appraisal and a new painless technique. *Obstetrics and Gynecology, 14,* 467-472.

Siegele, D.S. (1974). The gate control theory. *American Journal of Nursing, 74*(3), 498-502.

Silman, R.E., Chard, T., & Boyd, N.R.H. (1977). Fetal endocrinology. In E.E. Philipp, J. Barnes, & M. Newton, (Eds.), *Scientific foundation of obstetrics and gynaecology,* (ed. 2). Chicago: Year Book.

Smith, B.A., Priore, R.M., & Stern, M.K. (1973). The transition phase of labor. *American Journal of Nursing, 73*(3), 448-450.

Smith, P.B., Wait, R B., Mumford, D.M., Nenney, S.W., & Hollins, B.T. (1978). The medical impact of an antepartum program for pregnant adolescents: A statistical analysis. *American Journal of Public Health, 68*(2), 169-171.

Smyth, C.N. (1974). Biomechanics and human parturition. *Proceedings of the Royal Society of Medicine, 67,* 189-194.

Snider, G., & Snider, E. (1978). Personal communication.

Sokol, R.J., Stojkov, B.S., Chik, L., & Rosen, M.G. (1977). Normal and abnormal labor progress: I. A quantitative assessment and survey of the literature. *Journal of Reproductive Medicine, 18*(1), 47-53.

Sokol, R.J., Zador, I., & Rosen, M.G. (1976). Slowing of active labor associated with internal fetal monitoring. *American Journal of Obstetrics and Gynecology, 124*(7), 764-765.

Sousa, M. (1976). *Childbirth at home.* New Jersey: Prentice-Hall.

Steffenson, J.L., Shnider, S.M., & de Lorimier, A.A. (1970). Transarterial diffusion of mepivacaine. *Anesthesiology, 32,* 459-462.

Steinfels, M.O. (1978). New childbirth technology: A clash of values. *The Hastings Center Report, 8*(1), 9-12.

Steinfels, M.O., & Levine, C. (Eds.). (1977). The teaching of ethics: A preliminary inquiry. *The Hastings Center Report, 7*(6, Suppl.), 1-20.

Stewart, D., & Stewart, L. (1976). *Safe alternatives in childbirth.* Chapel Hill, North Carolina: National Association of Parents and Professionals for Safe Alternatives in Childbirth.

Strauss, A., Fagerhaugh, S.Y., & Glaser, B. (1974). Pain: An organizational-work-interactional perspective. *Nursing Outlook, 22*(9), 561-566.

Sweeney, W.J. (1963). Perineal shaves and bladder catheterization: Necessary and benign, or unnecessary and potentially injurious? *Obstetrics and Gynecology, 21,* 291-294.

Tanzer, C., & Block, J. (1972). *Why natural childbirth?* New York: Doubleday.

Taylor, E.S. (1976). *Beck's obstetrical practice and fetal medicine.* Baltimore: Williams & Wilkins.

Taylor, G., & Pryse-Davies, J. (1966). The prophylactic use of antacids in the prevention of the acid pulmonary aspiration syndrome. *Lancet, 1,* 288-291.

Teabeaut, J.R. (1952). Aspiration of gastric contents: An experimental study. *American Journal of Pathology, 28,* 51-53.

Theobald, G.W. (1968). Nervous control of uterine activity. *Clinical Obstetrics and Gynecology, 11,* 15-33.

Thompson, H.O., & Beebe, J.E. (1976). Nurse-midwifery and ethics...a beginning. *Journal of Nurse-Midwifery, 21*(4), 7-11.

Toppozada, H.K., Gaafar, A.A., & El-Sahwi, S. (1967). The urinary bladder and uterine activity. *American Journal of Obstetrics and Gynecology, 98*(7), 904-912.

Tritsch, J.E. (1930). Another plea for the prophylactic median episiotomy. *American Institute of Homeopathy, 23,* 327-328.

Tryon, P.A. (1968). Assessing the progress of labor through observation of patients' behavior. *Nursing Clinics of North America, 3*(2), 315-326.

Twiss, S.B., Jr. (1977). The problem of moral responsibility in medicine. In J.M. Gustafson (Ed.), Consent and responsibilities in medicine. *The Journal of Medicine and Philosophy, 2*(4), 330-373.

United States Department of Health, Education and Welfare. (1970). *Your child from 1 to 12.* New York: New American Library.

Vaccarino, J.M. (1978). Consent, informed consent, and the consent form (editorial). *New England Journal of Medicine, 298*(8), 455.

Vellay, P. (1975). Psychoprophylaxis and its evolution. *Birth and The Family Journal, 2,* 19-21.

Walker, J.L. (1974). Complete perineal incision for delivery. *Southern Medical Journal, 67*(3), 265-268.

Wall, P.D. (1976). Modulation of pain by non-painful events. In J.J. Bonica & D. Albe-Fessard (Eds.), *Advances in pain research and therapy* (Vol. 1). New York: Raven Press.

Ward, C., & Ward, F. (1976). *The home birth book.* Washington, D.C.: Inscape.

Weed, L.L. (1971). *Medical records, medical education and patient care.* Cleveland: The Press of Case Western Reserve University.

Wente, A.S., & Crockenberg, S.B. (1976). Transition to fatherhood: Lamaze preparation, adjustment difficulty and the husband-wife reltionship. *Family Coordinator, 25*(4), 351-357.

Willson, J.R., Beecham, C.T., & Carrington, E.R. (1975). *Obstetrics and gynecology* (ed. 5). St. Louis: Mosby.

Winner, W., & Romney, S.L. (1966). Cardiovascular responses to labor and delivery. *American Journal of Obstetrics and Gynecology, 95,* 1104-1108.

Witzig-Boldt, E. (1972). Retarded exhaling instead of holding the breath during expulsion. In Morris, N. (Ed.): *Psychosomatic medicine in obstetrics and gynecology.* London: Karger.

Wonnell, E.B. (1971). The education of the expectant father for childbirth. *Nursing Clinics of North America, 6*(4), 591-603.

Wood, C. (1976). Perinatal asphyxia, acidosis reduced by speeding delivery. *Obstetrical Gynecological News, 11*(22), 16.

Woodbury, W.J., van Wagenen, G., Csapo, A., Marshall, J.M., & Jung, H. (1963). Physiological principles of contraction in uterine muscle. In J.M. Marshall, & W.M. Burnett (Eds.),

Initiation of labor: Proceedings of Interdisciplinary Conference on the Initiation of Labor, no. 1390. U.S. Department of Health, Education and Welfare, Public Health Service.

Youngs, D.D., Niebyl, J.R., Blake, D.A., Shipp, D.A., Stanley, J., & King, T.M. (1977). Experience with an adolescent pregnancy program. *Obstetrics and Gynecology, 50*(2), 212-216.

Zax, M., Sameroff, A.J., & Farnum, J.E. (1975). Childbirth education, maternal attitudes, and delivery. *American Journal of Obstetrics and Gynecology, 123*(2), 185-190.

Zelnik, M., & Kantner, J.F. (1978). First pregnancies to women aged 15-19: 1976 and 1971. *Family Planning Perspectives, 10*(1), 11-20.

Chapter 7 | Birth

Carmela Cavero

It just felt like giving birth is such a pure, eternal thing always happening somewhere, always holy (Gaskin, 1978).

SECOND-STAGE LABOR is signaled by an abrupt change in the expectant mother's consciousness. Her senses and strength rally, even after many hours of "working to relax." In contrast to first-stage labor, this new activity promises immediate rewards. She is called upon at last to do something aimed at successfully concluding months of preparation and anticipation. She is approaching the culmination of her fantasies and fears, the realization of a dream. Responding to internal cues, she radiates a contagious intensity, which is the harbinger of birth.

This intensity is also the nurse's signal of the parents' increased dependence on her or his experience and knowledge. Having assessed their level of confidence and training, the nurse will know whether to demonstrate, instruct, assist, encourage, or simply to provide them with a steady flow of information.

By the time labor begins, the woman and her partner or coach will have developed a precise set of expectations. They will be counting on the nurse to help them realize their ideal birth experience by supporting their choice of environment, procedures, and position. This preplanning of the birth experience means that each delivery is unique, custom designed, never routine.

THE ROLE OF THE OBSTETRICAL NURSE

The obstetrical nurse's efforts to meet the needs and wants of the expectant parents must be smoothly integrated with many clinical and professional responsibilities. The nurse must manipulate the environment, minimize noise and activity, and shield the laboring woman from disruptive interferences. While dispelling fears and providing reassurance, she or he must monitor progress by observing clinical and behavioral signs of both the woman and the fetus and must be prepared to recognize and respond to any indication of a problem. She must gain the trust of the parents and be a constant source of energy while communicating any changes to them and to other members of the staff. At times, the nurse will have to support the supporting person, as well as coach the woman in relaxation, breathing, and pushing techniques. Without contributing to the tension of the birth moment, she must be ready to make and execute critical decisions in a manner least disruptive to the continuity of labor. While assisting the attending physician, she maintains close contact with the woman and her partner and continues to extend physical and emotional support as needed and wanted.

The nurse's job is to constantly empathize, evaluate, and act with regard not only for the patient's needs and her own duties, but also with regard for the physician's

175

guidelines, the institution's policies, and her own professional standards and philosophy.

Philosophies of Birth

It is not unusual for a nurse's philosophy of birth to be at variance with that of the institution where she works, the physicians she works with, or the people she cares for. It is, in fact, quite natural. All of the people involved have had different training and experiences, which have generated different perspectives and feelings which, in turn, dictate different standards and priorities.

In order for the nurse to function in these conflicting situations and relationships, and achieve a reasonable degree of personal and professional satisfaction, she must closely examine her basic feelings and attitudes about childbirth, the right of others to self-determination, and her security with tradition or longing for innovation. She must confront and respond to questions such as: Who does the birth belong to? Who should be in control? Is childbirth a normal physiological function? Or is it a potentially dangerous event? Are parents generally ignorant about birth and inclined to jeopardize the welfare of the mother and baby? Or are they generally responsible and therefore entitled to respect and as much freedom as possible? Is the nurse's primary duty to be a dependable ally of the physician or a guardian of the woman's safety?

The nurse must understand her own feelings about childbirth before attempting to reconcile them with those of other people.

The Nurse as Consumer Advocate

The current trend is to assign decisions surrounding the birth to the pregnant woman and her partner or family. This allows them to accept, modify, or refuse available plans of care. Some expectant parents clearly state their goals and desires; they can define the degree of responsibility they are able and willing to accept because of careful study. Others have given little thought to the process, usually out of ignorance or fear.

The nurse must seek to understand the expectations of the parents and try to assist them in their decision-making process by explaining the options of a particular institution. Areas for consideration may include the following:

- *Place of birth:* Labor bed, special maternity bed, or delivery table. Will the woman deliver in the unit where she has labored or will she be transferred to a delivery room?

- *Attendant at birth:* Private obstetrician, obstetrician on call from a group practice, general practitioner, family practitioner, resident, intern, medical student, nurse-midwife, OB/GYN nurse practitioner, husband.
- *Presence of others at birth:* Husband, labor coach, other children, parents, friends.
- *Position for delivery:* Lithotomy, squatting, hands and knees, left lateral, semireclining, with or without stirrups, dorsal-recumbent, no preference.
- *Procedures:* Draping, prepping, use of cap, masks, gloves, scrub outfits, restraints, intravenous fluids, oral fluids, episotomy.
- *Analgesia-anesthesia:* Which drug or anesthetic, if any; time of administration.
- *Oxytocics-ergotrate:* Is this routine? What timing and route are preferred?
- *Photographs:* Are they permitted? In the labor room? Delivery room?

The Nurse as Change Agent

As mentioned earlier, the parents, nurse, physician, and institution will probably have different opinions about the desirability and safety of these and other options. Standards of care are generally relative. What is considered safe practice in this country may not be acceptable elsewhere in the world, and vice versa. While most of these standards of safe care were introduced following careful research, others were initiated only for the convenience of the attendant or in keeping with social customs and traditions.

With experience, the nurse will come to question certain standards of practice. For instance, she knows enough about anatomy and physiology to conclude that a woman cannot push effectively while flat on her back, and that it is extremely uncomfortable and disruptive to move the woman to a delivery room in late second stage. With the wisdom to apply sound nursing principles will come the confidence to challenge standards and change priorities as required. The experienced nurse will conclude that no procedure should be routine. Whether it is an accepted practice or modification of one, whether its authority lies in scientific research or passing fad, she will find herself continuously evaluating all procedures according to criteria that reflect common sense and responsible practice.

A thorough evaluation of a given procedure will include the answers to such questions as: What prompted the initiation of this practice? Is there a consumer demand for it? Is there any documentation that the practice, or omission of the practice, is harmful to the mother or infant? Is there a more attractive alternative?

If the nurse is willing to work as an agent for change, she can effectively demonstrate that nontraditional methods are safe or can be adapted to comply with institutional policies. Her chances of success may be improved with an understanding of the principles of change (Bennis et al., 1964; Gassett, 1976). This approach to change focuses on patience, persistence, and good communications. It emphasizes the importance of involving those who will be directly affected and the effectiveness of a cooperative effort. It also employs various problem-solving techniques for settling differences of opinion.

Accomplishing desired changes may also save the nurse from assuming the distasteful role of manipulator in her attempts to overcome the discrepancies between a woman's birth goals and the available birth choices found in most hospitals. Having to present situations in exactly the right way to elicit the desired response is awkward and frustrating, necessarily involves some loss of self-esteem, and is rarely conducive to personal or professional satisfaction.

One common manipulative role assumed by an obstetrical nurse is that of "conspirator." As a conspirator, she may pull the attending physician aside and whisper sarcastically, "Look, Doctor Pal. These people are a little nutty...a couple of those hippy types, I guess. Anyway, she wants to deliver in a squatting position and I know it's silly but they really want to give it a try so why don't we just let them go along and see what happens."

Of course, the game will vary depending on the attending physician; with another, the same nurse may assume a "kind-hearted little-helper" stance. This time, she grovels and whimpers innocently, "Gee, Doctor Wonderful. This couple is really committed to delivering in a squatting position and they've worked so hard preparing themselves for it. They're just so together on the whole experience, can't we just go along with them?"

Even if the nurse simply lies for a woman preferring to deliver in the labor bed by saying there was no time to transfer her, it is a demeaning routine, but until nurses, physicians, patients, and hospital administrators can work together more openly, with mutual respect and greater cooperation, the manipulation will continue, and the obstetrical nurse will have to demonstrate and redemonstrate competence, good judgment, and trustworthiness.

The ultimate resolution will be an integrated approach that respects the patient's wishes, motivates physicians to provide individualized care, and allows greater flexibility in complying with institutional policies.

PHYSIOLOGY OF BIRTH

The second stage of labor requires a great expenditure of energy to overcome the resistance of the frictional force of the birth canal and the pelvic floor musculature. Thus the name *labor* was applied to the act of giving birth.

A convenient, though simplistic, aid in understanding the labor process is to visualize it as the "dynamic interchange of three P's": the *Powers* (expulsive forces); the *Passage* (resistive forces); and the *Passenger* (the fetus).

The Powers (Expulsive Forces)

As a result of the retraction of the uterine musculature, the upper contractile portion of the uterus is notably thickened, and the capacity of the uterine cavity is decreased. The passive lower uterine segment is thinned out and has undergone longitudinal shortening. The cervix is fully dilated, and the cervical lips are at about the level of the pelvic inlet.

With each contraction, the uterus changes in shape, increasing in length while diminishing in the transverse and anteroposterior diameters. This is due to the stretching of the lower uterine segment and is partially attributable to the straightening of the fetal vertebral column. The upper pole of the baby is being pressed against the uterine fundus and the fetal head is directed down into the pelvis.

The woman's bearing-down efforts utilize the abdominal muscles and the respiratory diaphragm to increase intra-abdominal pressure. This force, combined with the uterine contractions, assists in the spontaneous completion of labor.

The Passage (Resistive Forces)

As the fetal head descends, it displaces soft tissue layers and muscular structures, following a curve along the pelvic floor. The levator ani muscle and surrounding fascia are stretched in a downward and backward direction by the descending fetal head. As a result of this stretching, the passage becomes extremely thin-walled as the head reaches the pelvic floor. The perineum is reduced to a thin membranous structure approximately 2-4 mm thick (Figures 7-1 and 7-2).

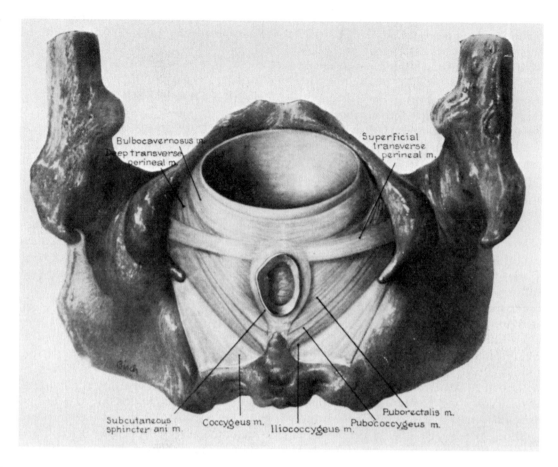

FIGURE 7-1   The muscles of the pelvic floor when head is crowning. (From Hellman, L.M., & Pritchard, J.A. (1971). *Williams obstetrics* (ed. 14). New York: Appleton-Century-Crofts, p. 366. With permission.)

The Passenger (Fetus)

During second-stage labor, the baby is being driven down and out through the birth canal. Molding of the fetal head allows adaption to the shape of the pelvis as the baby descends, flexes, and rotates. When the baby's head reaches the pelvic floor, it is flexed so that the base of the occiput impinges upon the subpubic arch. Extension occurs as a result of the trough formed by the resistive levator ani and the downward pressure of the uterus (Figure 7-3). The head follows an anteriorly directed arc as it distends the vulva. Progressively, the vaginal opening distends and the head "crowns" as the coronal sutures have passed through the vulvovaginal ring. The head is born as the brow, nose, mouth, and chin pass over the perineum.

Once the head is delivered, the shoulders and body follow fairly rapidly; the mechanisms of labor are completed.

ASSESSING THE PROGRESS OF LABOR

It is important to identify the onset of second-stage labor, which can be confirmed by vaginal examination. Repeated vaginal examinations, however, should be avoided because they are uncomfortable and because they involve unnecessary manipulation of the tissues and expose the woman to infection. There are a number of clinical signs that will help the nurse to recognize the end of first-stage-labor:

- The uterine contractions will change in character. Sometimes this causes the woman to experience an involuntary pushing movement; other times the only sign will be a "catch" in the breathing pattern.
- The amount of "show" increases, or there is a small trickle of bright red blood due to the rupture of capillaries as the cervix stretches.

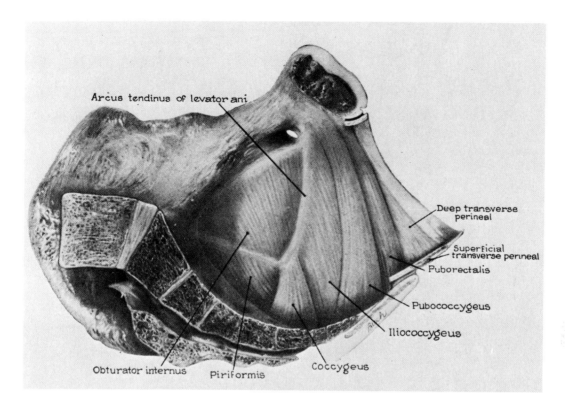

FIGURE 7-2 Lateral view of the muscles of the pelvic floor when the head is crowning. (From Hellman, L.M., & Pritchard, J.A. (1971). *Williams obstetrics* (ed. 14). New York: Appleton-Century-Crofts, p. 366. With permission.)

• If the membranes have not ruptured before this, they often do so now. The exact time and color should be noted and recorded.

There is a significant difference in the duration and pattern of descent between nulliparas and multiparas. In nulliparas, the vertex is usually engaged before the onset of labor. In multiparas, this engagement does not usually occur until active labor is in process. As a reference, Friedman (1978) gives an average descent rate of 3.3 cm/hr for nulliparas and 6.6 cm/hr for multiparas.

Observing the pattern of descent plotted against time on a graph helps to identify developing problems at an early stage. It then becomes critical to correctly assess the station of the fetal head in relation to the ischial spines. The usual method of charting the findings is −1 to −4 if the head is above the spines and +1 to +5 if it has passed the spines. It is also important to recognize when caput succedaneum is forming; the leading edge palpated on vaginal examination does not in fact represent the true descent of the fetal head.

Besides charting these findings, it is essential to record the frequency, duration, and strength of the contractions. There is usually a longer interval between contractions in second-stage labor. These findings constitute the data base on which managerial decisions must be made.

The fetal heart tones should be auscultated after each contraction. Auscultation during a contraction may also be useful. If the mother is in a position that makes this difficult, an electronic stethoscope or Doppler unit should be used instead of the fetoscope. The fetal heart rate can be more easily located in the suprapubic area at this stage.

ASSISTING NORMAL PROGRESS OF SECOND STAGE

Because the nurse is the most visible and accessible member of the health care team, the patient will rely on her or him most heavily for her needs and comfort. Meeting the physical and emotional needs of the woman in labor will contribute as much to the success of her birth experience as meticulous monitoring of her vital signs, fetal heart tones, and progress of labor will contribute to a healthy outcome for mother and baby.

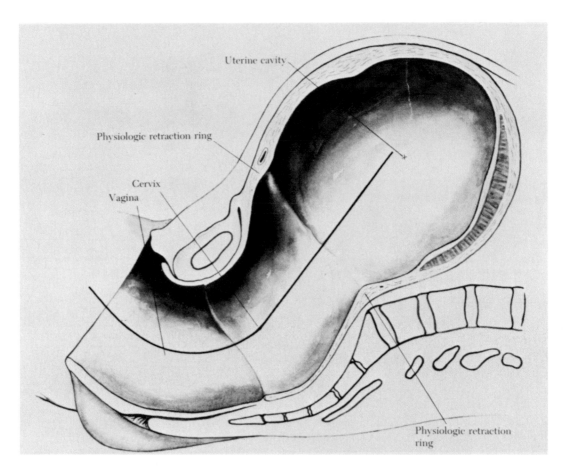

FIGURE 7-3 The complete parturient canal at maximal distention of all parts. The central curved heavy line indicates the axis of the canal. Note the sharp curve at the midpelvic plane. Above the retraction ring is the actively contracting portion of the uterus, and below it is the passively dilating portion. (From Greenhill, J.P., & Friedman, E.A. (1974). *Biological principles and modern practice of obstetrics.* Philadelphia: W.B. Saunders Co. With permission.)

A classic study by Lesser and Keane (1956) identified five needs expressed by most laboring women:

- To be sustained by another human being
- To have relief from pain
- To be assured of a safe outcome for both herself and her baby
- To have attendants accept her personal attitude toward, and behavior during, labor
- To receive bodily care*

The nurse will be ultimately responsible for providing or facilitating these needs.

*From Lesser, M.S., & Keane, V.R. (1956). *Nurse–patient relationships in a hospital maternity service.* St. Louis: The C.V. Mosby Co. With permission.

Another Human Being

Women do not like to be alone during labor. For safety reasons alone, they should not be left unattended during second stage. Hopefully, there will have been some continuity of care so that the nurse has been able to establish a relationship with the woman. The nurse's presence is a vital part of maintaining a supportive environment, which will enhance the progress of labor.

Fortunately, maternity care providers have heeded the importance of support from the partner or coach. Those who have witnessed parents sharing the birth experience see that it is an unequalled opportunity for mutual growth. A bonding can occur not only between the infant and parents but between the parents themselves and among all three as a family unit.

It is helpful if the couple have attended childbirth preparation classes together, but it is not essential. The nurse can coach the woman in breathing and relaxation techniques and offer some on-the-spot training.

As does the laboring woman, the father or coach will require support and encouragement. By the time second-stage labor is in progress, the father or coach should be oriented to the maternity unit, and familiar with the rest areas, bathroom, and eating facilities. The support person should be encouraged to take breaks for rest and nourishment without guilt. Ideally, the nurse has created a nurturing environment that allows the couple freedom to vacillate between a dependent–independent relationship as their needs change and the birth experience evolves.

Hopefully, the nurse and parents will have discussed what will be done in the event of an emergency. If no plans have been made, or if the plans made are suddenly inappropriate, the nurse must make decisions and act quickly. It is best to share the progress and plans for birth step-by-step with everyone involved, especially if the role of the father or coach must be altered.

Relief From Pain

The contractions of second-stage labor seem to cause less pain and discomfort than those of transition. There are, nevertheless, many sensations experienced by the woman that may be interpreted as pain. Pressure is felt on the bladder, urethra and rectum as the fetus descends. The perineum is stretched and displaced. Backache, if present during first-stage labor, sometimes continues into second stage, particularly if the position of the fetus is occipitoposterior.

Since excessive pain can be detrimental, it is necessary for the nurse to assess the woman's reactions to these sensations. Paying attention to nonverbal signals will help the nurse to anticipate the need for support measures (Angelini, 1978). Analgesics and anesthetics may be considered after carefully weighing the possible effects on the mother and baby. The expressed preferences of the mother and responsible attendant must, of course, be taken into consideration as well. Possible supportive measures may include the following:

- Comfortable and appropriate pushing efforts, rest between contractions, and heavy doses of praise and encouragement will contribute greatly to the laboring woman's comfort.
- Expressions of empathy through touch will greatly alleviate the woman's tension and pain. Back-rubbing is probably the most effective manner of

reducing the pain, which centers in the sacral area and radiates to the thighs and buttocks. Using the palm of the hand to exert firm pressure, deep circular massage should be applied to the sacral region or whatever area identified by the woman. Hot or cold packs may also be helpful.
- Women often complain of a cramplike sensation over the suprapubic area following strong pushes. Warm packs and a temporary change in the pushing position will eliminate compression over that area and relieve this sensation.

A Safe Outcome

Assurance and encouragement are the most effective solutions to the anxieties common to women in this stage of labor. Sensations such as stretching and pressure in the perineum may trigger fears of tearing, internal injuries, or being too small. The woman may also fear losing control and begin to doubt her ability to complete the task before her. She may feel helpless and suffer a loss of self-esteem. She may also worry that the baby will be unhealthy, deformed, or injured during expulsion.

Every action of the nurse will affect these anxieties. Her tone of voice, interpretation and explanation of each examination, and the confidence with which she performs every procedure are vital to the laboring woman's comfort. Anything the nurse can do to control the environment by keeping activity in the area to a minimum, arranging comfortable lighting and furniture, and by speaking in low, soft tones will reinforce the woman's ability to cope with the intense emotional and physical strains of second-stage labor.

Acceptance During Labor

"It was ridiculous the way I acted, screamed myself hoarse! I don't know why really. The pain wasn't that bad...the nurse was an angel. She kept telling me if I had to holler, it was all right. Then she'd talk to me in such a soft way. After a while, I just got quieter. I'll never forget her."

If the professional is bothered by the piercing scream often emitted at the birth moment, she might consider that many noisy women report that the actual birth "felt good." In fact, Newton (1955) has compared unmedicated childbirth and the physiology of sexual excitement and formed some interesting conclusions. There are, she notes, great similarities between the two, in the manner of breathing, facial expression, contractions of the uterus and abdominal muscles, body position, central nervous system reactions, sensory perception, and emotional response. One might conclude that making noise is quite natural for the uninhibited person in either situation. A nurse-midwife was told by one woman, following a very boisterous moment, "It felt so earthy to let out those sounds. It wasn't pain or fright at all."

Making a woman in labor feel that she doesn't have to "keep up a front" is one of the greatest services the nurse can provide. Self-consciousness and vanity should be put aside for the moment. The nurse might even encourage her to yield to her feelings. There are already many things the laboring woman is worrying about without having to put on a show for the people in attendance.

Bodily Care

Although the laboring woman may not acknowledge it at the time, she is acutely aware of, eminently refreshed by, and sincerely grateful for the nurse's attention to comfort needs, such as wiping the perspiration from her face and neck with a cool, damp cloth; applying lip emollient; relieving her thirst with mouth rinses, sips of water, or ice chips; cleansing the perineal area; providing clean bed linen; and handling her body with tenderness.

OBSERVING SIGNS OF IMMINENT DELIVERY

Current practice usually involves a move from the labor room to a delivery room. To minimize disruption of the laboring process, the decision to transfer should be made early enough to avoid rushing and excitement. On the other hand, the woman will not appreciate spending too much time on a delivery table in this stage of labor, thus, the timing of any transfer is critical to the woman's comfort and safety. Clinical signs signaling imminent delivery include the following:

- Gaping vulva.
- Tenseness between the anus and coccyx. As descent of the head progresses, the head can be palpated by gentle pressure against the perineum.
- Gaping of anus, with the anterior wall of the rectum visible.
- Presenting part is visible at the introitus. This immediately precedes a bulging of the perineum.

The nulliparous woman is usually transferred when 3-4 cm of caput is showing at the introitus; the multiparous woman toward the end of first stage if the vertex is at +2 station.

As soon as the nurse has determined that delivery is imminent, and moved the woman if necessary, she or he will prepare required equipment, supplies and oxytocics, and baby care items, and will assist the physician or nurse-midwife who is attending the delivery. The nursing assignment will generally include continuous monitoring of fetal heart tones after each contraction or every five minutes, administration of oxytocics, and charting the time of birth and subsequent procedures.

Pushing

Many well-intentioned nurses and attendants are inclined to instruct the woman to initiate vigorous pushing efforts as soon as the cervix is fully dilated. However, personal and professional experience has prompted others to modify this practice (Kitzinger & Litt, 1977; Noble, 1976). Beynon (1957) found that women who are not actively encouraged to push do not begin to do so until the baby's head distends the pelvic floor. She also noted that pushing efforts did not always coincide with the onset of contractions and that the urge to push varied from one contraction to the next. My approach is to wait until the urge to push is overwhelming before beginning active encouragement. This advice is based on the belief that a woman who is tuned in to her body is really the best judge of when and how hard to push. Forcing her to bear down does not allow for differences between women and their contractions. Further, the insistent commands of those around her will distract the laboring woman from controlling the delivery according to the type and intensity of the contraction she is experiencing.

Most women will eventually have the desire to push and will feel better when doing it. Generally, it takes several pushes for her to feel control over her efforts, and the nurse's assistance will be required while the woman and her partner or coach adapt to the rhythm of the contractions.

Position

Comfort should dictate the position for actual pushing: semisitting, back rounded with pillows, partner's or coach's arm for support. The head should be slightly forward because backward extension places strain on neck muscles. Elbows should be bent out from the body and the legs should be relaxed, with knees drawn up and rotated outwardly. Women often pull back on their legs as they push; grasping side rails or the partner's or coach's arms can be an alternative method to pulling on legs. Some women prefer a side-lying or squatting position.

Coaching

Throughout the baby's journey into being, the woman should be encouraged to rest, relax her entire body (with legs down), and breathe regularly between contractions in order to maintain her energy.

For effective pushing, the maximum intensity of the pushing effort should match the woman's inner urge to push. She should be coached to breathe in and out slowly until this pushing point is reached, at which time she will automatically hold her breath as she pushes down. She should then take several more breaths in and out until the next urge comes, and so on until the end of the contraction. The pattern of holding onto deep breaths as long as possible is not conducive to adequate oxygenation for the woman or her baby.

The words used for coaching should be consistent and repeated as necessary or planned. Only one person should do the coaching. Words of encouragement and praise should follow the completion of each push. The instruction to push as for a bowel movement is incorrect. The direction of such a push is different, and the association may inhibit her efforts since most women are already concerned about the embarrassment of defecating.

A mirror held above the perineum allows the woman to watch the gradual appearance of her baby's head. This will also relieve the woman who is resisting the urge to push the baby's head out because of burning and stretching sensations. Gentle reminders for her to "let go" and push through the sensation will help to alleviate fears of injury. Her ability to relax the pelvic floor muscles will reduce the amount of the expulsive force required and reduce discomforts and fears.

Once she is comfortably settled in a position for delivery, the woman should be assisted by *one* person in "breathing the baby's head out." This requires the woman to breathe through a contraction and gently push in the interim. It also allows for a gentle final stretching of the perineum and a slow, controlled delivery of the baby's head.

When the baby's head emerges, there is generally a collective holding of breath as those in attendance anticipate the baby's first cry. The expressions of intensity that persisted from the beginning of second-stage labor are replaced by incredulousness and joy. Within moments, the shoulders and hips are delivered, and the exultant mother receives her precious offspring, climaxing the birth moment.

REFERENCES AND ADDITIONAL READINGS

Angelini, D. (1978). Non-verbal communications in labor. *American Journal of Nursing, 78*(7), 1221–1222.

Bennis, W., Beene, K.D., & Chin, R. (1964). *The Planning of Change*. N.Y.: Holt, Rinehart & Winston.

Beynon, C.L. (1957). The normal second stage of labor: A plea for reform in its conduct. *Journal of Obstetrics and Gynaecology of the British Empire, 64*, 815–820.

Crawford, M.T. (1968). Physiological and behavioral cues to disturbances in childbirth. *Bulletin of the Sloane Hospital for Women, 14*, 132–142.

Cronenwett, L., & Newmark, L. (1974). Father's response to childbirth. *Nursing Research, 23*, 210–217.

Friedman, E.A. (1978). *Labor: Clinical evaluation and management* (ed. 2). New York: Appleton-Century-Crofts.

Friedman, E.A., & Sachtleben, M.R. (1970). Station of the fetal presenting part. IV. Slope of descent. *American Journal of Obstetrics and Gynecology, 107*, 1031–1034.

Gaskin, I.M. (1978). David and Carolyn's birthing. In *Spiritual midwifery*. Summertown, Tn.: The Book Publishing Company, p. 181.

Gassett, H. (1976). Participative planned change. *Supervisor Nurse, 7*(3), 34–40.

Greenhill, J.P., & Friedman, E.A. (1974). *Biological principles and modern practice of obstetrics*. Philadelphia: Saunders.

Hott, J.R. (1976). The crises of expectant fatherhood. *American Journal of Nursing, 76*(9), 1436–1440.

Jennings, B. (1982). Childbirth choices: Are there safe options? *The Nurse Practitioner, 7*(7), 26–37.

Kitzinger, S., & Litt, B. (1977). A fresh look at second stage. *Nursing Mirror, 145*, 17–20.

Lesser, M.S., & Keane, V.R. (1956). *Nurse–Patient relationships in a hospital maternity service*. St. Louis: Mosby.

Newton, N. (1955). *Maternal emotions*. New York: Hoebner.

Noble, E. (1976). *Essential exercises for the childbearing year*. Boston: Houghton Mifflin.

Chapter 8 | Emergency Delivery

Cathryn L. Anderson

I N THESE TECHNOLOGICAL TIMES, pregnancies can be planned; that is, conception and some aspects of birth can be planned. Babies, however, have always made appearances according to their own time schedules and not necessarily those desired by the expectant parents or the official birth attendants.

Many emergency births result from either premature labor (less than thirty-seven weeks' gestation) or precipitate labor (less than three hours in length). Sometimes a birth is both premature and precipitous. Such a birth is usually classified as medium- to high-risk, as both the baby and mother may need sustained special care after the birth.

EQUIPMENT

All public facilities that might be the site of an unexpected birth should have emergency delivery equipment available. The prenatal care offices, the emergency or admitting rooms of a hospital, and every room in the birthing suite should have emergency delivery packs. These sterile packs should include

- Bulb syringe: to suction baby's nose, mouth, and pharynx
- Plastic DeLee trap: more effective than bulb syringe in cases of meconium stained fluid
- Two Kelly clamps: for clamping umbilical cord

- Scissors, two pairs: one pair for emergency episiotomy; the other to cut umbilical cord
- Four towels: two to provide clean space on which the baby can be born; two to dry baby immediately after birth
- Baby blanket: to help keep baby warm, in addition to skin-to-skin contact with mother
- Blood tube: to obtain sample of cord blood for infant blood typing and Coombs' testing

ATTENDANTS

All health care personnel working with pregnant women should be fully prepared for an emergency birth. Registered professional nurses working in birth suites are likely to be attending unscheduled births and certainly should be given sufficient training in managing such occurrences safely until additional assistance can be obtained (Jennings, 1979).

Unexpected births can be unsettling to everyone; they often alter plans made regarding a birth, and may introduce serious health problems for the mother and/or the baby. Despite the potential for problems, the nurse must remain calm and transmit this feeling to the woman, her family, and friends. A technique for remaining calm is to slowly and simply describe the events of the birth and the behavior desired from the

TABLE 8-1   Problem-oriented framework

Problem	Prevention
Infection of the woman (perineal, uterine, systemic)	Don't put your fingers or hands into the woman's vagina or uterus unless it is necessary for life-saving management. Sterile gloves should be worn, and appropriate vulval preparation should be performed before the examination.
Infection of the baby (usually systemic)	Don't cut the cord with unsterile instruments unless the dangers of tight nuchal cord outweigh those of tetanus or systemic *Staphylococcus* infection.
Hemorrhage of the woman (lacerations of birth canal or third stage factors)	Promote slow, controlled birth by helping the woman to pant, not push, during contractions. Use proper hand maneuvers.
Hemorrhage of the baby (subdural hematoma or umbilical bleeding)	Don't accelerate the normal delivery of the head in a breech birth. Be sure any clamps or ties are tight before cutting the cord.
Meconium aspiration	Brown, yellow, or green amniotic fluid is a signal that recommends the use of a DeLee trap to clear the nose, pharynx, and oral cavity before the baby takes the first breath.
Cardiopulmonary distress in the baby secondary to nonpatent airway or cold stress	Place the baby on his or her side, on the mother's abdomen for skin-to-skin transfer of heat. (Position promotes drainage of fluids and maintains baby's temperature.) Use bulb syringe or DeLee trap to suction material from airway. Dry and cover the baby to prevent evaporative heat loss.

woman and her partner or coach. Talking keeps the face from freezing into a countenance that frightens observers.

PLACE AND POSITION

Many emergency births occur in the birth suite, with the woman in bed, on a stretcher (guerney), or in the bathroom (toilet) while she is undressing or emptying her bladder or bowels. The woman who is not already in a clean bed does need to be in the cleanest, most private space available when it is discovered that birth is imminent. The nurse should not increase the risk for the woman and baby by moving the woman. to a delivery room, or even onto a bed, if the baby is already emerging. If the woman is already in a bed, she should stay in that bed and that room. The woman who is not should be helped to lie down on the floor on a clean sheet or towel on which the baby can be born. A left lateral (Sims) position, or a hands and knees position provide maximum room for delivery of the baby with minimum tension on the perineum.

PROCEDURE

Nature usually does not need intrusive assistance, which in fact can cause problems rather than preventing them (Table 8-1).

When the birth is imminent, *don't run away. Stay with the woman and deliver the baby.* Call for assistance by activating an emergency call system or send someone to get help; call for help if help is nearby, but do not scream at the top of your lungs. Keep in mind that we are talking about the emergency management of spontaneous birth, not about the management of births requiring operative assistance of some type. In the case of the sudden, rapid birth, the first point to remember is that a slowing or controlling of the rate of birth is a major objective. This can often be accomplished by helping the woman to breathe short, quick breaths instead of holding her breath and straining down. Demonstrate the exact way, saying "Pant! Breathe as I am doing." Inevitable births should not be delayed by dangerous procedures such as crossing the laboring woman's legs, giving her general anesthesia in an attempt to delay the birth until a physician is in

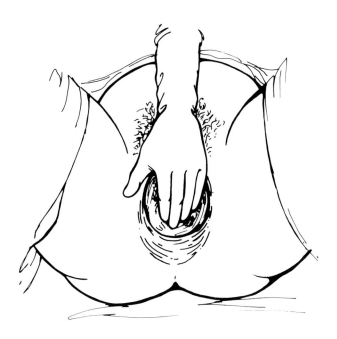

FIGURE 8-1 As the head is born by a process of extension, help slow the birth by maintaining a gentle pressure on the head with a flat palm. Coach the woman to breathe through contractions, allowing the force of the uterine activity to deliver the head as the forehead, nose, and chin pass over the perineum.

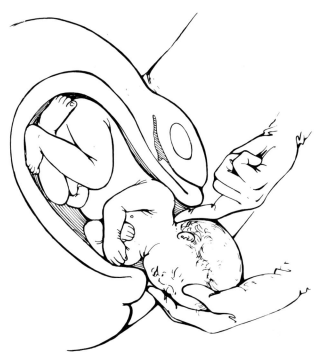

FIGURE 8-2 After birth of the head, support it in your hand as restitution and external rotation occur. Look and feel for the cord around the neck.

attendance, or forcibly preventing the emergence of the presenting part. Such behavior is gross malpractice.

The position of the baby determines maneuvers for assisting with the birth. Ninety-seven percent of all births are vertex, but in premature births, the incidence of breech births increases, especially in births of less than thirty-two weeks' gestation.

Vertex

If it is a vertex delivery, the largest part of the baby delivers first and the rest follows quickly. As the head becomes progressively more visible, gentle pressure on the occiput will slow the baby's advance (Figure 8-1). This allows maternal tissues time to gradually expand and accommodate the emerging head. As the head delivers, quickly check for a cord around the neck, which occurs in twenty to twenty-five percent of deliveries. (Oxorn, 1980) (Figure 8-2). If this is the case, slide the cord over the shoulder or head. To ease the

shoulders out, guide the head down and then up over the perineum (Figure 8-3A, B). Support the total slippery baby with a firm hand cradling the head and shoulders (Figure 8-3C). The baby can be placed on the mother's lower abdomen or on the bed between her legs, taking care not to place undo stress on the umbilical cord. A patent airway and establishment of respiration by the baby are the next objectives. Gently rub the baby dry with a towel to stimulate respiratory efforts and help prevent chilling from evaporation of amniotic fluid.

Breech

Breech deliveries are more difficult than vertex deliveries, as the largest part of the baby is born last and the cervix may not be fully dilated. The shoulders or head of the breech baby could have difficulty traversing the inlet or midpelvis, even with feet or buttocks already peeping from the introitus, or even with the body born

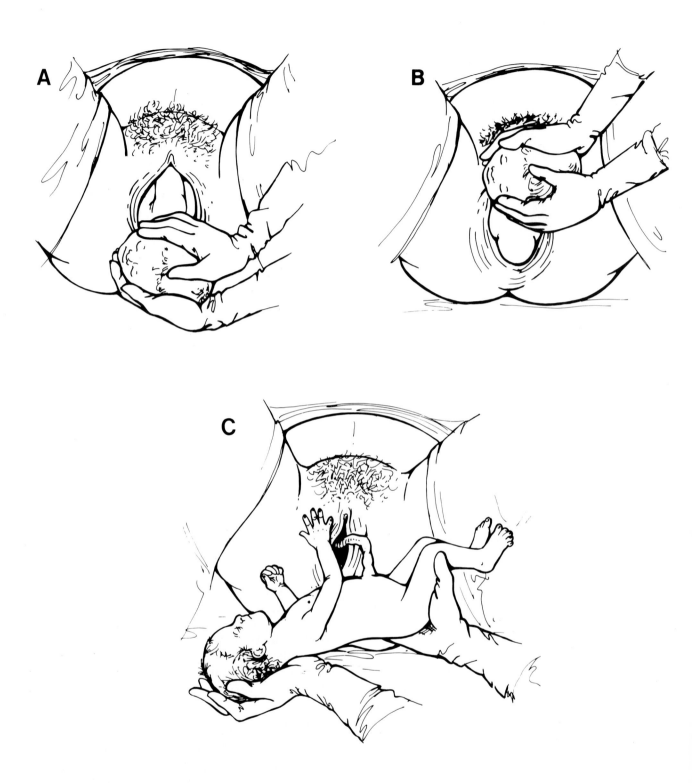

FIGURE 8-3 (A) To assist birth of the shoulders, place your palms over each side of the baby's head, over the ears. Apply gentle traction downward until you see the anterior shoulder appear fully. (B) To assist birth of the posterior shoulder, lift up on the baby's head to allow the shoulder to pass over the perineum. (C) At this point the baby will slip out easily. As the body emerges, slide your hand down the baby's back, holding the buttocks in one hand and the head and shoulders in the other.

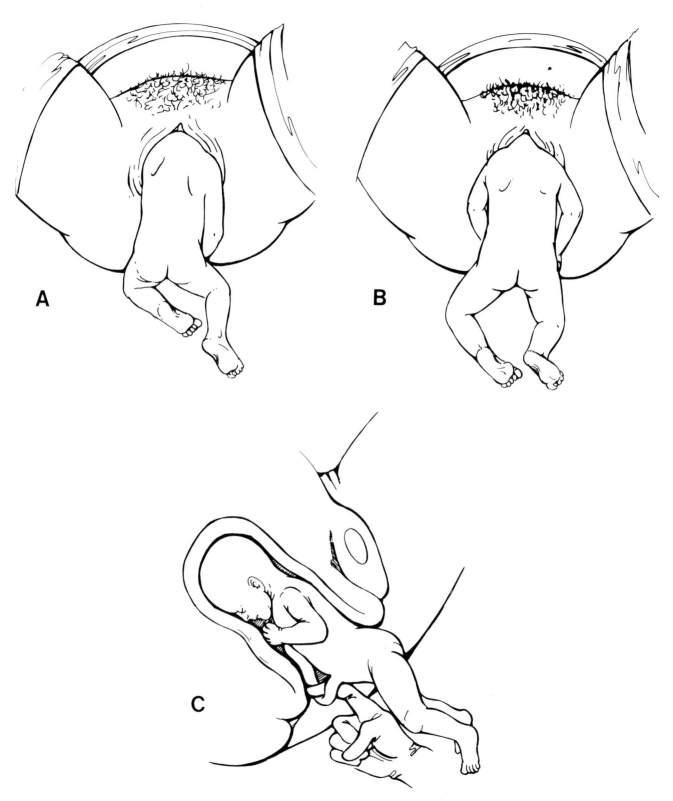

FIGURE 8-4 (A) Allow for spontaneous birth of the legs and hips. Do not attempt to assist the birth. (B) Allow for spontaneous birth of the arms. (C) When the baby's body is born to the umbilicus, gently pull down a loop of umbilical cord.

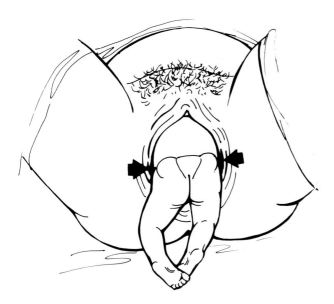

FIGURE 8-5 If any support or movement of the baby's body is necessary, the contact points on the baby are the sacrum and anterior iliac crests. The extremities, chest, or abdomen should not be manipulated at the risk of interfering with the normal mechanisms of labor or damaging the baby's soft tissue and organs.

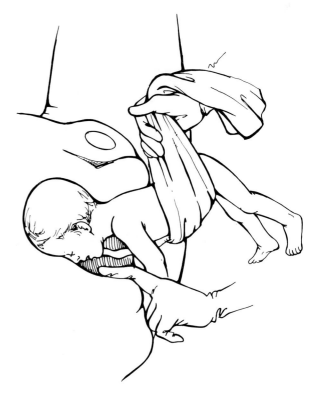

FIGURE 8-6 An airway may be established by depressing the posterior vaginal wall with a gloved hand. The baby may be wrapped in a towel to prevent heat loss.

to the umbilicus. There are seven major points to consider before assisting at a breech birth:

• The birth will occur in three mechanisms: the hips, the shoulders, the head (Figure 8-4A). Remember that the baby's back should be kept anterior, especially after delivery of the shoulders; if it is not, delivery of the head may be extremely difficult as the proper mechanism of birth is flexion, not extension.

• Don't attempt to assist with the birth until the baby is born to the umbilicus. Allow for spontaneous birth of the arms (Figure 8-4).

• Support or movement of the baby's body should be done by placing your thumbs on the sacrum and fingers on the iliac crests (Figure 8-5). Grasping the baby around the abdomen or chest should be avoided to prevent injury to soft tissue, such as rupture of the liver.

• When the baby's body is born to the umbilicus, gently pull down a loop of umbilical cord (Figure 8-4C) so that pulsation can be monitored and traction on the cord can be minimized if it is caught between the head and the pelvic wall.

• Wrap the baby's body in a dry towel to reduce heat loss (Figure 8-6).

• Delivery of the head should be accomplished at a moderate rate of speed, as rapid passage of the head

through the pelvis causes sudden compression and decompression of the cranial contents and can cause the ligaments of the brain (tentorium) to tear, leading to cerebral damage or death, secondary to hemorrhage. If delivery is prolonged, asphyxia may also cause cerebral damage or death. Positive outcomes are increased by calm and deliberate delivery rather than frantic attempts. Monitor oxygen supply to the baby by palpation of umbilical pulsation. Try to establish a patent airway through the baby's mouth within three to five minutes after birth of the umbilicus (Figure 8-6). Depress the posterior vaginal wall with a sterile gloved hand or a vaginal retractor, and wipe fluids away from the baby's mouth. Do not attempt to visualize the mouth by lifting the body high, as this interferes with birth of the head by flexion, and it is possible to lift the body so high as to hyperextend the neck and cause cervical damage.

• Constant suprapubic pressure (Kristellar maneuver) by the delivering woman or another person maintains flexion of the head and aids in delivery (Figure 8-7). It is usually necessary for the laboring woman to push more vigorously with a breech birth than with a

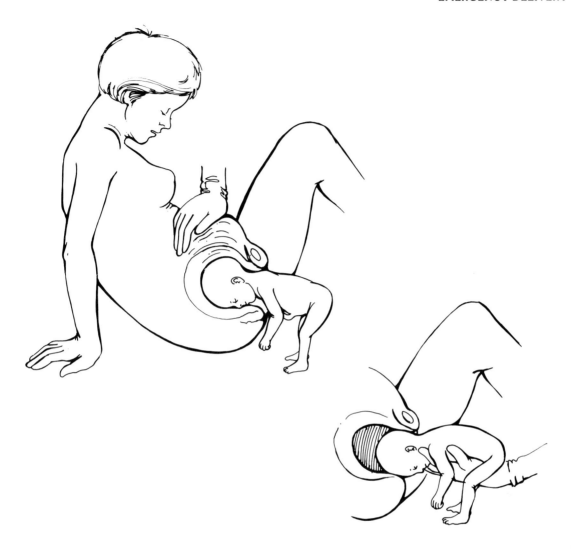

FIGURE 8-7 Suprapubic pressure may be used to maintain flexion of the head. The head will be born by a process of flexion. The body may be cradled in your hand astride your arm. Take care not to grasp the baby, thereby causing soft tissue injury. Don't lift the baby's body much beyond the horizontal plane.

vertex, using the abodminal muscles to move the head through the lower uterine segment.

As with the vertex delivery, firm support of the baby, while suctioning mucus from his or her nose and mouth is indicated immediately after the birth. Dry the body and get respiration going; use the Apgar scoring system to assess the baby. For infants in trouble, utilize sophisticated equipment and techniques rapidly and safely. Running 50 yards with a wet baby is not safe. Dry the baby, establish cardiorespiratory activity with CPR techniques, wrap him or her in a warm blanket, and then *walk* to the infant resuscitation unit. If any significant distance is involved; transport the baby in a heated unit with oxygen.

All of the psychological, social, and emotional aspects of birth remain important even when the birth is unexpected; support measures appropriate to labor and birth remain essentially unchanged (see Chapters 6 and 7).

REFERENCES

Jennings, B. (1979). Emergency delivery: How to attend to one safely. *MCN: The American Journal of Maternal Child Nursing, 4*(3), 148–153.

Oxorn, H. (1980). *Human labor and birth* (ed. 4) N.Y.: Appleton-Century-Crofts.

Chapter 9

Newborn Resuscitation

Patricia J. Johnson

RESUSCITATION OF THE NEWBORN has evolved over hundreds of years of trial and error, and has included methods and techniques that often resulted in trauma, tactile forms of deep pain stimuli, sphincter dilation, cold stimuli, tracheal milking, carbon dioxide inhalations, the Schultz grand swing, and respiratory stimulants, to name a few. Many of these techniques seem ridiculous from our current perspective, and most have been abandoned because their potential deleterious effects outweigh their therapeutic effects. Still, the purpose of resuscitative intervention for the newborn has remained the same through the years: to prevent and treat asphyxia neonatorum.

It seems logical to expect that improved obstetrical care over the past few years would decrease the number of infants requiring emergency resuscitation at delivery. However, these same improvements have also presented us with an additional group of compromised infants who, in the past, would theoretically have died prior to or at the time of delivery. Therefore, approximatley ten to twenty-five percent of all newborns remain candidates for some degree of acute supportive intervention or resuscitation at birth. The end result of ineffective or inadequate resuscitation of the significantly compromised infant is progressive asphyxia leading to brain damage and death.

Asphyxia of the fetus or newborn is defined as progressive hypoxia, hypercarbia, and acidosis resulting from inadequate gas exchange. The primary causitive factors are decreased or interrupted placental circulation, intra-uterine events leading to depressed or obstructed respiration, absent or ineffective respiration in the newborn, or a hypotensive episode leading to shock in the newborn. Ultimately, all major body systems including the brain, heart, liver, and kidneys, face potential irreversible injury, resulting in death or severe disability.

NORMAL PHYSIOLOGICAL CHANGES AT BIRTH

Even the normal birth process is a stressful event for the infant. Numerous physiological changes must take place at or around the moment of birth for the newborn to adequately adapt to his or her new extra-uterine environment. The fetus moves from a parasitic existence within the warm, moist, dark, controlled intra-uterine environment; through a relative compression chamber; into a light, cold, air-filled, noisy extra-uterine environment in which she must newly maintain her own pulmonary gas exchange, temperature regulation, waste excretion, and digestive processes, independent of her maternal host. The stimulus for this multisystem transition is only partially understood.

The first breath is probably stimulated by a combination of many interrelated occurrences. Normally, the maternal–fetal oxygen gradient is very narrow, and the fetus survives on PaO_2 of approximately 30 mm Hg, leaving little margin for variations (James, 1966). During the final phase of labor, the infant develops a mild acidosis, hypoxia, and hypercarbia because of the repetitive "breath holding" or decreased gas exchange caused by the interrupted uterine blood flow with each contraction. These biochemical stimulants, coupled with cord compression, temperature changes, tactile stimuli, and the passive rush of air into the lungs due to the elastic recoil of the chest wall as it exits the vaginal canal, have all been shown to have some cause–effect relationship to the initial respiration of the newborn.

The intricacies and interrelationships among all the factors thought to initiate newborn respiration are yet to be clearly defined. With the first breath the Po_2 rises, the Pco_2 decreases, and the pH increases, leading to a decrease in pulmonary vascular resistance and a three- to tenfold increase in pulmonary blood flow. Thus, perfusion of the newly inflated lungs occurs. The pressure required for the infant's first breath of life is 10–70 cm H_2O, usually accomplished with the initial cry, which allows the incoming air to overcome the viscous fluid in the tracheal bronchial tree, as well as the high surface tension in the alveoli. Some of this lung fluid drains out the mouth and nose, but much is probably absorbed by the pulmonary vascular system and lymphatic circulation. After 4–5 breaths, a functional residual capacity necessary to stabilize blood gases is reached, and the alveolar surface tension is lowered, so that the work of breathing is significantly decreased (Avery & Fletcher, 1974).

Simultaneous with the changes in the pulmonary system at birth, the cardiovascular system is also undergoing dramatic change (Figure 9-1). When the cord is clamped, the low resistance placental circuit is removed and the infant's systemic vascular resistance increases; aortic and left arterial pressures increase, closing the foramen ovale, and resulting in increased pulmonary blood flow. As the Po_2 increases, the patent ductus arteriosus begins to constrict, completing functional closure by fifteen to twenty-four hours. The umbilical arteries spasm, and the ductus venosus closes. A short time after birth, other body systems begin to function, often as they are challenged by their specific substrates or stimuli.

ASPHYXIA OF THE FETUS AND NEWBORN

With understanding of the basic physiology of birth, it becomes even more clear how vulnerable the fetus-newborn is during the process of birth. Should the placental unit suffer from either a chronic or acute decrease in its nutritional or gas exchange functions, the fetus would have little reserve for toleration of stress and would be at significant risk for physiological compromise during even the normal birth process. Likewise, the normal fetus faces potential risk of significant compromise if the birth process is complicated by one of many problems that could present additional stress (Table 9-1). These situations lead to the major causes for intrapartum asphyxia.

TABLE 9-1 Factors contributing to or associated with fetal and neonatal asphyxia

Contributing maternal factors
  Associated with fetal asphyxia
      Hemorrhage
      Placenta previa
      Abruptio placenta
      Increased maternal age
      Grand multiparity
      Toxemia
      Diabetes
      Prolonged pregnancy (>42 weeks from last menstrual period)
      Prolonged labor (primiparas > 24 hours; multiparas > 12 hours)
      Hypotension
      Hypertension
      Severe anemia
      Cardiorespiratory disease
  Associated with neonatal asphyxia
      Excessive analgesic agents
      Excessive anesthetic agents
      Excessive antihypertensive agents
      Prolonged labor
Problems during labor and delivery
  Cephalopelvic disproportion
  Malposition
  Shoulder dystocia
  Difficult forceps delivery
  Fetal rotations
  Cord accidents
  Multiple pregnancies
Fetal disease associated with asphyxia
  Severe isohemolytic disease
  Intra-uterine infections
  Meconium passage and aspiration
  Congenital malformations
  Pulmonary immaturity
  Fetal tachycardia, bradycardia, or arrhythmias

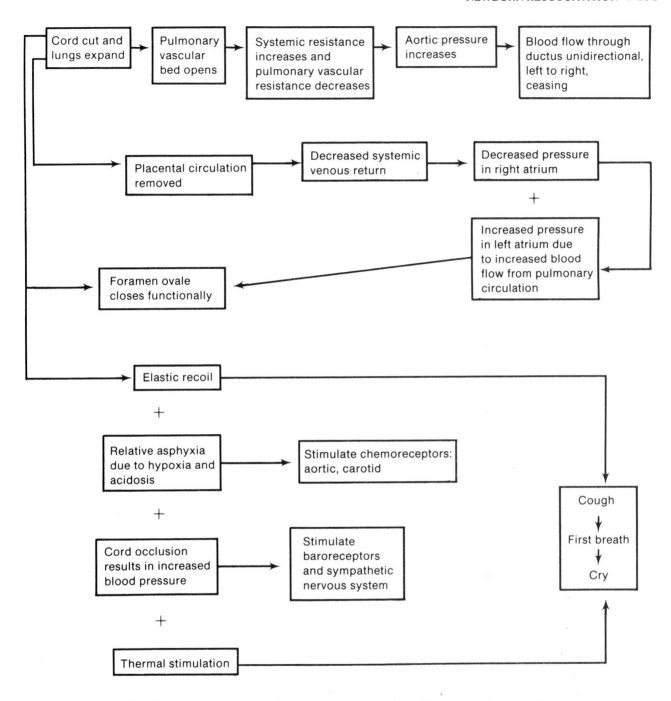

FIGURE 9-1 Relationship between pulmonary and cardiovascular changes at birth.

Most infants who present with significant respiratory depression at birth have suffered some degree of asphyxia prior to or during birth, although the degree and duration of the insult is often unknown. One can usually identify signs of fetal distress that indicate potential neonatal compromise (Table 9-2). The response of the human fetus-neonate to asphyxial insults is dependent on her nutritional state and blood sugar level prior to the insult, as well as the gestational age of the infant, the effect of maternal medications, and the degree and characteristics of the trauma caused by the birth process.

In the past, when mothers were heavily medicated prior to delivery, it was common to expect a one- to two-minute period of apnea in the newborn after birth. Today, medications are used more cautiously during

TABLE 9-2 Prenatal indications of fetal distress

Fetal tachycardia (> 160 beats/min)

Fetal bradycardia (< 120 beats/min)

Loss of baseline variability in fetal heart rate

Fetal acidosis (pH < 7.20–7.25)

Severe variable or late decelerations

Meconium-stained amniotic fluid

the intrapartum period to prevent additional chemical depression on the newborn. Nevertheless, maternal medications given intrapartum for either vaginal or Cesarean deliveries have the potential to cause respiratory depression of varying degrees (Table 9-3). The infant may or may not have an initial respiratory effort, followed by apnea, which can persist and result in significant asphyxia if the infant is not supported.

Asphyxia in the neonate generally presents as respiratory depression or apnea. The acute management of asphyxia, if it is to be successful, must be both efficient and effective, but not excessive. Therefore, one must be able to recognize the degree of asphyxia. Shock may be a precursor of the asphyxial insult or a late sign of more

progressive asphyxia (Dorand, 1977). Without an obstetrical history indicating evidence for an etiology of hypotension, it is difficult to use shock as an indicator of degree or duration of asphyxia. This does not, however, preclude the need to effectively treat shock. Treatment may, in fact, reverse some of the effects of asphyxia.

Following an asphyxial insult, the infant proceeds through two phases of apnea (Figure 9-2). Initially, she responds with one to one and a half minutes of increased respiratory effort, with respirations that are greater in depth and frequency. This is then followed by *primary apnea*, in which respiratory efforts cease for about one to one and a half minutes. Then the infant proceeds into a phase characterized by rhythmic deep gasping at a rate of 5 breaths/min; these become progressively weaker and slower, depending on the acid base status of the fetus, the effect of maternal drugs, and the temperature of the environment. After about eight and a half minutes, the gasping ceases, marking the onset of secondary apnea—the terminal phase (Dawes, 1968).

During primary apnea, the infant's respiratory activity is responsive to many forms of stimulus, including tactile stimuli. These stimuli will interrupt primary

TABLE 9-3 Fetal-neonatal effects of common pharmacological agents administered shortly before birth

Drug or Agent	Effect on Fetus
Barbiturates	Increases duration of primary apnea; possibly prolongs time to last gasp; may increase the infant's response to resuscitation suring secondary apnea
Halothane (and other similar general anesthetics)	Respiratory depression
Local anesthetic agents administered for paracervical blocks and epidural procedures	Fetal hypotension, bradycardia, acidosis; fetal death; respiratory depression (less respiratory depression than with general anesthetics)
Narcotic analgesics	Respiratory depression; prolongs duration of primary apnea
Meperidine (Demerol)	Prolongs time to last gasp; maximal depression of fetus is 1–3 hours following administration, with variation dependent on maternal metabolism and route of administration
Alphaprodine	Maternal and fetal effects similar, but peak and duration of effect shorter
Magnesium sulfate	If given before anoxia, prolongs time to last gasp and renders experimental animal more responsive to resuscitation; no effect on primary apnea; slows infant's gut motility, resulting in mild constipation to ileus

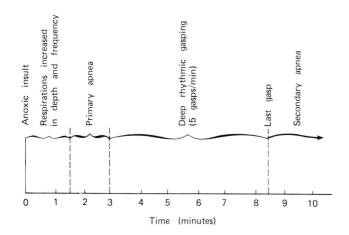

FIGURE 9-2 Approximate time sequence of primary and secondary apnea (documented in rhesus monkeys). (From Adamsons, K., Jr., Behrman, R., Dawes, G.S., James, L.S., & Koford, C. (1964). Resuscitation by positive pressure ventilation and tris-hydroxymethylaminomethane of rhesus monkeys asphyxiated at birth. *Journal of Pediatrics* 65:807–818. With permission.)

apnea and will usually initiate gasping. Following the phase of primary apnea, such stimuli are ineffective, and only intervention with effective artificial ventilation, and normalization of the acid–base status will successfully resuscitate the infant and reestablish respiratory effort. Each minute after the last gasp without ventilation of the infant will delay the onset of spontaneous rhythmic respirations by four minutes (Adamsons et al., 1964). Although the time sequences in progressive asphyxia are extrapolated from original work in rhesus monkeys, the human neonate can be expected to respond similarly. Variable temporal responses to asphyxia are species dependent, as well as postnatal and gestational-age dependent (Kabat, 1940; Mott, 1961).

At birth, it is often difficult to recognize which progressive phase of apnea the infant is in. Certainly, unequivocal response to tactile stimuli would indicate that the infant is in primary apnea, and the asphyxial or hypoxic insult was probably either recent or not too severe. Potentially traumatic stimuli such as pain or cold should not be used: They are no more effective than gentle but vigorous tactile stimulation. These methods of excessive stimulation are generally contraindicated in all cases of neonatal resuscitation, as are analeptics. Cold is particularly stressful to the already compromised neonate. Analeptics are of variable effectiveness and would be best replaced by successful supportive measures with more clinical efficacy.

RESUSCITATION

Successful resuscitation of the newborn depends on preparation of the team, adequate assessment of the infant's need for resuscitation, and, of course, one or more skilled individuals available as needed. Between fifty and seventy-five percent of those high-risk infants who are potential candidates for resuscitation can be anticipated through identification of the high-risk pregnancy. Nevertheless, twenty-five to fifty percent remain unexpected prior to labor and delivery. Although the characteristics of the newborn population may dictate the sophistication of the newborn services in general, any delivery room staff is obligated to maintain an optimal state of readiness at all times for resuscitating the newborn in need.

Area for Resuscitation

The delivery room or suite, including the operating room used for Cesarean sections, should be equipped to manage the newborn as well as the mother. This means arranging a specific area for the care of the newborn in either the delivery room or an adjacent room. This area needs to be large enough for two staff members to resuscitate the infant. It should be well lighted, warmed if possible to between 75° and 80°F with minimal drafts, and equipped with adequate electrical outlets for the necessary equipment. Oxygen must be available for the infant, as well as wall or portable suction. A radiant heat source over a workable, flat surface for the baby to lie on is essential (Figure 9-3). Although commercial radiant warmers are ideal, other forms of radiant heat can be devised for less cost, and are generally acceptable as long as safety precautions are built in. For example, a covered flat surface, approximately 36 inches from the floor with 200-watt screened flood lights 36 inches above the surface will suffice.

Equipment

Isolettes and Armstrong warmers are less effective as they make instrumentation of the infant nearly impossible if heat loss is to be prevented. A bassinette under a radiant heat source can be used if a flat surface is readily available to place over the bed when needed. A nearby cart should be available for storage of the following equipment and supplies:

- Stethoscope.
- Hand ventilator such as the Hope Resuscitator,

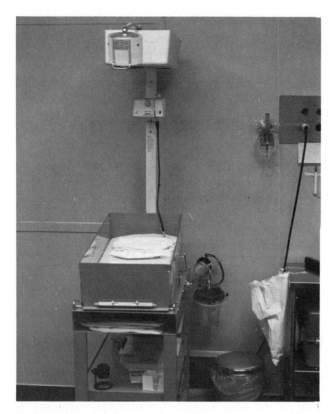

FIGURE 9-3 An adequate area for resuscitation of newborn in the delivery room, with oxygen outlet, suction, warmer, and electrical outlets.

preferably with the 100 percent oxygen adapter and/or an anesthesia bag with pressure manometer (Figures 9-4 and 9-5).

• Endotracheal tubes (2.5, 3.0, and 3.5 mm) with appropriately sized 15-mm adapters (Table 9-4). Use of cuffed endotracheal tubes is generally con-

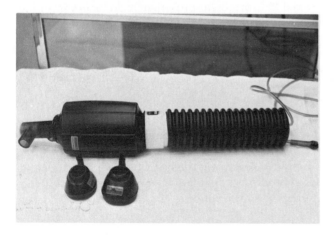

FIGURE 9-4 Hope resuscitator (Ohio Medical) with 100 percent oxygen adapter and face masks.

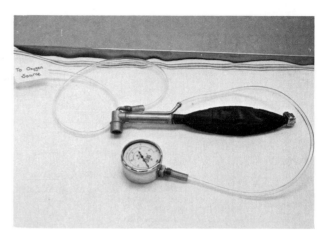

FIGURE 9-5 Anesthesia bag resuscitator with face masks.

TABLE 9-4 Endotracheal tube size for orotracheal intubation

Size of Infant (g)	Tube Diameter (mm)	Tube Length (cm)
<1000	2.5	7–8
1000–1500	3.0	8–9
1500–2500	3.0–3.5	8–10
2500–3500	3.5	9–11
3500–4000	3.5–4.0	10–11

traindicated because of pressure trauma to the larynx or trachea at the level of the cuff. Also, Cole (or tapered) endotracheal tubes are less effective because the narrowed lumen inhibits adequate suctioning and adds unnecessary resistance to air flow. Straight Portex or silastic tubes are more widely used. Portex tubes should not be resterilized as they become stiff and can cause trauma.

• Stylets or obturator for the endotracheal tubes (sterile pipe cleaners can be used) (Figure 9-6).

• Hand laryngoscope with 00 (premature blade for infants under 2500 g) and 01 blades, both with working, bright lights. It is important to have additional lightbulbs and batteries available.

• Suction catheters (size 5–6 French for suction down 2.5 endotracheal tubes; size 8 French; size 10 French for nasal and oral suction of copious secretions).

• Nasogastric tube (size 8 French).

• Infant airway.

• Magill forceps, if nasal tracheal intubation is preferred.

• Adhesive tape for securing the endotracheal tube (compound tincture of Benzoin can be applied to

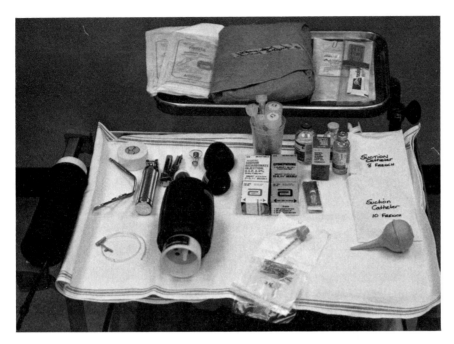

FIGURE 9-6 Resuscitation cart for delivery of a high-risk infant.

the skin under the tape to facilitate adhesion and protect the skin).

- 3.5 and 5 French end-hole umbilical catheters.
- Small sterile tray for umbilical catheterization, which includes one iris thumb forceps, two mosquito forceps, gauze 4×4, cord ties, scalpel, needle holder, a 4-0 silk suture, prep solution, sponges, and drapes (Figure 9-7).
- Needles and syringes: one TB syringe, 1.3 cc syringe, 1–2 and 5–6 cc syringes, and two large syringes, approximately 20–30 cc in size.
- Medications (Table 9-5).
- DeLee suction catheters (Bard-Parker) can be used for oral and nasal suctioning, but are less effective than wall or portable suction for thick or excessive mucus.
- Bulb syringes are useful for oral and nasal suctioning but must be used with caution because the excessive negative pressure produced (360 cm H_2O) can traumatize the mucosa.

Personnel

For additional readiness, one individual should be assigned to accept, evaluate, and, if necessary, stabilize and resuscitate the infant. This individual should be responsible solely for infant care and should be familiar with objective evaluation of the newborn by use of the Apgar score. In addition, he or she should be capable of at least initiating the resuscitation process, with additional assistance readily available to intervene. If a multiple birth is expected, at least one individual should be available for each infant anticipated.

The neonatal person or team should be aware, before delivery, of any significant factors or problems in the

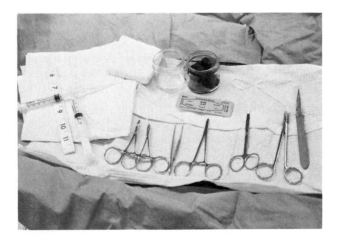

FIGURE 9-7 Umbilical catheter tray. Top (left to right): drapes, gauze, saline, Betadine prep solution and swabs, 4-0 silk suture, cord tie. Bottom (left to right): tape measure, catheter with stopcock, two mosquits forceps, one iris thumb forceps, needle holder, iris scissors, scalpel.

TABLE 9-5 Resuscitation medications

Drug	Indication	Dose	Instructions
Adrenalin Chloride (epinephrine), 1:10,000	Cardiac resuscitation	1 cc per endotracheal tube or 0.1 ml/kg IV or IC	More effective if severe acidosis is corrected
Albumin, 25%	Volume expansion	0.5–1.0 g/kg/dose IV as 5–10% solution	Mix with Ringers lactate (not stable if mixed with $D_{10}W$) 5% = 4 cc albumin/16 cc Ringers/g 10% = 4 cc albumin/6 cc Ringers/g
Calcium gluconate, 10%	Hypocalcemia; asystole	200–400 mg% in maintenance IV; 100 mg/kg IV push	Caustic—avoid infiltration; give through central line; clear line of sodium bicarbonate before administering
Dextrose, 50%	Hypoglycemia	1–2 cc/kg as $D_{25}W$ IV or dilute to $D_{10}W$ to avoid bolus infusion	Hyperosmolar glucose infusions ($> D_{12.5}W$) should be given through central line only
Narcan, 0.4 mg/ml (adult strength) or 0.02 mg/ml (neonatal strength)	Narcotic antagonist	0.01 mg/kg = 0.025 cc/kg/dose (adult) or 0.5 cc/kg/dose (neonatal)	Adult strength: may dilute as 0.1 cc narcan in 0.3 cc sterile water = 0.01 mg/0.1 cc. Give 0.1 cc/kg/dose
Sodium bicarbonate, 1 mEq/ml	Acidosis	2–4 mEq/kg/dose	Dilute 1:1 in sterile water
Atropine sulfate*	Sinus bradycardia	0.01 mg/kg dose IV or IM	Rarely used
Isuprel (1:5000), 0.2 mg/cc = 200 μg*	Shock	0.1 μg/kg/min IV drip	1 vial in 100 cc at 3 cc/kg/hr = 0.1 μg/kg/min

*Optional.

maternal history that could affect the status of the infant. In this way, problems can be anticipated and adequate preparations can be made for any special intervention. In certain high-risk situations, the involvement of the high-risk team may be indicated at the delivery. This service is often available to even the level 1 and level 2 centers through the regional perinatal center transport team.

The Apgar Score as an Indicator of Resuscitation

The degree of resuscitation needed by the compromised newborn in the delivery room can be facilitated by careful use of the Apgar scoring assessment tool. The one-minute and five-minute Apgar scores are important indicators of the infant's ability to cope with her new environment. More specifically, the one-minute Apgar score indicates the extent of resuscitative intervention required, and the five-minute Apgar indicates how effective that resuscitation has been.

Setting aside the value of a subjective, experienced assessment, the Apgar score, used appropriately, enables one to make rapid, sound judgments despite the often chaotic atmosphere. It is important that the score-keeper be responsible only for the baby's evaluation and care. Optimally, this individual is methodical, familiar with the scoring technique, and unbiased.

The system requires evaluation of only five signs, at one and five minutes after delivery of the whole baby, and should take only five seconds to do each time. A score of 10 is maximum and 0 is minimum. A score of 10 at one minute is unlikely, and score of 0, 1, or 2 at five minutes is ominous (Table 9-6).

The Apgar score of one minute is best utilized to direct the neonatal team toward the appropriate intervention. Obviously, the majority of infants with Apgars

TABLE 9-6 Signs associated with Apgar scores

Sign	Score		
	2	1	0
Heart rate	≥ 100	< 100	Absent
Respiratory effort	Crying	Irregular or gasping	No respiratory effort
Muscle tone	Well flexed	Slightly flexed extremities	Limp
Reflex activity	Grimace and cry to noxious stimuli*	Grimace only	No response
Color	Completely pink	Body pink, extremities blue	Blue, pale

*Catheter in nares or slap of feet.

Remember:

• If the infant appears obviously depressed, begin necessary resuscitative efforts before 1 minute.

• If the infant appears vigorous, don't insult her with unnecessary tubes and stimulation.

• Avoid swinging the infant by the feet, hot and cold baths, carbon dioxide inhalations, or other traumatic stimulation.

• Always attempt to keep the infant warm.

• An initial cry followed by apnea or an Apgar that deteriorates after 1 minute may indicate depression from maternal analgesia or anesthesia.

of 8–10 will need little more than gentle handling and preventative measures to avoid unnecessary cold stress. Excessive manipulation of these babies may result in stress and deterioration. Deep suctioning, gastric emptying and lavage, and thorough examinations can be deferred until later. These infants are generally stable within moments of birth and should be offered to the alert and accepting mother and father (if possible) to begin the acquaintance process. Circumcision is never indicated in the delivery room.

The neonates with evidence of minimal depression (Apgar 7) will generally recover with little manipulation as well. These babies respond well to the tactile stimulation from drying and a low flow of oxygen to the face. Assisting the infant with clearing of the upper airway is often necessary, but excessive deep suctioning of the pharynx should be avoided because it may result in a vagal stimulation with reflex bradycardia. The mouth should always be suctioned before the nose, since the reflex response to a catheter in the nares is normally a gasp, which could result in aspiration of oral pharyngeal contents.

The next group of infants benefit greatly from efficient and effective early intervention. They are moderately depressed, with Apgars of 4–6 at one minute. The intervention should begin with vigorous drying of the infant and strict attention to avoiding additional cold stress. The airway must be cleared of secretions, and the character and amount of the secretions noted. Many of these infants respond without positive-pressure ventilation, but by one minute, need for this should be evident. If the infant has no spontaneous respirations, she is positioned in the neutral-extended position (Figure 9-8) and ventilated with a positive-pressure hand ventilator bag and mask for one to five breaths (Figure 9-9). If the infant has no response, the nasogastric tube is inserted and regular ventilation begun with oxygen by mask at 30–40 breaths/min. After one to two minutes, if the artificial ventilation renders no response (i.e., onset of spontaneous respirations) or the heart rate is falling, the infant is intubated and ventilation continued. Many of these infants will respond within five minutes and can be extubated before leaving the delivery room. They should be closely watched during their transition period for signs of infection, oxygen dependency, and other signs of respiratory distress, hypoglycemia, or hypotension. Their transition will often exceed the usual six to eight hours, but they are usually well on their way to a recovery from their compromised birth by twelve to twenty-four hours.

The last group of infants would be considered severely depressed with a one-minute Apgar of 0–3. It is difficult to know whether their degree of depression reflects a prolonged asphyxic insult prior to birth, a severe insult, or the preinsult status of the infant. It must, however, be assumed that the asphyxial insult was enough to put the infant in or near the secondary apnea phase. Thus, most of these infants will not resume spontaneous respiratory effort without a significant amount of assisted ventilation, which is best accomplished with an endotracheal tube. After drying the infant, the nurse should proceed to vigorous oro-

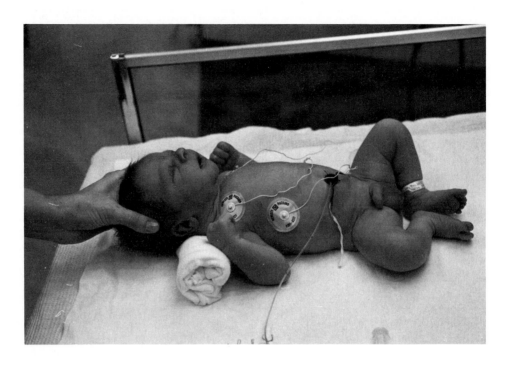

FIGURE 9-8 Neutral position of infant for successful mask ventilation and intubation.

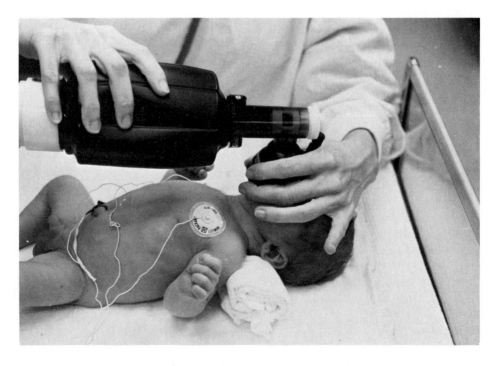

FIGURE 9-9 Proper technique for mask ventilation.

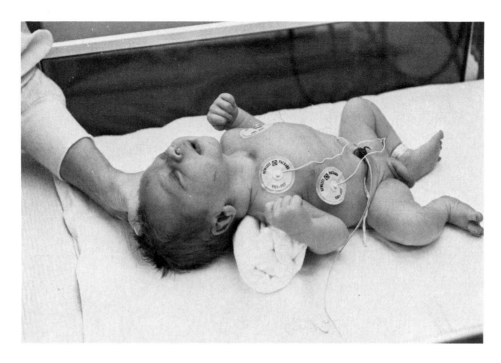

FIGURE 9-10   Hyperextended position—incorrect.

pharyngeal suctioning and immediate intubation. The endotracheal tube is suctioned, and ventilation with 100 percent oxygen is begun. Auscultation of adequate aerations should be checked with repositioning of the endotracheal tube as necessary, followed by securing the tube with tape.

Endotracheal Intubation

Endotracheal intubation of the newborn is no more difficult than intubation of any other individuals, and as long as the intubator is familiar with neonatal intubation and maintains the necessary confidence and calm, the procedure can be performed with ease and safety. Injury to the infant is caused only by haste and inexperience; therefore,the technique should be performed, or at least supervised, by the most experienced individual.

Essential to successful intubation is proper positioning of the infant. The infant should be placed supine on a flat surface at a workable level. The neck must not be hyperextended (Figure 9-10), as this will hinder intubation (the glottis is one to two cervical vertebraes higher in the newborn than in the adult). The infant should be placed in the "sniffing" position by extending the neck into a neutral position. This may be facilitated by a thin diaper roll under the occiput to prevent dependent

flexion of the head (Figure 9-8). The assisting team member can then immobilize the head by grasping it biparietally (Figure 9-11). The laryngoscope, held in the left hand, is inserted gently into the right side of the infant's mouth, between the tongue and the palate (Figure 9-12). After insertion, the blade is slowly moved to the midline while it is advanced 2 cm. Next, the tip of the blade is elevated slightly to visualize the thin, pink, curved rim of the epiglottis below the blade. The epiglottis can be lifted by gently advancing the blade further while lifting more on the scope and exposing the glottis. The epiglottis must not be hooked, as this may result in unnecessary trauma. If necessary, the pharynx can be suctioned to clear debris and secretions, which can easily impair visualization. The glottis will appear as an eliptical, vertical hole bordered laterally by the vocal cords. If the esophagus is seen, the scope should be pulled back slightly until the larynx drops into view.

The adapter end of the obturated endotracheal tube is grasped with the right hand and inserted down the right side of the mouth toward and through the cords (Figure 9-13). If the glottis seems high in the visual field, the infant's head should be flexed slightly, or the assistant should apply gentle downward pressure to the neck over the trachea. Intubation must not be attempted simultaneously with external cardiac massage.

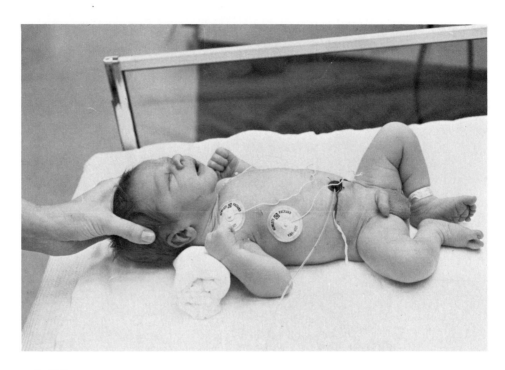

FIGURE 9-11 To immobilize the infant for intubation, the infant's head is grasped biparietally.

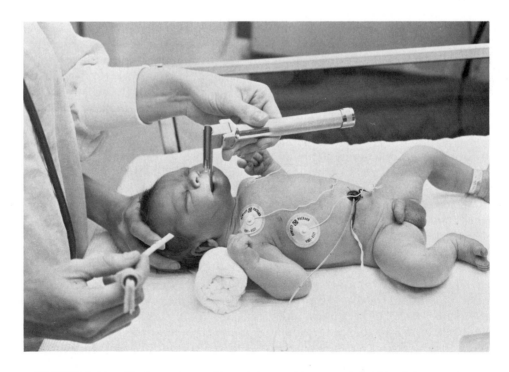

FIGURE 9-12 The laryngoscope blade is inserted into the right side of the mouth.

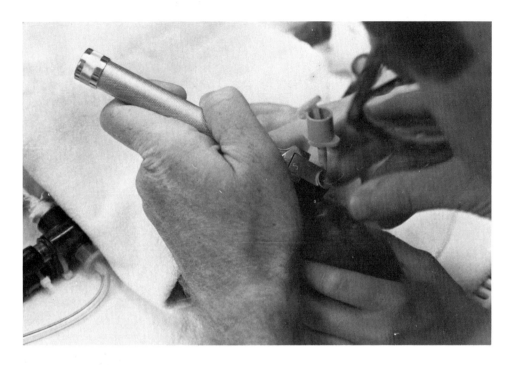

FIGURE 9-13   The endotracheal tube is inserted to the right of the laryngoscope blade.

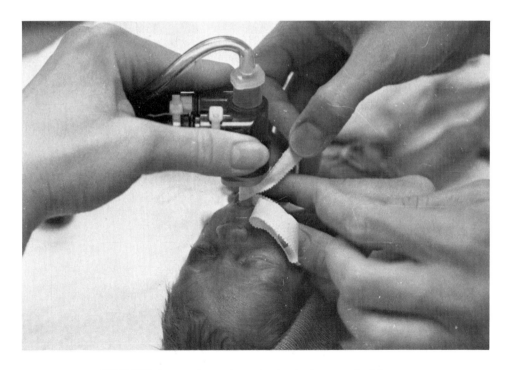

FIGURE 9-14   The endotracheal tube is secured with tape.

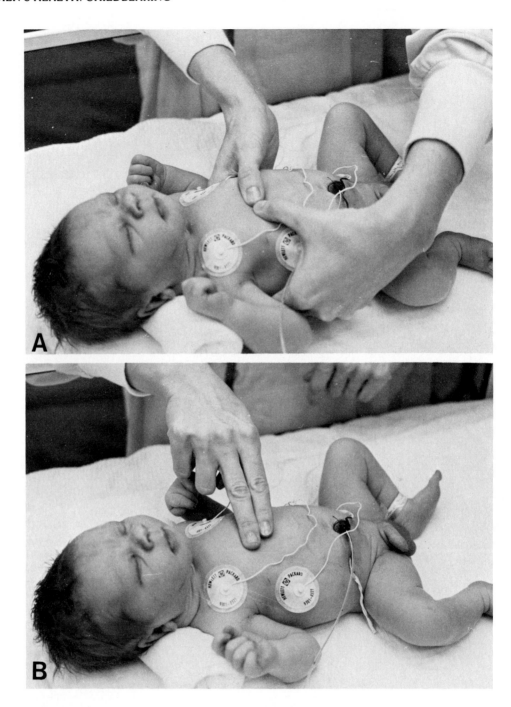

FIGURE 9-15 (A) External cardiac massage with two hands. (B) External cardiac massage with two fingers.

After insertion of the tube, the scope is removed while the tube is held in place. The obturator is then removed, and ventilation begun while auscultation is performed over peripheral lung fields bilaterally.

Intubation of the esophagus will be evident by one or more of the following signs:

- Response to ventilation (i.e., improved color and increased heart rate)
- Gurgling noises from tube with the onset of ventilation
- Auscultation of air movement over stomach
- Increased size of stomach

- Capability of deep insertion of suction catheter with removal of gastric contents from endotracheal tube
- Lack of aerations in chest

If the tube is within the trachea and equal breath sounds are auscultated bilaterally, the tube is secured with tape (Figure 9-14). The infant's cardiovascular status must be continuously evaluated. Following intubation and ventilation, a marked improvement in heart rate and color should be noted. If heart rate is not heard or is below 60 beats/min external cardiac massage should be begun (Figure 9-15). Most of these infants require pharmacological correction of a significant metabolic acidosis and may require volume expanders and vasopressor agents for hypotension. Pharmacological agents used in resuscitation with their specific indication, recommended route of infusion, and dosage are listed in Table 9-7. In general, these agents are most effective if given by a central route. Peripheral sites are usually difficult to establish and maintain during resuscitation. The umbilical vein is recommended as a readily accessible site for central infusion. It can usually be cannulated and maintained with ease using a 5

TABLE 9-7 Pharmacological agents used in resuscitation

Apgar	Degree of Depression	Predicted pH	Clinical findings	Appropriate resuscitation
9–10	None	7.30–7.40	Heart rate > 100; vigorous respirations with strong cry; active movement, good tone; cough or sneeze; ± acrocyanosis	• Dry and keep warm • Position on side with head slightly dependent • ± Minimal and shallow pharyngeal suctioning • *Do not elicit vagal response* • Less than 15% of infants will deserve a score of 10 at 1 minute
7–8	Mild	7.20–7.29	Heart rate > 100; shallow, irregular respirations with weak or absent cry; good to moderate tone with some flexion of extremities; cough or sneeze; Acrocyanosis or cyanosis	• Dry and keep warm • Position on side with head slightly dependent • Gentle, shallow suctioning of pharynx (mouth, then nose) • Gentle tactile stimulation (flicking sole of foot) • May need minimal oxygen to face • *Do not elicit vagal response*
4–6	Moderate	7.05–7.19	Heart rate ≤ 100; gasping respirations → apnea; moderate tone with some flexion → limp; grimace; cyanosis or pallor	• Dry vigorously and keep warm • Position supine with head slightly dependent and neck extended • Suction airway, mouth, then nose • Ventilate with 1–2 breaths using positive pressure mask with oxygen • If no response (i.e., spontaneous respirations), insert nasogastric tube and continue bagging at 30–40 breaths/min • If adequate aerations after 1–2 minutes cannot be maintained and/or heart rate falls, proceed to intubation • Correct metabolic acidosis
0–3	Severe	< 7.04	Heart rate ≤ 100 or absent, little or no respiratory effort; limp; absent reflex responses or grimace; cyanosis and pallor	• Dry and keep warm • Position supine with head slightly dependent • Suction airway through direct laryngoscopy • Intubate and begin positive-pressure ventilation with max FiO_2 30–40 breaths/min until spontaneous respirations; ensue if heart rate is 60 and doesn't respond promptly • Begin cardiac massage at rate of 120 beats/min, alternate 4:1 with ventilation • Correct metabolic acidosis

EXHIBIT 9-1 Problem-oriented approach to newborn resuscitation

Hypothermia

- Definition: core temperature below 97°F (36°C)
- A potential problem for all newborns as some degree of heat loss occurs by evaporation
- Prevention
  - Keep room temperature of delivery room or operating room at 75°–80°F, with minimal drafts
  - Immediately dry newborn thoroughly (especially head)
  - If normal-term infant:
    - Wrap in warm, dry blankets
    - While exposed for assessment, keep out of drafts and under radiant heat source
    - Place in warmer—i.e., isolette, incubator, or wrapped in a warm blanket in mother's arms
  - If high-risk infant:
    - Place on warm, dry blankets under radiant heat source
    - Maintain in neutral thermal environment
    - Transfer to isolette prewarmed to 88°–92°F
- Management
  - Warm slowly, approximately 1°F/hr, by one or more of the following methods:
    - Increase environmental temperature
    - Cautiously use *warm*-water-filled gloves or *warm* packs
    - Place under radiant heat source
    - Decrease drafts
    - Cover as many exposed areas as possible without deterring observation
- Resultant complications
  - Increased oxygen consumptions→↑hypoxia
  - Increased anaerobic metabolism→↑metabolic acidosis
  - Increased glucose consumption→hypoglycemia
  - Increased peripheral vasoconstriction→hypotension

Hypoxia and Hypoventilation

- Definition: hypoxia—inadequate oxygenation; hypoventilation—inadequate ventilation.
- May reflect short-term asphyxia (primary apnea) or more prolonged asphyxia (secondary apnea), which can be differentiated by the infant's heart rate and response to initial stimulation; color is not necessarily a good indicator at birth due to decreased peripheral perfusion
- Prevention
  - Clear oropharynx on delivery of head; the bulb syringe used properly is usually most readily available and adequate
  - Place infant on side with head slightly dependent (reverse Trendelenburg)
  - If normal-term infant:
    - Apply gentle tactile stimulation (flicking sole of foot or vigorous drying) if respiratory effort is less than adequate
    - Shallow suction the oropharynx, then nasopharynx as necessary to further clear airway
    - Provide minimum oxygen flow to face as necessary to facilitate improved oxygenation and color
  - If high-risk infant:
    - Vigorously dry infant, which may provide adequate tactile stimulation to initiate spontaneous respirations
    - If no immediate response, suction oronasopharynx
    - Ventilate 1–2 breaths with mask and positive-pressure bag; if no response, continue mask breathing, or, if Apgar less than 3, proceed to immediate intubation and continuous ventilation
- Management
  - Continue ventilation with 100% oxygen until spontaneous respirations are established; note: for every minute of apnea following the last gasp and onset of secondary apnea, 4 minutes of resuscitation are required to restore respirations
  - Provide warm, humidified oxygen sufficient to keep pink and observe closely; if concentrations greater than 35% are needed, blood gas monitoring is indicated
  - Consider maternal narcotic depression; administer Narcan (Endo Pharmaceuticals), 0.01 mg/kg IV or IM; repeat every 15 minutes as necessary
- Complications
  - Brain damage after about 10 minutes of hypoxia or anoxia
  - Increased metabolic acidosis, in addition to respiratory acidosis
  - Cell death, resulting in irreversible systemic complications that lead to death

Hypoglycemia

- Definition: serum glucose level of less than 20 mg% in the premature infant and less than 30 mg% in the term infant;

however, in most clinical settings, a serum glucose level of less than 40 mg% represents an abnormal level, especially in the sick or high-risk infant
- Specific risk for:
  - Infant of diabetic mother
  - Intra-uterine growth-retarded infant
  - Premature infant (especially if stressed)
  - Moderately or severely depressed infant
  - Cold-stressed infant
- Prevention
  - For most newborns: provide immediate and adequate environmental control (warmth) and respiratory support, followed by close monitoring of serum glucose levels as indicated after birth
  - For specific risk groups: provide continuous infusion of $D_{10}W$ 60–75 cc/kg/day for first 24 hours until adequate oral feedings are tolerated
- Management
  - Infuse (through umbilical vessel) $D_{25}W$ 1–2 cc/kg over 2 minutes
  - *Or* infuse $D_{10}W$ 3–5 cc/kg over 2–5 minutes, followed by continuous $D_{10}W$ infusion at 3 cc/kg/hr minimum
- Complications
  - Seizures
  - Brain cell damage
  - Death

Acid–Base Imbalance

- Definition: both metabolic and respiratory acidosis with pH less than 7.2
- Acidosis of mild degree is common in the normal newborn (pH 7.2–7.3); largely due to initial hypoventilation and inadequate gas exchange just prior to delivery; may be significant in the compromised infant
- Prevention
  - Establish respirations or adequate ventilation with necessary amounts of fractional-inspired oxygen to prevent hypoxemia
- Management in the infant with Apgar less than 4
  - Maintain adequate ventilation
  - Infuse (through umbilical vessel) $NaHCO_3$ diluted in equal amounts with D_5 or sterile water 1–2 mEq/kg 2–5 minutes
  - Repeat as necessary to correct persistent metabolic acidosis
  - Treat persistent hypotension
- Complications

Increased depression
Systemic cell damage
Death

Hypotension

- Definition: inadequate tissue perfusion, as evidenced by poor peripheral perfusion and pallor
- Uncommon if adequate heart rate is maintained, unless associated with acute hypovolemia or acute or severe anemia
- Specific risk:
  - Erythroblastosis fetalis
  - Maternal bleeding (placenta previa, abruptio)
  - Multiple pregnancies
  - Cardiac arrest
- Prevention
  - Keep baby at level of placenta until cord is clamped
  - Double-clamp cord with twins
  - Monitor for deterioration in heart rate, peripheral pulses (femoral), and color
- Management
  - If peripheral pulses diminish and heart rate is less than 60/min, initiate cardiac massage to maintain circulation at 120/min, alternating with ventilation with max Fio_2; heart rate usually responds to adequate ventilation
  - Infuse 1 g/kg of 5% albumin in Ringer's lactate or freshest O negative whole blood if available
  - Epinephrine (1:10,000) may be indicated; give 1 cc via endotracheal tube, or 0.1 cc/kg IC; usually not as effective given IV or via low UVC when an immediate effect is desired
  - Ventricular fibrilation is extremely rare in the newborn; asystole is more common; after correction of acidosis with no response to epinephrine ×2 IV, calcium gluconate may be successful in reversing a short-term asystole; give 10% calcium gluconate through a central line free of $NaHCO_3$ in a dose of 100 mg (1 cc)/kg while monitoring the EKG or heart rate
  - Infusion of pharmacological agents should only interrupt cardiac massage and artificial ventilation momentarily, at most
  - Reevaluate adequacy of ventilatory assistance
- Complications
  - Multisystem cell damage and death (e.g., renal failure, hepatic failure, disseminated intravascular coagulopathy)

French end-hole catheter. Placement should be distal to the portal circulation (approximately 2–5 cm) unless radiographic confirmation of placement above the diaphragm is timely. Once inserted, the catheter should be sutured securely in place and kept clamped or occluded (using a stop cock) when not infused.

The decision to administer epinephrine or other vasopressors in the delivery room is a serious one and must often be made with little time for forethought. The neonate with an absent heart rate at birth is either stillborn or has suffered a massive asphyxic insult. This infant may respond to extreme resuscitative efforts, but she certainly has little chance of totally intact survival. The resuscitation team must maintain an ongoing awareness of the infant's response or lack of respose to their intervention and follow some preset guidelines to direct the duration of their efforts. This is not to say that any infant displaying even minimal signs of life at birth does not deserve an all-out effort at resuscitation, possibly including the use of vasopressor agents. The neonate is an extremely resilient organism, capable of withstanding anoxic insults better than her adult counterparts, probably due in part to the healthy status of all organ systems and regenerative tendencies of some. Nevertheless, asystole in the neonate is an ominous sign of defeat, since the myocardium is one of the final organs to totally cease function in the newborn. The objective decision to abandon or defer resuscitation efforts is always difficult. It is a decision that all neonatal resuscitation teams will face at some time and should be anticipated and prepared for.

Complications of Resuscitation

The health care provider must be aware of the many common complications of resuscitation, as well as the possible methods for preventing the resulting iatrogenic problems (Tooley et al., 1977).

Umbilical Catheter Complications

Potential problems related to umbilical catheters are many. The following are the most common associated with resuscitation.

BLOOD LOSS Excessive blood loss during and after catheter insertion is usually avoidable by using a cord tie before cutting the umbilical stump and clamping or occluding the inserted catheter. Catheters should be kept visible and sutured in place.

LIVER TRAUMA Trauma to the liver by infusions of hypertonic resuscitation drugs directly into portal circulation can be somewhat prevented by using low venous lines inserted only until a blood return is obtained, and injecting diluted resuscitation medications slowly to allow some time for intravascular dilution. Umbilical artery catheters and high umbilical venous catheters are not generally used for resuscitation in our institution unless confirmation of acceptable placement has been made by x-ray. Epinephrine is never given through the umbilical arterial catheter.

INFECTION Infection from unsterile catheter insertion can be prevented by adherence to aseptic techniques.

Ventilation Complications

PNEUMOTHORAX Overventilation of the infant, and thus, pneumothorax, can be avoided by using hand ventilators with safety "pop-off" valves, provided these ventilators are used as recommended. Also, ventilation using an anesthesia bag is more safe if pressure manometers are applied and excessive inspiratory pressures are avoided.

ALKALOSIS OR ACIDOSIS Respiratory alkalosis may result from overventilation, and underventilation may impede the infant's spontaneous respiratory efforts or cause additional respiratory acidosis. Both problems can be prevented by ventilation of the infant at the appropriate rate of 30–40 breaths/min and with attention to adequate chest excursion and the onset of spontaneous respirations.

Oxygen Concentrations

Inadequate, as well as overadequate, oxygen concentrations should be monitored to prevent hypoxia or hyperoxia. The infant's color is generally a good indicator of oxygen delivery. Arterial blood gas monitoring is the best indicator of hyperoxia and should be employed if high concentrations of inspired oxygen are used for longer than fifteen minutes, especially in the premature infant.

Toxicity

Excessive and possibly toxic amounts of resuscitation medications can be avoided by administering medication according to specific clinical and, when possible, laboratory indications.

For example, correction of metabolic acidosis for moderately and severely depressed infants has traditionally been managed by infusion of sodium bicarbonate. Simmons et al. (1974) have documented the dangers of hypernatremia resulting from sodium bicarbonate administration. These researchers believe even severe metabolic acidosis in the newborn will usually resolve after the establishment of adequate ventilation, oxygenation, and perfusion.

Meconium Aspiration

Aspiration of meconium can be nearly prevented if appropriate steps are taken during resuscitation. Although meconium staining of the amniotic fluid occurs in about nine percent of births, not all of these infants require invasive intervention (i.e., intubation). About sixty percent will have meconium below the vocal cords that could be aspirated into the periphery of the lung with the onset of respirations. (Gooding et al., 1971; Gregory et al., 1974). To prevent aspiration of meconium, vigorous suctioning of the airway *prior to the onset of respiration* is indicated. The current recommendation is to suction the nose and mouth after delivery of the head and prior to delivery of the shoulders and chest. Then, if the infant demonstrates any significant degree of respiratory depression (Apgar lower than 5 or 6), with thick meconium staining, she should be intubated and tracheal suctioning begun. The endotracheal tube is used as a straw, and the intubator sucks on it, with his or her mouth covered

with a mask or gauze, while withdrawing the tube (Figure 9-16).

Mask ventilation must not be instituted before the airway is completely clear of meconium. The tracheal bronchial tree should not be lavaged in the delivery room, and the cords should not be visualized under direct laryngoscopy unless the intubator intends to, and is prepared to, intubate. The vigorous infant with thin meconium does not require aggressive suctioning (Gregory et al., 1974) or laryngoscopy and such manipulation could result in severe bradycardia and apnea.

Resuscitation of the Low-Birth-Weight Infant

The morbidity and mortality for the extremely low-birth-weight infants (less than 1000 g) have improved drastically in the past few years. These improved statistics are largely due to advancements in both obstetrics and neonatal medicine. Today fifty to eighty percent of these infants survive, and their preliminary followup is becoming more favorable. Nevertheless, their survival depends on expensive long-term care, and outcome is much less predictable than for other groups of high-risk infants.

One of the primary factors affecting both the morbid-

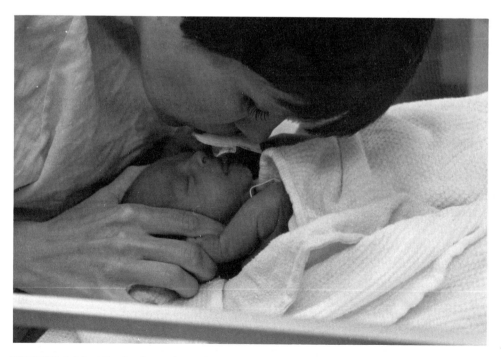

FIGURE 9-16 Tracheal suction of aspirated meconium by mouth-to-endotracheal-tube suction technique.

ity and mortality of these infants is effective resuscitation and support immediately following birth. However, effective intervention at such a premature stage often requires an ethical decision to salvage a potentially nonquality survivor or nonsurvivor. Obviously, no text can dictate a sound universal policy directing the resuscitation team to an appropriate goal or intent for supporting survival of each infant. However, the team must have acceptable guidelines to facilitate their decision-making process in order to proceed with effective resuscitation efforts or abandon them if so decided.

Even the guidelines for this decision are not very specific; nevertheless, they may serve as practical aids to delivery-room teams that more frequently face the difficult decision for salvage of the extremely low-birth-weight infant.

Before delivery it is important for the team to be aware of:

- Prenatal information, which may facilitate more accurate dating of the fetus and indicate significant complications that could affect fetal outcome
- The results of fetal evaluation during labor, which may provide some indication of fetal tolerance to the actual delivery process
- The parents' understanding of the gravity of the situation, their feelings about quality of life, and the value of the child to the family
- The current accepted predictors of lower limits for survival in terms of size and gestational age, such as 750 g and twenty-four weeks' gestation, or whatever limits the perinatal staff assigns
- The status of the infant immediately following delivery

The intrapartum assessment of the infant may complicate the decision for salvage because of clinical problems, such as the following:

- The prenatal and intrapartum information about mother and fetus is often scarce.
- The fetal tolerance to labor is often difficult to adequately monitor.
- The infant caretakers may be unable to communicate with the parents or obtain even secondhand information about their status and feelings.
- Apgar scores for these infants are not necessarily predictive of immediate or long-term outcome.
- Size determination of the infant is usually a gross estimate.
- Guidelines for clinical estimation of gestational age less than twenty-eight weeks' are unreliable.

Thus, the decision remains a difficult one.

Once the decision to salvage an infant has been made, however, all members of the obstetrical and resuscitation team should be aware of the intent, and their performance should reflect this functional agreement. The infant should be afforded every protective effort available during labor and delivery, including arrangements for delivery in a perinatal center when possible, to avoid the additional stress of transporting the newborn postnatally. The team should utilize the Apgar score as an indicator of supportive intervention requirements. The infant must be handled gently, and with maximum precautions to avoid cold stress or added trauma. Artificial ventilation of the infant should be introduced in the most efficient and least traumatic manner possible, with use of the most experienced personnel and of adequate oxygen, and avoidance of excessive suctioning. Finally, special attention to size of equipment and dilution of hyperosmolar solutions is essential. With these precautions, the infant will have the best available support early, which is likely to significantly affect survival and long-term outcome.

Resuscitation in the Nursery

The nursery in all institutions delivering infants should be as prepared as the delivery room for resuscitation and stabilization of an infant. The first six to twenty-four hours of an infant's life are a critical time for continued physiological stabilization. Therefore, normal newborn care services must incorporate a close observation period of a minimum of six hours during which nursing staff members monitor the infant's functional transition (Desmond et al., 1966). This observation does not preclude rooming-in for the normal-term infant who is at no apparent risk for a compromised transition; however, observation of these infants should not be solely the new mother's responsibility during this time. Obviously, infants at significant risk for morbidity will require extended observation and acute intervention.

Resuscitation of the infant in the nursery may be required at any time and, although it is often anticipated, signs and symptoms of a potential acute deterioration may go unnoticed.

Respiratory arrest is, by far, the most common problem requiring resuscitation of the neonate. Therefore, as in the delivery room situation, the initial goal of resuscitation will be establishing respiration and supporting circulation, with the end goal of preventing asphyxia.

To begin resuscitation in the acutely apneic infant, the resuscitator documents the apical heart rate and institutes tactile stimulation. If this stimulation results in some spontaneous respiratory effort, but with persis-

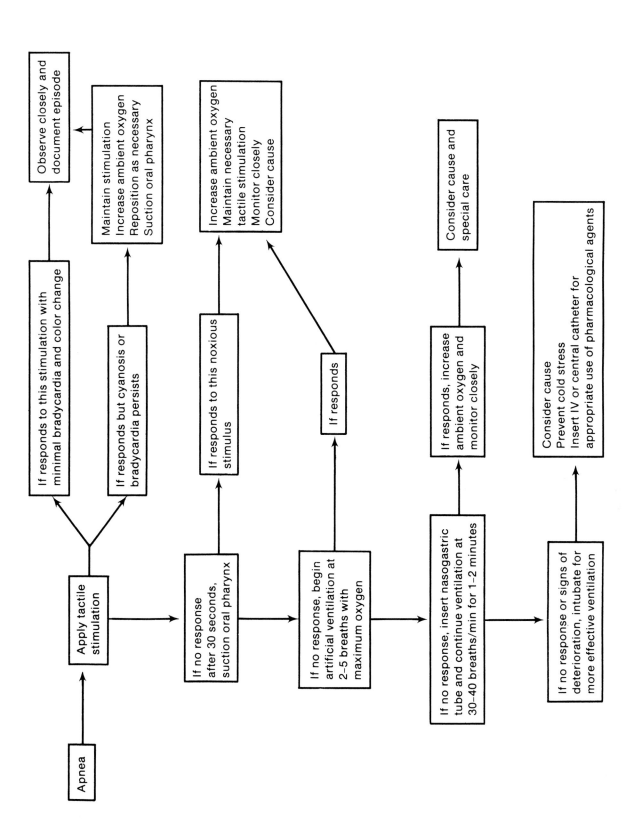

FIGURE 9-17 Management of acute neonatal apnea.

213

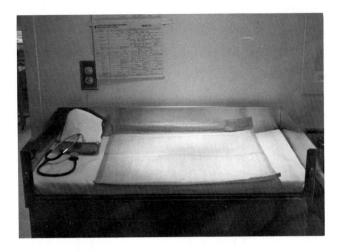

FIGURE 9-18   An example of a flat working surface with a radiant heat source for necessary interventions in the nursery.

tent cyanosis, the ambient oxygen is increased, the infant is repositioned to facilitate respiration (i.e., raising the head of the bed with infant supine or on her right side), and the oral pharynx is gently suctioned. If tactile stimulation does not result in some spontaneous respiratory effort and there is persistent or further deterioration in the infant's color and heart rate after a maximum of thirty seconds, the oral, then nasal, pharynx is suctioned. This alone may effectively stimulate respiration. If there is still no response, artificial ventilation is begun with maximum oxygen for two inspirations; if apnea persists, a nasogastric tube is inserted for gastric decompression and artificial mask ventilation is continued for one to two minutes. If the heart rate and/or color do not improve or further deteriorate, endotracheal intubation is indicated for more effective ventilation. In addition, external cardiac massage is indicated for heart rate lower than 60 beats/min, with insertion of an infusion line (preferably central) for infusion of sodium bicarbonate for correction of metabolic acidosis and infusion of colloid or vasopressor agents for hypotension and shock (Figure 9-17).

During the resuscitation, the infant should be on a flat working surface to facilitate the necessary interventions; some form of radiant heat should be provided to assure prevention of cold stress (Figure 9-18). Also, monitoring of EKG and blood pressure should begin early in the process. Additional resuscitation efforts should be directed toward treatment of the underlying etiology of the arrest whenever possible. The use of various pharmacological agents may be necessary:

- If a constant glucose infusion has not been maintained, glucose should be infused intravenously at 5 cc/kg of $D_{10}W$ or 2 cc/kg of $D_{25}W$.
- For asystole, *either* epinephrine (1:10,000) is given— through the endotracheal tube, 1 cc, or intracardiacly, 0.1 cc/kg; *or* calcium gluconate, 100 mg/kg, is given intravenously.
- For persistent sinus bradycardia, atropine is given intravenously, 0.01–0.03 mg/kg.
- Finally, for ventricular fibrillation (although extremely rare in the neonate), the heart is initially defibrillated with 2 watt-seconds/kg, and if there is no response, the dose is doubled up to 25–50 watt-seconds.
- Additional pharmacological agents are listed in Table 9-5.

Continuous reevaluation of the infant's response to the resuscitation efforts is necessary, as is documentation of drugs given and time lapsed. Also, intermittent assessment of the adequacy of ventilation should be made. At some point, the resuscitation team will have to abandon unsuccessful efforts. Most consider twenty minutes a reasonable length of time, after which reversal of asphyxia is unlikely if not impossible.

REFERENCES AND ADDITIONAL READINGS

Adamsons, K., Jr., Behrman, R., Dawes, G.S., James, L.S., & Koford, C. (1964). Resuscitation by positive pressure ventilation and tris-hydroxymethylaminomethane of rhesus monkeys asphyxiated at birth. *Journal of Pediatrics, 65,* 807–818.

Adamson, J.K. (Ed.) (1978). *Resuscitation of the newborn infant.* St. Louis: Mosby.

Auld, P.P. (1974). Resuscitation of the newborn infant. *American Journal of Nursing, 74,* 68–70.

Avery, M.E. & Fletcher, B.D. (1974). *The lung and its disorders in the newborn infant.* Philadelphia: Saunders.

Bacsik, R.D. (1977). Meconium aspiration syndrome. *Pediatric Clinics of North America, 24,* 463–479.

Dawes, G.S., Hubbard, E. & Windle, W.F. (1964). The effect of alkali and glucose infusion on permanent brain damage in rhesus monkeys asphyxiated at birth. *Journal of Pediatrics, 65:* 801–806.

Dawes, G.S. (1968). Fetal and neonatal physiology—A comparative study of the changes at birth. Chicago: Year Book.

Desmond, M.M., Rudolph, A.J., & Philaksphraiwan, P. (1966). The transitional care nursery: A mechanism for preventive medicine in the newborn. *Pediatric Clinics of North America, 3,* 651–668.

Dorand, R.D. (1977). Neonatal asphyxia: An approach to physiology and management. *Pediatric Clinics of North America, 24,* 455–461.

Drage, J.S., & Bernedes, H. (1966). Apgar scores and outcome of the newborn. *Pediatric Clinics of North America, 3,* 635–643.

Gregory, G.A. (1975). Resuscitation of the newborn. *Anesthesiology, 43,* 225–237.

Gregory, G.A., Gooding, C.A., Phibbs, R.H., & Tooley, W.H. (1974). Meconium aspiration in infants—A prospective study. *Journal of Pediatrics, 85,* 848–852.

Gooding, C.A., Gregory, G.A., Tabor, P., & Wright, R.R. (1971). An experimental model for the study of meconium aspiration of the newborn. *Radiology, 100,* 137–140.

James, L.S. (1966). Onset of breathing and resuscitation. *Pediatric Clinics of North America, 3,* 621–634.

Kabat, H. (1940). The greater resistance of very young animals to arrest of brain circulation. *American Journal of Physiology, 130,* 588–599.

Klaus, M.H., & Fanaroff, A.A. (1973). *Care of the high risk neonate,* Philadelphia: Saunders.

Llewellyn, A., & Milligan, J.E. (1976). Anoxia and resuscitation in the newborn. In J.W. Goodwin, J.A. Godden, & G.W. Chance (Eds.), *Perinatal medicine: The basic science underlying clinical practice.* Baltimore: Williams & Wilkins, pp. 546–557.

Mott, J.C. (1961). The ability of young mammals to withstand total oxygen lack. *British Medical Bulletin, 17,* 144–148.

Simmons, M.A., Adcock, E.W., & Bard, H. (1974). Hypernatremia and intracranial hemorrhage in neonates. *New England Journal of Medicine, 291,* 4.

Tooley, W.H., Phibbs, R.H., & Schluetar, M.A. (1977). Delivery room diagnosis and immediate management of asphyxia. In L. Gluck (Ed), *Intrauterine asphyxia and the developing fetal brain.* Chicago: Year Book.

Chapter 10

The Immediate Postdelivery Period

Cathryn L. Anderson

T HE PROCESS OF BIRTH has traditionally been divided into stages identified by the occurrence of certain significant events. Think of a play with four acts and no intermissions: Act I of this drama called Birth is the time between the beginning of contractions and the time of complete dilation of the cervix. During Act II, the baby travels from the uterus to the perineum, and emerges into the hands of attendants and parents. Act III is that time from the birth of the baby until the delivery of the placenta and membranes. This period is possibly the most hazardous time of the drama for the woman, as she is at serious risk of fatal hemorrhage until the uterus is completely empty and firmly contracted on its large blood vessels (Danforth & Hendricks, 1977). It is also the time of the beginning of the family relationship: mother–infant, father–infant, siblings–infant. During Act IV, the time from delivery of the placenta and membranes until approximately two hours later, this budding family relationship has time to blossom into a real bouquet for the family.

If the preceeding sounded a bit poetic, that's good. It was meant to set the stage, declare a philosophy of birth, and establish a mood of respect, awe, and joy for birth. On occasion, the birth process can fail to proceed normally and appropriate interventions are required to return the process to a state of normalcy. A recognition of normal and abnormal is necessary to help prevent problems.

THIRD STAGE OF LABOR

During Act III, the performers in this drama must concern themselves with the baby and with the placenta, sometimes almost simultaneously. At the beginning of Act III, the baby has just made his or her appearance and must rapidly adjust to room temperature, which is usually quite different from the body temperature of the uterus (approximately 37°C, or 98.6°F). Room temperatures vary, depending on the climate, the season, and the efficiency of a heating or air conditioning system. The baby must also begin to breath, as the placental source of oxygen ceases. In approximately twenty-five percent of all births, active babies manage to play with the umbilical cord in such a fashion that it becomes wrapped around their necks (Pritchard & MacDonald, 1980). One or two loose coils are easily slipped over the baby's body during birth. Two or more tight coils of nuchal cord require clamping and cutting before birth of the baby's body. This baby needs to breathe on his or her own a bit quicker than the infant who is still receiving oxygen from an intact, pulsating cord.

In an absolutely normal and prepared birth, the mother is aware of the movements of the baby at birth and is facilitating the birth process through relaxation of perineal muscles and control of breathing and pushing. Positions for birth vary with the preferences of the woman and the birth attendant. The best position is one in which no undue stress is exerted on the perineum, and in which maximum relaxation of the perineum and support of the baby's body during birth are possible. A clear view of the emerging baby is also requested by many expectant mothers. Touching, holding, or nursing a baby immediately after birth is desired by most women who have had normal labors, and is often desired even by women who are exhausted and uncomfortable from difficult labors (Gaskin, 1978; Lang, 1972).

Newborn Care

The baby who is normal, with an Apgar score of 7 or greater should be dried with a warm towel and given to the mother to hold against her warm body. Additional warm towels and perhaps the use of an overhead heating unit facilitate the baby's transition from uterine to room temperature (Britton, 1980; Fardig, 1980; Gardner, 1979). In a normal, prepared birth, the mother's hands and arms are free to hold and support her newborn, but it is the responsibility of the circulating nurse to help the mother and father in supporting their baby in a safe manner. The circulating nurse must also constantly observe the baby and be ready to gently suction mucus from the baby's nose and mouth if necessary.

If the mother is unable to hold the baby, he or she should be safely held in the arms of the father or other family member in attendance or placed in a suitable infant bed. If placed in a bed, it should have a firm mattress, clear glass sidewalls for an unobstructed view of the baby, an overhead heating unit that can be thermostatically controlled, and oxygen and suction immediately available.

Assignment of Apgar scores at one and five minutes of life should be done at all births. (Korones, 1981). Often, the circulating nurse has the responsibility of assessing the baby and assigning the score. In some settings, the physician or nurse-midwife delivering the baby does the assessment and assignment of the Apgar score, especially the first one. In other settings, where an anesthesiologist or nurse anesthetist is part of the delivery team, he or she assesses the baby and assigns the Apgar score. As long as the score is assigned after careful assessment, according to Dr. Apgar's system, at one and five minutes after birth, and appropriate intervention made for those babies with low scores, any qualified member of the delivery team may make the assignment. The circulating nurse is customarily responsible for recording the scores.

To promote family-centered care and safeguard the infant's well-being, maternity nurses should be skillful in newborn assessment. Apgar scoring, gestational age assessment, the initial physical examination, and seeing the baby safely through the early transition period are essential to newborn well-being. These evaluations should be made without separating mother, father, and baby.

Response of Parents to Newborn

Recording the initial response of the parents to their baby has become an important way to document the quality of the beginning relationship or to assist in identifying potential problems in the developing relationship. The technique is simple and should not be used as an absolute predictor, but it does give clues to a situation in which a mother or father may need encouragement, praise, and support in relating to the baby. The important questions to be answered and documented are:

- How does the mother (father) *look?*
- What does the mother (father) *say?*
- What does the mother (father) *do?*

Warning signs of a possible developing problem in the parent–child relaitonship include (1) a passive reaction in which the parent doesn't touch, hold, examine, or talk in affectionate terms or tones about the baby; or (2) a hostile reaction in which the parent makes inappropriate verbalization, glances, or disparaging remarks about physical characteristics of the baby, or makes no eye contact with the baby; and nonsupportive interaction between the parents (Gray et al., 1979).

Allowing the parents to express feelings about the sex and appearance of the baby is very important. The nurse should accept parents' feelings of disappointment regarding sex of the baby, being afraid to, or not wanting to touch the baby. Observations must be recorded at birth and throughout the recovery period. Postpartum and nursery personnel must continue to observe the parent–infant interaction. A therapeutic plan to facilitate adequate parenting could be initiated during postnatal hospitalization of the mother and her infant. The services of the entire health care team may be required. A coordinated plan for follow-up care for mother and baby must include information about birth and following days.

Case Study

Not all expressions of negative feelings at the time of the birth indicate future parenting problems. It is a time when intense, deep-seated emotions surface, thus it is important for all present at the delivery to remain observant and supportive. Although important observations can be made about potential problems at this time, participant-observers should avoid making immediate conclusions, except in the most blatant of circumstances. A case example may be made of a 23-year-old woman who gave birth to her second child. Had the birth attendants made hasty conclusions, the situation would have been grossly misinterpreted.

Louise had an extended breast-feeding experience with her first child (a 20-month-old boy). Both she and her husband wanted their second child to be a girl. Her health status during pregnancy was excellent and her labor progressed well.

After giving birth she cradled the baby, looking at him, saying nothing. Disappointment was evident by her facial expression and body language. By contrast, her husband showed much joy, hugging the two of them and crying. It was apparent that he may have preferred a girl but was not at all disappointed with the baby. The nurse-midwife asked the woman if she would like for her husband to hold the baby as she inspected the perineum for lacerations. The transfer was made and the husband held and cuddled the baby. The woman's mother had also been present during the birth. She praised her daughter for a job well done and demonstrated positive feelings about her grandson.

During the third stage of labor, the new mother did not verbalize about the baby or his birth. She remained quiet with tears in her eyes. She was told of how well she had done during labor and birth. After placental expulsion and perineal inspection, the mother was cleansed and clean sheets were placed on the bed. The nurse-midwife asked if she wanted to hold the baby. The woman responded affirmatively, taking the baby in her arms. At this time she began to inspect the baby, gain eye contact with him, and put him to breast. She verbalized that it would "take getting used to," but she thought two boys would be all right. As she went through her recovery period visited by more family members, she welcomed their praise and affection. She continued to breast-feed, hold, cuddle, and examine the baby. She and her husband had a name for a boy, which she began using. She made the statement that she was disappointed about not having a girl but was pleased to have a healthy, beautiful baby. She demonstrated positive mothering behaviors throughout her hospitalization. This woman and her family with two sons continue to do well.

The situation just described could have evolved very differently. Very important was the continuity of care provided by the nurse-midwife. The young woman was known to mother well. Her positive feelings during pregnancy were apparent. She had some concerns as to how her 20-month-old son would respond to a new baby, as the two of them were very close. It was apparent that this woman had a supportive husband. The prenatal information is essential when interpreting the events of the intrapartum and postpartum periods.

Following the birth, the attendant nurse and nurse-midwife provided care and support and observed the family's interactions. To have made statements such as, "At least he's healthy," or "You should be proud of a second son," would have been inappropriate. The message would have been clear to this woman: you are a bad mother to feel as you do. Instead her feelings and responses were respected. Efforts were made to meet her needs as well as those of her family members. The emotional climate surrounding the birth of a child creates a lasting impression on the woman and her family. It is important for the professionals in attendance to facilitate a positive emotional experience. Even in the presence of a response that warns birth attendants of parenting problems, every effort should be made to convey respect, warmth, and caring.

Delivery of Placenta

Usually, by the time the baby is snuggled in the mother's arms, the placenta and membranes are ready to appear. Cord blood samples have been obtained for any necessary tests. Separation of the placenta usually occurs within a few minutes (Jensen et al., 1979; Pritchard & MacDonald, 1980), but can take as long as twenty-five minutes. As long as bleeding is minimal, it is safe to wait for spontaneous separation. Monitoring for minimal bleeding is a two-step activity: observing the introitus for any blood flow, and keeping a hand gently on the uterine fundus. As the placenta separates and moves into the lower uterine segment, the fundus rises and becomes globular in shape. Partial separation of the placenta and internal bleeding will also cause a change in the uterus: from firm to boggy, an increase in size, and a possible rise toward the surface of the abdomen. Classic signs of placental separation are (1) the uterus becomes globular and more firm; (2) a gush of blood usually appears at the introitus; (3) the uterus rises in the abdomen as the separated placenta passes into the lower uterine segment, where its bulk pushes the uterus upward; and (4) the visable part of the umbilical cord lengthens as it protrudes from the vagina.

Spontaneous delivery of the placenta occurs in eighty-five to ninety-five percent of deliveries (Sorbe, 1978) and is facilitated by prudent management of the third stage; that is, by avoiding techniques that may entrap the placenta (Oxorn, 1980). When the baby leaves the uterus at birth, the evacuation causes the uterus to contract. Contraction of the uterine muscles accom-

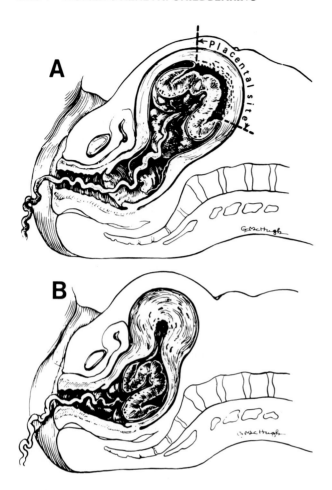

FIGURE 10-1 Uteroplacental relations in the third stage of labor. (A) Immediately after the baby has been expelled from the uterus, and the placenta has separated from its uterine attachment. Note the great decrease in the surface area of the placental site, the thickened uterine wall, and the change in the uterine contours. (B) After expulsion of the placenta into the lower uterine segment and vagina. The uterine corpus has become globular and has risen, and the lower uterine segment is distended by separated placenta. (From Danforth, D. (1982). Physiology of uterine contractions. In Danforth, D. (Ed.), *Obstetrics and gynecology* (ed. 4). Philadelphia: Harper & Row, p. 596.

plishes two major physiological processes: separation of the placenta from the uterine wall, and compression of the major blood vessels of the uterus, especially at the site of placental attachment (see Figure 10-1).

To further facilitate efficient compression of these blood vessels and prevent hemorrhage, the uterus needs to be completely empty. The contractions of uterine muscle fibers, which separate the placenta, are perceived as similar to contractions during labor and birth of the baby. As the placenta moves into the lower uterine segment, the woman often feels sensations similar to

that of birth and responds as she did for that event, by bearing down. The birth attendant carefully supports the uterine fundus with one hand to prevent inversion of the uterus, while applying gentle traction on the umbilical cord as the placenta and membranes pass through the introitus, taking care not to tear the membranes.

Immediate and careful examination of the placenta and membranes is indicated. Any pieces left in the uterus can interfere with uterine compression of blood vessels and lead to hemorrhage. Products of conception left in the uterus can also lead to postpartum endometritis (Oxorn, 1980). If the placenta and membranes are intact, the uterus usually contracts and stays firm, with only gentle massage of the fundus.

If the bladder is distended, it will push the uterus toward the umbilicus and interfere with maximum contraction of the uterus. Emptying the bladder by early and frequent voiding is necessary to prevent excessive uterine blood flow. If the woman is unable to void, catheterization is indicated, but all methods of encouraging spontaneous emptying of the bladder should be employed first as catheterization can force bacteria from the urethra into the bladder and lead to urinary tract infection.

Contraction of the uterus is also facilitated by the baby licking or sucking at the woman's breast. Stimulation of the nipple causes the release of natural oxytocin, which makes the uterus contract. It is thus advisable to put the baby to breast as soon as possible after birth.

Delivery of the placenta before it separates is an operative procedure and is not accomplished by massage of the fundus or pulling on the umbilical cord. Massage and pulling usually cause contraction of the cervix and trapping of the placenta, and may cause avulsion of the cord. Manual removal of the placenta is indicated only for the management of hemorrhage due to a partially separated placenta, an atonic uterus, or when the placenta has failed to separate by the thirty-minute time limit. Since it is an invasive and painful procedure, a fresh, long, sterile glove for the internal hand, and anesthesia or analgesia for the woman are needed. An intravenous solution, preferably Ringer's lactate, should be started immediately, using a No. 18 intracath, so that analgesia, oxytoxics, and fluid and blood replacements can be given as indicated.

Oxytocic Medications

American obstetrics has become highly technical over the years, and procedures developed to manage problems caused by other procedures are common in the management of third-stage labor. The routine use of oxytocic drugs given intravenously, intramuscularly, or subcutaneously with delivery of the anterior shoulder, or immediately following delivery of the placenta became popular in the era of general anesthesia, bottle-feeding, and elective induction of labor. Local or regional anesthesia is now more common than general anesthesia, only medically indicated inductions are done (*Facts and Comparisons,* 1982), and breast-feeding is gaining in popularity. In light of this climate, the use of oxytocic drugs should probably be reserved for those situations of actual need. As the nurse is personally responsible for any medications that he or she administers (Murchison & Nichols, 1970), a discussion is indicated.

Oxytocin

In the United States, three oxytocic preparations are available for obstetric use: oxytocin, ergonovine maleate, and methylergonovine maleate. *Oxytocin* is marketed under the brand names of Oxytocin (Invenex), Pitocin (Parke-Davis), and Syntocinon (Sandoz). All are synthetic oxytocin, as naturally derived oxytocin is no longer commercially available. Oxytocin can be used for *medically* indicated induction of labor and for control of postpartum bleeding.

As oxytocin has an intrinsic antidiuretic effect and acts to increase water reabsorption from the glomeruler filtrate, the possibility of water intoxication should be considered whenever oxytocin is given, especially when administered by continuous infusion. To decrease the possibility of water intoxication, it is recommended that a physiological electrolyte solution be used as the vehicle for administration of intravenous oxytocin. Intake and output should be carefully monitored, as decreased production of urine is a beginning sign of water intoxication.

Oxytocin appears to act primarily on uterine myofibril activity by increasing the permeability of cell membranes to sodium ions, thus augmenting the number of contracting myofibrils, thereby causing the uterus to contract. Uterine contractions stimulated by oxytocin are rhythmic in nature and are thought to primarily affect the upper uterine segment (Sorbe, 1978). Oxytocin is metabolized rapidly; its biological half-life is approximately three to four minutes. When given intramuscularly, uterine effects are noticed in three to five minutes; by intravenous infusion, within two to four minutes (Danforth & Hendricks, 1977). A bolus of oxytocin of 5 units or greater may cause transient but profound hypotension and thus is contra-indicated (Hendricks & Brenner, 1970). Electrocardiographic changes have also been reported (Mayes & Sherman, 1956). It seems that the safest way to give oxytocin intravenously is in a diluting solution. If a woman is at risk for postpartum hemorrhage, an intravenous catheter should be in place before delivery of the placenta, making it easy to add oxytocin to the solution after delivery.

Ergonovine Maleate/Methylergonovine

Ergonovine maleate, marketed as Ergonovine (Vitarine) or Ergotrate (Lilly), and methylergonovine maleate, marketed as Methergine (Sandoz), are similar agents. Although methylergonovine is perhaps a more purified drug than ergonovine, the two are usually considered interchangeable. They are *for postpartum use only* as they cause a sustained contraction of the uterus that could cause fetal demise or uterine rupture if used before delivery of the baby (*Facts and Comparisons,* 1982). The sustained contraction of the uterus includes contraction of the lower uterine segment, unlike the rhythmic contraction of oxytocin, which does not (Bryant & Danforth, 1977). Neither ergonovine nor methylergonovine should be given to women with hypertensive tendencies as the drug may precipitate sudden hypertension or even a cerebrovascular accident, especially if given intravenously (Table 10-1).

Controversy exists regarding the administration of oxytocics during third- and fourth-stage labor and the immediate postpartum period. Many families, opposed to the use of drugs, feel that for the normal woman, the natural oxytocin released by the baby's licking or suckling the breasts, on a demand-feeding plan, is quite sufficient to maintain uterine tone, prevent postpartum hemorrhage, and hasten involution of the uterus. In addition, these families do not want the infant exposed to any drugs transmitted through breast milk, (Gaskin, 1978; *Compulsory Hospitalization, or Freedom of Choice in Childbirth,* 1978; Lang, 1972; *Safe Alternatives in Childbirth,* 1976; *21st Century Obstetrics Now,* 1977). If the baby will not be breast-fed, and certainly if there are third-stage problems, the use of oxytocics will continue to be a valuable part of obstetric technology.

FOURTH STAGE OF LABOR

After the placenta and membranes have delivered and the uterus is firm, the birth attendant will examine the cervix, vagina, and perineum. Any lacerations will be identified and carefully and promptly repaired. This repair decreases blood loss and restores the integrity of the woman's genitals. If an episiotomy was necessary for the birth, it will also be repaired at this time.

Repairs are frequently done under local anesthesia. Those for obstetric use should not contain vasocon-

TABLE 10-1   Postpartum oxytocics

Drug	Dosage	Recommended Route
Oxytocin	10 U	Intramuscularly p̄ delivery of placenta
	or	
	10–40 U/1000 cc	Intravenous drip p̄ delivery of placenta
	5% Dextrose in Ringer's lactate solution	
Ergonovine maleate	0.2 mg	By mouth, as a series, p̄ delivery of placenta
or	q4h for 6 doses	
Methylergonovine maleate	*or*	
	0.2 mg	Intramuscularly p̄ delivery of placenta

Data from *Facts and comparisons,* 1982, pp. 118–118e. With permission.

strictors (e.g., epinephrine), as an interaction of an oxytocic drug and the vasoconstrictor may cause severe persistent hypertension. Drug allergies should be determined prior to the time of birth, as the excitement of the new baby may interfere with communication. Persons allergic to *p*-aminobenzoic acid derivatives (e.g., procaine, tetracaine, benzocaine) have not shown cross sensitivity to lidocaine (*Facts and Comparisons,* 1982), but equipment and medications to treat allergic reactions should be immediately available.

While the physician or nurse-midwife is repairing any lacerations, the new mother and father can continue to get acquainted with their baby, assuming, of course, that anesthesia is adequate for the repair. If for some reason anesthesia is not adequate, the mother will probably prefer to have the baby in the infant bed or the arms of another family member. Anesthesia may be supplemented by additional local or intravenous analgesia, as long as these drugs do not exceed recommended dosages. The nurse can also help the woman to cope with painful sensations by getting her to use the special breathing-relaxing techniques used during labor.

Parent–Infant Bonding

The baby has arrived and is doing well, the placenta has also arrived, uterine contractions are diminishing or ending, the fundus is firm, vaginal bleeding is minimal, the woman's blood pressure and pulse are normal, and she is not uncomfortable. Now is a time when the nurse can help the parents in the bonding process (Klaus & Kennell, 1982). As the nurse does an initial examination of the baby, the parents can be assured of the baby's normalcy and minor anomalies, such as an extra digit, can be identified and explained to them. Fingerprints of the mother and footprints of the

baby can be taken, identification bracelets for mother and baby put on, and weight and measurements of the baby obtained. Prophylactic eye care, such as silver nitrate drops, can be deferred until the end of the fourth stage. By that time, the baby will have had a chance to see and relate to the parents. Silver nitrate drops or their equivalent; such as antibiotic ointments, are required by state law for prevention of opthalmia neonatorum, but can be delayed until the baby has had an opportunity for an unblurred look at his or her parents.

Eye-to-eye contact for a period of time in the immediate postpartum period, plus opportunity for prolonged eye-to-eye contact in the first days of life, are important in establishing the parent–child relationship. (Klaus & Kennell, 1982) "Open your eyes. Look at me and let's get acquainted" or "Open your eyes and let me see who you are," are frequently heard statements made to a new baby. Bright lights shining in the baby's face discourage a baby from opening his or her eyes. Persons who have had minimal experience with babies think they are like kittens and puppies and that eyes remain closed until a period of time after birth. But the nurse can easily shade the baby's eyes with a hand and then the baby will open his or her eyes and look around, usually to the delight of all observers.

Care of the woman during fourth-stage labor is a continuation of observational activities and interpersonal skills begun in Act I of the drama. After repair of lacerations, hygiene becomes a consideration. Cleansing of the perineal area is usually welcomed. A sterile perineal pad to the vulva will absorb lochia. Ice bags applied to an episiotomy or perineal lacerations for six to twelve hours after birth will reduce the swelling and discomfort of the area. A sponge bath, a clean gown, and a warm, dry bed are indicated too.

Many women are hungry and thirsty at this time, and

cool fruit juices are welcomed. New fathers are also likely to be hungry and thirsty and should be offered juice. Fresh water should be available, and now is the time to make certain the woman knows she will need a high fluid intake over the next several days to help her body go through the dramatic changes of involution, such as diaphoresis. Some women prefer hot fluids to cold ones; arrangements should be made to respond to her requests. In some institutions, oral fluids are withheld during the fourth stage in case the woman needs an emergency procedure requiring general anesthesia. Providing oral fluids is a matter of professional judgment, but in any event, stomach acid diluted by juice, tea, or water is less caustic to the lungs than undiluted stomach acid (Pritchard & MacDonald, 1980).

In many facilities, families move from the birth room to another room for the remainder of the period labeled fourth-stage labor. Regardless of the location, the major activities of the fourth stage are centered on bonding between infant and parents (see Chapters 2, 15, and 16) and assuring the physical stability of the mother and baby.

Fourth-stage bonding activities include those begun in the third stage or initiation of activities that were not feasible then. If either the mother or baby is having problems, the developing relationship needs to be worked into the plan. Eye-to-eye contact, touching, holding, feeding, and minutely examining the baby are basic bonding activities. If the baby is having problems that require being in the special nursery and the mother is doing well, the mother can go to the baby. If the mother is having problems, the father can feed and hold the baby. Early and sustained contact of the baby with his or her parents enhances the growth of the relationship.

Nurse's Role

The nurse should continue observations of parent–child interaction begun during the third stage. Parents should be encouraged in their demands to have the baby with them. Even the woman who is exhausted from a difficult labor and birth usually wants to hold and feed her baby. Parents who are disinterested in their baby during the fourth stage are parents who may need further evaluation and counseling. A recent study at the University of Colorado (Gray et al., 1979) describes early identification of parents who need help, and the positive effects of early intervention. Observations of the parent–newborn interactions begun during third-stage labor should be continued during the fourth-stage and the postpartum period. If necessary, plans for

additional intervention can be made for the duration of the confinement and following discharge.

Mother and baby are expected to stabilize in the fourth stage of labor. Stable physical condition for the mother is defined as normal temperature, blood pressure, pulse, and respiration; a firm fundus; minimal vaginal bleeding; the absence of hematomas in the vagina or perineum; the ability to spontaneously empty the bladder; and the ability to ambulate with minimal assistance. A slight elevation in temperature could be due to dehydration during labor, so the nurse should make sure the woman is well hydrated with oral or intravenous fluids possibly obviating an expensive fever workup entailing blood cultures, etc. Changes in blood pressure and pulse reflect the integrity of the cardiovascular system. Changes secondary to pre-eclampsia or shock are the most common for women in the immediate postpartum period. Women with masked hypertension of pregnancy who have received regional anesthesia such as a continuous epidural may suddenly demonstrate hypertension when the anesthesia wears off and may even become eclamptic.

Fundal assessment is a major nursing responsibility of the fourth stage. Proper fundal assessment is *gentle* palpation of the uterus. Excessive vigor does not firm up the uterus any faster than gentle massage, but it does cause a lot of pain to the woman. The normal, firm uterus immediately postpartum is somewhere between a baseball and a softball in size and has that consistency. A boggy fundus may be difficult to locate due to relaxation and when found, feels like mushy, overripe fruit.

The woman should be taught to massage her fundus to keep it firm, and should also be taught that if she begins to feel cramping of the uterus at a non-breast-feeding time, she should immediately rub the fundus to help it contract. The fundus should be in the midline and below the umbilicus at all times. Deviation to one side, or a rise above the umbilicus may mean a uterus full of blood clots, but is most likely a full bladder displacing the uterus. This could lead to decreased uterine tone and excessive bleeding. Palpation of the full bladder feels like what it is—a hollow organ filled with fluid—imagine a balloon filled with water. The obvious response is to empty the bladder: spontaneous emptying is best, but if the woman cannot void, catheterization is indicated.

Excessive vaginal bleeding (saturation of a perineal pad in any period of time less than one hour) when the fundus is boggy or increasing in size indicates that the uterus needs help in contracting. Fundal massage will usually expel any clots from the uterus and allow it to contract firmly. There are exceptions that require more vigorous intervention and deem it necessary to call the physician or nurse-midwife.

Excessive vaginal bleeding that occurs when the fundus is extremely firm; pain of an increasing nature in the vagina or perineum, apart from the sensation of raw tissues; or discoloration or induration of the episiotomy area or in the vagina often indicate an unrepaired, or partially repaired laceration. The physician or nurse-midwife should be called to examine the woman and perform needed repairs or make other management decisions. Examination requires stirrups to support the woman's legs in lithotomy position, adequate lighting, sterile gloves and examining equipment, materials for suturing, anesthesia as needed, etc. Such an examination is usually done in a delivery room or a room specifically equipped for such procedures.

Most women are able to spontaneoulsy empty their bladders. If unable to get up to the toilet and the use of the bedpan is necessary, assisting the woman to sit up with her legs crossed tailor-fashion may help her to void. A dripping water faucet and privacy for the woman who is not severely dizzy, also facilitate spontaneous emptying of the bladder. Catheterization should be done only when absolutely necessary. If a woman has continuing difficulty in voiding and needs to be catheterized a second time, a Foley catheter connected to a closed drainage system may be necessary for twenty-four to forty-eight hours. A schedule of intermittent clamping and drainage may be necessary to restore normal bladder tone. Urethral lacerations, and sometimes periurethral lacerations, require a Foley catheter as edema or even pain interfere with voiding.

Ambulation with minimal assistance is usually possible for the woman who received little or no anesthesia. Regional blocks such as epidurals or caudals often last for thirty to sixty minutes after birth and the woman should wait until full sensation has returned to her feet and legs before ambulating.

Stable physical condition for the baby is defined as continuing Apgar scores of 9 or above, skin temperature of 36.0°–37.0°C, Dextrostix reading of 45 or greater, and the ability to nurse actively at breast or bottle. The normal baby (no serious congenital anomalies, uninfected, with a normal bilirubin and hematocrit) who is kept warm and fed as soon as possible after birth will usually remain stable. (See Chapter 15 for details of newborn assessment and care.)

In many institutions, the nurse is required to make observations and record the findings on a specific timetable, e.g., every ten to fifteen minutes. Documentation of the state of health is certainly important, and complete, accurate records play a significant part in accreditation of institutions. It is suggested, however, that record keeping might be modified when a modification is clearly in the best interests of the family's physical and psychosocial health. It is a little silly to interrupt a nursing infant and the mother at precise intervals to examine the mother's uterus. The examination can be safely deferred for a few minutes, since the nursing infant will be causing the release of natural oxytocin in sufficient quantities to keep the uterus firmly contracted. On behalf of complete and accurate records, the nurse could note "infant at breast, nursing well," in the space that requires entries at precise times for fundal height and consistency.

The role of the professional nurse during the third and fourth stages of labor is one that includes the ability to transfer knowledge of anatomy, physiology, and psychosocial phenomena into a personalized care plan for a specific family during a special time in their lives. Although some tasks performed on behalf of families may be the same, the nursing care is never routine; the drama of birth is always unique and special to each family as well as to the care provider.

REFERENCES

Bryant, R., & Danforth, D. (1977). Conduct of normal labor. In D. Danforth (Ed.), *Obstetrics and gynecology* (ed. 3). Hagerstown, Md.: Harper & Row, pp. 583–604.

Britton, G. (1980). Early mother infact contact and infant temperature stabilization. *Journal of Obstetrical and Gynecological Neonatal Nursing, 9*, 84–86.

Compulsory hospitalization, or freedom of choice in childbirth. (1978). Chapel Hill, N.C.: National Association for Parents and Professionals for Safe Alternatives in Childbirth (NAPPSAC).

Danforth, D. Hendricks, C. (1977). Physiology of uterine contractions. In D. Danforth (Ed.), *Obstetrics and gynecology* (ed. 3). Hagerstown, Md.: Harper & Row, pp. 522–564.

Facts and comparisons. (1982). (May). St. Louis: Facts and Comparisons, Inc., pp. 289–294.

Fardig, J.A. (1980). A comparison of skin to skin contact and radiant heaters in promoting neonatal thermoregulation. *Journal of Nurse-Midwifery, 25*, 19–28.

Gardner, S. (1979). The mother as incubator—After delivery. *Journal of Obstetrics, Gynecology, and Neonatal Nursing, 8*, 174–176.

Gaskin, I.M. (1978). *Spiritual midwifery* (rev. ed.). Summertown, Tn.: The Book Publishing Co.

Gray, J.D., Cutler, C., Dean, J.G., & Kempe, H.C. (1979). Prediction and prevention of child abuse. *Seminars in Perinatology, 3*(1), 85–90.

Hendricks, C.H., & Brenner, W.E. (1970). Cardiovascular effects of oxlytoxic drugs used postpartum. *American Journal of Obstetrics and Gynecology, 08*(5), 751–758.

Jensen, M.D., Benson, R.C., Bobak, I.M., (1979). *Maternity care.* (January). St. Louis: Facts and Comparisons, Inc.

Klaus, M.H., & Kennell, J.H. (1982). *Parent–infant bonding*. St. Louis: Mosby.

Korones, S.B. (1981). *High risk newborn infants* (ed. 3). St. Louis: Mosby.

Lang, R. (1972). *Birth book*. Palo Alto, Ca.: Genesis Press.

Mayes, B.T., & Shearman, R.P. (1956). Experience with synthetic oxytocin: The effects on the cardiovascular system and its use for the induction of labor and control of the third stage. *Journal of Obstetrics and Gynecology of the British Commonwealth, 63*, 812–818.

Murchison, I.A., & Nichols, T.S. (1970). *Legal foundations of nursing practice*. New York: MacMillan, p. 241.

Oxorn, H. (1980). *Human labor and birth* (ed. 4). New York.: Appleton-Century-Crofts.

Pritchard, J.A., & MacDonald, P.G. (1980). *Williams obstetrics* (ed. 16). New York: Appleton-Century-Crofts.

Safe alternatives in childbirth. (1976). Chapel Hill, N.C.: National Association for Parents and Professionals for Safe Alternatives in Childbirth (NAPPSAC).

21st Century obstetrics now. (1977). Chapel Hill, N.C.: National Association for Parents and Professionals for Safe Alternatives in Childbirth (NAPPSAC).

Sorbe, B. (1978). Active pharmacologic management of the third stage of labor *American Journal of Obstetrics and Gynecology, 52*(6), 694–697.

Chapter 11

Alternatives to Traditional Birth Settings and Practices

Margaret A. Emrey
Karren Mundell Kowalski

"TRADITIONAL" CAN BE DEFINED in as many ways as there are eras and cultures; it may refer to a field, a jungle hut, a plantation mansion, a small rural hospital, a maternity hospital, or a university medical center. For the purposes of this discussion, *traditional setting* is defined as a modern hospital maternity department, with specific rooms set aside within a restricted area for laboring women and for delivering women, separate nurseries for the newborn, and rooms reserved for women during the first few days postpartum. The physical layout and dimensions may vary, but the appearance of the area is usually functional, cold, sterile, and exudes efficiency. Labor and delivery rooms frequently have no windows; light is provided by fluorescent fixtures burning at the same intensity twenty-four hours a day. It is similar to other areas of the hospital that are reserved for those who are ill, injured, or dying.

Traditional birth practices are typified by the common procedures in use in virtually every hospital in the early 1960s. Laboring women were isolated in rooms where supportive family members were not allowed. Nurses managed the majority of labors with standing orders and telephone consultation with the physician who expected to arrive in the delivery room just as the baby's head was crowning. Women were placed in the supine position with feet in stirrups. Most women received considerable quantities of analgesia and anesthesia, making it difficult to push effectively in second-stage labor. Thus, the majority of deliveries were operative, employing forceps and episiotomies. Hospital routines were quite structured and employed every-four-hour infant-feeding schedules, limited maternal–infant contact, and no infant interaction for fathers or other family members except through the nursery windows.

Alternatives to traditional settings include renovated and redecorated areas within hospitals where more flexible care concepts are carried out; freestanding birthing centers where families remain only for the duration of their labors and deliveries; and the oldest setting of all—the home.

Likewise, alternatives to traditional practices include the presence of the father and significant others (including prepared siblings) during normal labor and birth; greatly decreased use of analgesia and anesthesia; use of forceps only for complications; use of various positions for birth including lateral, squatting, and sitting; infants staying with the mother and family immediately after delivery and for the duration of the hospital stay; immediate breast-feeding and demand-feeding thereafter; open visiting for families including siblings; and early discharge.

HISTORICAL PERSPECTIVE

In colonial times, childbirth was a social event in which women expressed caring and concern for one another. The term *lying in* was used to describe this event and included both the physiological aspects of birth and recuperation and the psychosocial aspects of women helping other women. The management of lying-in was the exclusive domain of women; the midwife and female friends and relatives were the source of skillful attendance, support, and comfort. These women not only attended the birth but, for at least a month, they also took care of siblings and all the household chores while the new mother stayed in bed and cared for the new baby (Wertz & Wertz, 1979).

During the last half of the nineteenth century, most midwives were replaced by physicians. In an attempt to establish themselves, physicians promised quick and painless childbirth through the use of forceps and chloroform. The Protestant ethic supported the use of science and technology to "improve" childbirth practices. As physicians became the predominant childbirth attendants, the sociocultural aspects of childbirth began to disappear. They assumed control over the birth, and the female support group was eliminated in favor of the nurse.

By the twentieth century, legislation had been passed forbidding midwives (this included trained nurse-midwives) from practicing. Childbirth was gradually moved from the home to the hospital where several laboring women could receive care by one physician. It was presumably safer to use forceps and anesthesia in hospitals. Thirty-six percent of births occurred in hospitals in 1935, eighty-eight percent in 1950 and ninety-six percent in 1960 (Devitt, 1977).

However, there were problems. Because there were no antibiotics and few immunizations prior to World War II, efforts to control infection and disease in hospitals focused on prohibiting family and friends from visiting parturant women. Babies were isolated in nurseries and had minimal contact with their mothers. These practices continued into the 1970s.

What began in the 1920s and 1930s as a joint effort by physicians and patients to pursue safe, comfortable, and efficient births, was recognized in the 1960s as an unpleasant and alienating experience for many women. Increased technical interventions to control natural processes, compounded by an impersonal, "assembly line" system for processing the patient, prevented a humane, dignified, and meaningful birth experience for the mother. Emphasis was placed on the improved statistics in maternal–infant survival of difficult births while the iatrogenic effects of labor intervention were ignored.

During this period, midwives had practically disappeared, except where they were needed to provide care to patients unable to pay a physician. Mary Breckenridge began the Frontier Nursing Service in 1925 in the mountains of Kentucky, with nurse-midwives who had been trained in Great Britain. Mortality and morbidity rates for both mothers and infants rapidly declined despite the fact that most of the births were in the homes (Breckenridge, 1952).

With the exceptions of the Frontier Nursing Service and a few large city programs such as those at the Maternity Association of New York, and the Chicago Maternity Center, most out-of-hospital births were assisted by untrained "granny" midwives, and showed a high incidence of perinatal mortality and morbidity (Devitt, 1977). These data reinforced the convictions of most professionals that out-of-hospital births were dangerous and should not be allowed. On the other hand, many consumers believe hospital data do not reflect the incidence of iatrogenic problems resulting from medical intervention in normal births. This group believes that birth is safer at home where intervention is less likely.

One compromise in the consumer–professional battle over the "right" place for birth has been the out-of-hospital birth center for low-risk pregnancies. In 1975, the Maternity Center of New York opened its childbearing center for low-risk women with the backing of the New York State Department of Health. The Center is staffed by nurse-midwives who provide patient care throughout the childbearing cycle and have consulting obstetricians and pediatricians available, as well as arrangements for emergency transfer to a nearby hospital if there are complications. Contrary to the predictions by opposing medical groups, of high morbidity and mortality, the maternity center statistics compare favorably with those of local hospitals.

ALTERNATIVE BIRTHING PRACTICES

Trends in Consumer Demands

With the advent of analgesia and anesthesia, consumers began requesting complete freedom from pain, involvement, and responsibility during labor, and placed complete control of the process in the hands of the health care professionals. While many women still choose this kind of care, other women are seeking to regain control. This diversity of demands can be confusing to care providers. This discomfort often causes resistance and rationalization.

In an increasing number of hospitals the "traditional" picture is changing, as concerned clients and staff raise questions, evaluate practices and behaviors, and demand changes to increase family involvement and minimize mother–infant separation. Animal breeders have known for centuries about the importance of creating a stress-free environment for labor, and minimizing mother–infant separation, as well as encouraging bonding and breast-feeding; this information is finally being recognized as valid for humans. Studies of deleterious catecholamine effects on both mother and fetus resulting from stress—physical, psychological, and environmental—are being confirmed and may greatly influence hospital practices and care (Read, 1959; James, 1969; Schnider et al., 1979). New environments for birthing within the institutional setting are evolving and becoming more and more accepted.

The first major breakthrough of traditional hospitalized birth practices occurred on two fronts. The first, rooming-in, was the product of a few committed professionals and of necessity. The second, husbands attending their wives during labor and delivery, was the result of collective pressure on the institution and physicians by expectant parents who had participated in childbirth preparation classes such as Lamaze, Bradley, and Grantly Dick-Reed methods. Once parents began to regain control of the birth experience, other changes followed.

Rooming-In

The concept of *rooming-in* is an alteration in traditional hospital practices that allows for normal newborns to remain with their mothers during their hospital stays as opposed to spending all of their time, except for feedings, in the nursery. The infants are cared for by both the mother and the father while the nursing staff provides support and teaching. This concept promotes the postpartum adjustment of the parents and infant prior to their being at home, where only minimal professional help is available.

Arnold Gesell, Edith Jackson, and others were among the first to advocate rooming-in. During World War II, this concept was seen as a solution to the nursing shortage (Olds et al., 1980), and after the war, there was a return to the traditional ways. However, psychiatrist John Bowlby (1953) was an early advocate of establishing immediate mother–infant relationships and his research motivated other professionals to advocate change. Research in the early 1970s by Klaus and Kennel substantiated the need for families and infants to remain together. In spite of this knowledge, many hospitals still take infants to mothers every four hours for feeding and then bring them back to the nursery. Parents need to be assertive to help change this practice. At the same time, other hospitals no longer require special rooming-in units with their accompanying nurseries. Any new mother, regardless of where she is on the postpartum unit may have her baby with her for as long as she wishes.

The increase in rooming-in has lead some nurses to consider alternative staffing patterns that view the mother and her infant as a unit. The mother and baby have a nurse who takes care of both of them rather than having a postpartum nurse for the mother and a nursery nurse for the baby.

Fathers and Significant Others in Labor and Delivery

Fathers were first admitted to labor rooms because they had taken a series of classes and were trained to help their wives during labor. Grantly Dick-Read's natural childbirth method was the first method to gain popularity in this country. However, in the 1960s, the Lamaze method was introduced on the east coast; it spread across the United States like a prairie fire. From the labor rooms, fathers pressured professionals to also be allowed in the delivery room. Shortly after the fathers who had been to classes gained entrance to labor and delivery, fathers who had not been to classes were also admitted. Nurses began to see that part of their role was coaching and supporting husbands so that they in turn, could coach and support their wives.

There were still many women delivering babies who did not have husbands. This lead hospitals to allow the significant person of the mother's choosing to be the person who coached and supported her. This person could be a friend or a family member.

The latest issues address whether the woman can have more than one support person during labor and birth, and whether the father should be allowed to accompany his partner to surgery for Cesarean births. With the dramatic rise in Cesarean deliveries over the last decade, this becomes an important issue. The objections raised are quite similar to those that originally came up when fathers first asked to be present in the delivery room: they will faint, they will be a problem for the professional staff, and lawsuits will increase. In the hospitals that do allow fathers to be present for Cesareans, none of these objections have proved valid (Donnovan, 1978).

Siblings at Birth

A most emotionally charged issue is whether siblings should be allowed to be present during labor and delivery. Significant numbers of parents are now requesting that their other children be allowed to attend the birth. Numerous case examples indicate that siblings have had a marvelous experience (Perez, 1979), although there are, no doubt, instances where children have had a negative experience. Many psychiatrists are convinced that male children will be impotent because of the experience, and female children will be afraid to bear children. However, there are no longitudinal studies at this time to confirm or denounce such convictions.

What appears to be important to assuring a good experience for children attending a birth is preparation and flexibility (Anderson, 1979; Kowalski, 1980; Perez, 1979). Of foremost importance in preparation is selecting a coach for the child. The coach should have no responsiblity at the birth except for the welfare of that child. The coach need not be a professional person but should be someone who is warm and supportive, known to the child or who can spend time getting to know the child, comfortable with sexuality and the birth experience, and flexible enough to encourage the child to deal with the situation in whatever way is most comfortable for him or her (Kowalski, 1980). If there are several children it may be appropriate to have more than one coach.

Actual preparation should include sex education and instruction about conception and birth, preparation to meet the child's physical and activity needs during the labor, experiential understanding of what the child will see, and birth setting orientation.

Sex Education Children are naturally curious about where babies come from. Parents differ in their comfort levels and abilities to talk about conception. The best approach seems to be a direct one in which information is presented in a straightforward manner. Many children enjoy pictures of the fetus at various stages of gestation. Of course it must be done in an age-appropriate way. However, once children are nearing school age, some helpful books include: Mayle's *Where Did I Come From?* (1973), Sheffield and Bewley's *Where Do Babies Come From?* (1977), Nilsson et al.'s *A Child Is Born* (1981), the Carnation Company's *Pregnancy,* and pictures of birth from *The Birth Atlas* (1968). A childbirth movie is a possibility but should be used with discretion as some adults even have difficulty with these movies.

If the children have never seen their parents without clothing, this may be appropriate preparation. If the mother is uncomfortable being nude with her children, these children may not be good candidates for attending birth.

Meeting the Child's Needs During Labor Since children need reassurance that they will not be left behind if labor begins at night, in the last month before delivery the child could pack a sleeping bag and a suitcase or backpack full of toys and snacks to take along. Labor is boring for children because it seems long and slow. They should feel free to watch TV, or play with toys and games. They should also feel free to come and go in the labor room. The role of the coach is to stay with the child whether he or she is with the mother or outside of the labor or birthing room. Children can make appropriate choices for their own well-being if they feel free to do so, rather than being pressured by adults to participate in something they cannot handle. Many children become anxious during the advanced stages of labor and need to feel free to leave if they want to.

Some children like to have a special task to do, such as taking the first picture or holding the baby or giving the baby a present. In spite of the concerns expressed by psychiatrists, many parents report a very close relationship and little sibling rivalry between siblings and the new baby when they attend the birth (Anderson, 1979).

Experiential Understanding Children can be helped to understand advanced stages of labor through
preparation. Some children can help in counting
during contractions, and can practice these exercises
with their parents. Children can participate in strenuous exercise such as running, and can learn to
recognize what hard work it is, and that people become
red in the face, perspire, and breathe rapidly and heavily
when doing hard work. They can then gain some
appreciation of what hard work their mothers will do
during labor. Her behavior will then be less "scary."

Birth Setting Orientation Some institutions are
now offering sibling classes, which familiarize children
with the birth setting. For example, in a hospital the
class might include a tour of labor and delivery in
which they see a fetal monitor and hear a fetal heartbeat.
They might also see a postpartum room, play with the
electric bed, and of course look into the nursery and see
all the babies. They might practice putting on cover
gowns, play with disposable diapers and dolls, and try
on disposable caps and masks, which they could take
home. Of course a treat such as cookies and milk makes
a strange environment seem quite nice.

Special Concerns Perhaps one of the greatest concerns for parents and professionals about siblings at
birth is the chance of complications to the mother or the
baby. This is a normal concern and needs to be
considered carefully. If there is a problem, it is the
responsibility of the children's coach to remain with the
children and to talk about what is happening and to
reassure them. The coach might be prepared to take the
children to the corner of the room, out of the way of the
various activities, and hold them and talk quietly to
them.

Another concern is the appropriate age for siblings
attending birth. Although there are many opinions
about age, it is a highly individual question. Some
children, of course, are ready for such an experience
before others. If the child still has difficulty differentiating between him- or herself and the mother, or has
difficulty understanding labor, birth, and such concepts
as pain and blood, the child is probably too young.

Open Visiting on Postpartum Units

One of the biggest objections to traditional hospital
care has been the restrictions on visitors to the postpartum unit. These restrictions stem from the efforts to
control infections in mothers and babies in the earlier
part of this century.

Visiting hours for father and grandparents have
slowly relaxed, so that in many settings they can visit
when they want and stay as long as they want. In
situations where the baby is ill or dies, fathers can
remain overnight.

Visiting for children has been more difficult. The
primary objection has been that children bring disease
into the hospital and increase the incidence of infection
in the newborn nursery. Yet Umphenour (1980) found
that bacterial colonization was no greater in babies
whose siblings had unrestricted contact at the bedside
than those babies who had no sibling contact.

Sibling visitation seems most important to younger
children who are still quite dependent on their mothers.
Anxiety about her absence is coupled with the adjustment to the loss of her full attention when she returns
home (Kennell & Bergen, 1966), and can lead to intense
sibling rivalry. The optimum length of a visit seems to
be two to three hours and might include a meal or
snack. In situations where there are several mothers in
one room, a family visiting room could be established
and mothers could sign up for a specific time (Kraus,
1979).

Care Providers

One of the major concerns of pregnant women, as
reported by Mehl (1977), was to avoid unfamiliar and
nonsupportive caretakers, and to be attended by supportive women attendants—midwives, monitrices or
physicians—who would remain with them throughout
their labor *and* birth. Due in part to the economic
realities and time constraints, many physicians delegate
the management of labor to the nursing staff and arrive
for delivery in time to "catch the infant." Many women
are objecting to this kind of care. Some opt for home
births. Others select nurse–midwives because the nurse-
midwife is with the mother throughout her labor and
delivery. The use of nurse-midwives has increased considerably in the past decade as more of them are trained,
and state laws allowing them to practice have been
modernized.

BIRTH ENVIRONMENTS

Observation of births at the hospital, at home, at
hospital-based, alternative birth centers, and at out-of-
hospital birth centers provides the setting for a provocative comparison of attitudes, practices, and behaviors of
health care providers and recipients.

Hospital Births

In the hospital, the laboring woman is called a "patient" as are sick persons in the facility. She and her support persons are guests in the health care establishment, which has planned and created the environment, policies, and procedures, in order to best meet its own needs of cost-effectiveness, economy, efficiency, and safety in caring for large numbers of patients. Personnel time must be divided among all patients and other management tasks essential to running the unit smoothly. Tasks are organized into routines to assure that each patient receives the same basic level of care, and that necessary procedures and observations are made in a timely and appropriate manner. At any given time, the obstetrical staff may be caring for a wide variety of women—from those who are normal and healthy to those with serious complications or those who expect unfortunate outcomes. The frequency of complications in a hospital reinforces the perceived importance of routines and precautions, and the emotional drain of coping with intense, sometimes tragic, situations on a daily basis leaves the staff less able to become personally involved with each patient's experience. This is frequently reinforced by staffing patterns that, for many reasons, may be inadequate to meet patient needs on a one to one basis. The result may be impersonalized care and rigidly structured procedures for admission (including perineal shave and enema), restricted ambulation, limited oral intake, routine intravenous fluids, standard delivery position (for the convenience of the care provider rather than the comfort of the mother), and separation of mother and infant for medical management of the newborn in the transition period.

Traditional hospital protocol has developed over many years, and although a given procedure may have been valid at one time, current research has rendered many of the procedures unnecessary. For example, several years ago women were usually heavily sedated for labor and anesthetized for delivery. For safety reasons, this required that the woman remain in bed in a recumbent position, and that she deliver on a table that would hold her limbs immobile and her body in a position that would allow her caretakers access to her perineum. Forceps were frequently needed because she was unable to push, and an episiotomy was required to allow for the use of forceps. The newborn was quickly removed to the nursery because the sedated mother was unable to hold or relate to the infant, and because the baby frequently needed special care to recover from the medication given to the mother. Sterile draping and an extensive array of instruments were needed because of the hazards of infection and the need for intrusive or surgical procedures to facilitate the delivery. Each of these procedures may still be necessary and valid in certain circumstances today, but for the healthy, well-prepared, cooperative woman, they are obsolete.

Of primary importance in the continuance of rigid, sometimes unnecessary hospital routines is the fact that so many health care providers have been trained and socialized to these routines as a way of life. They know no other way of functioning, nor have they observed labor without these routines. Delivery, which is a technical skill, has often been learned with the woman in the supine position; a change in her position means relearning certain aspects of the technical skill, such as positioning of the hands. Many care providers are uncomfortable in a "learning" role and so resist changes in accustomed procedures and techniques. Furthermore, their training has been to ignore "new" care concepts until valid research data are provided (i.e., they are published in an established journal) and the alternative concepts of care have frequently not yet undergone such research.

Another aspect of this resistance revolves around the issue of litigation. Because of the frequency of complications, regardless of cause, and the increased incidence of litigation, care providers have become sensitized to the possibility of complications and thus, practice defensively. Though the risks and benefits of practices and procedures may be weighed, the decision is frequently on the side of action or intervention rather than inaction, or waiting.

Home Births

In contrast to the practices and behaviors observed in the traditional hospital setting are those seen during births at home. Here the care provider is the guest at the home of the woman. The environment is familiar to her; she knows where things are, and everything is her own. There are no strange or unfamiliar sights, sounds, or persons intruding on her privacy. Usually she has met and developed a relationship with the care providers during her pregnancy, and they have agreed upon the care and management of her labor. In the home the care provider has no responsibility for tasks unrelated to direct support of the laboring woman, and he or she can direct undivided attention to this one person, rather than several The woman is never left unattended because of other patients' needs, and she has considerable freedom to walk about and occupy herself in any way she chooses until the labor consumes her entire attention. Positions during labor and delivery are usually chosen by the woman as her comfort dictates; after the birth, the infant remains in the mother's arms or immediate presence. Medication is not usually used in the home setting, nor are other interventive procedures; if these are deemed necessary, the woman is usually transferred to a hospital. The care provider's role in the home setting is to observe and support the woman's progress and management of her own labor and to detect abnormalities should they occur. Prior to labor, accurate assessment of the woman's risk status, suitability for laboring in the environment chosen, and potential for an uncomplicated delivery and postpartum period is critically important to the safety and well-being of the mother and her infant. Beyond these assessments and observations, through much of the labor the care provider takes a back seat to the woman's own support persons. The role is more passive and supportive than that of the hospital care provider. The role of the woman herself in the home setting is less dependent, more responsible, and more active. She has chosen the components of her environment and perceives the situation in terms of wellness, rather than illness. The care providers are seen and behave as facilitators, rather than managers.

Hospital-Based Alternatives

The other alternative birth settings, which comprise components of both hospital and home settings to varying degrees are the hospital-based, alternative birth center, hospital birthing rooms, the out-of-hospital birth center, and the maternity home. These also are designed for the woman who is expected to develop no complications and who wishes more active participation in the birth process. The care provider may need to attend more than one woman at a time in these settings, but she or he generally has fewer extraneous responsibilities and less simultaneous contact with complicated deliveries than in the traditional maternity unit. The atmosphere is oriented to normal births, but back-up resources in case of trouble are more visible. The settings here belong to the care providers, though the woman has freedom to adapt them to her own needs while she is there.

The hospital-based, alternative birth center has rapidly increased in popularity over the past few years. These birth centers are usually adjacent to, but not necessarily within, the traditional labor and delivery units and are furnished in a style much like a bedroom. Homestyle furniture, drapes, wall decorations, comfortable chairs, washable throw rugs, and double beds are most commonly seen, with plants and stereo frequently added. The atmosphere is calm and relaxing, with support persons of the mother's choice welcomed. Siblings are frequently permitted to remain for the labor and the birth, as long as each child has his or her own adult support person to provide explanations and reassurance and to remove the child if he or she becomes tired or upset. Analgesia is seldom used; mothers are usually required to attend birth preparation classes. If intervention is needed, the mother is usually transferred to labor and delivery. The mother in the birth center delivers in the same bed in which she experiences labor, and provision is usually made for immediate and continuing skin-to-skin contact with the newborn. The baby is not removed to the nursery but remains with the family until discharge. Early discharge is usually allowed, and the family goes home six to twelve hours after birth. Home follow-up is arranged for the first few postpartum days to help the new family care for their newborn and to assess for any complications or abnormalities that may develop.

Hospital birthing rooms are similar to alternative birth center rooms but are converted labor rooms located in the labor and delivery area. Where space allows, furnishings may be much like those in the birth centers. Policies regarding adult support persons are usually similar as well, though siblings may not be accepted. Complications are more likely to be handled without transfer because of the close proximity of emergency resources, though a mother may be moved to the delivery room if indicated for the birth. As in the birth centers, immediate rooming-in and early discharge are usual. The key to successful use of birthing rooms is not the amount of money spent on furnishings, but rather the promotion of the kind of birth experience desired by the woman and her family.

Out-of-Hospital Birth Centers

Out-of-hospital birth centers are reappearing in this country in response to the needs of well prepared, uncomplicated childbearing families who wish to deliver outside the disease-oriented institutional setting, but who are still seeking the support and security of the health care team with basic emergency resources. These centers have best been described as "maxi-homes" rather than "mini-hospitals" (Lubic et al., 1978). They offer homelike surroundings and atmosphere, family support, parent education, and primary care throughout the childbearing process by nurse-midwives with physician back-up. They encourage active family participation and self-support, and involve parents in the decision-making process perhaps more than in any birth setting other than the home. These centers usually have a reception area, areas for educational and group meetings, examining areas, rooms for labor and delivery, lounging areas for early labor, and space for maintenance and storage of supplies and equipment. They have resources to cope with nonsurgical emergencies, such as resuscitation equipment, IVs, emergency drugs, and oxygen, and have established procedures for emergency transportation to a back-up facility if that should become necessary. Careful screening of families reduces the risk potential; no one with any foreseeable complication is accepted for delivery in such centers. Care practices are extremely flexible and other than basic monitoring of progress are dictated by the needs and comfort of the mother. Ambulation, choice of position for labor and delivery, and oral fluids of choice are encouraged. There are usually no "routines" as in traditional settings. Mother and infant are not separated, and both are usually discharged within twenty-four hours of admission. Faison et al. (1979) demonstrated that the mortality-morbidity statistics for the Maternity Association are comparable to institutions in the area with similar patient populations.

The Choice of Birth Settings

There are several considerations in choosing a setting for a birth expected to be uncomplicated: convenience, economics, availability of a desired birth attendant, availability of assistance or other resources, and—very important—the comfort and confidence of the pregnant woman. The family who decides on the nontraditional birth setting solely because it is close to home, costs less, allows children and friends who wish to be there, despite the mother's secret desire to be alone, or only because it allows for the presence of a specific caretaker, is unlikely to have a positive, satisfying experience.

There are many qualities, not usually considered in the traditional birth setting, that are essential to the mother's comfort and ability to relax and allow the birth to proceed spontaneously without need for intervention. These include the mother and her family's degree of self-sufficiency and self-confidence, degree to which their lifestyle depends on outside resources or technology, birth experiences of family or friends, and the attitudes of the cultural group to which they belong. If the choice is made solely as a result of peer pressure or economics without regard to her personal needs and comfort, the mother is likely to experience considerable anxiety and discomfort during the labor, with the

frequent result of the labor process being inhibited or complicated in some way. Many women instinctively know where they prefer to labor and deliver, but many still make their choices for practical or impersonal reasons. It is the responsibility of the astute nurse or birth attendant to assist the woman and her support persons with this process of introspection before labor, and to adapt the chosen environment of the birth as far as possible to meet their needs.

Another major consideration in the choice of an appropriate birth environment is the establishment of the mother's risk status. Risking is usually considered in terms of what intervention is needed, rather than what is unlikely to be needed. Some clinicians maintain that a low-risk pregnancy can only be diagnosed in retrospect; all women are high risk until proven otherwise. There is, however, a slowly growing trend, spurred on by consumers who are unhappy with what they consider to be the misuse or overuse of technology, to consider risk in a more positive light. There are many high-risk lists, and systems for categorizing low-, and high-risk women. Lacking however, is a system defining risk in terms of specific outcome or purpose, or answering the question, High risk for what, when? Most high-risk lists include factors that pose risk only until or at a certain point in pregnancy, only for the mother, only for newborn, or only during the postpartum period. Likewise, most lists mix factors that can be cured or treated with those that cannot, and factors of simple management along with those requiring complex management. Examples relevant to consideration of an alternative birth setting include the woman with a history of premature deliveries who has reached term gestation without incident and thus, could be likely to experience a normal and uneventful delivery in an alternative birth center. The woman with nutritional anemia that responds appropriately to counseling and supplements is unlikely to be at risk at the time of delivery. A well-adjusted, unmarried woman with a good support system may opt for an alternative birth setting and have a positive experience. Mothers with certain risk factors may deliver more safely in a hospital-based birth center with closer and easier access to high-risk care than in an out-of-hospital setting. These might include older primigravidas, teens, mothers with history of prolonged labors, or other conditions that require anticipation or observation rather than action, and where development of the condition does not present an emergency. Presence of other risk factors may allow the mother to participate in some parts of an alternative birthing program but not other components, such as early discharge. This may especially be true with certain neonatal problems such as mild blood incompatability, history of certain congenital problems, or maternal class A diabetes.

Development of risking criteria for acceptance into an alternative birthing program, for admissions at the time of delivery, for transfer during the intrapartum, postpartum, and neonatal periods, and for early discharge are essential parts of planning for safe care in an alternative birth setting. These criteria must, however, reflect consideration of the question, High risk for what, when? They must also take into account the availability of, and proximity to, high-risk and emergency resources. The out-of-hospital maternity care facility with Cesarian delivery capability and nursery facilities may safely accept mothers with very different risk status than the one who opts to transfer all mothers needing any level of intervention or technology. It is clear, then, that there is no single list of risk factors that can meet the needs of all alternative birth settings, or even all those of one type. Each service must design its own criteria to fit its own situation. For an example of the criteria used for admission by a few birth centers, see Table 11-1.

Most care providers who have worked closely with pregnant women have developed an instinctive ability to predict how various women will handle their labors and which ones are more likely to develop unforeseen complications, or to do well in spite of known complications. Much research has been done on risk factors, but little on this instinctive predictive ability, yet risk factors of themselves are considerably inaccurate in predicting problems or outcomes. In a birth setting where modern technologies and equipment, specialist staff, and highly developed resources are readily available, accurate prediction of complications may be less critical. However, in an alternative birth setting without such resources, the safety of mother and infant demands a high level of accuracy in assessment of risk and prediction of problems. Birth attendants who practice in alternative settings rely both on the commonly accepted risk factors, and on their instinctive predictive ability when assessing their clients for delivery in such settings. They have observed that those who tend to do well in alternative settings are women at low risk by usual standards who are also highly self-sufficient and self-confident in other areas of their lives. These are women who tend to rely on their own resources rather than on outside assistance, whose associates have had positive birth experiences, and who accept responsibility for their own lives. They tend to see the care provider as a resource or assistant rather than as a caretaker or manager of the labor process. They have

confidence that birth is a normal life event and they they as individuals are uniquely designed to cope with it. These attributes must be present in the woman before she becomes pregnant; it is rarely possible for her to reverse her life patterns during a time of such intense change and adaptation.

The various alternative birth settings discussed here vary in their access to interventive procedures and back-up resources, and the women who choose them vary accordingly in their needs or desires for such back-up. The mere availability of resources may be all that is necessary to instill the confidence needed to proceed smoothly with the task of labor, even though the woman may have no desire to utilize the resources.

The phenomenon of contractions decreasing in frequency and intensity when a woman arrives at the hospital or when she is transferred from the labor to the delivery room is commonly, if not usually, seen. Depending on the stage of labor, pitocin augmentation is often employed, but even without it, most often, progress resumes normally within the hour as she becomes accustomed to her new surroundings. This phenomenon almost never occurs when there is no change of setting or environment. Observations of animal mothers in labor reveal a similar experience. Mares, for example, rarely drop their foals in the presence of a human or when they feel they are being observed, unless they have an unusually close attachment to their owner or handler. For this reason, breeding stables devise elaborate means, such as darkened apartments with glass floors above the foaling stalls, for the handlers to observe the proceedings in case of trouble. Bitches attached to their owners become quite anxious and decrease their contractions when the owner leaves the room or moves them to different surroundings during labor. If strangers are present or there is commotion in the environment, delivery of the pups may be noticeably delayed.

Presumably, similar mechanisms are at work in the mothers of many species that allow their young to be born easily only in environments perceived to be safe or nonthreatening. The life experience, cultural background, and belief system of each mother dictate what she defines as safe, and what the components of a safe environment should be. In the United States today, there is simultaneous movement both toward and away from technological intervention in childbirth, with a demand for birth settings to accommodate both philosophies. The dilemma is to provide the best of both alternatives with maximum comfort and safety to the mother and her infant. This is possible only with highly developed and accurate risking mechanisms and

TABLE 11-1   Criteria for determining whether a woman is at low risk and can use a birth center

Score	Problem Description	Score	Problem Description
	INITIAL DATA BASE	2	Previous Rh sensitization
		2	Term pregnancy of five or more
	Sociodemographic Factors		Infertility problems
2	Chronological age: 40 and over, nulliparous 45 and over, multiparous	1	Workup and counseling more than 3 years prior to this pregnancy
2	Permanent residence outside specified target area	0–2	Use of fertility drugs to achieve this pregnancy
	Documented Problems in Maternal Medical History		Previous abortions
	Cardiovascular	2	Three or more spontaneous (<28 weeks)
2	Chronic hypertension	2	One septic
2	Heart disease		Uterus
2	Pulmonary embolus	2	Previous uterine surgery including Cesarean section (if previous tubal pregnancy and enrollment before 16 weeks, accept conditionally)
2	Congenital heart defects		
	Urinary System		
2	Renal disease moderate to severe including nephritis and/or one episode of chronic renal disease	0–2	Cone biopsy at discretion of M.D.
		2	Previous placenta abruptio
1	One episode of pylonephritis prior to this pregnancy	1	Previous placenta previa and/or significant third-trimester bleeding
	Psychoneurological	2	Severe hypertensive disorder during previous pregnancy
1	Previous psychotic episode adjudged by psychiatric evaluation and/or required use of drugs related to its management	2	Postpartum hemorrhage apparently unrelated to management
			History of prolonged labor
2	Current mental health problem adjudged by psychiatric evaluation	1	Primipara: stage I > 24 hours; stage II > 3 hours; and/or stage III > 1 hour
1	Epilepsy or seizures	1	Multipara: stage I > 18 hours; stage II > 2 hours; and/or stage III > 1 hour
2	Required use of anticonvulsant drugs		
2	Drug addiction (heroin, barbiturates, alcohol), current use of addicting drugs, or therapy related to these addictions		*Documented Physical Findings*
		1	Stillbirth (>28 weeks' gestation)
2	Severe recurring migraines		Birthweight:
	Endocrine	1	< 2500 g
2	Diabetes mellitus and/or gestational diabetes	1	> 4000 g
	Thyroid disease	1	Major congenital malformations
1	History of thyroid surgery	1–2	Genetic-metabolic disorder (genetic counseling)
2	Enlarged thyroid gland with symptoms of thyroid disease based on T3 or T4		
1	Current use of thyroid-related medications		*Maternal Physical Findings*
	Respiratory		Gestation
1	Asthma and/or chronic bronchitis within the last 5 years	2	> 22 weeks (nullipara) > 28 weeks (multipara) if had previous classes and current prenatal care
	Other Systems		
2	Bleeding disorder and/or hemolytic disease	2	Weight for height outside the averages on chart below
1	Sensitivity to local anesthetics ("caines")	2	Clinical evidence of uterine myoma* or malformations, abdominal or adenexal masses
2	Previous radical breast surgery		
2	Other serious medical problems	2	Polyhydramnios or oligohydramnios
	Documented Problems in Maternal Obstetrical History	2	Cardiac diastolic murmur, systolic murmur grade III or above and/or cardiac enlargement
0–2	Expected date of delivery less than 12 months from date of previous delivery (evaluated individually)	2	Pelvimetry indicative of inadequacy to delivery an infant of 3100 g

Score	Problem Description	Score	Problem Description
	Laboratory–Radiological Findings	2	Consistent nonattendance at classes and/or office hours
	Hematocrit		
1	< 31%		*Intrapartum-Postpartum Transfer Factors*
2	< 28%	2	Premature labor (< 37 weeks' gestation)
2	SS Hemoglobin	2	Premature rupture of membranes (> 12 hours before onset of regular contractions)
2	Pap smear class of 3 or greater with positive colposcopy	2	Nonvertex
2	Evidence of active tuberculosis		Evidence of fetal distress
		2	Abnormal heart tones
	Antepartum Referral Factors	1–2	Meconium staining
2	Hematocrit of less than 34% if entering the 37th week of gestation	2	Estimated fetal weight < 2500 g or > 4000 g
2	Evidence of fetal chromosomal disorder in amniotic fluid	2	Development of hypertension
2	Multiple gestation affirmed by sonogram		Failure to progress in labor:
2	Development of symptoms of preeclampsia	2	First stage: lack of steady progress in dilation and descent after 24 hours in primipara and 18 hours in multipara
2	Intra-uterine growth retardation		
2	Thrombophlebitis	2	Second stage: more than 2 hours without progress in descent
2	Pylonephritis		
2	Symptoms of gestational diabetes affirmed by abnormal glucose tolerance curve	2	Third stage: more than 1 hour
			Soft tissue problems
2	Development of unexplained vaginal bleeding	2	Severe vulvar variosities
1	Abnormal weight gain (< 12 or > 50 lb)	2	Marked edema of cervix
1	Nonvertex presentation persisting past 37th week of gestation	2	Intrapartum blood loss > 500 cc and/or postpartum hemorrhage
2	Laboratory evidence of sensitization in Rh-negative women	2	Prolapse of the cord
		2	Development of other severe medical or surgical problems
2	Postmaturity: 42 weeks' (294 days') gestation		
2	Development of genital herpes affirmed by culture	2	Evidence of active infectious process
		2	Any condition requiring more than 12 hours of postpartum observation
2	Documented asthma attack		
2	Development of any other severe obstetrical, medical, and/or surgical problem		*Infant Transfer Factors*
		2	Apgar score less than 7 at 5 minutes
	Circumstantial Factors	2	Signs of pre- or postmaturity
	Medical team staff decision, after taking into account and review of all of the family circumstances, including composition, general physical condition, and total situation, that the childbearing in this case would best be accomplished under the supervision of a physician in a more traditional medical setting, i.e.:		Weight:
		1	<2500 g pediatrician to determine whether hospitalization is necessary
		2	Jaundice
		2	Persistent hypothermia (less than 97°F rectal after 2 hours of life)
		2	Respiratory problem
		2	Exaggerated tremors
2	Lack of available support person to be in the home during the first 3 postpartum days	2	Major congenital anomaly
		2	Any condition requiring more than 12 hours of postdelivery observation
2	Lack of source of follow-up after (1) pediatric 34 weeks, (2) obstetrical 28 weeks of gestation		

(continued)

TABLE 11-1 *(continued)*

Height Without Shoes		Acceptable Weights (lb) for Women Over 25† at Last Menstrual Period		
		Type of Frame		
		Small	Medium	Large
4 ft 8 in	(56 in)	92–98	96–107	104–119
4 ft 9 in	(57 in)	94–101	98–110	106–122
4 ft 10 in	(58 in)	96–104	101–113	109–125
4 ft 11 in	(59 in)	99–107	104–116	112–128
5 ft 0 in	(60 in)	102–110	107–119	115–131
5 ft 1 in	(61 in)	105–113	110–122	118–134
5 ft 2 in	(62 in)	108–116	113–126	121–138
5 ft 3 in	(63 in)	111–119	116–130	125–142
5 ft 4 in	(64 in)	114–123	120–135	129–146
5 ft 5 in	(65 in)	118–137	124–139	133–150
5 ft 6 in	(66 in)	122–131	128–143	127–154
5 ft 7 in	(67 in)	126–135	132–147	141–158
5 ft 8 in	(68 in)	130–140	136–151	145–163
5 ft 9 in	(69 in)	134–144	140–155	149–168
5 ft 10 in	(70 in)	138–148	144–159	153–173
5 ft 11 in	(71 in)	142–152	148–163	157–177
6 ft 0 in	(72 in)	146–156	152–167	161–181
6 ft 1 in	(73 in)	150–160	156–171	165–185

Developed by the Medical Team Staff of the Childbearing Center and approved by the Medical Advisory Board, Maternity Center Association, New York, N.Y. Published with permission.
Note: These criteria will be applied to all women by professional staff during antepartum, intrapartum, and postpartum periods. A cumulative score of 2 points on the initial score sheet indicates that the woman is at a risk incompatible with project care. Accepted women will be continuously evaluated for the presence of any listed antepartum, intrapartum, and postpartum criteria and for possible referral or transfer.
*Clinical uterine myoma (evaluated by M.D.); score 0–2.
†Subtract 1 lb for each year under 25. Underweight: prepregnant weight 10% or more below standard weight for height and age (Pitkin, 1975); overweight: prepregnant weight 20% or more above standard weight for height and age (Pitkin, 1975).

a wide variety of options available to the mother and the care provider.

DEVELOPING AN ALTERNATIVE BIRTH SETTING

Essential to the task of developing an alternative birth setting is an understanding of and appreciation for some basic principles of the process of change (Welch, 1979). These principles are applicable to any desired change in birth practices as well as in developing the birth setting.

Change Takes Time Health care professionals have been trained to research, test, and evaluate new ideas and practices. Experiences with alternative birth practices in the past were associated with high mortality and poor outcomes in general. Modern technology has dramatically reduced many former risks, however, the concept that these life-saving technologies may in some instances actually *introduce* risks is still evolving, and the knowledge of when to utilize them is still imperfect. The identification of risk status and accurate prediction of outcome are still in the developmental stages. Huge malpractice settlements and the broadening legal definition of "standard of practice" strongly enourage the defensive practice of medicine with utilization of any support technologies available. Relatively little valid research has been done to document the safety, cost-effectiveness, and feasibility of alternative birthing methods and settings. The health care professional is caught between the popular demand for change, the legal and ethical demand for practicing safe and well-accepted care, and his or her own unfamiliarity with the practices and techniques requested. The natural response is to delay action until the requested change can be evaluated, a difficulty with the lack of sound, published data.

Change Requires Patience The process of change begins with a need or discomfort with the status quo. This must then be transmitted or translated to others needed to effect the change. Each of these others must in turn experience that same need or discomfort in order to be motivated to develop the necessary plan of action. Each must become convinced that the suggested change is an appropriate one, and that it will improve or reduce the need or discomfort being experienced without introducing another of equal intensity. Those involved must feel that both they, and the program or service that they represent have something to gain from the change. This process can be lengthy and frustrating for the one who is initiating the change; it may involve seemingly constant repetition, extensive documentation of various features of the change, and many apparent backslides as others with opposite ideas attempt to prove their position. Anger and hostility are seldom effective; they merely serve to reinforce and unite the opposition. Calm, logical discussion, liberally laced with facts and valid data, stand the greatest chance of ultimate success (Olson, 1979).

Change That Happens Overnight Seldom Lasts If the process discussed above is short-circuited, the change effected is not likely to be a lasting one. The twig that bends with the wind will just as easily and quickly bend with the breeze from another direction. Change requires careful planning and foresight; problems or complications must be anticipated and avoided or met with well-developed contingency plans. Program development must be based on all related events, and expected outcomes. Anticipating problems is not a sign of negativity; it can be the basis for logical and constructive planning. A mechanism for ongoing evaluation is an essential component of any program plan; without it there can be no justification for change.

Basic Steps

There are certain basic planning steps for the development of an alternative birth setting, in or out of the hospital. The first essential is a review of the available literature covering such topics as physical, socioeconomic, psychological and emotional risk factors, alternative birthing techniques and procedures, home birth, alternative birth centers, family-centered care, psychoemotional aspects of pregnancy, bonding, consumer

evaluations of maternity care services, midwifery and nursing roles, and evaluation techniques. Also essential is a review of maternity care resources and bed utilization for the area involved; statistical data relating to perinatal mortality, out-of-hospital births, and such prevalent risk factors as lack of prenatal care, prematurity and low birth weight. These data should be available from local and state health departments, regional health-planning agencies, libraries or some local health care institutions. A review of the area's geographic characteristics relevant to the utilization of health care resources is also essential, with such factors as distance, transportation, road and weather conditions, and population centers considered. The actual needs and wishes of the consumers should be specifically surveyed and documented; the general statement that "Mothers want _____" is inadequate at best and could result in development of a program that would be underutilized because it would not include specific features desired or needed by the target population identified. Finally, the number of families expected to use the new birth setting should be determined and documented. This is essential for developing cost data, space allocations, and staffing patterns.

Once the above information is obtained and evaluated, a statement of need should be prepared. This should include statistical data relevant to the community and the target population, a summary of currently available maternity care resources and their limitations in relation to the need for a new birth setting, and documentation of consumer needs and desires. This statement of need can be used for presentation of the concept to other persons whose support is needed.

Once the decision has been made to establish an alternative birth setting, and support has been obtained from key persons, the next step should be to establish a planning committee. This committee should represent all departments or groups that will have some level of responsibility for implementing the new service; members of the committee should be those who can speak for, and make decisions for the groups they represent. For example, a hospital-based birth center planning committee might include someone from administration, nursing administration, department of obstetrics, nursing staff from labor and delivery, postpartum and nursery, infection control committee, hospital auxiliary or volunteer staff, housekeeping, and consumer representatives. Additional services could be involved as indicated. An out-of-hospital birthing center planning committee might include key persons from the agency or organization sponsoring the center, supportive persons from the medical and nursing communities,

EXHIBIT 11-1 Developing an alternative birth setting: Initial functions of the planning and advisory committees

- Overall development of the philosophy, goals, and objectives, and details necessary for implementation of the plans
- Investigation into local facility licensing, bed use, zoning; use, building, and occupancy regulations and requirements; and health and safety, fire, and sanitary codes
- Interpretation of the proposal to the local health systems agency or other health-planning groups
- Development of a budget, plan for economic self-sufficiency, and sources of start-up funds
- Investigation into relevant legal and malpractice issues
- Responsibility for development of a physical facility in accordance with the stated philosophy of care, budget, and necessary codes and regulations
- Development of an evaluation plan based on the established philosophy, goals, and objectives
- Dissemination of information about the proposed service to other agencies, institutions, and professional and consumer groups
- Development of formal agreements for back-up, transportation, and follow-up with relevant agencies and institutions
- Selection of appropriate staff to implement the service

EXHIBIT 11-2 Developing an alternative birth setting: Areas requiring detailed planning

- Philosophy of care or underlying principles
- Goals
- Objectives
- Financial plan: budget, revenue sources, fee scales, etc.
- Staffing plan to cover primary care, nursing support, medical records, pharmacy, billing and accounts, and administrative functions, including plan for call schedules
- Organization chart showing lines of authority and communication
- Back-up facilities and personnel: identification, location, procedures for utilization, copies of written agreements in the case of persons, agencies, or institutions outside the agency or institution sponsoring the service, list of telephone numbers for emergencies or essential services.
- Provisions for communication with staff, such as telephone numbers and paging procedures
- Informed consent forms and policies relating to their use
- Parent-education plan, including orientation of families to use of the facility, its policies and procedures, childbirth education, provisions for peer support, and policies related to the requirement of each component of the patient-education plan
- Staff continuing-education plan and requirements for updating on emergency procedures
- Staff personnel policies
- Fire and disaster evacuation plan
- Supplies and equipment, including lists of items to be stocked or located in certain areas, cleaning, and sterilization procedures
- Patient care policies, procedures, and protocols: criteria for acceptance into program; criteria for admission to birth facility; criteria and procedures for transfer to back-up resources during intrapartum, postpartum, or newborn periods; criteria for discharge of mother and infant; policies and protocols for home follow-up of mother and infant; infection-control policies and procedures; procedures for disposal of wastes; patient management procedures and protocols, including specific emergency situations
- Program evaluation plan

persons familiar with financial and fund-raising activities and with legal concerns, and consumer representatives. If possible, supportive key persons from other agencies or institutions for back-up or other services should be involved. This may be difficult in the case of the out-of-hospital birthing services, because such services are still not widely accepted as safe and valid alternatives. Consumer representation in any planning activity is extremely important to provide input on what prospective mothers really want, to assure communication surrounding potential limitations on services to be offered, and to facilitate the dissemination of information about the new service to the public. Key groups to be considered include pregnant and recently delivered mothers who utilize the agency or facility, childbirth educators, parent-support groups, breast-feeding groups, and other parents- or infant-oriented groups.

In many situations, separate planning and advisory committees may facilitate involvement of a greater number of persons, and may increase the resources available to the proposed service. This may also promote long-term involvement of these key people and

assure cooperation and communications as the program develops.

The initial functions of the planning and advisory committees may include activities such as those listed in Exhibit 11-1.

Considerable assistance in program development is usually available from consultants in state or local health departments and from others already implementing similar programs. These persons can identify key factors to be considered, potential barriers and ways. to overcome them, and resources that might strengthen the program. Their support can be invaluable in overcoming seemingly insurmountable bureaucratic obstacles, and may be essential to obtaining necessary approvals.

All components of the proposed program and its plan for implementation, including a timetable, should be in writing. Accurate minutes should be kept of all meetings, and notes should be made of each committee member's responsibilities so that nothing gets overlooked. Specific areas requiring detailed planning are listed in Exhibit 11-2. These should be included in a written manual for the service.

An essential component of any service and one which too frequently receives last consideration is the plan for evaluation. This should be based on the program's stated philosophy, goals, and objectives, and should include both statistical and descriptive data. It should reflect provider and consumer input and provide information on relative safety, feasibility, acceptability, and cost-effectiveness. Because of the scarcity of published information about alternative birth settings, the evaluation component should ideally include a plan for specific research studies to be conducted, and a plan for publishing or disseminating the data. As these programs become more widespread and their results more widely known, acceptance of birth alternatives in both the professional and lay communities will be greatly facilitated.

REFERENCES AND ADDITIONAL READINGS

Anderson, S. (1979). Siblings at birth: A survey and study. *Birth and the Family Journal, 6*(2), 80–87.

Arms, S. (1975). *Immaculate deception: A new look at women and childbirth in America.* Boston: Houghton Mifflin.

Bowlby, J. (1953). *Childcare and the growth of love.* Baltimore: Penguin Books.

Breckinridge, M. (1952). *Wide neighborhoods.* New York: Harper Brothers.

Caldeyro-Barcia, R. (1975). Some consequences of obstetric interservice. *Birth and the Family Journal, 2*(2), 34–38.

Chard, T., & Richards, M. (Eds.) (1977). *Benefits and hazards of the new obstetrics.* Lavenham; Spastics International Medical Publications.

Devitt, N. (1977). The transition from home to hospital birth in the United States, 1930–1960. *Birth and the Family Journal, 4*(2), 47–58.

Donovan, B. (1978). *The Cesarean birth experience.* Boston: Beacon Press.

Dunn, P. (1976). Obstetric delivery today: For better or for worse? *Lancet, 2,* 790–793.

Epstein, J., & McCartney, M. (1977). A home birth service that works. *Birth and the Family Journal, 4*(2), 71–75.

Faison, J., Pisani, B., Douglas, R.G., Cranch, G., & Lubic, R.W. (1979). The childbearing center: An alternative birth setting. *Obstetrics and Gynecology, 54,* 527–532.

Ferris, C. (1976). The alternative birth center at Mount Zion Hospital. *Birth and the Family Journal, 3*(3), 127–128.

Gaskin, I.M. (1978). *Spiritual midwifery.* Summertown: The Book Publishing Company.

Haire, D. (1972). The cultural warping of childbirth. *ICEA News Special Report.* Seattle: International Childbirth Education Association.

Hosford, E. (1976). Alternative patterns of nurse–midwifery: The home birth movement. *Journal of Nurse-Midwifery, 21*(3), 27–30.

James, W.H. (1969). The effect of maternal psychological stress on the fetus. *British Journal of Psychiatry, 115,* 811–825.

Kennell, J., & Bergen, M. (1966). Early childhood separations. *Pediatrics, 37*(2), 291–297.

Kitzinger, S., & Davis, J.A. (Eds.). (1978). *The place of birth.* New York: Oxford University Press.

Kowalski, K. (1980). Siblings attending birth, Letters to the Editor. *MCN: The American Journal of Maternal Child Nursing, 5*(2), 80.

Kraus, N. (1979). Postpartum hospital visits for children. *Issues in Health Care of Women, 1*(4), 27–39.

Lubic, R.W. (1975). The effects of cost on patterns of maternity care. *Nursing Clinics of North America, 10*(2), 229–239.

Lubic, R.W., & Ernest, E.K.M. (1978). The childbearing center: An alternative to conventional care. *Nursing Outlook, 26,* 754–760.

Mayle, P. (1973). *Where did I come from?* Secaucus, N.J.: Lyle Stewart.

Mehl, L. (1977). Options in maternity care. *Women and health, 2*(2), 29–42.

Mehl, L.E., Peterson, G.H., Shaw, N.S., & Creevy, D.C. (1975). Complications of home birth. *Birth and the Family Journal, 2*(4), 123–135.

Mehl, L., Peterson, G., Sokolosky, W., & Whitt, M. (1978). Outcomes of early discharge after normal birth. *Birth and the Family Journal, 3*(3), 101–107.

Moawad, A.H. (1977). Some problems of professionally attended home births. *Journal of Reproductive Medicine, 19*(5), 248.

Mullaly, L., & Kervin, M.C. (1978). Changing the status quo. *The American Journal of Maternal Child Nursing, 7,* 25–80.

Nilsson, L., Furuhjelm, M., Ingelman-Sundberg, A., & Wirsen, C. (1981). *A child is born,* (ed. 11). New York: Delacorte Press/ Seymour Lawrence.

Olds, S., London, M., Ladewig, P., & Davidson, S. (1980). *Obstetric nursing.* Menlo Park, Ca.: Addison-Wesley.

Olson, E.M. (1979). Strategies and techniques for the nurse change agent. *Nursing Clinics of North America, 14*(2), 323–336.

Perez, P. (1979). Nurturing children who attend the birth of a sibling. *MCN: The American Journal of Maternal Child Nursing, 4*(4), 215–217.

Pitkin, R.M. (1975). Risks related to nutritional problems in pregnancy. In S. Aladjem (Ed.), *Risks in the practice of modern obstetrics* (ed. 2). St. Louis: Mosby, p. 168.

Pollinger, A.C. (1977). Diffusion of innovations in childbirth: An analysis of sociocultural factors associated with traditional, natural, and home birth. (Ph.D. Dissertation, Fordham University, Department of Sociology).

Read, G.D. (1959). *Childbirth without fear.* New York: Harper Brothers, pp. 58-71.

Richardson, S.A., & Guttmacher, A. (1967). *Childbearing: Its social and psychological aspects.* The William & Wilkins Company.

Scaer, R., & Korte, D. (1980). MOM Survey: Maternity options for mothers—What do women want in maternity care? *Birth and the Family Journal, 5*(1), 20-26.

Schnider, S.M., et al. (1979). Uterine blood flow and plasma norepinephrine changes during maternal stress in the pregnant ewe. *Anesthesiology, 50*(6), 524-527.

Sender, N. (1977). Changing from orthodox to family-centered obstetrics. *Journal of Reproductive Medicine, 19*(5), 295-297.

Shaw, N.S. (1974). Forced labor: Maternity care in the United States. In *Pergamon studies in critical sociology* (Vol. 1). New York: Pergamon Press.

Sheffield, M., & Bewley, S. (1977). *Where do babies come from?* New York: Knopf.

Stanton, M.E. (1979). The myth of "natural" childbirth. *Journal of Nurse-Midwifery, 24*(2), 25-29.

Stewart, D., & Stewart, L. (Eds.). (1976). *Safe alternatives in childbirth.* Chapel Hill: NAPSAC, Inc.

Stewart, D., & Stewart, L. (Eds.). (1977). *21st century obstetrics now* (Vol 1). Chapel Hill: NAPSAC, Inc.

Stewart D., & Stewart, L. (Eds.) (1977). *21st century obstetrics now* (Vol. 2). Chapel Hill: NAPSAC, Inc.

The birth atlas (1968, ed. 6). N.Y.: The Maternity Center Association.

Timberlake, B. (1975). The new life center. *The American Journal of Nursing, 75*(9), 1456-1461.

Umphenour, J. (1980). Bacterial colonization in neonates with sibling visitation. *Journal of Obstetric, Gynecologic and Neonatal Nursing, 9*(2), 73-75.

Ward, C., & Ward, F. (1976). *The home birth book.* Washington: INSCAPE Publishers.

Welch, L.B. (1979). Planned change in nursing: The theory. *Nursing Clinics of North America, 14*(2), 307-321.

Wertz, R., & Wertz, D. (1979). *Lying-in: A history of childbirth in America.* New York: Schoeken Books.

White, G. (1977). A comparison of home and hospital delivery based on 25 years experience with both. *Journal of Reproductive Medicine, 19*(5), 291-292.

Part 4 The Family Postpartum

POSTPARTALLY, there are many areas on which health care providers must focus. There is the need to assess and determine the health of the infant, and the need to facilitate a woman's adjustment to a nonpregnant state, both emotionally and physiologically. There is the need to facilitate the new family's understanding of their child's behavior and to incorporate the child into the family system. Finally, the infant's nutritional needs must be met, and parents provided the assistance they require to adequately breast- or bottle-feed their child. Part 4 deals with all of these issues, with emphasis on the family who is basically healthy.

Chapter 12

Two Psychological Aspects of the Postpartum Period

Reva Rubin

An individual's body concept, and the boundaries prescribed to it, establish one's perception of self and the ability to perform effectively.

Diane Angelini (1978) noted that "body image is closely entwined with ego formation" and is one of three interdependent aspects of self-concept, the other two being ideal body image and self-image. Jacqueline Fawcett (1977) defined body image as "the picture of our own body which we form in our minds...the way which the body appears to ourselves" (p. 228). Dianne Moore described it as follows:

As humans our body image is determined in several ways. One of these is through the experiences of the body's muscles, organs, and nerves, and how they respond to the environment. Another is how we master the world around us and still another is how others respond to our body. Body image is a combination of many things, only part of which is the physical appearance.*

*From Moore, D.S. (1978). The body image in pregnancy, *Journal of Nurse Midwife, 22*(4), 17–18. With permission.

Body boundary is one facet of bodily concerns and body image. It fluctuates with varying situations, so that the extent of any one individual's body boundary is difficult to ascertain. Angelini (1978) noted that "there is no sharp border between the body and the surrounding space within the environment." Nonetheless, individuals conceptualize their own body boundaries, and thus define for themselves where their body starts and ends. Angelini pointed out that disturbances result when body boundaries do not function as imagined, or do not maintain the established integrity defined by the individual.

Pregnancy, labor, birth, and postpartum, therefore, may threaten established boundaries, body images and self-concepts. New boundaries may need to be constructed as the body swells during pregnancy and then gradually diminishes again in the months after birth. Such alterations may leave a woman more vulnerable and susceptible to criticisms of her body's ability to function adequately.

The significance of body-boundary formation for the childbearing woman is obviously tremendous; it affects her view of herself as a woman. It may, however, be more difficult to understand the meaning of body boundary to the development of maternal-infant attachment.

Reva Rubin provides, in the following sections, a theoretical framework describing the importance of body boundaries for the woman's body image as she moves through the childbearing experience, as well as for the fetus and newborn. Jacqueline Fawcett (1977) has further demonstrated that body-boundary changes are evident during childbearing in the male partner as well. Professionals must be aware of the significance of body-boundary formation and incorporate such an understanding into the care provided the childbearing family.

Rubin also discusses her theory on the binding-in process during the postpartum period. She provides a brilliant role model as well as valuable insight regarding the need for future analysis and research in maternal–infant attachment, self-concept formation, interdependence, dependence, and independence.

The Editors

BODY IMAGE AND BOUNDARY

Body Image

The body image is the self-concept of a person in action and in engagement with his experiential world. As such, the body image of our patients, expressed verbally or in body language, is a most useful indicator of their biopsychological condition: the problems they confront, their capacities and their limitations in coping with the many situations within an experience requiring health care.

The body image comprises three subjective, interchanging, and interpenetrating areas: the *appearance,* the *functioning,* and the *intactness* of one's body. In an obstetrical setting, the intactness of the body has special meaning.

The desire for wholeness and intactness of the body is universal and necessary to the human condition. Emotions generated by the loss, threatened or actual, of wholeness or intactness serve to mobilize energy and resources for self-preservation. Gestalt theory proposes that this need for wholeness and completeness dominates perception and behavior. To effect a good whole in configuration of form or concept, there must be a good fit of subject and context, good continuance within and between systems, good symmetry, and good, satisfying closure. When tracing the history of words

such as *hale, hail,* and *health,* we find that they derive from the word *whole.*

Infant Intactness

The significance of intactness, completeness, wholeness—the integrity of the body—is manifest by the newly delivered mother in relation to her newborn child. The question, "Is he all right?" encompasses appearance, function, and intactness of his body. In subsequent sessions with her baby, however, the intactness and wholeness of the infant's body dominates her observations.

All the external body parts must be present in the baby to make him or her an integral and whole individual. Incompleteness, such as a harelip, a nubbin instead of an ear, or spina bifida, has a double effect on the mother: first, the difficulty everyone has of not knowing how to relate to an extraordinary individual, and second, the personal disaster of functional inadequacy in creating a whole baby.

There is a maternal drive, fortunate for the baby, to make the child whole, to fix whatever body part may not be whole; to effect the integrity of the child's body. This is true whether the defect is internal or external. Although a mother will be eternally grateful to the surgeon who fixes a defect, and to those who care for her infant in the interval, hostility and self-hate remain because she has to be dependent on others to complete what she was unable to make whole.

The complete, "perfect" baby is seen not only as testament to her functional adequacy as a woman, but also as a gift, a generous blessing of her hopes and caring efforts, and as a complimentary response of her baby to her.

Intactness is seen by the new mother as being necessary to wholeness. Abrasions, swellings, and supernumerary parts on the body of the infant rouse deep maternal concerns of the baby's intactness. Caput, hematomas, hernias, blebs, and even milia, are seen, quite correctly, as eruptive growths of the baby's body boundary. Scratches and cracks on the infant's skin are seen as discontinuities in the body surface, a surface that serves as a boundary, separating and delineating the baby as a separate entity from the surroundings.

An intact body boundary keeps inner contents inside the body. During the phase of initial identification of her newborn, in the primacy of the significance of intactness, all extrusions from the infant are viewed with alarm. The loss or expulsion of inner contents of the baby's body arouses maternal anxiety and concern. A wet burp to a new mother is as frightening as projectile vomiting. It takes second thoughts on her part to realize that urination and defecation by her infant really are normal behaviors. The first thought or image is of a damaged or inoperable body boundary. The second thought draws her attention to the orifices in the body boundary.

Crying, vomiting, hiccoughing, and sneezing, however, retain their significance, and continue to cue alarm: something is not right. Bleeding from the navel, circumcision, venipuncture, or any orifice of the body is never acceptable. Blood is equated with life, and belongs inside, protected and encapsulated by the body boundary.

Intactness and completeness of the body boundary is significant for everyone, but for the newly delivered mother, there are cogent experiences of body imagery in wholeness and intactness during childbearing and childbirth of both the baby and herself.

The underlying image of the infant's body during pregnancy is quite different from the baby a mother hopes will be born to her. The image of the unborn baby is as conceptus; somewhat like an internal organ, without skin, nails, or hair, and without shape or extremities. Pregnant women often display revulsion at the cannibalistic suggestion that she prepare or eat internal organs, such as calf's liver. Her experiences with bodily productions, such as excreta, discharges, exudates, and sometimes even words have been formless, without unity, and foul in character and odor. Thus, women dread seeing their babies immediately after the baby is born, though at the same time, they can hardly wait out of unsatisfied curiosity and desire. The rapturous delight in the sweet smell, the hair, skin, fingernails, and feet of the newborn are not just because the baby is beautiful, but also because the baby, as delivered from her body, is so unlike the characteristic body productions that she dreaded and half expected.

The experience of childbearing is largely one of preserving body intactness and stability. After delivery, the subjective need is for restoration and recovery of wholeness, completeness and integrity; the reconstitution and reaffirmation of her body and ego boundaries.

Wholeness is a consideration of body imagery that goes through drastic changes antepartum, intrapartum, and postpartum.

Particularly in the third trimester, though to a lesser extent in the first trimester as well, the image of the body giving birth is one of explosively splitting open. Striae on the abdomen are not seen only as a cosmetic infringement on the body, but also as an awesome threat to the body. As one woman, looking at her own abdominal striae, phrased it, "It's like a chick trying to break out of the egg." Fetal movement is pleasureable most of the time, but the forceful kicking of the fetus at term is disturbing, not because it hurts, since it does not, but because of the threat of the aggression to her body, in its quiet wholeness.

Maternal Intactness

Women's bodies are perfectly designed for nurturing their infants in utero. But, as their expected due dates approach, women can and do have an unrealistic and frightening image of a 20–35-lb mass coming through two small orifices and one narrow canal. Objectively, the prospect is very simple, even normal. But subjectively the prospect, and sometimes the actual experience, is a searing, splitting, and destructive experience. Subjectivity makes the women more reality bound, more prescient, and more prepared (or is it courageous?), than their objective and uninvolved caretakers. Lacerations of the cervix, vagina, and perineum; cystoceles and rectoceles; protrusion of the rectum into hemorrhoids; forced displacement of the coccyx posteriorly; marked blood loss; and Cesarean delivery are all within the norm, obstetrically. There are a few possibilities, such as paralysis, inverted uterus, massive infection, bleeding of hemorrhagic proportions, and death, that are outside the norm. Normal or abnormal, every one of these occurrences is possible, many of them are probable, and none of them is subjectively desirable.

Being reality bound, the pregnant woman may be sick to her stomach in anticipation. She plans and arranges not to be unattended when the baby comes out of her body. She arranges her home, her affairs, and the placement of her other children for a departure that might not be temporary. The appearance of blood at the vaginal orifice, the perineum, or rectum is an alarm cue; the image is one of ongoing destruction inside her body. Facts are used with inferential logic: If slight bleeding is a sign of early labor, how much bleeding will there be in advanced labor? She knows fear, and even panic, in labor as the baby comes "barreling down" through her body.

Immediately after delivery, there is relief and joy in being alive and whole. The ensuing fatigue and sleep hunger are caused by the cumulative effects of carbon dioxide and lactic acid, not only in the uterine muscles, but throughout the body in response to the tension of alertness to danger sustained over a long period of time. The completion of birth is a signal to drop the guardedness against accidental destruction.

Postpartum Intactness

This highly exercised and developed capacity for alertness and guardedness against accidental destruction is extended and transferred to her infant, and is further developed to become the dominant and pervasive characteristic of maternal behaviors. Maternal protectiveness is anticipatory alertness to the accidental, unintentional dangers, as well as those dangers everyone else recognizes. She worries about little things, because her observations and awareness are highly developed and if nothing happens, it is because she takes successful measures to prevent them from happening.

The postpartum experience is characterized not by impending possible or probable loss of wholeness and intactness, but by actual loss. There is a loss of well-developed motor skills, of the level of energy and effectiveness by which a woman knows and identifies herself as a whole, intact, and active person. The "gappiness" in the body boundary at the lacerated, sutured, or edematous sites makes it feel as though the contents of her body are falling out by gravitational pull, or by explosive, extrusional push in coughing, sneezing, laughing, urinating, or defecating.

Primiparas are unprepared for the subjective experience of loss of body boundaries, and with it the loss of ego. Labor and delivery seem so overwhelmingly dangerous that there is no capacity to cope with any more. Multiparas, however, are not so euphoric when delivery is accomplished; they instead prepare themselves for the puerperium phase of childbirth by recruiting help, and taking as many relief or avoidance measures as possible.

The Protective Response

The phenomenon of the body boundary was first described by Schilder (1964). It is readily seen in the common protective response to intrusive approach to, or through, the body. The protective response is reflexive and consists of mobilization and constriction of tissues, a spontaneous recruitment to reinforce the site of penetration of the body boundary.

In the normal, intact skin surface of the forearm, for example, a neutral object approach will elicit the protective response at 2-cm distance from the skin surface; the hair on the skin will become erectile. If the approach is arrested and the object is held at 2 cm, the response will recruit additional tissue: there will be a sensation of creeping skin around the site; the muscles, skin, and hair follicles of the neck will constrict; the face, arm, back and leg muscles will constrict; and the breath (and speech) will be held still or constricted. At the orifices of the body, eyes, nostrils, ear canals, and rectum, the protective response occurs 3 or more cm

from the actual opening, providing a greater boundary. Approach to the eyes causes the eyelids to close, the forehead wrinkles, the mouth purses, the facial muscles constrict, and the shoulder muscles constrict to elevate the shoulders. The rectal sphincter constricts on approach; if there is hovering in the approach at the body boundary, the gluteal muscles constrict to cover the rectum.

If the object approaching is sharp or forceful, or if the rate of speed of approach is accelerated, the normal body boundary is increased, possibly by an "additive buffer zone" or by recruitment and enlargement of the boundary. The protective response is increased to involve motor muscle responses, increasing the distance between the approaching object and the subjective body boundary.

When the body boundary is not intact as with an open wound, the defensive response is elicited 6 inches to two feet away from the body surface. There is little differentiation between a sharp or dull, a hard or soft object, a fast or slow advance; any penetration becomes a threat when intactness is lost; the defensive response is set in action sooner, more energetically, and with more motor responses.

Intrusions or penetrations of the body boundary are in themselves painful, even without skin penetration. A breast examination does not require penetration of the skin, but it elicits a sustained constriction of movement, of respirations, and of muscles of the face, eyes, shoulders, and hands. The vaginal speculum elicits more of a defensive response before it is actually inserted because the body boundary is larger at that zone. Each further poke in a vaginal examination, whether by speculum or by finger, is a further penetration. It is the penetrations, not the examinations, that are painful. Blood tests are more painful and harder to endure than urinalysis, x-ray, and the like.

Because medical examinations and lab tests are "legitimate," they are endured with a great deal of self-control involving a lowering or a pass through of the body boundary by an increased recruitment of body tissues, an increase of muscle tension to rigidity, a "holding-on." Prolonged muscle tension, or an onslaught of multiple experiences of sustained tension is painfully exhausting. The same woman who can easily cope with a vaginal examination and can endure the painful constriction in her body during pregnancy or early labor, can be overwhelmed by the same demands of her in advanced labor, when she is tired and still aching from the last contraction.

There are real, subjective problems in maintaining a stable body boundary in the normal course of pregnancy. Until the third trimester, the growing fetus and the enlarged uterus are contained very nicely in or above the pelvis and in alignment with the axis of the maternal body. Beginning in the seventh month of pregnancy, however, the fetal mass does not remain in alignment with the maternal body but hangs forward in upright and bending positions, and hangs back when the pregnant woman turns from side to side. The progressive thinning of the woman's abdominal wall reduces her sense of fetal containment. There is a righting reflex against the forward tilt, and the pregnant woman redistributes her body backwards to provide a wider base for standing, walking, or sitting. Normal movements and positioning of the body become increasingly labored and slow.

From this position, people and objects in the world often appear too close and too fast in their approach. The pregnant woman is acutely aware of, and on guard for, sudden and forceful movements of people and objects around her because she needs more lead time now to take care of herself. When providing an adequate postural base takes so much effort, she is particularly aware of such things as loose boards in steps, escalators, and broken sidewalks. The constant guarding and alertness is in itself fatiguing, but more important is her heightened sense of vulnerability.

Diffusion of Body Boundary

The vulnerability of pregnancy is at its height in the last half of the seventh month when the boundary separating the self from the world tends to diffuse. Body images of appearance and functional inadequacy produce a lowered self-respect. In the folklore of femininity (usually correct) the eighth month is the dangerous time. It is not just coincidence that the time of onset of toxemia or premature labor coincides with the heightened vulnerability in pregnancy. Toxemia is a disease of involuntary muscle constriction. Uterine muscle contractions are quite common in the eighth month of pregnancy. To call uterine contractility "uterine irritability" or false labor fails to explain the reasons for it.

In the dissipation of body boundaries a woman protects herself in two ways. One measure of care involves distancing herself from intrusive or penetrating forces by avoidance or curtailment. The other measure is to set up a protective "buffer zone," either within her home or through the quiet, sustained presence of another person.

Diffusion and dissipation of body boundaries also occur with pain. Persistent or sharp pain floods the body, spreads out from the local area to adjacent areas. The reflexive response to pain is to recruit one's hand to the affected area, to provide counterpressure, or counter-temperature, or to contain or encapsulate the pain from

erupting the body boundary. With pain, however, there is generalized muscle weakness; a diffusion of energy, of body parts and zones, and a general diffusion of body boundaries in the diffusion of pain.

A woman in advanced labor hurts all over: there is pressure in the sacrum and coccyx, but there is also headache and pressure in the eyeballs. There is pressure on the perineum, but also on the diaphragm. Relief given for the headache or eyes reduces pain there, and in the general musculature and disposition. Pain and relief have a spread effect.

Without body boundaries or buffers, the woman in pain is more vulnerable to external assaults such as loud noises or screams outside the room, a quick and loud opening or closing of the door to her room and forceful speech or forceful intrusions or probings into her body. She uses other people as buffers, since she cannot recruit her own protective responses.

In the recovery and restoration of body boundaries, she yearns for contact with the body of her baby or her partner. The caregiver's touch, gentle and unhurried, localizes the area of pain and provides reconstruction of the body's boundary.

A newborn does not have a body boundary. There is no protective response; in fact, there is delay of a few seconds between the insertion of a needle and the infant's response to pain. Newborns do experience pain, but they feel it as a total flooding of their bodies; infants cannot localize pain. There are no boundaries between their bodies and the world around them; they are vulnerable to all assaults.

Somehow the new mother realizes her baby's lack of body boundaries. She uses her own body ego to provide the infant a buffer zone. Her touching, handling, and caressing of the outer surfaces of his or her body promotes the construction of a body boundary, a body image, and a self-concept. A part of this construction is the second aspect of the postpartum period to be considered here: the process of binding-in that occurs between the mother and her infant.

BINDING-IN IN THE POSTPARTUM PERIOD*

Binding-in is a somewhat clumsier term than attachment or bonding, perhaps because it is a direct translation from the German *ein bindung,* but it is more accurately descriptive of the formative stages of the maternal–child relationship as a process, not a state.

*Modified from Rubin, R. (1977). Binding-in in the postpartum period. *Maternal–Child Nursing Journal, 6,* 67-75. With permission.

The process is active, intermittent, and accumulative, and occurs in progressive stages over a period of twelve to fifteen months. The origin and endpoint of the process are in the maternal identity itself.

Maternal identity and binding-in to the child are two major developmental changes, each dependent on the other, in the three trimesters of pregnancy and the two trimesters following delivery of the child. Developmental progress in maternal identity and in binding-in is promoted or retarded on the one side by the infant itself and on the other side by society, particularly closely related family members.

A conceptual model of the binding-in process might well be like the weaving of a tapestry. Not a cord, nor a bond, nor a welding job, but rather a large creative work, framed between the child and the mother's own significant social world, systematically and progressively developed for durability against time and stress to form the substance of her own personal identity and the fabric of her relationship with this particular child.

The initial stimulus for maternal binding-in is a physical one provided by the infant itself. The internal, enteroceptive stimulus of fetal movement produces an awareness of "Another." The awareness is continued and augmented during pregnancy by the varied movements of the infant, his growing size and weight, the idiosyncrasies of his behavior in response to hers, and her accommodative changes in activities and preferences in terms of the infant. There is a psychosocial as well as a biological interdependent reciprocity, or symbiosis, between mother and child during pregnancy.

After delivery, the maternal binding-in changes in form and accelerates markedly. Instead of the symbiotic oneness of pregnancy, there is an identification of the infant as an objective human entity with his or her own form, appearance, and behavior. Instead of the complete and exclusive possession of the infant in pregnancy, there is a claiming of her infant in a social context. Instead of the very significant incorporation of the infant into her self-system during pregnancy, there is a polarization of selves in the postpartum period.

Identification

The infant during pregnancy has no gender and no objective form or appearance, only an incorporated presence subject to indirect verification in the form and appearance of the woman's own body, her own appetite and interest changes, her different affective and ideational style, form, and content (Rubin, 1970, 1972). After the birth of the child, there is an intense need, almost a drive, to identify the child by direct verification. The modalities of sensory information about the child change from the enteroceptive sensations of pressure and movement during pregnancy to the predominantly proprioceptive sensory modalities postpartum: visual, tactile, auditory and olfactory (Rubin, 1961). After the birth of a child, there is an object, a child, to see, to touch, to hear, and to smell. The varied hypothetical fantasies of the child during pregnancy are eagerly replaced postpartum by hard empirical data to identify the child.

The purpose of identification of the infant is to define one's self and one's behavior in relation to that child. Identification organizes maternal behavior and maternal attitudes. Sex, size, and condition of the infant are paramount. Each mother, each time she becomes a mother, must know the sex of the child in order to begin to relate. Disappointments take time to overcome and the identification and other binding-in measures are delayed or limited. A bigger child is easier to relate to and interact with than a very small child. Even the tone of voice will change in addressing even the normally small infant and there is almost complete silence in addressing the still smaller baby. The condition of the baby, particularly its wholeness and intactness, is essential to determine before acting or interacting in relation to the child. From antepartum fantasies of the unborn child and her own misgivings about being able to produce anything desirable or perfect out of her own body, each mother has an expectancy of an imperfect or deformed child. In the same way people avoid a doctor when they are ill lest he confirm a dreaded suspicion, many women cannot bear to watch the birth of their child and prefer to have the news of whether the baby is "all right" filtered through their husbands' or partners', their doctors', or their nurses' report on the condition of the baby.

If sex, size, and condition are all fine, each one of these attributes of the child is received by the mother as a gift to her, a contribution by the infant itself to her. Binding-in through identification then accelerates and continues with intensity. The appearance and function, including behavior, of the child are ascertained through all sensory modalities, and inventoried and memorized. Identifying the appearance and function of the infant is done through experiences with the infant, establishing the permanence of the characteristics and qualities of the child already identified, and making new observations and identifications in greater extent or detail. In the presence of a supportive adult, the cyclical experiences of infant identification increase in duration, in extent, and in delightful discovery. With supportive adults and a normal, healthy baby, the identification process is operationally complete by four weeks. Complete identification of the infant by the mother can be said to occur when the mother "knows" by looking, touching, hearing, or smelling whether her baby is well or not, hungry or satisfied, comfortable or uncomfortable.

Claiming

At the end of pregnancy a strong attachment to the unborn infant has developed. The pregnant woman's ego is involved with the child, and there are narcissistic gratifications, as well as misgivings, in creating and possessing a child. If the pregnancy is carried to term, the pregnant woman also has a highly developed identification with the child's vulnerability and need for protection (Rubin, 1975).

There is a progressive investment and commitment of the maternal self in the child during pregnancy, and an inordinately high cost of investment and commitment in labor and delivery. In the pleasure of the birth of a perfect child, she will assert that the high cost "was worth it." There will be many times, particularly in the first postpartum month, when she will reconsider and be dubious about the value of that investment. However, the bonds created by involvement, identification, and commitment formed during pregnancy secure the fabric of the relationship.

There is an extension postpartum of the exclusive possession during pregnancy to an inclusion of the child in the social sphere of those persons she claims as her own and who, in turn, claim her as their own. This is done through identification of the child's characteristics and qualities in appearance and behaviors. She observes and examines the newborn, and identifies items in appearance or in behavior that are "like" her husband's, "like" her other child's, "like" her own. The linking in association binds the newborn into the exclusive and intimate social sphere of her significant others.

The reciprocal claiming behaviors of the significant persons in her personal social sphere anchor the claiming bonds. Without this reciprocal claiming of the child by others who claim her, further investment and commitment by the mother to the child is severely restricted.

Identification and claiming are part of the polarization stage in neomaternal identity and binding-in to the child. However, all parents—paternal, adoptive, grandparents—identify and claim the newborn to some extent. Only biological mothers, however, display the phenomenon of polarization.

Polarization

Helena Deutsch (1945) first identified the important and difficult process of polarization following delivery. The term *polarization* is descriptive of a stage in cell reproduction before final separation of mother and daughter cells. An analogous process of polarization, physically and conceptually, occurs in the reproductive process of the human mother.

The physical unity of one being within the other achieved during pregnancy, through adaptation and accommodation of the mother to the constant enlarging presence of her infant, is an embedded, nested, and contained stage of mothering and nurturing. The concomitant incorporation of the infant into the self-system (the ideal-, self-, and body-image) of the mother during pregnancy, consolidates the unity psychosocially as well as psychobiologically, so that there is no difference between what is within and the self. It is only in the realm of imagery and fantasy, valuable cognitive capacities, that the pregnant woman can conceptualize the infant within as a projected individual in outer, external space. Imagery and fantasy are transitory and highly variant projections, dependent on inner experiences at the particular moment.

Polarization is the physical and conceptual separating-out process of the incorporated infant of pregnancy into a separate, external, and constant entity postpartum. Labor and delivery are necessary but not sufficient for polarization. In fact, polarization begins late in pregnancy and seems to be a necessary condition for spontaneous birthing of the infant.

Physical separating-out of the infant from the stage of unity starts with labor, is heightened with delivery, and continues through postpartum involution, a period of four to six weeks.

Restitution of her own intactness, completeness, and wholeness as an individual seems to be an essential precondition to the maternal conceptualization of her infant as a complete, whole individual. Tissue healing of the placental site and the episiotomy is usually complete by the third week. The abdominal incision of the woman with a Cesarean delivery will take longer.

Until involution is completed, the enteroceptive sensations of abdominal mass and weight, the difficult and laborious gait, and the slow rate of physical activity postpartum are experientially continuous with being pregnant. The extensive fatigue of the postpartum period adds to the sensation of being burdened, as in pregnancy. The appearance of the body postpartum is essentially unchanged from that of pregnancy.

Feeling, looking, and functioning as though one is

pregnant, although one is patently not pregnant, is disconcerting. In her dislike and aversion to the incongruous body image of residual pregnancy, the postpartal woman will describe her body as flabby, empty, fat, or useless. She may use equally hostile and uncomplimentary remarks about her infant's bodily appearance: he is hers, there remains a oneness, a unity.

Dysfunctions or inadequacies in simple body function or body maintenance such as urination, defecation, lactation, standing, and walking serve to further alienate and disorient her body image from her self-image of functional adequacy and competence. If the baby should have difficulty sucking, grasping the nipple, or burping, she perceives this as more of the same, a continuation of self, another blow to her self-image.

There is often an attempt to get rid of the pregnant body image. The new mother may dress to go home from the hospital in decidedly nonpregnant clothing. When the clothes do not fit, despite her wishes and the fact that she has delivered her baby, the disconcerting and confusing loss of identity typical of the involution period really starts. There is a characteristic neglect in dress and grooming of the unloved and unwanted maternal body image; these feelings about her own body image are extended to that of her infant's body. The dress and grooming of the infant are direct reflections of her own dress and grooming. The infant is an extension, a part of herself, still incorporated, not quite separate.

An unloved and unlovable body is not typically nourished. Characteristically, most women become apathetic or even aversive to food for at least one month postpartum. The apathy is reinforced by her relative isolation and abandonment by adults in the second and subsequent weeks postpartum. In these situations, there is a tendency to underfeed, to disrupt feedings, or to force-feed the infant. The child is an extension of herself and she feeds him just as she does herself. The infant's cries are not objectively perceived; the crying either does not make any sense, because she is not hungry, or simply is an echo of her own feelings and her own situation.

A phenomenon similar to that of the "phantom limb" persists through the first two to three weeks postpartum. In addition to the anachronistic body image of pregnancy, the sensations of enteroceptive contact and movements of the infant in utero continue, like the perceptual after-image or the limb sensations of the amputee. Few women talk about the phenomenon, but most avoid lying on their abdomens. When this position is suggested, the postpartal mothers are startled and then embarrassed when they realize there is really no baby inside any longer. That this is not merely habit, is supported by early postpartal dream content. The dream content is a continuation of the late pregnancy dreams. Most dreams are of labor and delivery, remnants of her fears of dismemberment or explosion in childbirth, with the child still unborn. Dreams of the infant are single scenes in which the child appears and disappears again.

The continued after-image sensations in utero are not disturbing. On the contrary, they are as enjoyable as early fetal movement is during pregnancy. What is important is that what is still sometimes inside is not always outside. It takes awhile to adapt to the child "outside." Everyone else is very much aware that the child is outside, but that is the only experience available to all others than the biological mother. The biological mother is bothered by the need to consciously learn that the baby is external. In the hospital, the day is organized around the coming and going of the baby, the appearance and disappearances. At home, in the organization around family needs, the mother concentrates on the reorganization of the family to include the baby. But when it is not "time" to feed, bathe, or visit with the baby, a mother may forget there is a baby. If the baby is not within visible proximity, the mother might startle when reference is made to the baby; or when the baby cries, remember and then say, "Oh, the baby." One mother forgot her quiet newborn baby for ten hours in the usual vortex of a day with her three preschool-aged sons. She was still shaking with fear, fear of herself and for her baby, when she told of the incident a month later. Most mothers set the alarm clock, so that they do not sleep through or forget. When polarization progresses and there is object constancy, with the child outside, permanently and consistently in the external world, there is an inner clock and an inner awareness of the child outside. As the child becomes more active, as in the two- or three-month old, responsive baby, there is no question of the stability of the mother's awareness of the child's presence externally and constantly.

Externalization of the infant conceptually and experientially has its own orderly progression: from within, enteroceptively; to around and in direct contact with the surface of the maternal body, proprioceptively; to within personal space, proximity in the same room; and then to social space, distally in the same or adjoining rooms, perceptually and apperceptively. The order of progression in the spatial relationship of mother to child is most vivid in the feeding progression: antepartum, she feeds the infant internally; postpartum, for breast- or bottle-feeding, she enfolds and draws the baby to her body for full surface contact; later, for spoon and cup feeding, she sits directly in front of the baby, permitting more activity space; and still later, she will eat lunch on the table at the other end of the kitchen and tell the child to go eat lunch.

Externalization seems to be the singularly important aspect of polarization to the new mother. At delivery, the experience of feeling the baby outside her body, on the surface of her body, across her abdomen or in her arms, is particularly meaningful. A woman who has not had this experience does not seem to feel that she has given birth to a child or that she has been given a child.

Beyond this initial experience, there is a need to hold—to just hold—the child in her arms. There is a cradling in the arms and across the breasts. The weight and gravitational pull of the infant enfolded in her arms enables her to make an orderly transition in embeddedness and containment from the internally passive to the externally active. The weight and gravitation pull provide her a substantial sense of the infant's reality and stability.

The holding is of relatively short duration. Prolonged holding becomes painful in the fatigue and achings of the early puerperium. After repeated holding experiences, the proprioceptive experience of the infant replaces the enteroceptive experience of the fetus and the phantom-limb sensation disappers. Holding promotes identification and claiming, but beyond the early and initial holdings, proprioceptive pleasure wears thin. Until the child by his or her own activities can renew pleasure and interest in the holding, maternal holding will decrease markedly after the first week postpartum.

The natural tendency is for the new mother to want the baby in close spatial proximity, in the same room if possible, present but not necessarily in direct contact continuously. This enables her to make many observations of the child who is close by, to know what he does in the long intervals between feedings and care taking, and to establish a continuity in her knowing him perceptively. The frequent observational sampling of his behavior and personality promote the experience of his constancy, of his existence in space and time.

Polarization proceeds slowly for the first three to four weeks postnatally. The new mother is taken up with the slow rate of physical and psychological recovery from pregnancy, labor, and delivery. Recovery takes longer than three to four weeks, but characteristically at this time there is a healthy revolt against the feelings of apathy, depression, and void in identity.

The new mother "bursts out" of her home into a wider world, away from the baby to adult society, away from social isolation into social participation, away from the routine and monotony to the unusual and interesting. It is as though she needs to renew and reassert herself as an integral, individual person.

The forms of bursting out vary considerably. The preferred form seems to be a gala evening on the town: well dressed and escorted by her husband to a big reception or to a dinner and movie. If there is no husband to escort her, she will go alone to meet and interact with adults. The beauty shop, a bar, the supermarket are all used when there is no escort and little money. There is a determined, justified taking of time for herself. When the event includes extra measures of body care, such as dressing up, having her hair done, or eating and drinking special foods and having these foods served to her, the event becomes more satisfying.

Other forms of the same behavior occur later by one or two weeks: the mother will return to work or leave the baby with a trusted caretaker such as her mother. Hospitalization of the child serves the same purpose sometimes. These measures are more permanent than the single, short burst out and have a strong element of quiet desperation.

The outcome of this bursting out in the third week is not only a self renewal but effects polarization. There is a pull back to the child after the escapade. The more gratifying the experience is to the new mother, the more guilty she feels. It is this guilt at having been self-indulgent that turns her with renewed and accelerating love to her infant. Her warmth for her helpless, dependent, and abandoned infant wells. She mothers her child instead of just performing caretaking acts. But more important in terms of polarization, she addresses her child in the second person, singular "you," in a strongly affectionate tone.

The separation at the third to fourth week, out of deliberate choice and with positive reinforcement in her self-worth, serves to disengage the unity that made the infant only an extension of herself, and effects the polarization where there is a "You" and a restored "I." She reidentifies anew the "You" as well as the "I." The possessive and historical bond of "We" is fortified by her guilt and the infant's acceptance and forgiveness.

REFERENCES

Deutsch, H. (1945). *Psychology of women* (Vol. 1). New York: Grune & Stratton.

Fawcett, J. (1977). The relationship between identification and patterns of change in spouses' body images during and after pregnancy. *International Journal of Nursing Studies, 14*(4) 199–213.

Moore, D.S. (1978). The body image in pregnancy. *Journal of Nurse Midwife, 22*(4), 17–27.

Rubin, R. (1961). Basic maternal behaviors. *Nursing Outlook, 9.*

Rubin, R. (1963). Maternal touch. *Nursing Outlook, 2*(11).

Rubin, R. (1970). Cognitive style in pregnancy. *American Journal of Nursing, 70*(3).

Rubin, R. (1972). Fantasy and object constancy in maternal relationships. *Maternal–Child Nursing Journal, 1*(2), 101–111.

Rubin, R. (1975). Maternal task in pregnancy. *Maternal–Child Nursing Journal, 4*(3).

Rubin, R. (1977). Binding-in in the postpartum period. *Maternal–Child Nursing Journal, 6,* 67–75.

Schilder, P. (1964). *Contributions to developmental neuropsychiatry* (L. Bender, Ed.). New York: International Universities Press.

Chapter 13 | Education for Parenting

Betty Lia-Hoagberg

There are only two lasting bequests we can hope to give our children. One of these is roots; the other, wings (Carter, 1977).

Once you think of parenting, rather than mothering or fathering, you are free to question some of the basic assumptions about the nuclear family, to consider some of the economic underpinnings beneath life styles, and most important, you are free to think about how to divide the task of parenting in new ways that might develop the growth potential of all concerned.*

THE AMERICAN FAMILY has been changing in the last century; family roles have become more complex and flexible, there is an increased level of family income, increased educational attainment of parents and children, a tendency toward smaller nuclear families, more remarriage, and changes to more permissive childrearing practices (Duvall, 1977).

Bronfenbrenner (1976) notes other changes in the family, such as more working mothers, fewer adults in the home, more single-parent families, more unwed mothers, and more adoptive, foster, blended (as stepparents), single, or surrogate parents. He also notes the

---

*From McBride, A.B. (1973). *The growth and development of mothers.* New York: Harper & Row, p. 130. With permission.

lack of family support systems such as quality day-care, fair part-time employment practices for parents, and a need for enhancing the status and power of women in the home and in the marketplace.

The social pressure and stress on parents is also supported in the Report to the President from the 1970 White House Conference on Children:

> In today's world, parents often find themselves at the mercy of a society which imposes pressures and priorities that allow neither time nor place for meaningful activities involving children and adult, which downgrade the role of parents and the functions of parenthood and which prevent the parent from doing the things he wants to do as a guide, friend and companion to his children. (Gilberg, 1975, p. 61)

Another important fact is that parents and families can be greatly affected by their socioeconomic or minority group status. LeMasters (1970, p. 97) states that "insofar as social class position involves a subculture or way of life it would seem to affect the parental performance in a variety of ways." He discusses factors pertinent to parenting in various social classes, and notes the many overwhelming problems facing lower-class parents, and the generic problems common to minority group parents in our society: poverty, residential segregation, slum housing, unemployment (or underemployment), inadequate schooling, poor health (mental as well as physical) and health care, prejudice, loss of civil rights, discrimination, and poor self-image.

Two other areas to be considered are the myths about parenting, and the ways in which parents and families are presented in the media. LeMasters (1970) has identified seventeen folk beliefs that exist about parenthood. A few of the most common are (1) all married couples should have children; (2) two parents are always better then one; (3) there are no bad children—only bad parents; (4) children always improve a marriage; and (5) American parents can be studied without interviewing fathers. Because of the romantic viewpoint and the myths, many people don't know what they are getting into until after they have children. Another myth in American culture is that parenting and *mothering* mean the same thing (Rapoport et al., 1977).

It should also be recognized that television, advertising, and other media often present unrealistic pictures of parents, children, and family life. It takes much effort to counteract these myths, and deal with parents who feel the pressures of these untrue portrayals.

PARENTHOOD AS A DEVELOPMENTAL PROCESS

Parenthood has been described as a developmental process. Benedek (1970, p. 135) states that "the basic assumption of our deliberation is that parenthood as a bio-psychologic experience activates and maintains a developmental process in the parent." The developmental process concept is also endorsed in the report on parenthood issued by the Group for the Advancement of Psychiatry (GAP, 1973).

McBride (1973, p. 130) argues that *parenting* should replace *mothering* or *fathering* as the description for this generative function. "It does imply sensitivity to the needs of the next generation, kindliness, protectiveness, continuity of care and respect for the dignity of children."

Rapoport et al. (1977) noted that the child-centered, mother-focused paradigm for parenting has been the most prevalent notion, and that it is in great need of revision.

For our current purposes, parenting is defined as the process in which an individual (mother, father, or another interested adult) provides for the basic physical, psychological and social needs of the child. It also denotes a reciprocal relationship between the parent and child through which the parents' healthy needs for growth can be met.

The process of parenting can be viewed as a continuing development, involving many changes. Basic to this process is the understanding that the development of parenting begins with the parents' own infancy and the way they were parented. Social and psychological components of a person's life are set in motion in infancy and further influenced by the individual's inner nature, and various social forces.

Duvall (1977) has identified ten categories of behavior "tasks" of the individual from birth to death. Some of the tasks are achieving an appropriate dependence–independence pattern, relating to changing social groups, and developing a conscience. The task on affection can be traced from infancy to maturity.

There may also be crisis factors in the child's life (such as death of a parent) that can alter this behavioral progression, and may later have an impact on their own parenting.

Normal Parental Growth and Development

There has been little systematic study of the growth and development of parents. Much of the research has focused on parenting from the vantage point of child-rearing. There is an abundance of material discussing ways to raise a child, but scant information on the experiences and feelings of parents as they undertake and perform this very complex and important job. More realistic information about parents and family life has begun to emerge in the last ten years (LeMasters, 1970; McBride, 1973; Rapoport et al., 1977; Skolnick, 1973).

In the past, the parenting process was portrayed as having a one-way direction: Parent → Child. Recent studies (Bell & Harper, 1977; Lewis & Rosenblum, 1974) support the relationship as a two-way process: Parent ⇄ Child.

The interaction of the parent and child can result in developmental growth for both individuals, and also extends into relationships with others. Parents often learn more about themselves as people through their experiences with their own and other children.

The health care provider must be aware that for some parents, the process does not move toward positive growth but rather in negative paths of frustration, hopelessness, and anger, which is often directed toward the child. Many factors can produce negative parenting; some are unwanted pregnancies, unwanted children, poor parenting in own childhood, lack of knowledge and understanding about children's growth and development; social factors such as no job, low economic status, poor housing; and deficits in self-esteem and self-image. It is difficult to give and care for a child or family when the parent's own needs are not being met.

Early Formative Years

Parenthood education begins in the family of origin—the family into which the child is born or adopted. In the past, the primary parent was usually the mother, with additional, and often a different kind of, parenting provided by the father. There may or may not have been extended family members, such as grandparents, aunts, uncles, and siblings, who also contributed to the parenting functions of child care, teaching, and playing. For some children, there were surrogate parents in foster homes, or institutions, who acted as or performed the functions of the parent for the child. These people become the earliest models for parenting; the quality of care received from them can have a significant effect on the child's later abilities and attitudes toward parenting.

Later Years

There are other individuals who also become influential role models, such as parents of friends, teachers, or other adults in the community. These role models exert an effect by their friendship, interest, and concern for a child. These can lead to increasing the child's self-esteem, as well as the child's ability to relate to others or to build trusting relationships with others.

An adolescent may have further experiences that can shape her or his later parenting skills; some examples would be caring for younger siblings, babysitting or child care jobs, or working in jobs such as camp counselor. Some high schools or colleges offer family life courses, which can provide additional information about child development and parenthood, although these classes often lack "laboratory" experience. Many people feel that this has been an underdeveloped area of education (Harris, 1977; LeMasters, 1970).

Decision to Parent

Many people still become parents because of an unplanned pregnancy, but today, many women and men are making conscious decisions about parenthood (Rapoport et al., 1977; Schaffer, 1977). For the first time in history, with the use of more reliable contraceptives, many people can choose parenthood. Many areas have discussion groups where couples can consider the pros and cons of parenthood. One organization for the voluntary childless is the National Organization for Nonparenthood (NON), which was founded in California in 1971 (Veevers, 1973). However, there is still considerable social pressure on couples to have children, and for women and men to be married if they choose to have children.

Psychological, Social, Cultural Considerations

Many people have recognized the lack of understanding of the social and psychological realities of parenthood (Biller & Meredith, 1974; Harris, 1977; Hoffman & Hoffman, 1973; Wuerger, 1976).

Often, the information comes after the child has arrived. There is a need for prospective parents to examine their motivation for wanting a child; is it to satisfy a selfish need of the parent, or to learn, grow, know, and experience the joy of a child?

There is a great need for more information on factors such as time demands, financial costs, child development needs, and possible effects on other aspects of life such as careers and marriages. Unfortunately, there is still a very romantic conception of parenthood in this society. Most people do not think about or discuss possible parenthood, and thus, many times the unconscious factors for unmet personal and social needs are the strongest motivations for having a child.

Parental Development During Pregnancy

The nine months of pregnancy can be viewed as an adjustment and growth period for the prospective mother or the prospective parents. For most people, including those who planned the pregnancy, there is a period of adjustment to the pregnancy and all of its ramifications (Coleman & Coleman, 1973; Jessner et al., 1970; Rapoport et al., 1977). Pregnancy is accompanied by many psychological experiences as well as physical changes. Often the expectant mother and father will review their own experiences as children. They will discuss or think about the ways they were parented and begin to sort out those aspects they want to retain and those they want to change.

The prospective mother begins to form her own unique mothering identity (Caplan, 1961). She will need to resolve her relationship with her own mother; it is a task that women do with varying degrees of success. This seems crucial in establishing her own separate, motherhood identity.

The prospective father, too, uses the period of pregnancy for reflections about and growth toward fatherhood; this phenomenon has been noted in the un-married and married father. He recalls and reconsiders his experiences and relationship with his own father or father figure. As the Colmans' note (1973, pp. 105–106), "pregnancy is more than simply a biological event; it is a time of crisis for those involved, a time when identities are changing and new roles are being explored."

These same reflective and integrative processes occur in many adoptive parents (GAP, 1973), who also have to deal with other factors such as their own infertility or different reactions they receive from others about being adoptive parents.

Childbirth and Early Postpartum Experiences: Effects on Parental Development

In the early years of this country, childbirth took place in the family home. The mother was usually assisted by a midwife or other family members. The father and other children were soon involved in the arrival of the new baby.

For reasons of safety and convenience, birth increasingly took place in the hospital in the 1920s through the 1940s. Much of the family atmosphere and support was lost or repressed by the bureaucratic rules of these institutions. Many parental rights were also abused in these settings.

Fortunately, in many parts of this country, there has been a change in birth practices and parental involvement within the last twenty years. Through the efforts of consumer groups such as the International Childbirth Education Association (ICEA), LaLeche League International, and some strong and persistent health professionals, parents today can be active participants in the birth and early parenting process. There are educational programs for couples and singles, that provide information on preparation labor and delivery and parenthood education. Hospitals provide family-centered care where the prospective parents can share the labor, birth, and early postpartum experiences.

There are also a number of parents who choose to have a home birth. They feel that the hospitals still do not provide a supportive environment either for birth or for family continuity (Arms, 1975).

Support for increased parental involvement came also from work by Klaus and Kennell (1976), whose studies strongly suggest that the immediate postpartum period is an important time in the development of the mother's bonding (attachment) to her child.

Parke's (1974) research with parents in hospital settings also shows that the father's role is one of active and responsive participation with his new baby. Greenberg and Morris (1974) focused on engrossment, or the link-up of father to his newborn. The results of their research suggests that fathers begin developing a bond to their newborn by the first three days after birth and often earlier.

The immediate postpartum period is an important period for the new mother and father and can be a vital period in strengthening family integration (Rising, 1974).

The outcome of pregnancy is usually a normal, healthy child. Unavoidably, however, a number of pregnancies result in a premature or sick child, an infant with a congenital malformation, or an infant who dies. These problems introduce stress and marked changes in the developmental growth of parents.

Transition to Parenthood

Becoming a parent, whether through birth, adoption, or stepparenthood, involves a major role change: from nonparent to parent. It involves a readjustment of other facets of life, such as relationships with family and friends, job, and marriage.

In studies of parenthood, the birth of a child (particularly the first), has been viewed as either a transition or crisis period in a parent's life (Hobbs, 1965, 1968; LeMasters, 1957; Meyerwitz & Feldman, 1966). Russell (1974) discusses the transition in terms of both problems and gratifications.

Rossi's (1968) sociological analysis describes parenthood in a developmental framework. She cites four factors as affecting preparation for parenthood: (1) scarcity of preparation for the role; (2) limited learning during pregnancy; (3) abruptness of the transition (no "apprenticeship" before, and then twenty-four-hour duty); and (4) lack of guidelines to successful parenthood.

Major and minor adjustments of the postpartum period are openly described by Rozdilsky and Banet (1972), along with helpful suggestions for coping with such problems as lack of sleep, feelings about babies and baby care, mental and marital stress, and pressures on the new parents.

PARENT–CHILD RELATIONSHIP

There are two distinct and separate parts to the parent–child relationship: the needs of the child and some of the effects of the parent on the child; and the needs of the parent and some of the effects of the child on the parent.

The Needs of the Child

The child has two basic categories of needs: physical and psychosocial. In the first category fall those requirements for physical growth and survival, such as food, clothing, sleep, safety and health care. In the second group fall those psychological needs for love, protection, acceptance, encouragement, education, and opportunities for satisfaction in work and play (Callahan, 1973; Talbot, 1976).

The Effects of the Parent or Caretaker on the Child

There is much that we do not know about the effects of the parent on the child. These effects are difficult to assess because of the many different personality and social variables involved. The mother has been the primary caretaker and has often been blamed for characteristics that emerge in later childhood or adulthood.

Studies show that babies do need loving relationships with familiar people who provide consistent care throughout the years of childhood, but the person does not need to be the biological mother (Schaeffer, 1977). In her cross cultural studies, Mead (1954) and others (Rapoport et al., 1977; Skolnick & Skolnick, 1977) note that the child's growth and development is facilitated when they are cared for by, interact with, and learn to trust many friendly, dependable people (adults and children). Talbot (1974) comments that when a difference of opinion arises regarding the rights and wishes of the parents or the child, the child's well-being is the most important factor.

The Needs of the Parent

Parenthood today is being reevaluated because of the number of social changes that affect parents and families, and thus need reconsideration. The old models for parents are no longer adequate and there are no new models for parents to follow. Our society as a whole has tended to have a negative model of parenting, as illustrated by such practices as isolation of the nuclear family, lack of social policies that support families and parents, and authoritarian and punitive childrearing practices.

Brim (1965) cites the six primary influences of parent behavior as ability factors, unconscious factors, cultural values, interpersonal and social controls, group structural determinants, and ecological or physical factors. Although some of these causes are external, a number are internal and relate to the parents' needs for personal growth and development. This seems to be especially true for women today. Many women are expanding their lives to include jobs or careers in addition to parenthood. Increasing numbers of men want to expand their lives to include growth in interpersonal relationship skills and in parenting roles in addition to their traditional career emphasis. An androgenous model would seem a more appropriate one for the full human development of both sexes.

Parents also have needs for knowing and understanding themselves in relation to their children. They need to feel good about being parents and about the ways they carry out their parenting roles. Much more discussion on the nurturing and support of parents is needed, as are more places for parents to openly discuss their honest feelings about being a parent, to freely relate their frustrations, fears, and misgivings as well as their joys and feelings of accomplishment. Society has readily supported the positive comments but turns a deaf ear to the negative. There is a need for social policies that provide active support and services to promote healthy parenting.

The Effects of the Child on the Parent

Recent research has demonstrated that the newborn begins to affect the actions of the parents in the early days of life (Lewis & Rosenblum, 1974), though some mothers will say the effects begin before birth! The effects continue to be experienced by the parents as the child moves through infancy and childhood (Bell & Harper, 1977).

Parents have known for a long time that their children have a profound effect on them. This belief is more recently being accepted and incorporated into the practice of professionals working with families.

The child affects the parents in many ways. Parents learn, through their experiences with their children, more about the kinds of people they are. Through their interactions, parents can learn to feel what the child feels, to examine their own attitudes, values, and beliefs about many facets of life, and to expand their definition of people and the world. In facing new stresses and crises involving their children or family life, parents face new opportunities for self-growth.

The reverse can also be true; the strains and demands of parenthood, in addition to the variety of other social forces impinging on the family, may result in family crisis and dysfunction. Child neglect, child abuse, other family violence, or parental illness can be the result of parental frustrations, overload, and unfulfilled expectations.

In the same way, the marital relationship may be either enhanced or may suffer as a result of parenting experiences. Unresolved stresses, or differences in child-rearing philosophies can produce additional pressure on a shaky or fragile relationship.

The relationship of the parents to their own parents may also be improved or changed. There is often a new perspective on their own upbringing, and an appreciation for the strength and wisdom of their parents.

EDUCATION AND NURSING INTERVENTION

An understanding of the development of the process of parenthood is important to nurses who work with parents and families at critical times during the parenting process. Nurses have unique opportunities for teaching, counseling, and supporting parents.

Parent Education

Some background information on education is helpful in understanding the parenting process and interventions. Brim (1965, p. 20) defines parent education as "an activity using educational techniques in order to effect change in parent role performance." He distinguishes *parent education* as directed to people already in the parent role and *preparental education* as that for people prior to their involvement in the parental role. Brim further designates three basic types of parent education as mass media, individual counseling, and group discussion. He notes that most of the parents involved in parent education efforts in the past have been middle-class mothers.

Parent education is separate from family life education, which is conducted for high school and college students and other young adults. Family life education concentrates on personality development and roles of family members (Duvall, 1970). It would appear that family life education could be a prerequisite to parent education.

There are a number of different approaches currently being used to help prepare people for parenthood, or to assist them while they are parents.

Parenthood education programs are being tested for use with young people, aged 13–18. Education for Parenthood projects have been launched by a joint effort of HEW's Office of Child Development and Office of Education, and also by groups such as the Salvation Army (Jones, 1975; Kruger, 1975; MacLachlan & Cole, 1978). These programs offer students the opportunity to learn about and work with children, and to learn more about themselves.

Another approach is the development of intervention programs to work with mothers and children from birth through early childrearing years (Gordon, 1973; Gross & Gross, 1977). Still other programs concentrate on helping parents understand children's behavior and use principles that foster more positive growth (Croake & Glover, 1977; Huber & Lynch, 1978). Two main approaches, based on democratic childrearing methods, are the Dreikurs-Adlerian approach and Gordon's Parent Effectiveness Training (Dreikurs & Soltz, 1964; Gordon, 1970). Other groups that seek to support and educate parents include MELD (Minnesota Early Learning Design) and Parents Anonymous. These groups have reached parents who would not otherwise have been informed. The nurse should try to be aware of other groups or programs in her or his community that provide educational services to parents and families.

Nurses have been involved in a variety of educational approaches with parents. They may work with high-risk parents on a one-to-one basis (Josten, 1978), with a peer teaching model used with minority parents (Johnston et al., 1977), in group teaching settings with a variety of client needs (Cooper, 1974; Spaulding, 1969; Thistleton, 1977) or as a member of an interdisciplinary health team working with families (Heinz, 1975).

One of the major problems in this educational area is that there has been a dearth of research on evaluation and effectiveness of educational methods. Hereford's study (1963) is one of a few carefully controlled studies using good experimental design. In his study he found the experimental parents showed a significantly greater change in attitudes than did the three groups of control parents. There is a definite need for more research and evaluation as well as an increase in educational interventions and programs for parents.

Educational-Nursing Intervention

The nurse working with families will be engaging in educational-counseling interventions with parents on a one-to-one basis or in group settings. Whatever the area of practice, there are some guidelines that may enhance the nurse's interactions and effectiveness with parents. These guides will be discussed through the use of a case study.

Case Study*

Susan and Mike Smith are beginning their parenthood years. Susan is 20, has had one year of college and has been working for two years as a secretary. Mike is 21 and has started his last year of college. He hopes to go into business with a friend when school is completed.

Susan is a middle child of a family with four children. Her father runs a hardware store and her mother is a housewife. Susan's parents live in the same town as the Smiths.

Mike is the youngest of three children. His mother is a teacher and his father works at a bank. Mike's parents live about 500 miles away.

Susan's pregnancy was confirmed three weeks ago, and she is scheduled for her first obstretrical visit. She is attending a hospital out-patient clinic where she will be seen by a nurse and an obstetrician throughout her pregnancy.

On her first visit, Susan is seen first by the nurse, Nancy, who introduces herself and welcomes Susan to the clinic. She talks informally with Susan and explains that she will be seeing her throughout her pregnancy. She gathers information on Susan's health history, obstetrical history, and personal data. The latter information is recorded on the *continuity of care* form. It is important that the prospective mother's entry into the health care system helps her feel comfortable in the setting, that she feels accepted by the staff, and that there be an open atmosphere for asking questions and receiving care. The continuity of care form is used to ensure that information assessed during the pregnancy will be used in planning for and supporting later aspects of care and parenting skills.

As a part of this program, Nancy teaches in the parent education program. She invites Susan and Mike to attend the early prenatal classes in the evening. Susan says she will attend but thinks that Mike will probably be too busy with school. Susan does attend the classes, which focus on the changes of pregnancy, nutrition, and physical and psychological well-being during pregnancy. Susan also borrows some books to read at home.

Nancy, who has a baccalaureate degree in nursing, has worked in the maternity department for two years; one year in the postpartum area and one year in the clinic. Nancy uses and expands on her basic nursing knowledge with her clients. It has been identified that the nurse needs knowledge of the teaching–learning process, of human behavior, of cultural norms and values, of family structure and function, and an understanding of group process (McCaffery, 1967).

Nancy reads materials pertinent to maternity care and parent education. She and the other nurses from the postpartum area, labor and delivery, and the parent education program meet bimonthly to discuss and evaluate their maternity care program and ways of improving themselves in their roles.

Nurses working with parents can continue to improve their education and practice with parents in many ways. There are many books available on different aspects of childrearing and parenting. Schools offer different levels of courses on family relationships and family sociology, which would provide more information on these areas.

The nurse's attitudes about parents and children emerge in her or his interactions with clients. Because some of these feelings may conflict with those of the parent, it is important for the nurse to acknowledge these factors. It is a clarifying experience for the nurse to write out her values, attitudes, beliefs and assumptions about parents and children. It can also be revealing for the nurse to analyze her own family background. How was she parented? Mothered? Fathered? What are the feelings about her child-rearing experiences? Being parented? What effect does she feel these have on her nursing practice with clients? The fact that the nurse had a very authoritarian father may have a bearing on the way she expects clients to follow all prenatal care directions.

Nancy continues to see Susan on subsequent visits to the clinic. As a part of each visit, in addition to obstetrical data, she continues to assess Susan's adaptation to the pregnancy as well as her readiness and preparation for parenthood. Susan and Mike had been dating seriously for a year and a half and Susan was over two months pregnant when they were married. Nancy understands that the couple is adapting to two new roles at the same time, wife and husband as well as prospective mother and father. She poses questions and comments to elicit some of Susan's feelings about these adaptations: What are some of the changes that have occurred in your life since your marriage? Since your pregnancy? How do you feel about the changes?

The nurse can assess the patient's reactions to the pregnancy by cueing-in to comments made about the baby's movements, her reaction to her changing body, and the ways the pregnancy changes are affecting her. Preparation for parenthood can be appraised by posing questions related to buying baby clothes, preparations for a place for the baby in the home or the feelings and concerns about getting ready to be parents.

Mike did accompany Susan on one clinic visit. He came into the examination room, but sat quietly throughout the time, often reading in his book. He did express an interest in listening to the baby's fetal heart tones when the experience was offered and commented with a smile, "I never knew it beat so fast."

Nancy spent time during this visit discussing some of the ways in which pregnancy changes a couple's relationship. Mike commented very little but did say that he felt "pregnancy is a woman's problem." He also mentioned that Susan was a lot more "grouchy" since she had become pregnant and

*The continuity of care and parent education approaches used in this case study are based on the program of the maternity department of the University of Minnesota Hospitals in Minneapolis. The author directed the parent education program and worked as a clinical specialist in the maternity department from 1972 to 1975. She wishes to thank all the nurses who have contributed so much to the success of this program.

that he didn't know pregnancy affected so many things. Susan talked quite openly about being tired, "getting fatter" and being afraid of labor. Nancy talked with them further and encouraged them to come to late pregnancy expectant parents classes.

The nurse needs to be aware of basic principles of learning, and resistance to learning when working with parents (Auerbach, 1968; Redman, 1976). (Some of the basic principles are listed next and some are interspersed in related parts of this case study.)

Effective educational approaches start with the parent. This includes an assessment of the client, as Nancy has been doing with Susan and Mike. What are the parents' goals in the learning process? What is their background—attitudes, values, beliefs? What educational approach would best meet their needs? Where is the parent in the parent development process?

Learning can be facilitated once the parent has an interest in an area or wants to learn about the experience. Susan and Mike did come to the expectant parents classes. Nancy used a small group discussion format. Introductions were relaxed and informal, with group members sharing information about themselves and planning and choosing what they would like to discuss in the sessions.

The parent's learning may be greater if there is an open, exploring environment. Different alternatives can be explored to encourage the parent to take responsibility for choices, and to be more committed to the decision or choice Parental learning can be greatly expanded in a group setting, where parents can learn from and support one another.

Although the classes stressed preparation for labor and delivery (information and exercises), much time was devoted to exploring areas and concerns about baby care and prospective parenthood. Nancy asked the parents to write out how they were parented, and how they felt about their parents. What kind of parents did they want to be? What did they see as obstacles to being that kind of parent? The prospective parents' comments were discussed in the next class, with interesting insights and many similarities.

The discussion pointed out that the prospective parents came from diverse backgrounds and were raised with a variety of parenting styles and family situations. Parent educators should embrace the belief that there are multiple conceptions of the good or effective parent. The basic physical, psychological, and social needs of the child can be met in a variety of ways; whether there is a single parent, an extended family, or a nuclear family.

In helping prospective parents to consider the kind of parents they want to be, it is also important to encourage them to think about their goals in having a child. What needs of their own do they expect the child to meet? Do they need someone to love, or someone to control? What does the child symbolize for them? Is the infant expected to carry on the family name? Hold their marriage together? The educator-nurse can help parents to examine the reality of these beliefs, and to better understand themselves and their situations.

Many nurses will be working with clients who will not come to classes, or with one parent when the other will not come. These same learning-sharing techniques of helping the parent review her or his own parenting, and also to begin thinking ahead to being at home can be adapted to one-to-one settings with patients. This may be difficult for some expectant parents whose regular behavior does not include planning ahead. Or, the parent may be a member of a sociocultural group with expectations that conflict with those of the health care provider. The nurse may want to use peer teachers from those cultural groups in that type of situation.

During the Smiths' visits to the clinic, Nancy also spent time assessing their support system. It was disclosed that, although her mother lived in town, Susan was not sure she wanted her around after the baby was born because they didn't "get along." Nancy asked about Mike's parents, and Susan mentioned that they lived in a distant city. Mike's father was an alcoholic and there were many negative feelings between the father and son. The couple got along well with Mike's mother, and she had said she could come and help out for a few days.

When Susan went into labor, Mike stayed and worked with her during labor but had decided not to be in the delivery room. Susan and Mike did spend time together after the delivery, talking with and holding their new baby son.

Susan's postpartum hospital period went relatively well. Susan had decided to bottle-feed the baby, because she planned to return to part-time work in six weeks. The primary nurse caring for Susan and the baby in the hospital was Jean. Nancy also stopped in to see Susan and the baby, and to leave a prenatal class evaluation form for Susan to complete.

Jean used the continuity of care information form (started in the clinic and added to by the staff from parent education and labor and delivery) for planning Susan's care. Jean planned Susan's hospital care and teaching after consulting with Susan and Mike. Readiness for learning was assessed and care planned accordingly.

Jean observed the Smiths' behavior and listened to their comments to assess their parenting development. Susan had the baby in the room with her during the day and wanted to learn how to care for her son. She seemed uncomfortable and awkward caring for her baby and remarked, "These little creatures sure scare me."

Mike spent about an hour each day at the hospital. Although there were open visiting privileges for fathers, Mike seemed somewhat hesitant about being involved; Jean encouraged his participation. He did come in and hold his son the first two days and watched Susan bathe him on the third day. That day he asked if he could give the baby his late afternoon feeding and was observed humming to and rocking the baby in his arms. Jean spent much time talking with them, reinforcing positive parenting behaviors, and discussing possible situations and problems that might occur at home.

The learning should be meeting some of the parents needs, either for more information, different ways of handling problems or issues, or in helping the parent find greater satisfaction in parenting. Parents may often be seeking support for themselves or their parenting behavior through educational experiences. Parents can also derive much satisfaction when they are helped to identify needed changes, and then are supported in this growth.

As a part of the continuity of care program for Mike and Susan, the primary nurse offered to make a home visit (as she offered to each of her patients) after discharge from the hospital. She also gave them the station phone number and encouraged them to call if any questions came up at home. Jean usually called all her patients on their second day home, to offer support and a familiar, caring voice.

Jean made her visit to the Smiths one week after Susan's discharge. She arranged to come in the late afternoon, when Mike would also be home from school and before he went to work. Susan met Jean at the door with a long list of questions and looking very tired. Jean spent an hour answering their questions on feeding, and sleeping. She also spent time assessing their parenting patterns; their reactions to their baby, the demands on their time, sharing of duties, their physical and psychological states; and reevaluating their support structure of friends and relatives Susan said her mother had been over to help but "she just took over the baby and I felt so incompetent." Jean spent time talking over alternative ways for Susan and Mike to handle this and other problems.

Mike had been gone a lot with school and work, and felt guilty about leaving Susan and the baby but not yet ready to babysit alone. They explored ways of sharing the responsibility of the baby, and yet getting out together. Susan had been calling her hospital roommate, who was a mother of three, as a support person.

Jean also taught a postpartum parenting class and invited Susan and Mike to come, and bring the baby. They were told that the group included other couples from their expectant parents classes.

Susan and Mike decided to attend the parenting classes and to bring their son. The groups were established as an optional part of the hospital's continuity of care program. The primary goal was to provide support and information for new parents. Susan and Mike learned that other couples were having many of the same experiences of adjustment, and feelings of insecurity and of wanting to know more about care and growth and development of their baby. Jean presented the most recent information and also some of the differences in childrearing philosophies.

Educational information must be shared with parents in language that makes it understandable to them. Parents also need to know that they are not the only ones having these types of problems. This is why groups work so well for many new parents.

Jean encouraged the couples to discuss their relationships with their own parents and to be aware of ways in which those feelings affect new parents in their interactions with their children. Both Mike and Susan said they were trying to deal with some of the negative feelings and experiences they had had with their parents. They realized that was an area that

they would need to continue to work on, because they each felt that grandparents should be an important part of their child's life. Jean thanked the Smiths for sharing such honest feelings and encouraged them to continue growing.

The continuity of care program used evaluation forms to ask the parents for comments and suggestions relating to all aspects of the program. These were reviewed by the staff and used as a basis for planning changes and making improvements in the program. Parents were provided with a list of continuing parents' groups, or other groups in the community, that provided for parent support and education.

Evaluation should be a continuous process in the teaching-learning experience. The parent needs to evaluate her or his learning to be able to identify growth areas and areas that will require continued help. The nurse should seek evaluation from the parents about the program; what was helpful, what was not, and what could be changed to provide better assistance. The nurse could also be using some systematic method of evaluating the program, such as changes in parent behaviors and attitudes. Criteria could be established in advance by the nurse, or a contract arrangement could be made with the parent. It is important to document this aspect of nursing practice, because it is an important part of working with families.

This case study has been presented to illustrate how nurses can support and guide parents through pregnancy, postpartum, and in the early weeks and months after birth. It shows that parenting is a process of development, which can be guided by nursing interventions.

Nurses can continue to assess, support, and educate parents during the preschool and school years as well. We have a very special and unique challenge to support the healthy development of parenting, and improve family life.

REFERENCES AND ADDITIONAL READINGS

Arms, S. (1975). *Immaculate deception: A new look at women and childbirth in America.* Boston, San Francisco: Houghton Mifflin.

Auerbach, A.B. (1968). *Parents learn through discussion.* New York: Wiley.

Bell, R.Q., & Harper, L.V. (1977) *Child effects on adults.* New York: Wiley.

Benedek, T. (1970). The family as a psychologic field. In J. Anthony & T. Benedek (Eds.), *Parenthood: Its psychology and psychopathology.* Boston: Little, Brown, pp. 109–136.

Biller, H. & Meredith, D. (1974). *Father power.* New York: David McKay Co.

Brim, O.G. Jr. (1965). *Education for child rearing.* New York: Russell Sage Foundation.

Bronfenbrenner, U. (1976). Who cares for America's children? In V.C.

Vaughan & T.B. Brazelton (Eds.), *The family—can it be saved?* Chicago: Yearbook, pp. 3–32.

Callahan, S.C. (1973). *Parenting: Principles & politics of parenthood.* Garden City, N.Y.: Doubleday.

Caplan, G. (1961). *An approach to community mental health.* New York: Grune & Stratton.

Carter, H. (1977). Quoted in L. Peter (Ed), *Peters' quotations.* New York: William Morrow, p. 103.

Colman, A., & Colman, L. (1973). *Pregnancy, the psychological experience.* New York: Seabury Press.

Cooper, I. (1974). Group sessions for new mothers. *Nursing Outlook, 22*(4), 251.

Croake, J.R., & Glover, K.E. (1977). A history and evaluation of parent education. *The Family Coordinator, 26*(2), 151–158.

Dreikurs, R., & Soltz, V. (1964). *Children: The challenge.* New York: Hawthorn Books.

Duvall, E.M. (1970). *Faith in families.* Chicago: Rand McNally.

Duvall, E.M. (1977). *Marriage and family development.* Philadelphia: Lippincott.

Gilberg, A. (1975). The stress of parenting. *Child Psychiatry and Human Development, 6*(2), 59–67.

Gordon, I. (1973). *An early intervention project: A longitudinal look* (ERIC ED 093498). Gainesville, Fl.: Florida University, Gainesville Institute for Development of Human Resources.

Gordon, T. (1970). *Parent effectiveness training.* New York: Peter H. Wyden, Inc.

Greenberg, M., & Morris, N. (1974). Engrossment: The newborn's impact upon the father. *American Journal of Orthopsychiatry, 44*(4), 520–531.

Gross, B. & Gross, R. (1977). Parent–child development centers: creating models for parent education. *Children Today, 6*(6), 18–22.

Group for the Advancement of Psychiatry (GAP). (1973). *The joys and sorrows of parenthood.* New York: Scribner.

Harris, B.G. (1977). Learning about parenting. *Nursing Outlook, 25*(7), 457–459.

Heinz, L. The nurse's role in a parenting process program. *Journal of Psychiatric Nursing and Mental Health Services, 13*(2), 27–30.

Hereford, C.F. (1963). *Changing parental attitudes through group discussion.* Austin: University of Texas Press.

Hobbs, D.F. (1965). Parenthood as crisis, a third study. *Journal of Marriage and the Family, 27,* 367–372.

Hobbs, D.F. (1968). Transition to parenthood: A replication and an extension. *Journal of Marriage and the Family, 30,* 413–417.

Hoffman, L.W., & Hoffman, M. (1973). The value of children to parents. In J.T. Fawcett (Ed.), *Psychological perspectives on population.* New York: Basic Books.

Huber, H., & Lynch, F. (1978). Teaching behavioral skills to parents: A preventive role for mental health. *Children Today, 7*(1), 8–10.

Hughes, C.B. (1977). An eclectic approach to parent group education. *Nursing Clinics of North America, 12*(3), 469–479.

Jessner, L., Weigert, E., & Foy, J.L. (1970). The development of parental attitudes during pregnancy. In E.J. Anthony & T. Benedek (Eds.), *Parenthood: Its psychology and psychopathology.* Boston: Little, Brown, pp. 209–243.

Johnston, M., Kayne, M., & Mittleider, K. (1977). Putting more pep in parenting. *American Journal of Nursing, 77*(6), 994–995.

Jones, P. S. (1975). Parenthood education in a city high school. *Children Today, 4*(2), 7–11.

Josten, L. (1978). Out-of-hospital care for a pervasive family problem—child abuse. *MCN: The American Journal of Maternal Child Nursing, 7*(4), 111–116.

Klaus, M.H., & Kennell, J.H. (1976). *Maternal–infant bonding.* St. Louis: Mosby, pp. 38–98.

Kruger, W.S. (1975). Education for parenthood and school age parents. *Journal of School Health, 45*(5), 292–295.

LeMasters, E.E. (1957). Parenthood as crisis. *Marriage and Family Living, 19*(4), 352–355.

LeMasters, E.E. (1970). *Parents in modern america.* Homewood, Il.: Dorsey Press.

Lewis, M., & Rosenblum, L.A. (1974). *The effect of the infant on its caregiver.* New York: Wiley.

MacLachlan, P., & Cole, E.P. (1978). Learning about children and family life; the salvation army education for parenthood program. *Children Today, 7*(3), 7–11.

McBride, A.B. (1973). *The growth and development of mothers.* New York: Harper & Row.

McCaffery, M.S. (1967). An approach to parent education. *Nursing Forum, 6*(1), 77–93.

Mead, M. (1954). Some theoretical considerations on the problem of mother–child separation. *American Journal of Orthopsychiatry, 24*(3), 471–483.

Meyerwitz, J.H., & Feldman, H. (1966). Transition to parenthood. *Psychiatric Research Reports, 20,* 78–84.

Parke, R.D. (1974). Father–infant interaction. In M. Klaus, T. Leger, & M. Trause (Eds.), *Maternal attachment and mothering disorders: a round table,* Sausalito, Ca.: Johnson & Johnson Co.

Rapoport, R., Rapoport, R., & Strelitz, Z. (1977). *Fathers, mothers, and society.* New York: Basic Books.

Redman, B. (1976). *The process of patient teaching in nursing.* St. Louis: Mosby.

Rising, S.S. (1974) The fourth stage of labor: Family integration. *American Journal of Nursing, 74*(5), 870–874.

Rossi, A.S. (1968). Transition to parenthood. *Journal of Marriage and the Family, 30,* 26–39.

Rozdilsky, M.L. & Banet, B. (1972) *What now? A handbook for couples (especially women) postpartum.* Seattle: Magic Machine.

Russell, C.S. (1974). Transition to parenthood: Problems and gratifications. *Journal of Marriage and the Family, 36*(2), 294–301.

Rutter, M. (1977). Dimensions of parenthood: Some myths and some suggestions. In R. Rapoport, R. Rapoport, & Z. Strelitz (Eds.), *Fathers, mothers, and society.* New York: Basic Books, p. 3.

Schaffer, R. (1977). *Mothering.* Cambridge, Ma.: Harvard University Press.

Skolnick, A. (1973). *The intimate environment.* Boston: Little, Brown.

Skolnick, A.S., & Skolnick, J.H. (1977). *Family in transition.* Boston: Little, Brown.

Spaulding, M.R. (1969). Adapting postpartum teaching to mothers' low-income life-styles. In B. Bergerson (Ed.), *Current concepts in clinical nursing.* St. Louis: Mosby, pp. 280–291.

Talbot, N. (Ed.) (1974). *Raising children in modern America.* Boston: Little, Brown.

Thistleton, K.S. (1977). The abusive and neglectful parent: Treatment through parent education. *Nursing Clinics of North America, 12*(3), 513–524.

Veevers, J.E. (1973). Voluntary childless wives: An exploratory study. *Sociology and Social Research, 19,* 356–365.

Wuerger, M.K. (1976). The young adult: Stepping into parenthood. *American Journal of Nursing, 76*(8), 1283–1285.

Chapter 14 | Fourth Trimester

Laura Duckett Newton

THE POSTPARTUM PERIOD has traditionally been defined as the time required by the body to return to its prepregnant physiological state (Clark, 1979; Easterling, 1977; Jensen et al., 1977; Pritchard & MacDonald, 1976; Ziegel & Cranley, 1978). Recently, the term *fourth trimester* has been coined (Donaldson, 1977; Edwards, 1973; Ziegel & Cranley, 1978). This conveys several meanings: The childbearing process involves one entire year; medical definitions have for too long guided nursing practice; and the three-month period following delivery is a time that is at least as crucial as each of the trimesters of actual pregnancy.

There is considerable documentation in the literature to support Rubin's (1975) assertion that maternity nursing care stops too soon, creating gaps in the health care that a family receives after the birth of a new baby. Traditionally, obstetricians have scheduled postpartum checkups six weeks after delivery, since major physiological restorative processes are usually complete by that time (Easterling, 1977). Some writers now recommend that a postpartum exam be done three weeks after delivery in order to detect any abnormalities that might be developing during the mid- to late-postpartum period (Barden, 1975; Pritchard & MacDonald, 1976). The mother's postpartum checkup and "well-baby" screening may be the only contact the family has with a health care provider after discharge from the hospital; but the postpartum needs are often far more complex than the mother's physical recovery and the infant's growth and development. Nurses are beginning to document, with research data, the need for more comprehensive services to the postpartum family, especially during the first six weeks after delivery (Gruis, 1977; Hill, 1978; Sumner & Fritsch, 1977; Williams, 1977).

BECOMING PARENTS—CRISIS OR TRANSITION?

LeMasters (1957) studied forty-six married, middle-class couples, whose first child was less than 5 years old, using an unstructured interview technique. Data were coded using a 5-point scale ranging from no crisis to severe crisis. Eighty-three percent of the couples were found to have experienced severe to extensive crisis while adapting to first time parenthood. Among these thirty-eight couples, thirty-five of the pregnancies were planned or desired, thirty-four rated their marriages as good or better, and crisis did not appear to be related to neurosis or other psychiatric disorder. However, these parents felt they were almost totally unprepared for their new roles as parents. The mothers attributed their problems to loss of sleep, chronic fatigue, confinement to home, giving up outside employment, additional laundry and declining housekeeping standards, guilt feelings related to not being better mothers, day and night care of infant, and worry over appearance and weight. The fathers were stressed by many of the above as well as by decreased sexual response on the part of their wives, economic pressures, decreased social life, concern about a second pregnancy, and disenchantment with the parental role. All eight professional women studied who had retired due to the birth of the infant, experienced extensive to severe crisis. LeMasters suggested two further reasons to explain the study findings: first, the arrival of the first child forces the parents to reorganize into a triangle group system, which falls into the volatile "pair and isolate" combination; and second, children and parenthood have been extremely romanticized in our society.

This exploratory study, despite its various methodological problems (retrospective, nonrandom sample, small study population, and no reliable method for coding of data) is especially significant because it served as a springboard for a series of studies.

Dyer (1963), using a sample of thirty-two couples and a Likert-type scale to measure crisis, replicated LeMaster's study. In this sample, the firstborn child of each couple was not over 2 years old at the time data were collected. Fifty-three percent of the couples were classified in the extensive and severe categories, and another thirty-eight percent in the moderate category.

Using a random sampling of white, urban first-time parents, Hobbs (1965) measured the degree of crisis related to new parenthood using an objectively scored twenty-three-item checklist, which was derived from LeMaster's description of difficulties experienced by new parents. On a 3-point scale (none = 0, somewhat = 1, very much = 2), subjects rated, the degree to which they were bothered by each item on the checklist. Total scores could thus range from 0 (no crisis) to 46 (severe crisis). There was a sixty-five percent return of useable questionnaires, which yielded a study population of fifty-three couples. The babies' ages ranged from 3 to 18 weeks (mean 9.8). The fathers' mean crisis score was 6.3 and the mothers' was 9.06; there was no correlation between husbands' and wives' scores. Eighty-seven percent of the couples were classified as experiencing slight crisis, and thirteen percent moderate crisis. None scored in the extensive or severe categories, in sharp contrast to the eighty-three percent of LeMaster's couples who did.

Of the twenty-three items on Hobbs's checklist, two items, interruption of routine habits and money problems, bothered seventy-five and sixty percent of fathers, respectively. Four items were scored as bothersome by mothers: interruption of routine habits by seventy-four percent of mothers, tiredness by sixty-eight percent, increased money problems by sixty-six percent, and feeling emotionally upset by sixty percent.

A second study by Hobbs (1968) of twenty-seven couples similar to those in his first study yielded findings very like those of his first study. In addition to using a checklist, an unstructured interview was also used to measure crisis. There was a significant correlation between scores obtained using the two tools.

Jacoby (1969) critiqued and discussed the four previously cited "parenthood as crisis" studies and one unpublished study, in an attempt to assess the state of accession research. He summarized certain methodological problems common to some or all of the studies: inconsistant, and possibly invalid, measurements of crisis; combination of husband and wife scores even though they might be expected to differ (as Hobbs reported); small samples; and nonrepresentative sampling except in the Hobbs studies. To this list can be added the basic problems of designs that use recall data. Referring specifically to the Hobbs checklist, one has to wonder if being "bothered" about a lot of the twenty-three items "very much" necessarily adds up to crisis as it was defined by LeMasters.

Jacoby also suggested the following reasons that might help to explain the great differences in the findings of the five studies:

- The differences in findings might be artificial—a result of the differences in scoring procedures. This is possible but not likely.
- The differences might be due to differences in the methods of data collection (i.e., unstructured interviews, Likert-type scale, and checklists). However, it is difficult to completely explain the magnitude of the differences this way, especially since LeMasters (using unstructured interviews) and Dyer (using Likert-type scale) reported similar findings.
- The age of the child at the time of data collection may be an important variable. In the five studies there seems to be a relationship between ages of children and crisis scores, with higher scores related to higher ages of children at the time of data collection.
- The differences in results may be partly explained by the differences in the study samples. Since the middle-class samples of LeMasters and Dyer had higher crisis scores than Hobbs's two predominantly working-class samples, it is possible that the transition to parenthood is more traumatic for middle-class parents than parents of the working-class.*

---

*For a discussion of related literature that provides theoretical support for this explanation, see Jacoby, 1969.

TABLE 14-1 Differences between a crisis and a transition phase

Characteristic	Crisis	Transition Phase
Time	Acute; ranges from very brief periods to longer; 6–8 weeks is usual.	Varies in length; tends to be much longer.
Marked behavioral change	Individual is less effective than usual. There is an attempt to discharge inner tension through activity. Usual methods of coping are tried without success. Frustration increases and effectiveness decreases.	Loss of effectiveness may not be as obvious to others; depends on the complexity of the situation and the person's coping ability.
Subjective aspects	Feelings of helplessness and ineffectiveness are experienced due to what seems to be an insoluble problem. Individual perceives a threat to major life goals. Anxiety, fear, guilt, or defensive reactions result.	Feelings result from person's "inability to function in a well-organized manner in the usual situations of every day life. At the time there doesn't seem to be any way to change one's own functioning" (Crummette, 1975, p. 70).
Relative aspects	Individual's perception of threat and crisis is unique to her or him. What constitutes a crisis for one person may not for another.	The intensity and duration vary depending on the number of tasks with which the individual is trying to cope.
Organismic	Individual will experience generalized physical tension, which may be expressed through a variety of symptoms.	

Adapted from Crummette, 1975.

Jacoby (1969) and Rossi (1968) suggested that there is a very basic problem with accession-to-parenthood research, which is oriented around crisis, since this provides only a partial picture of the adjustment to parenthood. Jacoby felt that such research had "allowed little opportunity or stimulus for the reporting of affectively positive or neutral attitudes toward the adjustments required by parenthood" (p. 722). Rossi stated that the time had come to "drop the concept of 'normal crises' and to speak directly, instead, of the transition to an impact of parenthood" (p. 28).

Crummette (1975) described crises and transition phases as similar, yet different. She listed five characteristics of crisis, and contrasted crises and transition phases in relation to these: Table 14-1 summarizes her points. On the basis of this comparison, one could conclude that becoming a parent is a major transition, which is perceived as a crisis in some cases.

Shereshefsky (1973), summarized findings of an interdisciplinary study of sixty-four couples and discussed the idea of a *first* pregnancy as crisis. She concluded that if crisis means "a stress involving threat or loss requiring resources beyond the ordinary" (p. 244), then their study data suggested that the first pregnancy was not a crisis in most cases. Those families in their sample who

experienced crisis, as defined above, had been predisposed to it. However, crisis, if defined as a transitional phase or turning point, was experienced by all of the couples in the study.

For a variety of reasons, the developmental transition to parenthood appears to be a more difficult role change than others (e.g., marriage and change of jobs). Rossi (1968) described four broad stages in a role-cycle and for each stage contrasted the parental role with the marital and occupational role. Table 14-2, which is based on Rossi's discussion, lists each role-cycle stage and its description and, for each stage, contrasts the parental role with the marital role.

Several factors, described by Rossi (1968), contribute to the uniqueness of the parental role and make the transition to parenthood particularly difficult, despite the potential rewards.

• The infant's need for the parents, particularly the mother, is absolute. The baby is *completely* dependent on them.

• There is cultural pressure to assume the parent role. (Despite a growing trend during the 1970s for nonparenthood, it is extremely probable that many couples still are somewhat pressured into parenthood despite having ambivalent feelings about the role.)

TABLE 14-2 Stages in a role-cycle: parental versus marital role

Role-Cycle Stages	Marital Role	Parental Role	Comment
Anticipatory stage	Engagement period	Pregnancy	A crucial difference here is that the man and woman each know each other as a unique real person during the anticipatory stage, so adjustment is based on reality. The child can only be fantasized during pregnancy.
Honeymoon stage: the time period immediately following the full assumption of the adult role.	Begins with marriage ceremony and continues through literal honeymoon into the psychic honeymoon, which is the extended post-marital period of close intimacy and joint activity. The onset of pregnancy can be viewed as marking the end of the honeymoon stage.	The period after childbirth when intimate and prolonged contact between parent and child occurs such that and attachment forms.	
Plateau stage: protracted middle period of a role-cycle during which the role is fully exercised.	This stage can be subdivided for both of the above roles. A couple will be in this stage of both of the above roles simultaneously for an indefinite number of years, if one or more children are born and reared.		The opportunity exists for conflict between these two roles.
Disengagement-termination stage; immediately precedes and includes the actual termination of the role.	Separation and divorce or death of spouse.	"A unique characteristic of parental role termination is the fact that it is not clearly marked by any specific act but is an attenuated process of termination with little cultural prescription about when the authority and obligations of a parent end" (Rossi, 1968, p. 30). Marriage of a child is often viewed as the psychological termination of the active parent role.	For the parental role the ambiguity related to this stage has the potential for producing or intensifying a variety of stressors.

Adapted from Rossi, 1968.

• Inception of the parental role may not be voluntary. Engagements can be consciously considered, freely entered, and freely terminated, if desired. Pregnancy may result from recreational rather than procreative sexual encounters. Despite advances in contraceptive technology, unplanned pregnancies still occur frequently. Abortion (though now legal) is still not fully socially sanctioned.

• Except in rare cases, parenthood once commenced is irrevocable. Divorce and remarriage are now widely accepted; unsatisfactory jobs can be terminated and more satisfying ones sought; but children cannot be "traded in."

• There are many deficits in the preparation for parenthood in our society: (1) the educational system in our country focuses on the cognitive development of children and youth and preparation for occupational roles, often at the expense of preparation for marital and parental roles; and (2) limited preparation for parental roles occurs during pregnancy. Although there has been a tremendous improvement in prenatal education during the last decade, the focus is still primarily preparation for labor and delivery. This is due in part to a belief, on the part of many childbirth educators, that parents are not ready to learn about parenthood before the child is born. However, many strategies can be used prenatally to help the parents think about coping with the demands of parenthood. The transition to parenthood is abrupt: The birth of the child is not followed by a gradual assumption of responsibility. While becoming more prevalent than in the past, guidelines for parenting—available from different sources—often suggest conflicting approaches and thus confuse vulnerable new parents.

EXHIBIT 14-1   Tasks for new parents*

- Attach to infant
- Plan activities to optimize the mother's physiological restorative processes and lactation
- Reconstruct and review the birth experience
- Work through any losses associated with the childbirth experience or new parenthood (e.g., pregnant body, ideal or perfect child, ideal birth experience, freedom, any role given up or changed, some of partner's attention)
- Develop infant caretaking skills
- Stimulate infant's growth and development
- Accept infant as a unique individual and encourage that individuality
- Develop a satisfactory relationship with partner that includes parenting:

  Maintain or improve the couple relationship (i.e., emotional and sexual intimacy, intellectual exchange, recreational activities)

  Facilitate the partner's development as a parent:

  Wife—promote the father–child relationship from the beginning (bonding, caretaking, enjoying infant's growth and development); recognize and reinforce husband's growth as a father

  Husband—share parenting responsibilities; recognize and reinforce wife's growth as a mother;

*The terms *husband* and *wife* are used in order to simply and clearly distinguish between the roles of partner-mate and parent. The tasks are also applicable to the unmarried couple living together as a family, and, to some extent, to the single-mother family where the boyfriend is somewhat involved.

attempt to decrease stressors impinging upon wife

Develop view of infant as "ours"

- Develop mutual conceptions of major roles
- Allocate time and energy to all roles (wife, mother, worker, or professional; husband, father, worker, or professional)
- Each partner has the task of maintaining his or her own identity as an individual
- Develop a sense of being a family:

  Learn about new things to do and places to go as a family with an infant

  Adapt some of previous couple activities so that they can be done as a family with an infant (e.g., biking, boating, camping)

- Alter environment to meet needs of infant:

  Obtain supplies and needed equipment

  Provide for safety of infant (see Duvall, 1977, pp. 233-235, for excellent suggestions)

  Allow for infant's exploration as his or her locomotion begins

- Plan for adequate income and housing to meet the needs of the expanded family
- Work out relationships with relatives
- Maintain relationships with friends
- Make decisions regarding having or not having another child; implement family-planning method as indicated
- Improve strategies for dealing with conflict:

  Accept conflict as a part of life that is neither good nor bad, but neutral

  Learn more effective conflict resolution skills

FAMILY DEVELOPMENTAL TASKS: THE FIRST YEAR OF NEW PARENTHOOD

The writings of Erik Erikson (1963) have accentuated the fact that human development is a lifelong process rather than one that ends with adulthood. According to his model of development, individuals who have become parents are dealing with the stage where the ego quality of generativity, rather than stagnation, will hopefully emerge. Becoming a parent does not, of course, mean that the developmental task has automatically been achieved. "Generativity...is primarily the concern in establishing and guiding the next generation.... [T]he concept...is meant to include such more popular synonyms as productivity and creativity" (Erickson, 1963, p. 267). New parenthood then provides the opportunity for developing generativity, although it can certainly be developed in many other ways as well.

Family stages as defined by Duvall (1977) have been used by a variety of disciplines for more than three decades. These stages and tasks have been criticized for being geared primarily to the traditional husband–wife–child nuclear family structure in which the husband takes on the role of sole breadwinner unless the woman must help supplement the family income. For example, task 8 for the wife with an infant includes "supplementing the family income when it seems wise or necessary, in ways that safeguard the well-being of all members of the family" (Duvall, 1977, p. 225).

While the tasks are, no doubt, intended to represent a high level of development at each stage, some tasks sound too idealistic and in some cases there seems to be some denial of the realities of being human.

Despite the criticisms that have been made, Duvall's family stages and developmental tasks can be a helpful tool for nurses working with childbearing and child-rearing families, if the tasks are adapted according to family structure, and if they are interpreted in light of the trend toward more liberated roles in some families. An example of such an adaptation is given in Exhibit 14-1.

EXHIBIT 14-2   Operations involved in the process of assuming the maternal role*

Rubin (1967a) studied the process of attaining the maternal role, and described the following operations as integral to this process:

Taking-on

- *Mimicry* is the adoption of simple behavioral manifestations (e.g., dress, speech affects, gestures) that are recognizable symbols of the status desired.
- *Role play* is similar to mimicry but "goes beyond the outward symbolic manifestations of status into an *acting out* of 'what a person of this position does in a situation like this.' The acting out is of short duration and situation specific" (p. 241). Objects for role play can be children of friends and relatives and even animals. In Rubin's study, if subject was already a mother, she role-played being the mother of two. "It seemed to be immaterial who the object was, as long as the role play took them into some function of the role" (p. 242).

Taking-In

- *Fantasy* is the internalization of role play. Possible situations are elaborated in fantasy.
- *Introjection-projection-rejection* resembles mimicry, where there is a taking-on of isolated acts. However, Rubin found that in introjection-projection-rejection,

"action began within the self, a model was found outside, and the behavior or event of the model was then matched for 'fit' with the behavior or event that the subject was experiencing. If the 'fit' was good, it served as reinforcement. If the 'fit' was unsatisfactory, it was rejected" (p. 242). Models can be the same for mimicry and introjection-projection-rejection, but the operations are different. The circular process seems to firmly bind-in role traits.

Letting-Go

- *Grief work* "is a letting-go of a former identity in some role(s) that are incompatible with the assumption of the new role" (p. 243). "Separating-out in grief work seemed to be dependent upon the extent of the taking-in, or binding-in to the new role" (p. 244). Multiparas have grief work to do related to changing their role with their other children. These mothers seem as bewildered by the task of dividing or changing their mother role as they were when assuming it with the first child.
- *Completion of grief work* comes only after role identification is fairly well established. "Most grief work was not finalized but was brought to some level of resolution" (p. 244).

*Quoted material is from Rubin, R. (1967a). Attainment of the maternal role, part I: Process. *Nursing Research, 16,* 237–245.

If the infant is not the first child, the parents will be dealing with the developmental tasks associated with being parents of older children as well as again coping with tasks associated with a new infant. One important new task for the parent having an additional child is to facilitate the adaptation of the older child (or children) to the new sibling. For some families this seems to be the most stressful task, and thus consumes the most energy.

THE POSTDELIVERY YEAR: RESEARCH

In a study by Rubin (1967a) designed to explore the process through which the maternal role is assumed, five primiparas and four multiparas were studied in depth, both prenatally and during the first postpartum month. Additional subjects from the same population were studied briefly prenatally or postnatally. Exhibit

14–2 provides a description of the operations involved in the process of assuming the maternal role (see also Figure 14–1). Achievement of the process led to the sense of being in the role.

Rubin's study is thought-provoking in several ways. There is no indication that nurses, other than the interviewers who had children, were used as models. Did women in the study sample really not use other nurse models or did something about the study methodology obscure the identification of nurse models? If the study were replicated, using random sampling and a large number of tracer subjects, would the same findings emerge? Additional questions about the validity of the tool used for coding data and about the reliability of coding would need to be answered prior to replication of the study. In a future study one could look for relationships between certain structural variables and the use of the various operations.

Although some mention is made of fathers engaging

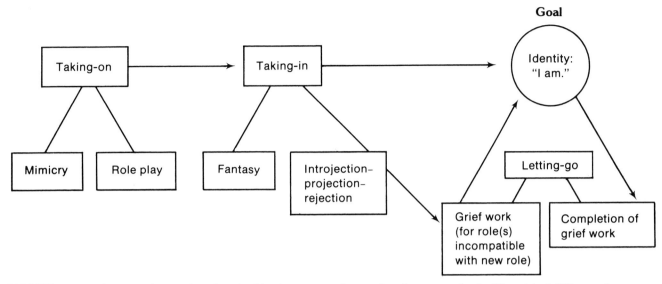

FIGURE 14-1 Diagram of operations involved in the process of assuming the maternal role. The critical difference between taking-on and taking-in is "the subject's question moves from how-does-one (stereotyped-one) behave in this position to how-will-it-be-for-me in this position, in this situation" (Rubin, 1967a, p. 242).

in the role assumption operations (Rubin, 1967b), they were not studied as subjects. One might question, then, whether fathers engage in operations similar to or like those described by the findings of this study.

If one makes the assumption that the study findings are valid, how can nurses facilitate the parents' progression through the operations so that role identity is achieved? Can nurses serve as models in the operations? Or are nurses rejected as models because they appear too competent?

In another study using role theory as the conceptual framework, Meleis and Swendson (1978) tested role supplementation as a nursing intervention. Role supplementation had been previously defined by Meleis (1975) as "the conveying of information or experience necessary to bring the role incumbent and significant others to feel awareness of the anticipated behavior patterns, units, sentiments, sensations, and goals involved in each role and its complement" (p. 267). The goal of role supplementation was role mastery; its process was communication; its components were role clarification and role taking; and its strategies were reference groups, role rehearsal and role modeling. (See Figure 14–2 for a diagramatic representation of role supplementation.)

Is there a relationship between the use of role supplementation and wives' postpartum reactions (a group of variables related to self and baby)? Data were collected at several points pre- and postdelivery, using a variety of tools (Meleis & Swendson, 1978).

Findings of the study included the following:

- Pretreatment role supplementation and study-group husbands and wives had more equalitarian perceptions of their marriage roles than control subjects.
- For husbands, the actual birth of the infant appeared to change role perception (to more equalitarian) more than did participation in study group preparation or role supplementation.
- Mean anxiety level, after the study, was lower for experimental wives than for controls, but the difference was not statistically significant.
- Husbands in the experimental group had significantly higher anxiety pretreatment than controls. Posttreatment experimental group husbands' anxiety had decreased significantly.
- Role supplementation did not affect mothers' posttreatment attitudes toward themselves.
- Posttreatment "experimental and Fam Cap [study] group mothers manifested less ignorance and more cognizance of the needs of their infants than did control group mothers. Control group mothers demonstrated more protective behaviors and more nonintegrative (nonappropriate) responsiveness to the infant than the others" (p. 17).

Limitations of the study include very small experimental group ($N = 12$), self-selection of experimental subjects, questionable reliability and validity of some of the tools, and participation of control couples ($N = 46$)

Strategies   Process   Components   Goal

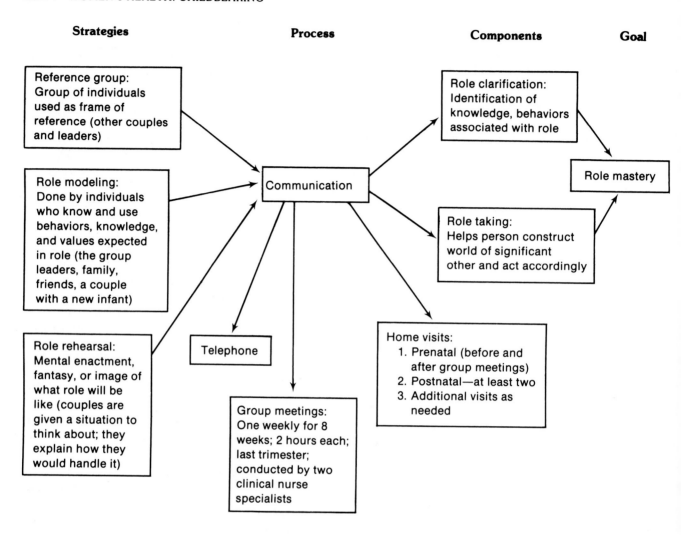

FIGURE 14-2 Role supplementation.

in other prenatal classes, which may have included some strategies of role supplementation (without being identified as such). The latter may have decreased potential differences between control and experimental couples.

Several nursing studies have focused on the expressed needs and concerns of families during the early postpartum period. Data from these descriptive studies can be useful as stimuli for (1) additional descriptive studies with larger and/or different populations: (2) experimental design intervention studies; and (3) planned changes in the delivery of nursing care to postpartum families.

In an early exploratory study of concerns about infant care activities, Adams (1963) interviewed forty first-time mothers three times each during the postpartum period—in the hospital, on the second postpartum day; at home, one week after the mother assumed care of the infant; and again when she had

been caring for the infant for one month. Twenty mothers had infants who were over 2500 g at birth and twenty had infants who were 2500 g or less at birth (premature by weight). Four premature infants remained in the hospital after their mothers were discharged (from six to twenty-one days). The mothers were heterogeneous with respect to age, race, religion, social class, and education; all were married.

For more than half of the mothers at two days and one month postpartum, and for over two-thirds at one week, feeding was the primary concern. One-third of the mothers, at each interview, were concerned about crying. Over one-half were concerned about cord and circumcision care before discharge but only a fourth were at one week. Other problems cited were elimination, hiccups, when to take the child out, rashes, weight, and sleeping.

Sumner and Fritsch (1977) documented the numbers of calls made and types of questions asked by new mothers during a one-month period. All calls made by mothers with infants 6 weeks old or less were recorded. Two hundred and seventy calls were made, sixty-two percent by primiparas and thirty-eight percent by multiparas. During the study period twenty-five percent of eligible multiparas and eighty-eight percent of eligible primiparas called.

During the first three weeks postpartum, parents of males had more questions than parents of females, and there was greater concern about feeding behavior among parents of males. Primiparas called three and a half times more frequently than multiparas but the latter asked more questions per call. The highest percentage of questions was about feeding (31 percent), especially breast-feeding. Next twenty-one percent were questions in the "gastrointestinal" category, and skin and "other" (stuffy nose, birth marks, blocked tear ducts) categories accounted for sixteen and fifteen percent of the questions, respectively. Nine percent of questions were in the "postpartum" category (anxious mother, breast problems, sexual relations, medication effect in breast milk); and eight percent in the "sleep/cry" category. Overall the purpose of the calls seemed to be more to seek validation from a reliable source than to obtain specific information. It was concluded that the study had served to document the existence of a gap in nursing service for the postpartum clients of that facility.

Williams (1977) asked graduates of her prenatal classes about their interest in a postpartum class for new parents. Sixty-three percent of the parents (mostly first-time) responded. Eighty-two percent felt that such a class would be helpful, and the most commonly suggested time was two or four weeks after delivery (choices of times ranged from before discharge from hospital to three months postpartum). The main problems mentioned by parents were feeding, crying, and the baby's schedule. Parents commented on their exhaustion and resentment of lack of predictability in their routines. They were interested in learning how other parents handled problems and in topics such as changes in family life, grandparents, dependency of the infant, tuning-in to infant cues, physical care, and child care literature. Seventy-four percent of parents were interested in bathing and feeding although these were covered during the postpartum hospitalization. When asked what parenting information they would have liked to have before delivery, fifty-eight responded "nothing."

Gruis (1977) sent questionnaires to mothers at one month postpartum in an attempt to discover which of four developmental tasks of the puerperium (physical restoration, relating with newborn, learning infant needs, and accommodating a new family member) had been of the most significant concern to new mothers during the first postpartum month. Forty mothers—seventeen primiparas and twenty-three multiparas—responded to the questionnaire; all had private obstetricians and delivered at private hospitals. Infants were all normal and no mothers or infants experienced postpartum complications. All mothers were living with the father of the baby. Maternal ages and amount of education completed varied. The five concerns reported with the most frequency for all mothers included three common concerns: return of figure to normal (ninety-five percent), regulating family demands (forty-eight percent), and emotional tension (forty percent). However, the other two for primiparas were infant behavior and infant-feeding in contrast to finding time for self and fatigue for multiparas. It seems significant that these data were collected at one month postpartum. By that time, basic infant-care tasks probably seemed less difficult. Maternal concerns, such as episiotomy discomfort, breast soreness, constipation, and hemorrhoids, were probably selected with less frequency because they were less acute or almost forgotten by one month postpartum. However, discrepancies between their ideal and actual figures would have been quite apparent to them by that time. It is also logical that fatigue, regulating family demands, and family planning would have emerged as concerns by one month postpartum.

For help, the mothers primarily used their husbands. None cited the nurse as a source of help, despite the fact that eight were visited at home by a public health nurse.

Using a modified version of the tool used by Gruis, Hill (1978) studied new mothers on their second to third postpartum day. Data were collected at a private hospital. All mothers were married Caucasians who had experienced an uncomplicated pregnancy, labor, and delivery, and who gave birth to a normal infant. Ages and amount of education completed varied. The questionnaire asked for the mothers' degree of concern and degree of interest in learning about a number of items related to self, baby, and family. Twenty-one primiparas and ten multiparas responded, yielding a seventy-eight percent return rate.

Hill asked the mothers to list, for each major category, the item of greatest concern to them and the item they were most interested in learning about. In the category "baby," the three highest ranking items, for both "concern" and "learning," for the total group were: feeding, physical care, and infant behavior.

Highest ranking concerns related to self were: for primiparas—changing role, diet and weight, and emotional changes; for multiparas—emotional changes, feeling tired, and figure to normal. Highest ranking learning interests related to self were: for primiparas—emotional changes, changing role, and figures to normal; for multiparas—emotional changes, exercises, and hemorrhoids.

In the category related to family the highest ranking concerns were: for primiparas—relationship with husband, and father's role; for multiparas—children's reactions, regulating responsibilities, and relationship with husband. Highest ranking learning interests related to family were: primiparas—relationship with husband, and father's role; for multiparas—children's reactions, and father's role.

Considering all of the studies of postpartum concerns, needs, and interests as a whole, several things become apparent:

- Some variability of concerns, needs, and interests is due to the exact time postpartum when studies are done.
- Some issues, such as return of the figure to normal, are of great concern to both primiparas and multiparas. Concern about many other issues varied, as one would expect, with parity.
- Differing responses are probably also dependent on variables, for which analyses are not reported.
- Much less is known about the postpartum concerns, needs, and interests of fathers than of mothers.
- Numerous and varied needs and concerns were expressed by the mothers (parents) who were studied.

MATERNAL ADAPTATION

Taking-In and Taking-Hold

Rubin's (1961) classic description of the adaptation a woman makes following childbirth was a unique contribution to the nursing literature at that time and has served for more than two decades as the basis for many nursing textbook discussions of maternal postpartum care. She succeeded in graphically describing, as no one had before, the many types of adjustments that the new mother must make.

Rubin described two phases of the early maternal adaptation: the taking-in phase and the taking-hold phase. The taking-in phase begins immediately after a deep, therapeutic sleep of several hours has refreshed the new mother, and continues for two to three days. During this phase the mother sleeps, eats heartily, and is concerned about the infant's oral intake. She is very talkative and exhibits excited, euphoric speech. She has a need to review labor and delivery and to search for missing details. Her behavior can best be characterized as passive and dependent. Thus, the mother accepts what is given, does what she is told, and awaits others' actions rather than initiating.

During the taking-hold phase that follows, the mother asserts her independence and autonomy and becomes the initiator. She is involved in the present and seeks help in meeting her needs. "there is a strong element of anxiety here in this phase. If she cannot control her own body, how can she expect to assume responsibility for anyone or anything else?" (Rubin, 1961, p. 754) It is during this phase that the mother "begins to take hold of some of the tasks of mothering" (p. 755). As she feels successful coping with mothering tasks, she has energy to focus on things at home. This phase lasts about ten days and is characterized by frequent, rapid, mood swings until equilibrium is reached.

Any guide to nursing practice should be periodically reexamined for pertinence to the present. Therefore several questions arise about Rubin's description of maternal adaptation:

What was the data base for the description? Since a formal descriptive research study is not mentioned, it can probably be assumed that the description was formulated from observations made while engaging in nursing practice and education. It would be helpful to know whether observations were made in predominantly one place or in many. Were the mothers observed a homogeneous group?

What hospital policies and practices prevailed in the institutions where the observations were made? Prior to 1961 there were few prepared deliveries, and more analgesia and anesthesia were used than is common today. Fathers usually were not present during labor and delivery, and babies usually were housed in a central nursery, except at feeding times, until discharge. Was this true where the observations by Rubin were made? If so, do mothers who attend childbirth classes, labor and delivery with their partner's support, breastfeed on the delivery table, insist on ample opportunity for bonding immediately postdelivery, and keep their infants in their postpartum room most of the time behave at all differently from mothers who were observed by Rubin?

To which populations of new mothers can the findings be generalized? The wise consumer of research findings recognizes the danger of overgeneralizing from study findings, and carefully reads the research report to determine the characteristics of the sample, how the sample was obtained, and the methodology used for data collection. In the case of this classic description of maternal adaptation, it is not possible to do that from the available information. It is implied that the description is true of all mothers.

In what ways has the description been used and/or misused in the past? If the description has been partly responsible for any of the following, then one might question the possibility of misuse: (1) bottle-feeding breast-babies in the nursery at night because the mothers are in the taking-in phase and need to rest more than to feed and bond to their infants; (2) assuming that teaching about infant care should wait until the third or fourth postpartum day; or (3) resisting a plan for flexible rooming-in on the assumption that new mothers need to mostly rest and be taken care of the first few days and should not have to worry about their infants except for feeding times. When the foregoing have occurred in nursing practice, the nurses involved have made a too literal interpretation of Rubin's description.

On the other hand, the description has helped many nurses to better appreciate the major adjustments mothers make postdelivery. It has probably helped nurses to understand why some new mothers are not immediately interested in baby care tasks, such as diapering and bathing. Hopefully, nurses are understanding of maternal mood swings, and use therapeutic listening skills as mothers relive their birth experiences. Rubin's description can continue to be useful to nurses as they carefully interpret collected, comprehensive information about individual women who are new mothers.

Reviewing the Birth Experience

Several nurses have stressed the important need of new parents to review their birth experience. Rising (1974) emphasized that a mother needs to hear later from someone who was there that she did a good job. The observations of Swendson et al. (1978) were essentially in agreement with what Rubin described about reviewing the birth event during the taking-in phase. "We have found that until mothers can describe these experiences in detail they are unable to focus on restoring themselves and accepting and caring for the infant outside the womb" (p. 85).

Rubin (1961) described the mother's need to "ferret out the missing details" (p. 754). A high percentage of the 150 mothers interviewed on the second and third postpartum days by Affonso (1977) were found to be "missing pieces" of their birth experiences. "It was found that many women cannot completely reconstruct their childbirth experience, and become 'stuck' on certain events that they either cannot understand or cannot remember from their labor or delivery" (p. 159).

Specific behavioral manifestations were found among mothers who had not integrated parts of their labors and deliveries:

- Verbalization of recurrent themes: the same question may be asked to the same or different persons over and over.
- The recurrent theme manifested in dreams: the mother may share the dream, or she may complain of not sleeping well or of fatigue upon awakening.
- Inability to focus on her present situation: the mother may not show interest in herself or the baby.

Affonso isolated factors that make women particularly vulnerable to missing pieces: (1) a long labor; (2) receiving minimal data during labor and delivery about their progress; (3) a rapid labor; (4) any high-risk situation; (5) unfulfilled expectations; and (6) predictions that distort perceptions or blur the memory.

It appears that nurses caring for women after childbirth should assist them in verbalizing about their labor and delivery experience, and should take seriously their need to look for missing information. Several specific factors could help prevent missing pieces, and might help each mother reconstruct the events of birth. These include (1) having a significant other with the mother at all times during labor and delivery, and keeping that person well informed; (2) encouraging the significant other to write down important events and the time they happen; (3) letting expectant families know ahead of time that still or motion pictures can be taken during labor and delivery; (4) using a system of primary nursing, so that the nurse who was with the mother during the birth experience cares for her during the postpartum period and can help her review; or (5) having the nurse who was with her during labor and delivery visit her during the postpartum period to discuss the birth event with her.

Postpartum Emotions

Mood swings in postpartum women, which Rubin (1961) described as part of the taking-hold phase, have long been recognized. The tendency for new mothers to cry easily, and without always having an immediately obvious reason, has been labeled by some as *baby blues* and often has been attributed to hormonal changes. The term *postpartum depression* is used by some professionals almost synonymously with baby blues, while others reserve its use to distinguish the minority of mothers who experience profound depression.

Nott (1976) reviewed previous investigations of postpartum emotional disturbance and then designed a study to test the relationship between maternal postpartum emotions and hormone changes. Twenty-seven married women, without psychiatric, medical or obstetrical, financial, social, or marital problems, were studied three times before delivery and sixteen times during the first six weeks postpartum. Emotional upset was found to be common before and after delivery, and to decline after the tenth day. Lability of mood was found among the subjects, but emotional upsets were found to be neither severe nor prolonged. "Fourteen subjects not only rated themselves most depressed during the ten days postpartum but also rated themselves most happy at some time during the same period" (p. 381). Overall, the study failed to provide strong evidence that hormones are related to postpartum emotions; however, hormone changes were weakly, but significantly, correlated with several specific symptoms: predelivery estrogen levels were high in those who were more irritable; the greater the progesterone drop, the more likely the subjects were to rate themselves as depressed within ten days but the less likely to report sleep disturbance; and the lower the postpartum estrogen level, the more sleep disturbance was reported.

Although much is yet to be learned about the role that hormones play in relation to maternal postpartum emotions, it seems clear that many other factors affect postpartum lability of mood.

Gordon et al. (1965) studied 435 women in order to analyze the social history factors associated with their postpartum emotional reactions. Two factors were found to be related to abnormal emotional reactions: *maternal role conflict factor,* which indicated that the mother was prepared for social, economic, and educational advancement but not for motherhood; and *personal insecurity factor,* which resulted from personal insecurity and inexperience, as well as events such as past losses, hurts, and failures. Emotional problems brought on largely by the personal insecurity factor were usually of shorter duration than those related to the role conflict factor. Women with high stress scores had longer-lasting emotional problems. Instruction about reorganizing activities and attitudes for the motherhood role decreased the likelihood of postpartum emotional problems. Mothers who made changes aimed toward reducing role conflict, and who were assisted in this effort by another person, had happier postpartum adjustments.

PHYSIOLOGICAL ADAPTATION

The physiological restorative processes that occur during the early postpartum period are numerous and profound (Rubin, 1961), yet for the great majority of women are an expression of health—of integrated system function. Tables 14-3 and 14-4 are included as a review of postpartum physiology and to offer references for further study.

Increasingly, nurses, as primary care providers, as primary nurses, and/or coordinators of the health team, are making decisions or providing major input for decisions that were traditionally regarded as medical decisions. Nurses in these roles need to base practice decisions on factual information and research findings from a variety of sources, including those not traditionally used by nurses.

Postpartum Physical Assessment

One of the essential nursing functions during the postpartum hospitalization is to perform periodic physical examinations to monitor the restorative processes and to detect any disruption early. The following skills, at a minimum, should be in the repertoire of the staff-level nurse and utilized in assessing the new mother:

- Overall inspection
- Vital signs, including auscultation of breast and lung sounds
- Breast examination
- Auscultation, percussion, and palpation of the abdomen to assess fundal height, position, and tone; bowel sounds; bladder; presence or absence of diastasis of the recti; and abdominus muscles
- Inspection of the perineum, lochia, and rectum
- Inspection of legs for signs of thrombosis, including pain; warmth; tenderness; swollen, reddened veins; Homan's sign (dorsiflexion of the foot causes muscles in calf to compress veins, which may cause pain if there is thrombosis)

Several articles (Clausen, 1972; Malinowski, 1978; Storr, 1978) concisely summarize the specific techniques of postpartum physical assessment and are useful to the nurse.

The frequency of postpartum examinations should be based on a wide variety of data and sophisticated interpretation of those data. Increasingly, highly skilled nurses are making decisions such as whether an examination can be postponed to allow an exhausted mother

TABLE 14-3 Postpartum physiology: The uterus

Parameter	Characteristics	References
Size and position	Immediately after delivery of placenta and membranes: • Weighs 1000–1200 g; 14 cm long, 12 cm wide, 10 cm thick; about the size of a 15- to 16-week gestation. • Apex lies approximately half way between umbilicus and symphysis or slightly higher. • Consists of a mass of tissue with a flattened cavity with anterior and posterior walls close together, each measuring 4–5 m thick. • Remains about the same size for approximately 2 days. After second postpartum day decreases rapidly in size (involution); weighs 500 g at 1 week postpartum. By 10–14 days postpartum: • Weighs about 300 g. • Lies in true pelvis, thus cannot be palpated above symphysis. By 6 weeks postpartum: • Nonpregnant size has been reached. • Weighs 100 g or less.	Barden, 1975; Easterling, 1977; Pritchard & Macdonald, 1976
Myometrium	Atrophy of myometrium during involution: • Total number of cells does not decrease. • Marked decrease in size of cells due to decrease in amount of cytoplasm (exact mechanism not fully understood). Contractility: • Immediately after delivery, uterine contractions of high intensity (often greater than 300 mm Hg and sometimes up to 400 mm Hg) occur. • These strong contractions are thought to be due to the contracting of the active uterus around the greatly decreased volume. • The high uterine activity present immediately postdelivery decreases smoothly and progressively in the first 1½–2 hours after delivery. • The decrease in intensity of contractions is less steady and predictable than the decrease in frequency of contractions. • Incoordinate contractions begin to appear several hours postdelivery, and these become increasingly incoordinate as time passes. • Coordination of contractions can be restored by administration of oxytocin or suckling of the infant at breast.	Barden, 1975; Easterling, 1977; Hendricks et al., 1962; Pritchard & MacDonald, 1976
Hemostasis	Immediately postdelivery, high myometrial pressures during contractions exceed systolic blood pressure, producing uterine ischemia lasting approximately 1 minute. These periods of uterine ischemia and the compression of blood vessels during contractions allow for thrombus formation and promote hemostasis. Changes in uterine vessels: • It is believed that large vessels are obliterated completely by hyaline changes and new and smaller vessels develop. • It is therefore possible to microscopically differentiate between uteri of parous and multiparous women.	Anderson & Davis, 1968; Easterling, 1977; Hendricks et al., 1962; Pritchard & MacDonald, 1976

(continued)

TABLE 14-3 *(continued)*

Parameter	Characteristics	References
Healing and Regeneration	Placental site: • Diameter of site: immediately postpartum—9 cm or less (average diameter of placental discs 18 cm); at 8 days—4.5 cm; at 8 weeks—a 2-cm zone of mucosa less resilient than surrounding endometrium. • Elevation of site: immediately postpartum—4 mm (irregular and nodular); at 8 weeks—no longer elevated. • Surface of the placental attachment site immediately postpartum consists of hemmorrhagic decidua of variable thickness (variably the decidua spongiosa or basalis). • Degenerative changes soon occur that convert part of decidua into necrotic slough. It appears that the entire decidual area does not become necrotic, rather viable decidua is maintained as a buffer zone between necrotic slough and intact deeper endomyometrium. • "Williams considered the placental site to be pushed off by regenerating endometrium. However, exfoliation seems best explained on the basis of a necrotic slough of infarcted surface tissue followed by a reparative process not unlike the repair of any superficially denuded epithelial area whether it be squamous or glandular" (Anderson & Davis, 1968, p. 32). • Process of placental site regeneration requires 6–7 weeks. Nonplacental-site endometrium: • Decidua is not completely shed at parturition with the placenta and membranes. Many of these cells are used in the reconstruction of the endometrium. • Pritchard and MacDonald's (1976) examination of first postpartum week specimens showed portions of degenerating decidua with blood clot, thrombosed blood vessels, and glands of varying size. • Eighth and ninth postpartum day specimens examined by Sharman (1953) had mitotic figures in the glandular epithelium, signifying proliferative changes. • Specimens examined on the 16th postpartum day and after had a structurally restored endometrium (Sharman, 1953).	Anderson & Davis, 1968; Easterling, 1977; Pritchard & MacDonald, 1976; Sharman, 1953; Williams, 1931 (considered the classic source by most textbook writers)
Cervix	Size of opening: • Remains open approximately 2 cm first 4–6 days postpartum. • Should admit only smallest size curet by end of second week postpartum. Appearance: • Edematous, thin, fragile for several days. • Lateral margins often appear lacerated. • External os does not return completely to its prepregnant appearance. • After a few weeks cervix has characteristic parous appearance, remaining wider with lateral depressions at laceration sites.	Easterling, 1977; Pritchard & MacDonald, 1976

some sleep. These decisions used to be dictated by hospital policy or physician's orders.

Usually the primary care provider orders a hemoglobin and hematocrit to be done on the second to third postpartum day and performs a pelvic examination prior to the client's discharge.

The nurse can play a major role in promoting the physiological restorative processes and in helping to modify any discomforts that occur during the postpartum recovery period. The following sections describe specific considerations of postpartum care.

Uterus

A major concern during the first twenty-four to seventy-two hours is that uterine tone and contractility is adequate to provide hemostasis and prevent excessive blood loss. Breast-feeding, which triggers oxytocin release, provides the ideal "natural" means for achieving the goals of hemostasis and involution. In the past, mothers were frequently given doses of an oral oxytocic drug during the early puerperium to achieve the same goals, and that practice continues to a lesser extent today. Clinical investigations have failed to document

TABLE 14-4 Postpartum physiology (excluding the uterus)

Parameter	Characteristics	References
Vagina	During the early part of the puerperium, is large and smooth walled. Gradually decreases in size; by sixth to eighth week approaches nulliparous dimensions. (Sources vary regarding extent to which nulliparous dimensions are regained. This probably varies greatly among individuals.) By end of fourth week rugae reappear and are less prominent than in nulliparous woman.	Easterling, 1977; Pritchard & MacDonald, 1976
Pelvic floor	After delivery, bloody serum infiltrates the pelvic floor. Muscle fibers often are overstretched or torn. Although blood and serum are absorbed quickly, scars resulting from damage to the perineal musculature may cause atrophy and weakness of the pelvic floor.	Clark, 1979
Perineum	Appearance during postpartum period will vary greatly, depending on type and extent of episiotomy and/or tearing, if any. Swelling, bruising, and/or a hematoma may be present. Episiotomies usually have healed and are asymptomatic by the third week postpartum. Following careful repair and restoration of the perineal body, the introitus should resemble that of the nulliparous woman.	Easterling, 1977; Pritchard & MacDonald, 1976
Lochia	Rubra: • Lasts 2–4 days, sometimes longer. • If lasts longer may indicate small portion(s) of retained placenta and/or imperfect involution. • Composed of erythrocytes, leukocytes, epithelial cells, shreds of degenerated decidua, and bacteria. Serosa: • Follows lochia rubra. • Because admixed with serum, appears pale and watery. Alba: • After approximately 10th day. • White to yellowish white color. • Marked admixture with leukocytes and epithelial cells. Microorganisms are found in lochia even when sample is obtained from uterus.	Barden, 1975; Easterling, 1977; Pritchard & MacDonald, 1976
Endocrine system	Hormonal control of lactation: • Prenatally high levels of progesterone and estrogen as well as increased levels of insulin, cortisol, prolactin, and human placental lactogen (HPL; also called human chorionic somatomammotropin, HCS) stimulate the development of the milk-producing components of the breast. The high levels of progesterone and estrogen appear to inhibit actual secretion by the alveoli. • Postnatally, levels of estrogen, progesterone, and HPL drop drastically, and levels of prolactins and insulin also drop. All have been said to decrease to or below nonpregnant levels (Easterling, 1977; Pritchard & MacDonald, 1976). Recently, however, Tyson et al. (1978) have demonstrated persistant elevation of basal prolactin in nursing mothers for up to two years postpartum.	Easterling, 1977; Gaspard et al., 1978; Pritchard & MacDonald, 1976; Tyson et al., 1978; Voherr, 1974

(continued)

TABLE 14-4 *(continued)*

Parameter	Characteristics

- Events of infant suckling cause variable increases in prolactin secretion by the anterior pituitary. The resulting increases in plasma prolactin levels appear to be more related to intensity of suckling than to frequency or duration of suckling.
- The sucking stimulus is also transmitted from areolar nerve endings to the nuclei of the hypothalamus, which results in an increase in the synthesis and transport of oxytocin to the posterior pituitary from which it is released into the circulation. Traveling to the breast, oxytocin causes contraction of myoepithelial cells resulting in milk ejection, or "let-down." Circulating oxytocin simultaneously causes uterine contraction.
- Once lactation is established, suckling appears to be the most important factor required to maintain it.

Resumption of cyclic function:
- Nonlactating mothers:

    Many textbook sources state that resumption of menstruation occurs 6–8 weeks after delivery.

    Summarized data reported by Voherr (1974) indicate the following rates of return of menses: within 6 weeks postpartum in 40 percent of nonlactating mothers; within 12 weeks postpartum in 65 percent of nonlactating mothers; within 24 weeks postpartum in 90 percent of nonlactating mothers.

    The first postdelivery cycle may be ovulatory or anovulatory.

- Lactating mothers:

    Tremendous variation in return of mensus occurs.

    Variables that affect the return of menses appear to include (1) frequency of suckling stimulation; (2) duration of episodes of suckling stimulation; (3) intensity of suckling stimulation; (4) quantity of milk removed from breasts; and (5) factors that affect (1) through (4), such as scheduled or demand-feeding, supplementary formula, and introduction of solid foods.

    The first postdelivery cycle may be ovulatory or anovulatory.

- Regulation:

    The hypothalmic-pituitary-ovarian function postdelivery is complex, not completely understood, and the subject of considerable current research.

    During the first 28 postpartum days, low basal levels of follicle-stimulating hormones (FSH) and luteinizing hormone (LH) are found in both nursing and nonnursing mothers. Administration of gonadotropin-releasing hormone intravenously does not stimulate a rise in either hormone during the first 28 days (Tyson et al., 1978). The exact cause of this phenomenon is controversial.

    Among nursing mothers, weaning is associated with a significant decrease in plasma prolactin (PRL) concentrations and significant increase in plasma LH. Decline of peripheral PRL correlates with resumption of cyclic function.

    From their findings, Tyson et al. (1978) concluded that LH and PRL secretion appears to be significantly influenced by nursing. This includes the loss of episodic LH secretion with demand-feeding. "What remains is to show the specific threshold for PRL secretion above which ovulation

Parameter	Characteristics	References
	is denied and below which the restoration of cyclic gonadotropin secretion occurs either as a result of the decrease in PRL or as the result of the decrease of a separate mechanism controlling LH secretion" (p. 161).	
Cardiovascular system	Cardiac output • After increasing during the first and second stages of labor, peaks during early puerperium. Normally there is little change in blood pressure. Bradycardia usually occurs regardless of type of anesthesia. Postpartum alterations in blood volume are affected by: • Blood loss, which causes immediate but limited decrease in blood volume. • Mobilization and excretion of extravascular water. Blood volume gradually returns to near nonpregnant levels by approximately 1 week postpartum. Blood: • For first 72 hours there is a greater decrease in plasma volume than in cellular components. Therefore, after the immediate postdelivery period there may be a slight increase in hematocrit. • For first few postpartum days there may be considerable variation in hematocrit, hemoglobin, and erythrocyte count. • Moderate to marked leukocytosis is present during first 24 hours postpartum: increase is predominantly granulocytes; there is relative lymphopenia and absolute eosinopenia. • The following pregnancy-induced changes persist after delivery: Elevated plasma fibrinogen is maintained at least through the first postpartum week; Sedimentation rate remains high during the early puerperium.	Barden, 1975; Easterling, 1977; Pritchard & MacDonald, 1976
Urinary tract	Renal pelves and ureters: • Dilation, which occurs during pregnancy gradually decreases unless infection has supervened. • Normal size and contour is regained within 4–6 weeks postpartum. Bladder and urethra: • Passage of infant through pelvis causes trauma. • Bladder wall is edematous and congested with blood, especially if labor is difficult and prolonged. • Bladder has increased capacity and is less sensitive to intravesical fluid pressure: urge to void may be absent or diminished and urinary retention may develop; incomplete emptying with residual urine may occur. • Conduction anesthesia, when it has been used, often contributes to postpartum bladder dysfunction. Diuresis: • Normal pregnancy produces an increase of 2–3 liters of extracellular water. • Between postpartum days 2–5, diuresis reverses above process. Sugar (lactose) may be found in urine during early postpartum, and longer if breast-feeding. During early hours postpartum, acetone may be present in urine, especially if labor was difficult or prolonged.	Easterling, 1977; Pritchard & MacDonald, 1976

(continued)

281

TABLE 14-4 *(continued)*

Parameter	Characteristics	References
Abdomen	The broad and round ligaments of the uterus are much more relaxed postdelivery than in the nonpregnant state. Considerable time is required for them to recover from being stretched and loosened.	Easterling, 1977; Pritchard & MacDonald, 1976
	During pregnancy there is distention of the abdomen by the enlarged uterus and rupture of elastic fibers in the skin. With time and exercise, skin elasticity and tones of the abdominal muscles can be regained, although there is considerable individual difference in the amount of time and exercise needed for these restorative processes to occur.	
	Occasionally the rectus abdominis muscle remains separated (diastasis recti abdominis), but should become less evident as time passes.	
	Silver striae, which frequently develop during pregnancy, do not disappear postpartum but do fade and become less noticeable. This is also true of those on breasts, thighs, and hips.	

the value of administering oral or intramuscular oxytocin to normal women after active third-stage bleeding has been controlled (Adams & Flowers, 1960; Pritchard & MacDonald, 1976). Furthermore, mothers who receive oral oxytocin frequently experience severe discomfort from uterine contractions. It therefore seems appropriate for nurses, as client advocates, to question any routine postpartum prescription of oral oxytocic drugs.

Although ongoing assessment of the uterus is a nursing responsibility, many mothers are interested in the involution process. Such women, if instructed adequately, are often willing and even eager, to check their fundal position and firmness, and to massage it if indicated. Such client participation should be a supplement to, not a substitute for, regular nursing assessment.

Lochia

According to some sources, clots of the lochia are definitely abnormal (Barden, 1975; Clark, 1979) and, in fact, they are sometimes indicative of retention of a small piece of placenta or fetal membranes. However, after a period of lying down, it is not unusual for a mother, upon standing, to experience a sudden heavy flow of blood and to expel one or more clots, due to lochia that has pooled and clotted in the vagina. Whenever the source of clots is questionable or bleeding seems excessive, it is wise to begin a pad weight and count to gather more information for assessment. Often an increase in activity causes an increase in the lochia, and new mothers should be taught, prior to discharge

from the birth center or hospital, to regard a significant increase in lochia as an indication that less activity and more rest may be needed.

Perineal Care

Over the years, postpartum perineal care has evolved from an elaborate nursing procedure to a more simplified activity that is taught to the mother as a self-care activity as soon as she is ambulatory. A number of different methods are currently suggested by various sources to increase cleanliness and comfort, promote healing, and prevent infection of the perineum. These methods include washing from front to back with soap and water, using a clean wash cloth; rinsing after each voiding or bowel movement with warm tap water, using a small plastic squeeze-bottle; sitz baths (110°F, 43°C); heatlamps; topical anesthetic sprays and ointments; and witch hazel compresses. Ice is recommended for the early postdelivery period. Usually some combination of the above is used in a particular agency, but there has been no nursing research to guide nursing practice in this area.

Some important questions can be asked concerning the therapeutic use of heat and cold postpartum. The basic principles for heat and cold application can help answer some of these questions. Because of their respective physiological effects, cold is used to decrease pain and muscle tonus, prevent edema, decrease circulation and oxygen supply to an area, decrease metabolism, and retard bacterial growth; while heat is used to decrease pain and muscle tonus, promote healing and suppuration, dilate veins, and relieve deep congestion. However, a phenomenon called *secondary effect,* which essentially reduces the therapeutic effect, occurs if heat is used continuously for more than twenty to forty-five minutes or cold for more than thirty to sixty minutes. To avoid a secondary effect, the heat or cold application should be applied for the therapeutic time and then discontinued for at least one hour (Dodd, 1979).

An ice bag applied to the perineum shortly after delivery can be very useful in preventing edema and decreasing pain. However, these ice applications are frequently ordered as continuous applications for a certain number of hours postpartum, which can lead to a secondary effect. Additionally, there are few data available to guide decisions about how many hours cold application should be continued; this varies tremendously among institutions. Certainly, individual factors such as extent of trauma to the perineum and amount of pain should be considered, but more definitive information is needed.

Heat is widely used postpartum to promote healing, relieve congestion, and relieve pain. Authors and institutions differ as to whether sitz baths alone, heat lamps alone, or a combination of the two is recommended. Dodd (1979) has contrasted the advantages and disadvantages of dry and moist heat applications and when this information is applied to the situation regarding the postpartum perineum, it appears that sitz baths offer more advantages and fewer disadvantages (especially less drying of skin and pulling at suture line) than heat lamps, if sitz baths can be implemented in an effective, comfortable manner. An installed porcelain sitz tub, which allows for a continuous flow of fresh hot water, is ideal for achieving maximum therapeutic effect. This type of tub should be considered when units are remodeled or new facilities are built. Mothers report considerable relief from this type of sitz bath and seem to need less pain medication. An investigation of these impressions would be helpful.

When given a choice, mothers often prefer use of a topical anesthetic ointment rather than a spray, since the latter often stings. Mothers report relief of both episiotomy and hemorrhoid pain with application of witch hazel compresses.

Kegel Exercises

The Kegel exercise, which is frequently taught prenatally, is also extremely important during the postpartum period and, for that matter, throughout a woman's life. For this isometric exercise, the pubococcygeal muscle (vaginal-perineal) is contracted and relaxed approximately ten or more times, several times daily. The exercise has many benefits, which include stimulation of circulation to the perineum, thus promoting healing; restoration of prepregnant size and tone of vagina; and strengthening of the pelvic floor, which improves support for the pelvic organs. Continuing the Kegel exercise indefinitely can help prevent stress urinary incontinence and can contribute to sexual pleasure.*

Breasts

Due to the hormonal mechanisms described in Table 14-4 the breasts begin to fill by the second to fourth postpartum day. Ordinarily, they become congested with blood and lymph which contribute to the engorgement. (See also "The Breast," *Women's Health: Ambulatory Care,* for information about breast care for the breast-feeding mother.)

For bottle-feeding mothers, interventions are geared toward minimizing engorgement and discomfort. Despite a 1977 ruling by the federal Food and Drug Administration that required that women be informed of the risks associated with estrogens, the hormone is still widely used for lactation suppression. Estrogen used alone is associated with increased risk of thromboembolic disease (Tindall, 1968; Turnbull, 1968). A combination of testosterone enanthate and estradiol (Deladumone OB, Squibb) has been shown to be more effective than estrogen alone, oral androgen–estrogen preparation (Tace, Merrell-National), or placebo in preventing postpartum engorgement and discomfort (Morris et al., 1970; Womack et al., 1962). Deladumone OB should be administered just before second-stage labor, or immediately following delivery.

A snugly fitting bra or a breast-binder should be worn to help suppress lactation. The breast should not be pumped since that would stimulate milk production. If needed, ice bags decrease discomfort and may help suppress lactation.

Pain

The new mother may experience pain from her episiotomy, especially if a third- or fourth-degree laceration occurred, or from engorged breasts. In mul-

---

*For further description of the exercise and several variations consult Bing, 1975, or write to the Sex Advisory and Counseling Unit, University of California Medical School, 624 Parnassus, San Francisco, CA.

tiparas painful, vigorous uterine contractions frequently occur at intervals for several days, especially when the infant nurses (Pritchard & MacDonald, 1976). The uterus of the primipara, however, tends to remain contracted unless blood clots or fragments of placenta are retained.

Nursing interventions can assist the new mother in coping with discomfort (e.g., appropriate application of heat and cold, breast massage and manual expression, and relaxation and breathing for uterine contractions). In addition, a mild analgesic is usually ordered for the mother to take every three to four hours as needed. In a recent double-blind study, for which subjects were randomly assigned to groups, Jain et al. (1978) found aspirin 800 mg with caffeine 64 mg to be significantly more effective than aspirin 650 mg or a placebo in relieving severe episiotomy pain. Aspirin 650 mg alone was not much more effective than the placebo in relieving severe episiotomy pain. For uterine pain, the results were less conclusive; for that part of the study the sample size was quite small.

This study suggests that even a mild drug, such as aspirin-caffeine combination, can be very useful in relieving postpartum episiotomy pain. Studies using similar methodology and tools for measuring pain, and comparing the relative effectiveness of other mild analgesics to placebo for their ability to relieve episiotomy and uterine pain would be useful.

Most new mothers on the postpartum-newborn unit at the University of Minnesota Hospitals participate in a self-medication program, which allows them to take and record their own drugs. Most women have an order for a mild analgesic with or without codeine. The self-medication drugs, excluding those with codeine, are issued from the pharmacy in safety-top containers. Initially, mothers are taught about the medication system and about each drug they are taking. Nurses continue to check with the mothers to see if they have questions about the system and to see if they have remembered to take their medications.

This approach is well accepted by both clients and staff and is especially effective in respect to drugs for pain relief. A mother can take a drug as soon as she feels the need (if a long enough interval has passed since the last dose) without having to wait for her nurse. In many cases, the mother can choose between a milder and stronger drug, depending on her perceived pain. Overall, pain-relief drugs tend to be taken sparingly by the mothers, whereas other relief measures (such as sitz baths) are used liberally.

Urinary Tract

Malinowski (1978) discussed several intrinsic and extrinsic factors that affect the functioning of the urinary tract during the early postpartum period. *Intrinsic factors* include (1) increased bladder capacity due to decreased intra-abdominal pressure and stretched, relaxed abdominal muscles; (2) diuresis, which occurs between postpartum days two to five, (3) reflex spasm of the urethra that may occur due to tenderness or edema of the vulva and perineum; and (4) the common fear among postpartum mothers that voiding may be painful. *Extrinsic factors* include (1) the common practice of forcing fluids; (2) desensitization, which may occur if conduction anesthesia is used; and (3) trauma to the urethra that can be caused by the fetus or by forceps. These factors contribute to bladder distention.

Harris et al. (1977) screened 667 postpartum women for urinary tract infections and confirmed asymptomatic bacteriuria in only four percent. Significantly more of bacteriuria occurred in women who had been catheterized than in those who had not been. Among those who had been catheterized for Cesarean section, preeclampsia, and tubal ligation, the incidence was not significantly different from those patients who had not been catheterized. The significant increase in bacteriuria was found among those patients who had been catheterized for postpartum urinary retention. Longer duration of catheterization was significantly related to bacteriuria. Harris et al. suggested the use of prophylactic antibiotics for women with urinary retention who are catheterized over twenty-four hours, but not for other postpartum patients who are catheterized. Ziegel and Cranley (1978) and Malinowski (1978) have described interventions the nurse can employ for bladder assessment and prevention of distention.

Gastrointestinal Tract

Unless a mother has had excessive analgesia or anesthesia, decreased motility of the gastrointestinal tract lasts only a short time after a vaginal delivery (Easterling, 1977). Many women are hungry and ready to eat a full meal, which is helpful in providing fluid and nutrients, shortly after delivery.

Anticipating the first bowel movement is a source of great anxiety to many mothers who have sore perineums, and especially to those who have third- and fourth-degree lacerations. Often mothers find that actually passing the stool is much less painful than they had feared, especially if they relax rather than strain. Mothers can be taught to use the relaxation techniques that were learned prenatally. The mother should go to the toilet promptly when she feels the urge to defecate, consciously relax until a peristaltic wave is perceived, and then bear down very gently in synchrony with peristalsis.

Due to several factors, a normal bowel movement may not occur during the first three postpartum days. These factors include decompressed abdomen and bowel dilation, perineal pain, enema during labor, and little or no oral intake during labor (Mundow, 1975).

While many sources suggest that a stool softener, laxative, or enema may be used, there has been very little research done in this area. Mundow (1975) reported on a double-blind study of 200 consecutive postpartum mothers in which a combination laxative and stool softener (Dorbanex, containing danthron and polox-alkol; Riker Laboratories, England) was compared with a placebo. Mothers who received the active drug had their first bowel movement significantly sooner than controls. Significantly more control mothers needed enemas and later developed hemorrhoids than mothers who received the active drug. Only one mother who received the drug experienced a side effect (crampy pain).

While danthron 75 mg used alone as a laxative may cause catharsis in a nursing infant, the quantity of danthron used in combination with a stool softener is not reported to have the same effect (*Physicians' Desk Reference*, 1979), although the possibility of this effect should be studied further.

Nutrition

The importance of good nutrition to the nursing mother and the nutritional requirements for lactation are discussed in Chapter 17. Eating a well-balanced diet, planned according to the nutritional and calorie requirements for a normal nonpregnant woman of comparable height and age, will promote the postpartum health of the nonnursing woman. Nurses who work with newly-expanded families can use the opportunity to assess family nutrition, and can plan with the family for improving it, if necessary.

Return of Weight and Figure to Normal

In the studies by Gruis (1977) and Hill (1978) cited earlier, figure, weight, and exercise were major concerns among new mothers studied. With all of the current professional interest in family bonding and role transitions, these important areas of maternal interest and concern may not be dealt with fully and effectively during the postdelivery period.

Mothers are often disappointed when they weigh themselves soon after delivery and find that their weight loss is much less than they had expected—usually less than 15 lb initially. Due to diuresis another 5 lb should be lost by the fifth postpartum day (Pritchard & MacDonald, 1976). Some nursing mothers find that their weight returns rapidly to normal in the early postpartum weeks. The frequency with which this happens is unknown and data related to this phenomenon have not been reported in the literature.

New mothers should have the opportunity to learn about postpartum exercises while they are in the hospital. Verbal descriptions of exercises can be reinforced by written instructions with pictures. There are many variations among the postpartum exercises suggested by professionals (Clark, 1977; Jensen et al., 1977; Ziegel & Cranley, 1978). Bing (1975) provides descriptions and photographs of postpartum exercises, some of which can be started as early as the first postpartum day. A teaching–learning situation which allows for discussion of the mother's feelings about her body will be more helpful than just giving information about specific exercises.

Fatigue and Sleep

Fatigue was also a major concern to mothers in the Gruis study (1977) who were studied at one month postpartum, and to multiparas in the Hill study (1978) who were studied two to three days postpartum. Although there is frequently sleep deprivation during labor, which results in a "sleep hunger" in early postpartum (Rubin, 1961; Williams, 1967), the mothers in the Hill study may have recovered somewhat by the second to third postpartum day. Multiparas, however, were probably anticipating more accurately what the early months at home with a new baby would be like—especially coupled with the demands of another child or children.

During the last fifteen years, sleep has been the focus of considerable research. Findings from sleep research have been summarized recently by Sanford (1979) and help explain why fatigue is such an important problem for a new mother. Two major types of sleep have been identified and studied.

Rapid-eye-movement (REM) sleep, also called active or paradoxic sleep, is accompanied by large muscle immobility, increased oxygen consumption by the brain, increased cardiac output and vivid, full-color dreams. REM sleep is felt to be necessary for the maintenance of mental and emotional equilibrium. NREM (non-REM) or quiet sleep consists of four stages and is a quiescent stage accompanied by decreases in the vital signs and metabolic activity. REM and Stage-4 NREM sleep are felt to be especially important for optimal physical and mental functioning. Loss of either of these types of sleep results in a rebound phenomenon (the type of sleep lost occupies a greater percentage of the total sleep time during the first subsequent night in which sleep is undisturbed). Unfortunately, for new parents, there are no nights of undisturbed sleep with a new baby.

In a study of endocrine influences on sleep, Petre-Quadens and DeLee (1974) documented sleep alterations in postpartum women. In women not breast-feeding, paradoxical sleep (PS) percentage (ratio of REM sleep to total sleep time) decreased gradually and was more abrupt between the tenth and fifteenth days postdelivery. Subsequently, rebound increase in PS occurred. The PS percentage remained higher in breast-feeding mothers and the possibility of a complex hormonal relationship was suggested by the investigators.

Sleep is of most benefit if it is synchronized to the individual's biological clock (circadian rhythm), which has an approximately twenty-four-hour cycle, with lowest mental and physical functioning occurring at night. Disruptions in the normal pattern of sleeping at night result in desynchronization and efforts to resynchronize. Unless the change in the sleep–wake schedule is fairly constant, resynchronization cannot occur. Continual efforts to resynchronize lead to chronic fatigue (Sanford, 1979).

With night feedings and sporadic naps, which accompany life with a newborn, it is easy to understand why new mothers report chronic fatigue! Nursing intervention cannot alleviate the problem altogether, but perhaps can modify it. Some anticipatory and concurrent discussion of the problem can help the mother to realize that she is not unique in feeling exhausted, and that her less-than-optimal physical and mental functioning has a physiological basis. Some nursing mothers find that keeping the infant's bed beside theirs, where they can easily reach for her when she cries is very helpful. The baby then nurses while the mother sleeps and may or may not be returned to bed. For many years this practice was discouraged by professionals on a cultural basis; they also claimed erroneously that the child might suffocate. Renewed interest in touching, bonding, and unrestricted breast-feeding have modified attitudes of some professionals and parents.

PATERNAL ADAPTATION

If adaptation to parenthood is difficult for mothers, then it is probably even more difficult for fathers, largely due to the ambiguity currently surrounding the role. Lamb (1975) stated that, although research has documented that many fathers and infants interact extensively, there has been a tendency in Western society to devalue the father's role by focusing intensely on the mother–child relationship. He also claimed that a "definition of the role of father is lacking" (p. 259).

At the beginning of this century things were much clearer. There were specific family functions, which were clearly divided between the two persons who enacted the roles of "mother" and "father" in traditional, patriarchal farm families. Mothers functioned as homemakers, nurturers, and caretakers of the children; fathers served as providers, protectors, disciplinarians, and teachers. Fathers rarely became acquainted with their children when they were infants. As industrialization occurred, and many families moving to towns and cities where fathers worked away from home during many of the waking hours of their children, role functions began to do some shifting. In order to fulfill some of the protecting and disciplining functions, mothers incorporated some aggressive and dominant behavior into the maternal role. World War II, with the entry of large numbers of women into the work force, helped to reinforce these new maternal behaviors. In a corresponding trend, some father began to take a larger part in caretaking and rearing of children (Benedek, 1970; Gollober, 1976). "The paternal role took on new qualities. These qualities (i.e., love, warmth, and compassion) which the father began to exhibit are now included in the term fatherliness" (Gollober, 1976, p. 18).

Since World War II, many changes have occurred that have affected how the essential family functions are divided between the male and female heads of various families. Such changes include the women's movement, rising inflation, more women entering professions, and more women working in general. The changes have not, of course, affected all families in the same ways, with the result that today there are infinite variations in essential role functions in families. One basic truth, stated by Benedek (1970, p. 167) remains however: "Fatherhood and motherhood are complementary processes which evolve within the culturally established family structure to safeguard the physical and emotional development of the child."

While some parents reach an agreement, verbal or understood, of the parental roles they will play, others find that they have reached the threshold of parenthood with a set of expectations about their roles that differs drastically from their spouses' view of the role. Some fathers prefer a traditional paternal role; others philosophically embrace the idea of fathering that includes a share of all of the important family role functions, but find themselves grossly unprepared for the nurturing and caretaking functions (Gearing, 1978), or find themselves blocked in their efforts to enact the role (e.g., paternity leave refused; Heise, 1975). Fein (1976) studied thirty-two middle-class couples before delivery and for six weeks after the birth of their first child. Fathers in the study adopted two different versions of the father role, either breadwinner or equal parent. Both of these approaches were effective for coping with the stresses of new parenthood, as long as both members of the couple agreed on the ways they would divide the basic family tasks. One father in Fein's study expressed very clearly what many contemporary fathers probably feel.

> I feel in a bind. When I was small my father never really took care of me. He was the breadwinner, and I guess he demanded respect more than he gave affection. But now the norms seem to have changed. Men are expected to take care of children. I feel like I want to take care of our baby, and I feel I ought to care for the child, but frankly I don't know how I'm afraid I won't be a good father.*

A common belief today seems to be that women attempt to push or pull their frequently resistant husbands into enacting a paternal role that includes more caretaking. However, Reiber (1976) concluded from her extensive study of nine couples that "some women choose to keep much of the child care to themselves and...men do have a deep interest in family involvement" (p. 371). It would be interesting to investigate this phenomenon using a much larger sample.

Manion (1977) found that among the forty-five couples she studied, new fathers were more likely to rock or walk the baby, give a bottle, or change a diaper than to bathe the baby. Fathers who remembered their parents as nurturant and who had high "participation in birth" scores also had significantly higher infant caretaking scores.

Less is known about the mechanisms used by fathers for assuming the paternal role than is known about the transition to the maternal role. Regarding the *couvade syndrome*, or pregnancylike symptoms experienced by

some men during their wives pregnancies, May (1978) suggested that "these symptoms, rather than being an overidentification with the female partner or a manifestation of parturition envy...may be an unconscious expression of the father's pregnant emotional state" (p. 9). Through interviews, May found that fathers who were most involved with preparations for parenthood were aware of and able to talk about their own tender and nurturant feelings aroused by the pregnancy. These men seemed to feel pregnant, and May hypothesized that there might be a relationship between the capacity to feel pregnant and the later capacity to feel fatherly. Some fathers shared that they and their partners had discussed "how it would be to be a family." This would correspond to one of the role taking-in operations described by Rubin (1967a, 1967b)—that of fantasy—except, rather than either parent fantasizing alone, both parents were participating in a type of joint fantasy.

Among the twenty expectant fathers she interviewed, Obrzut (1976) found evidence that they engaged in all of Rubin's five role attainment processes—mimicry, role play, fantasy, introjection–projection–rejection, and grief work. Eighty percent of these fathers were concerned about infant-care skills and sixty-eight percent about adequacy as a father.

Today the message seems clear that, while much has been done to help prepare couples for childbirth, much less has been done to help prepare parents—and especially fathers—for parenting. Gearing (1978) feels that childbirth educators, who are frequently nurses, are aware of paternal anxieties but are not always prepared with the counseling skills needed to effectively help fathers. She has proposed a model program for expectant and new fathers that involves (1) prenatal classes in child care, using real infants and male and female role models; (2) group counseling for the expectant fathers; (3) prenatal couple counseling sessions (to work out what their complementary mother and father roles will be); (4) active participation in the birth by fathers; (5) postpartum rooming-in, with fathers practicing baby care and staying overnight; and (6) postpartum continuation of group counseling for the fathers.

Resnick (1978) have described an existant model (psychoeducational) for helping men adapt to fatherhood. This model has been implemented by an interdisciplinary team, including nurses. The professionals, working in pairs, offer expectant parent and fathering classes. The expectant parent classes are similar to many offered around the country, but include several components that are not always present in such classes. These components include: occasionally breaking the class into same sex groups for discussion, stressing the

---

*From Fein, R. (1976). The first weeks of fathering: The importance of choices and supports for new parents. *Birth and the Family Journal, 3*, 53–57. With permission.

importance of developing decision-making skills, role playing of potentially difficult situations, and visits to the class by new parents. The fathering classes are organized so that groups of about eight fathers who have children the same age (infancy through preschool) meet together. These classes have the following features: (1) fathers attend with their children; (2) information and skills (e.g., physical development exercises) are taught; and (3) feelings of fathers are shared during group discussion.

Model programs offer promise for helping men deal with the uncertainty and stress involved with becoming a father. An important issue to consider is how can comprehensive programs become cost-effective and available to all fathers who can be encouraged to participate?

COUPLE ADAPTATION

It may seem obvious that two mature individuals who have developed an intimate, caring relationship, within which effective problem solving is used to resolve conflict, are likely to experience a satisfactory or optimal postdelivery adaptation. Yet all childbearing couples do not have the type of relationship described above. This may be a discouraging and unalterable variable in some cases, but there are reasons for suggesting that it probably should not be. A couple relationship that is already stressed will be particularly susceptible to the additional stresses that usually follow childbirth. These stresses may precipitate a state of crisis or near crisis for such a couple. Crisis intervention by a capable health care provider can help modify the stress state and promote growth. According to Baird (1979), crisis in Chinese means *danger, yet opportunity* and is defined as "a state of upset and disequilibrium, but also a time when an individual or family has the opportunity to grow" (p. 299).

Programs such as role supplementation and parenting classes, which can be useful to any couple, may also be useful to a less mature couple with a stressed relationship. At a time when crisis intervention is provided for such a couple, the two individuals may be more willing to consider a suggestion to attend a growth-oriented program than they might be otherwise. By the same token, the couple might be more willing to consider marriage counseling if it were recommended during the course of crisis intervention.

The literature suggests several additional variables that may contribute to parental adjustment after childbirth. In Fein's (1976) study, couples who agreed on how they would share family tasks coped better after childbirth than did other couples. Swendsen et al. (1978) found that skills with role taking facilitated couple adaptation. Individuals who developed the skill found that they could be more empathetic with their partners and that this ability eased difficult times in early parenthood.

Among the ninety-five Caucasians studied by Gilman and Knox (1976), paternal fantasizing about the "good old days" (before baby) was negatively correlated with postpartum marital happiness. However, "holidays" (going out alone as a couple) were positively correlated with postpartum marital happiness. Since the return rate of questionnaires mailed to the defined population of first-time fathers was only twenty-eight percent, the validity of the findings must be questioned.

One of the most difficult tasks of couple adaptation following childbirth is for both partners to continue to nurture each other while learning to nurture their infant. The potential is great for one or both partners to feel excluded. Fein (1976) found that postnatally the men and women he studied did not spend less time with each other, but they gave each other less attention. Couples frequently experience difficulty finding time to be alone together (Resnick et al., 1978). Some individuals manage, despite the demands of new parenthood, to find ways of saying "I love you" and "You are so special to me" to their partners. Others may need to be helped to recognize their spouses' needs for attention and to verbalize their own needs.

The couple's sexual relationship can be a source of stress or of great comfort during the months following childbirth. In the past, couples received little professional guidance in this area, other than some help with family planning and directions to refrain from intercourse until after the six-week checkup. According to Bing and Colman (1977), "one woman believed...that the professionals almost categorically do not willingly help a woman with intimate problems" (p. 6). Fortunately, the need for nurses to discuss needs of an intimate and sexual nature with clients is increasingly being recognized, and help is becoming more available for nurses who wish to gain the comfort and skill required to help clients with these needs. In addition to formal courses, continuing education programs, and numerous new textbooks, articles such as those by Adams (1976 a, 1976b) and Zalar (1976), offer specific realistic suggestions for effectively discussing sexuality with clients.

Only a limited amount of research related to postchildbirth sexual adaptation has been done—the best known being that of Masters and Johnson (1966). They interviewed 101 women during the postpartum period and studied the physiological responses of six women. At four to five weeks postpartum the six women had orgasms that were shorter and weaker, and their organs responded more slowly and less intensely during sexual activity, when compared with nonpregnant sexual responses. However, the women were subjectively satisfied, and reported sexual tension to be at their nonpregnant levels throughout the first six to eight postpartum weeks. Women had less vaginal vasocongestion and lubrication until ovulation resumed. Generally, the physiological sexual responses of the six women had returned to normal by three months postpartum. Among the women who were interviewed, the highest postpartum sexual interest and eroticism were reported by a group of breast-feeding mothers, despite the longer delay in the return of ovarian steroid production for these women.

Newton (1973) accentuated the fact that women have three acts of interpersonal reproductive behavior (coitus, parturition, and lactation), in contrast to males who have only one (coitus). She described seven psychophysiological similarities between lactation and coitus (1) uterine contractions occur during suckling and sexual excitement; (2) nipple erection occurs during both; (3) breast-stroking and nipple stimulation occur during nursing and foreplay; (4) sexual contact and breast-feeding both involve skin changes; (5) milk let-down may be caused by breast-feeding and sexual excitement; (6) emotions experienced during nursing and sexual stimulation may be similar (some women experience sexual stimulation, to plateau level or even orgasm, while breast-feeding); and (7) "an accepting attitude toward sexuality may be related to an accepting attitude toward breast-feeding" (p. 83). These similarities may help explain the Masters and Johnson findings related to breast-feeding mothers.

From a study of nineteen primiparas, Falicov (1973) reported findings relevant to postpartum sexual adjustment that were different in some respects from those of Masters and Johnson: Within two months after delivery two-thirds of the couples had resumed sexual intercourse, and of these, one-half had rapidly returned to their prepregnancy level of sexual functioning. The other half, however, experienced problems with maternal fatigue, breast engorgement, and sore episiotomy sites, which interfered with the couple's sexual interaction. Nursing appeared to have heightened breast eroticism for about half of the breast-feeding women. Of the five women in the study who were bottle-feeding, four were in the group who had not resumed intercourse by six to eight weeks postpartum. At seven months postpartum, sexual intercourse was considerably less frequent for ten couples than before pregnancy, largely due to fatigue and psychological tension.

Tolor and DiGrazia (1976) studied four groups of women, one group in each trimester of pregnancy and one group of fifty-five postpartum women. Compared to the other three groups, the postpartum group reported increased desire for sexual activity and had sexual intercourse more frequently. All of these women indicated a high need for close physical contact during pregnancy and postpartum. There was a greater preference for oral sexual activity among the postpartum women and less preference for clitoral stimulation. The increased potpartum sexuality was felt by the researchers to be the result of a genuine recovery of libidinal drive and not solely an effort to please husbands.

Sensitive and well-informed nurses can facilitate the sexual adaptation of couples during the weeks and months following childbirth partially by discussing the following points with new parents during the early postpartum period:

Resumption of Sexual Intercourse Intercourse can safely be resumed when lochia has ceased, when the episiotomy has healed, and when the new mother feels ready—usually after three to four weeks. (Isreal & Rubin, 1967; Kyndely, 1978; Zalar, 1976). Mothers who have had third- or fourth-degree lacerations may need to wait longer for the perineum to heal. The first postpartum intercourse will probably be somewhat uncomfortable, so patience and gentleness by the partner are very important. A position that puts less strain on the perineum than the missionary position should be tried at first (e.g., woman on top or side-lying). A water-soluble lubricant is helpful if there is diminished vaginal lubrication.

Alternatives to Intercourse Prior to the resumption of intercourse a couple can maintain sexual intimacy and relieve sexual tension by using pleasurable activities that are acceptable to both partners. The woman will likely not be interested in oral or manual genital stimulation until external perineal healing is complete, but is likely to desire to be held and caressed. The man can be helped to have satisfying orgasms manually or orally.

Breast-Feeding Women should know that many women experience sexual stimulation while breast-feeding. In fact, infant survival, long before the concept of "duty" evolved, was dependent on successful breast-feeding. It, therefore, had to be sufficiently pleasurable to ensure its frequent occurrence (Newton, 1973). Information and discussion can help mothers enjoy this aspect of their sexuality rather than to feel guilty about their feelings. Fathers have varied responses to breast-feeding. Some find their partner's enlarged, sensitive, lactating breasts and the act of breast-feeding to be extremely sensual. For them, the let-down of milk that often occurs during sexual arousal may be very erotic rather than troublesome or disgusting. Other fathers may resent the intimate breast-feeding relationship between the mother and infant and feel left out. No doubt the woman's comfort with her own sexuality and her approach to breast-feeding affect the father's response. Some women have reported becoming totally absorbed in breast-feeding to the point of not desiring intimate contact with their husbands (Bing & Colman, 1977). In these cases, naturally, the fathers are almost certain to feel excluded and resentful.

Family Planning The couple will need to have opportunities to discuss and make a decision about contraception prior to resuming intercourse. The nurse's role in helping the couple may be that of primary care provider or information giver (see "Method of Conception Control," *Women's Health: Ambulatory Care*), or she or he may simply answer or act as a sounding board or resource linker (e.g., referral to a natural family planning couples group).

SIBLING ADAPTATION

It has been widely recognized by professionals who work with children and parents that the birth of a sibling is a stressful event for a child. A number of prominent authors of parenting books (e.g., Brazelton, 1969; Salk, 1972; Spock, 1976) have included sections on how to help the older sibling adapt to a new baby. Increasingly basic nursing texts are including information on ways to promote sibling adaptation (e.g., Jensen, et al., 1977; Ziegel & Cranley, 1978). Often one of the primary, if not *the* primary, concerns of parents expecting a second or more child is sibling adaptation.

Legg et al. (1974), reviewed seven research reports on the reactions of preschool siblings to the birth of a new baby. The studies included three unpublished dissertations. Four of the studies, including one of the former, used the doll-play or wooden-toy techniques. Two major difficulties with the use of doll play, and perhaps with the use of wooden toys, is that attention getting and regressive behavior may not be seen as clearly as they occur in real life. From their review Legg et al. found some evidence in the literature for the following conclusions:

- Common reactions by the older child to the birth of a new sibling include regression, attention-seeking behavior (acting out), and aggression toward the infant.
- Children under 3 years tend to be more disturbed initially than older children. Older children may react more negatively when the baby is old enough to disrupt their play.
- The child may repress anger, in an attempt to use more acceptable behavior; diminished affect, creativity, and aggression, and greater rigidity may result.
- An imaginary playmate may be used by the older child to alleviate stress.
- A closer relationship between the mother and older child tends to be associated with greater disturbance and overt hostility on the part of the older child when a new baby is born.
- Initially, the older child's stress is probably primarily related to separation from the mother and loss of some of her attention. As time passes the older child associates these losses specifically with the baby and the baby becomes the object of rivalry. This is probably especially true when the age difference between the children is less than three years.
- First children seem to have a more difficult time adjusting than children who already have a sibling.
- When the father is very involved with the older child, the child's adjustment appears to be less difficult.

Legg et al. (1974) then did a pilot descriptive study of sibling reactions to the birth of a new baby. Twenty-one families were studied and in four families it was possible to collect data on more than one birth event, making the total number of children's responses studied twenty-five. Data were collected mainly by interview with mothers and two fathers, though naturalistic observation of the child was done also for part of study. All of the parents studied were college educated; ethnic backgrounds were varied. Ages of the children studied ranged from 11.5 months to 5 years. Some of the study findings are as follows:

- Except in the cases of five children who were 1½ or less at the time of the infant's birth, children were told about the baby at about the time of quickening. The five younger children were not prepared at all because the parents felt they were too young to understand.

- As ways of preparing the child some mothers referred to babies in the neighborhood and many encouraged the child to feel the fetus move.
- Children 1½–3½ years old were not very inquisitive about the pregnancy and were given simple, concise explanations by the mothers.
- Children aged 4–5 asked more questions about delivery, but most did not ask about how the baby got there.
- Several techniques used by parents to help prepare the child were apparently helpful: taking the older child along to a prenatal visit, making changes in sleeping arrangements before the birth of the baby, getting a special new bed for the older child, and planning ahead for the child care needed during the mother's hospitalization.
- Several parents looked for good children's books to help in preparing the older child but felt those available were poor.
- Greater involvement (prior and contemporary) of the father with the older child, seemed to be directly related to a better adjustment by the child to separation from the mother and to the baby.
- In every case where hospital policy allowed sibling visitations, it was viewed as very helpful by the parents.
- Gift giving to the older child at the time of birth, or at the mother and baby's homecoming had varied usefulness. In cases where it was most useful, the child was given something that he or she had wanted very much. "In each situation where dolls were given, invariably they were not accepted as cherished gifts" (p. 24).
- The most common regressions observed were demands for a bottle or pacifier, and interference with toilet training. Regression in toilet training was always accompanied by an additional stressor (over-protectiveness by mother, parental difficulty in managing aggressive impulses, or moving to a new home).
- Mothers who reported enhanced development on the part of the older child were also those who used a variety of supportive tactics.
- Direct aggression toward the baby tended to be delayed until the baby was more mobile, although some occurred earlier.
- In every case where the mother breast-fed, the older child responded with jealousy.

The minimal research that has investigated sibling adaptation to the birth of a new baby is too meager to serve as a basis for nursing intervention, but it does help point out the need for more research in this area and suggests variables that should be considered when studies are designed. Some questions that could be asked and researched are suggested below:

- What is the prevalence of various coping mechanisms (e.g. withdrawal, regression, acting out, and aggression) in a population of children who experience the birth of a sibling?
- In terms of each specific coping mechanism, is there a particular time postdelivery when the frequency and/or intensity of the coping mechanism peaks?
- What variables (e.g., other stressors such as moving, infant-feeding method, educational level of parents, degree of paternal involvement with older child) are associated with the use by older siblings of specific coping mechanisms?
- To what extent, or under what circumstances is the degree of overt disturbance on the part of older siblings correlated with the degree of covert disturbance? It appears that some parents are more comfortable with the idea that an older child may have negative feelings about the new baby than other parents. While some parents let children know that all feelings are okay—but that behavior will be limited—other parents convey to children that they should only have positive feelings. The latter children will probably resort to more covert ways of dealing with their feelings. This apparent phenomenon could be investigated.
- What types of prenatal and postpartum strategies are associated with healthy adaptation of older siblings to the birth of a new baby?
- What types of parental behavior are negatively correlated with healthy adaptation of young children to the birth of a new sibling?
- What nursing interventions are useful in promoting adaptation of younger children to the birth of a new sibling?

Sweet (1979) developed a unique program at the University of Minnesota for preparing siblings for the birth of a new baby. Families with children between approximately 2 and 10 years of age come by appointment to the prenatal clinic for a class session that is tailored to the needs of the particular family. There is discussion of what it will be like to have a baby in the family and about reproduction and the birth process. A variety of visual aids are used and children can handle life-sized models, which show the baby with umbilical cord in the uterus. Parents receive handouts that include suggestions on ways to help the child adapt, and a list of children's books that can be helpful. Although Legg et al. (1974) found that children in their study who were under 4 asked few questions about the pregnancy, children as young as 2 have been included in Sweet's individualized sessions. Parental evaluations of the program, which are completed immediately after the session and again at three weeks postpartum, have been unanimously positive.

NURSING STRATEGIES FOR FACILITATING FAMILY ADAPTATION

Family-Centered Care and Primary Nursing

In order to optimize the adaptation of all family members during the early days, weeks, and months following childbirth, a large repertoire of nursing strategies have been developed. Some, like primary nursing and family-centered health care have been widely accepted and employed by nurses across the country. Ciske (1979), who was one of the pioneers in the primary-nursing movement, has addressed common misconceptions about primary nursing and has attempted to clarify what it really is. Sonstegard and Egan (1976) have described the benefits of a program that combines the strategies of family-centered care and primary nursing.

Teaching–Learning During Postpartum Hospitalization

It is hard to imagine providing nursing care for newly expanded families without thinking of the many learning needs of the new parents. Both individual and group teaching–learning approaches have been widely used for a variety of specific purposes. Some specific learning needs of new parents and effective approaches for meeting these needs will be briefly described below.

Maternal Self-Care

When appropriate to the client's cognitive level and readiness, individual teaching about such things as breast care, use of the shower, perineal care, and uterine involution help the client maintain a sense of security and personal control, and can help her to better understand the restorative process, and how she can facilitate the process. This type of informal teaching is most effective when the nurse has time for questions and discussion.

Infant Characteristics and Infant Care

When the same nurse cares for the mother and infant there are many opportunities for teaching and learning to occur. Almost all infant care can take place at the mother's bedside with the father or other designated support person present. In such an atmosphere, it is easy to point out and discuss infant characteristics and behavior. The nurse can also observe parental responses to the infant and assess their attachment behaviors. Parents learn from observing the nurse as she works with the baby, from having the nurse demonstrate and explain specific skills, and from doing return demonstrations. When the nurse and the family mutually decide on the level of parental involvement at a given time, the amount of stress can be minimized and learning can be maximized. It is important for scheduling to be flexible enough so that the father or significant other person can be present.

When infant care is taught, it is helpful to stress to the parents that there is no right or wrong way to do each task, as long as a few basic principles are followed. For example, each nurse might demonstrate bathing the baby a little differently, but all will follow the "clean-to-dirty" principle. Knowing this may help the parents to develop flexibility in caring for their infant, to be less anxious when doing return demonstrations. An enjoyable alternative approach to infant bathing is the cuddle-bath which was researched and reported by Iles and McCrary (1976). During the cuddle-bath, the baby is completely covered with a folded, wet, warm towel. The cuddle-bath minimizes crying and often babies remain in the quiet–alert state during the bath. It is much easier to discuss principles of bathing with parents when the infant is not crying; it is also reinforcing to the parents to bathe an alert, calm baby who sometimes establishes eye contact during the bath process.

Family Planning and Resumption of Sexual Activity

Both individual couple and group instruction, or a combination of both, can be very effective if the instruction is appropriate to the individual clients, if expression of feelings and questions are encouraged, and if meaningful discussion takes place. As part of a group, couples learn that other new parents have similar concerns and questions; sometimes one person asks a question that another person could not verbalize. Sometimes, however, couples are more willing to discuss these intimate topics with one trusted nurse than within a group setting.

For family-planning discussions, it is helpful to use visual aids such as plastic models, diagrams, and examples of various types of contraceptives. Printed diagrams or slides of positions for sexual intercourse which reduce strain on the perineum can provide concrete help for clients. They also can help communicate matter-of-factly that the topic is important and can be discussed.

Return of the Figure to Normal

Since many new mothers are concerned about this topic, it deserves higher priority than it often receives during the postpartum hospitalization. Perhaps a specific "shaping-up" class, during which mothers discuss concerns about their bodies and see demonstrations of exercises, could be implemented. Mothers should be given printed diagrams and directions for any exercises that are taught.

Infant Massage

A growing number of postpartum newborn units offer a class on infant massage to new parents. These classes, which stress the importance of touching and stroking the infant, are usually extremely well attended by parents. Many parents are pleased to learn about something that can help them provide calming sensory stimulation to their babies. The massage technique described by LeBoyer (1976) can serve as a guideline for such a class and can be modified in order to be practical and appropriate for a given group of clients.

Feeding Techniques and Infant Nutrition

Much of the instruction about feeding takes place on an individual basis with the client. However, mothers can benefit from meeting together in small groups to discuss either bottle- or breast-feeding and related topics. Often, experienced mothers can be effective role models for new mothers and can share excellent pointers with the group. (See also Chapter 17 for more information about feeding techniques and infant nutrition.)

Going Home

At the University of Minnesota Hospitals, the "Going Home" class has been very well received by clients. The class serves as a method of providing anticipatory guidance for coping with new parenthood. Such a class can be especially effective if geared to the specific concerns and questions of each group of parents, and if a discussion approach is used. Topics covered may not always be the same but can include such common concerns as coping with crying, sibling adaptation, resumption of sexual activities, contraception, fatigue, relationships with relatives, maternal and infant symptoms that should be reported to the primary care provider, and resources for new parents that are in the individual communities.

A Learning Center

This approach to meeting postpartum learning needs has been tried, at least to some extent, in some hospitals. With some clever utilization of space and a lot of creativity, family-centered units could include a comfortable resource center for the families. Books on parenthood, infant care, infant growth and development, parenting, family planning, sexuality, and other topics could be used in the center or checked out and taken to the client's own room. Audiovisual materials on similar topics could be available for client self-instruction. This type of center would not replace individual and group teaching, but could reinforce it. Also clients could more thoroughly pursue topics of special interest to them.

Documentation of Teaching

Since teaching is such an important aspect of the nursing care provided on a new-family unit, it is important that it be documented carefully and systematically. Such documentation helps justify the staffing needed to carry out a comprehensive educational program, serves as a permanent record, and helps maximize the effectiveness and efficiency of client education. When teaching is documented on a teaching record or flow sheet it is more likely that needed reinforcement will occur, that random teaching by each different nurse will be eliminated, and that the family will have better opportunities for learning before discharge.

Sibling Visits

When prepared childbirth and various forms of family-centered labor, delivery, and postpartum care became available in so much of the country, some professionals and parents began to question whether family-centered care that left out older siblings really was family centered. Proposals for siblings to visit their mothers and look at the new baby through a glass partition were met with cries of concern that newborn infection would occur as a result—an echo of concerns that had been voiced when fathers were first allowed into labor and delivery areas, and were allowed to have postpartum contact with their infants.

Results of a two-year study by Mullaly and Kewin (1978), indicate that children are felt to benefit from early, hospital contact with their new sibling in the following ways: (1) they see their mother alive, well, and happy; (2) they are exposed to nurses and hospitals at a time when the focus is on wellness; (3) they gain a realistic perception of what the infant is like (i.e., not a playmate); (4) they see the baby prior to the important event of mother's homecoming; and (5) they can be reassured that mother still loves them.

Discharge Planning

Discharge planning begins soon after delivery and is coordinated by the primary nurse although she or he may not implement all aspects personally. Each part of the process is documented, and a permanent record of the discharge planning becomes a part of the client's record. It is helpful to develop some type of discharge planning guidelines or checklist. A checklist helps ensure that no part of the planning is omitted, and makes clear what has been accomplished. Discharge planning usually includes, but is not limited to: (1) assisting the client family with arrangements for follow-up appointments for the mother and infant; (2) planning with the family for desired educational experiences; (3) reviewing postpartum learning; (4) assessing the client's home situation and available resources; (5) assessing parent–infant bonding and the parent's infant caretaking skills; (6) coordinating or performing discharge examinations of mother and infant; (7) discussing community resources, such as parenting classes, with family; (8) referring to other agencies if indicated.

Early Discharge

Some parents, for a variety of reasons, desire to be discharged from the hospital or birth center within a few hours after delivery (Lubic, 1975). Some view childbearing as a healthy condition, feel that they can manage well at home, and perhaps have their own sources of support. They may oppose certain hospital policies. Mehl (1976) reported on outcomes of 130 early discharges and concluded that self-selected women who deliver without medication, and who meet specified criteria, can be discharged with their infants within a few hours after delivery without increasing maternal or neonatal risk. Close nurse–patient and doctor–patient relationships need to exist and a nurse should be available to make home visits if indicated. Mehl pointed out the methodological limitations of the study and the need for further research of early discharge.

Telephone Support, Home Visits, Referrals

Several strategies can make a difference in helping parents through the early, and sometimes difficult, postpartum weeks at home. One strategy is to make it clear to the parents at the time of discharge that they can phone the new-family unit when they have questions or concerns. They can either talk to a nurse that is working or leave a message for "their" nurse to call. A familiar nurse can often be helpful by just listening, answering questions for which there is a specific answer, helping the parent solve problems, or by referring the parent to

the primary care provider or another resource. Often parents ask questions as a means of seeking validation for what they are doing.

Another telephone strategy is for the nursing staff to contact client–families several days after discharge in order to offer support and assess the postdischarge adaptation. Haight (1977) reported on the value and efficiency of telephone follow-up. In addition to providing a needed service to clients, the telephone follow-up provided data for evaluating nursing services.

Few, if any, areas of our country have adequate public health nursing resources to provide for a postpartum follow-up visit to every newly expanded family. Sometimes it is impossible to determine at the time of discharge or before whether a family really needs a public health referral. A strategy that has been extremely helpful to families who deliver at the University of Minnesota Hospital, has been a follow-up home visit made one to two weeks after discharge by their primary nurse or another nurse from the new-family unit. As part of discharge planning, all clients who live within reasonable geographic boundaries are told about the service and encouraged to accept the visit. Some families are still referred to a community health agency at the time of hospital discharge. Others are referred after the nurse's home visit, if the assessment made in the home indicates that there is a need.

Parenting Classes

With prenatal education classes increasingly becoming available and being viewed as an integral part of prenatal care, attention has turned to the postpartum needs of families for education. Programs to meet these needs have been developed by nurses, psychologists, and at least one lay organization, although only a limited number of reports have appeared in the literature. While programs vary greatly in length and structure, all seem to share the philosophy that group discussion and peer support are as important as the specific information that is taught.

Smith and Smith (1978) reported on the Parent Education Project in Seattle, which was co-sponsored by the Junior League and Northwest Hospital and which included prenatal classes and five postpartum classes during the first three postpartum months. "The curriculum material was presented through small group methods. The small group classes were designed to enhance parents' problem-solving techniques and help parents gain self-confidence and security in their new roles" (p. 23). Well-qualified lay volunteers were trained to act as "follow-through agents." These persons assisted in classes and made follow-up phone calls and home visits. Although some parental cognitive changes were documented, the most impressive findings of the evaluation were parental comments about how the classes had decreased their anxiety, helped them to share feelings, and helped them to establish friendships.

Another approach to parenting classes has been developed by the Minnesota Early Learning Design (MELD), which received funding from the Lilly Foundation. MELD uses a parent self-help approach, with parents who have been trained by MELD serving as group facilitators. Groups are formed prenatally and continue for two years.

A Center for Parents

Miller and Baird (1978) described a nursing organization, called the Young Family Resource Center, that opened in 1977 and is jointly sponsored by the University of Texas at San Antonio and two community volunteer organizations. The organization has been funded by grant monies since its inception. To collect data for the original grant proposal, questionnaires were sent to 750 new parents. "In the 225 returned responses both mothers and fathers indicated significant deficits in information regarding baby care, expressed a great need to discuss their feelings following the birth of their baby, and felt the existing support systems in the community allowed many of their needs to remain unmet" (p. 118).

The aim of the organization is to provide primary prevention by offering information and support to parents of young children and by assisting them to use community resources effectively. The center staff includes: the director, a masters prepared nurse; the codirector, a Junior League member who coordinates the volunteers; and two clinical nurse specialists. All positions are part-time. Services offered by the organization include: parent discussion groups; workshops for parents; individual consultation, using the nursing process, with parents who have problems, a library of educational material covering a wide range of topics related to child care and family life; and referral. The center has been used as a clinical site for graduate nursing students and a pediatric resident. Miller and Baird feel that the center has provided a new role for nursing and is helping to meet the needs of the young families it serves.

REFERENCES AND ADDITIONAL READINGS

Adams, G. (1976). Recognizing the range of human sexual needs and behavior. *MCN: The American Journal of Maternal Child Nursing, 1,* 166–169. (a)

Adams, G. (1976). The sexual history as an integral part of the patient history. *MCN: The American Journal of Maternal Child Nursing, 1,* 170–175. (b)

Adams, H. & Flowers, C. Oral oxytocic drugs in the puerperium. *Obstetrics and Gynecology, 15,* 280–283.

Adams, M. (1963). Early concerns of primigravida mothers regarding infant care activities. *Nursing Research, 12,* 72–77.

Affonso, D. (1977). "Missing pieces"—A study of postpartum feelings. *Birth and the Family Journal, 4,* 159–164.

Anderson, S. (1979). Siblings at birth. *Birth and the Family Journal, 6,* 80–87.

Anderson, W., & Davis, J. (1968). Placental site involution. *American Journal of Obstetrics and Gynecology, 102,* 23–33.

Baird, S. (1979). Crisis intervention strategies. In S. Johnson (Ed.), *High risk parenting: Nursing assessment and strategies for the family at risk.* New York: Lippincott, pp. 299–311.

Barden, T. (1975). Perinatal care. In S. Romney, et al. (Eds.), *Gynecology and obstetrics: The health care of women.* New York: McGraw-Hill, pp. 704–712.

Benedek, T. (1970). Fatherhood and providing. In E.J. Anthony & T. Benedek (Eds.), *Parenthood: Its psychology and psychopathology.* Boston: Little, Brown, pp. 167–183.

Bing, E. (1975). *Moving through pregnancy.* New York: Bantam Books.

Bing, E., & Colman, L. (1977). *Making love during pregnancy.* New York: Bantam Books.

Brazelton, T. (1969). *Infants and mothers: Differences in development.* New York: Dell.

Cahill, A. (1975). Dual-purpose tool for assessing maternal needs and nursing care. *Journal of Obstetric, Gynecologic, and Neonatal Nursing, 4,* 28–32.

Cameron, J. (1979). Year-long classes for couples becoming parents. *MCN: The American Journal of Maternal Child Nursing, 4,* 358–362.

Campbell, S., & Smith, J. (1977). Postpartum assessment guide. *American Journal of Nursing, 77,* 1179.

Ciske, K. (1979). Accountability—The essence of primary nursing. American Journal of Nursing, 79, 890–894.

Clark, A. (1979). The postpartal period. In A. Clark & D. Affonso (Eds.), *Childbearing: A nursing perspective.* Philadelphia: Davis, pp. 471–535.

Clausen, J. (1972). Efficient postpartum checks. *Nursing 72, 2,* 24–25.

Crummette, B. (1975). Transitions in motherhood. *Maternal–Child Nursing Journal, 4,* 65–73.

Dodd, M. (1979). Caring for persons requiring applications of heat and cold. In K. Sorensen & J. Luckmann (Eds.), *Basic nursing: A psychophysiologic approach.* Philadelphia: Saunders, pp. 1145–1172.

Donaldson, N. (1977). Fourth trimester follow-up. *American Journal of Nursing, 77,* 1176–1178.

Donaldson, N. (1981). The postpartum follow-up nurse clinician. *Journal of Obstetric, Gynecologic, and Neonatal Nursing, 10,* 249–254.

Duvall, E. (1977). *Marriage and family development*. Philadelphia: Lippincott.

Dyer, E. (1963). Parenthood as crisis: A re-study. *Marriage and Family Living, 25*, 196–201.

Easterling, W. (1977). The puerperium. In D. Danforth (Ed.), *Obstetrics and gynecology* (ed. 3). New York: Harper & Row.

Edwards, M. (1973). The crises of the fourth trimester. *Birth and the Family Journal, 1*, 19–22.

Erikson, E. (1963). *Childhood and society*. (ed. 2). New York: Norton.

Falicov, C. (1973). Sexual adjustment during first pregnancy and post partum. *American Journal of Obstetrics and Gynecology, 117*, 991–1000.

Fawcett, J. (1977). The relationship between identification and patterns of change in spouses' body image during and after pregnancy. *International Journal of Nursing Studies, 14*, 199–213.

Fein, R. (1976). The first weeks of fathering: The importance of choices and supports for new parents. *Birth and the Family Journal, 3*, 53–57.

Fishbein, E. (1981). The convade: A review. *Journal of Obstetric, Gynecologic, and Neonatal Nursing, 10*, 356–359.

Gaspard, U., Remacle, P., Van Cauwenberge, J.R., Colin, C., Hendrick, J., Reuter, A., Legros, J., & Franchimont, P. (1978). Simultaneous evaluation of the serum levels of estradiol, prolactin, casein and neurophysins in gestational and nursing women. In C. Robyn & M. Harter (Eds.), *Progress in prolactin physiology and pathology*. Amsterdam: Elsevier, pp. 233–241.

Gearing, J. (1978). Facilitating the birth process and father–child bonding. *The Counseling Psychologist, 7*, 53–55.

Gilman, R., & Knox, D. (1976). Coping with fatherhood: The first year. *Child Psychiatry and Human Development, 6*, 134–148.

Gollober, M. (1976). A comment on the need for father–infant postpartal interaction. *Journal of Obstetric, Gynecologic, and Neonatal Nursing, 5*, 17–20.

Gordon, R., et al. (1965). Factors in postpartum emotional adjustment. *Obstetrics and Gynecology, 25*, 158–166.

Gruis, M. (1977). Beyond maternity: Postpartum concerns of mothers. *MCN: The American Journal of Maternal Child Nursing, 2*, 182–188.

Haight, J. (1977). Steadying parents as they go—by phone, *MCN: The American Journal of Maternal Child Nursing, 2*, 311–312.

Hames, C. (1980). Sexual needs and interests of postpartum couples. *Journal of Obstetric, Gynecologic, and Neonatal Nursing, 9*, 313–315.

Harris, R., Thomas, V., & Hui, G. (1977). Postpartum surveillance for urinary tract infection: Patients at risk of developing pyelonephritis after catheterization. *Southern Medical Journal, 70*, 1273–1275.

Havinghurst, R. (1972). *Developmental tasks and education* (ed. 3). New York: David McKay Co.

Heise, J. (1975). Toward better preparation for prepared fatherhood. *Journal of Obstetric, Gynecologic, and Neonatal Nursing, 4*, 32–35.

Hendricks, C.H., Eskes, & Saameli. (1962). Uterine contractility at delivery and in the puerperium. *American Journal of Obstetrics and Gynecology, 83*, 890–906.

Hill, M. (1978). A descriptive study of the concerns and educational interests of women during the immediate postpartum period. (Unpublished Master's thesis, University of Minnesota, Minneapolis, Mn.).

Hill, R. (1949). *Families under stress*. New York: Harper & Brothers.

Hobbs, D. (1965). Parenthood as crisis: A third study. *Journal of Marriage and the Family, 27*, 367–372.

Hobbs, D. (1968). Transition to parenthood: A replication and extension. *Journal of Marriage and the Family, 30*, 413–417.

Iles, J.P., & McCrary, M. (1976). Cuddle bathing can be fun. *MCN: The American Journal of Maternal Child Nursing, 1*, 350–354.

Inglis, T. (1980). Postpartum sexuality. *Journal of Obstetric, Gynecologic, and Neonatal Nursing, 9*, 298–300.

International Childbirth Education Association, Inc. (1978). *Position Paper on Planning Comprehensive Maternal and Newborn Services for the Childbearing Year*. Milwaukee: ICEA. (Available from ICEA, P.O. Box 20852, Milwaukee, WI 53220.).

Interprofessional Task Force on Health Care of Women and Children. (1978). *Joint Position Statement on the Development of Family Centered Maternity/Newborn Care in Hospitals*. (Available from Interprofessional Task Force Secretariat, ACOG, 1 East Wacker Drive, Suite 2700, Chicago, IL 60601.).

Israel, S.L., & Rubin, I. (1967). *Sexual relations during pregnancy and the post-delivery period*. New York: Siecus, 1967.

Jacoby, A. (1969). Transition to parenthood: A reassessment. *Journal of Marriage and the Family, 31*, 720–727.

Jain, A., et al. (1978). Aspirin and aspirin-caffeine in postpartum pain relief. *Clinical Pharmacology and Therapeutics, 24*, 69–75.

Jensen, M.D., Benson, R., & Bobak, I. (1977). *Maternity care: The nurse and the family*. St. Louis: pp. 413–446, 689–702.

Kyndely, K. (1978). The sexuality of women in pregnancy and postpartum. *Journal of Obstetric, Gynecologic, and Neonatal Nursing, 7*, 23–32.

Lamb, M. (1975). Fathers: Forgotten contributors to child development. *Human Development, 18*, 245–266.

Leander, K., & Grassley, J. (1980). Making love after birth. *Birth and the Family Journal, 7*, 181–185.

LeBoyer, F. (1976). *Loving hands*. New York: Knopf.

Legg, C., Sherick, I., & Wadland, W. (1974). Reaction of preschool children to the birth of a sibling. *Child Psychiatry and Human Development, 5*, 3–39.

LeMasters, E.E. (1957). Parenthood as crisis. *Marriage and Family Living, 19*, 352–355.

Lubic, R. (1975). Developing maternity services women will trust. *American Journal of Nursing, 75*, 1685–1688.

Malinowski, J. (1978). Bladder assessment in the postpartum patient. *Journal of Obstetric, Gynecologic, and Neonatal Nursing, 7*, 14–16.

Malinowski, J. (1979). Answering a child's questions about sex and a new baby. *American Journal of Nursing, 79*, 1965–1968.

Manion, J. (1977). A study of fathers and infant caretaking. *Birth and the Family Journal, 4*, 174–179.

Marecki, M. (1979). Postpartum follow-up goals and assessment. *Journal of Obstetric, Gynecologic, and Neonatal Nursing, 8*, 214–218.

Masters, W., & Johnson, V. (1966). *Human sexual response*. Boston: Little, Brown.

May, K. (1978). Active involvement of fathers in pregnancy: Some further considerations. *Journal of Obstetric, Gynecologic, and Neonatal Nursing, 7*,(2), 7–12.

Mehl, L. (1975). Complications of home birth. *Birth and the Family Journal, 2*, 123–134.

Mehl, L. (1976). Outcomes of early discharge after normal birth. *Birth and the Family Journal, 3*, 101–107.

Meleis, A. (1975). Role insufficiency and role supplementation: A conceptual framework. *Nursing Research, 24*, 264–271.

Meleis, A., & Swendsen, L. (1978). Role supplementation: An empirical test of a nursing intervention. *Nursing Research, 27*, 11–18.

Mercer, R. (1979). She's a multip...She knows the ropes. *MCN: The American Journal of Maternal Child Nursing, 4,* 301–304.

Mercer, R. (1981). The nurse and maternal tasks of early postpartum. *MCN: The American Journal of Maternal Child Nursing, 6,* 341–345.

Merrill, S., & Olson, K. (1979). Nurses' attitudes toward allowing siblings to have contact with the newborn. (Unpublished clinical study, University of Minnesota, Minneapolis, Mn.).

Miller, D., & Baird, S. (1978). Helping parents to be parents—A special center. *MCN: The American Journal of Maternal Child Nursing, 3,* 117–120.

Morris, J., Creasy, R., & Hohe, P. (1970). Inhibition of puerperal lactation. *Obstetrics and Gynecology, 36,* 107–114.

Moss, J. (1981). Concerns of multiparas on the third postpartum day. *Journal of Obstetric, Gynecologic, and Neonatal Nursing, 10,* 421–424.

Mullaly, L. & Kerwin, M. (1978). Changing the status quo. *MCN: The American Journal of Maternal Child Nursing, 3,* 75–80, 124.

Mundow, L. (1975). Danthron/polxalkol and placebo in puerperal constipation. *The British Journal of Clinical Practice, 29,* 95–96.

Newton, N. (1973). Interrelationships between sexual responsiveness, birth, and breast feeding. In J. Zubin & J. Money (Eds.), *Contemporary sexual behavior: Critical issues in the 1970's.* Baltimore: John Hopkins University Press.

Norr, K. (1980). The second time around: Parity and birth experience *Journal of Obstetric, Gynecologic, and Neonatal Nursing, 9,* 30–36.

Nott, P.N. (1976). Hormonal changes and mood in the puerperium. *British Journal of Psychiatry, 128,* (1976), 379–383.

Obrzut, L.A.J. (1976). Expectant fathers' perception of fathering. *American Journal of Nursing, 76,* 1440–1442.

Olson, M. (1981). Fitting grandparents into new families. *MCN: The American Journal of Maternal Child Nursing, 6,* 419–421.

Perez, P. (1979). Nurturing children who attend the birth of a sibling. *MCN: The American Journal of Maternal Child Nursing, 4,* 215–217.

Petre-Quadens, O., & DeLee, C. (1974). Sleep-cycle alterations during pregnancy, postpartum, and the menstrual cycle. In M. Ferin (Ed.), *Biorhythms and human reproduction.* New York: Wiley, pp. 335–341.

Petrowski, D. (1981). Effectiveness of prenatal and postnatal instruction in postpartum care. *Journal of Obstetric, Gynecologic, and Neonatal Nursing, 10,* 386–389.

Physicians' Desk Reference. (1979). Oradell, N.J.: Medical Economics Co., p. 1391.

Pritchard, J., & MacDonald, P. (1976). *Williams obstetrics* (ed. 15). New York: Appleton-Century-Crofts, pp. 374–384.

Reiber, V. (1976). Is the nurturing role natural to fathers? *MCN: The American Journal of Maternal Child Nursing, 1,* 366–371.

Resnick, J. (1978). Fathering classes: A psycho/educational model. *The Counseling Psychologist, 7,* 56–60.

Rising, S. (1974). The fourth stage of labor: Family integration. *American Journal of Nursing, 74,* 870–874.

Rossi, A. (1968). Transition to parenthood. *Journal of Marriage and the Family, 30,* 26–39.

Rubin, R. (1961). Puerperal change. *Nursing Outlook, 9,* 753–755.

Rubin, R. (1967). Attainment of the maternal role, part I: Process. *Nursing Research, 16,* 237–245. (a)

Rubin, R. (1967). Attainment of the maternal role, part II: Models and referrants. *Nursing Research, 16,* 342–346. (b)

Rubin, R. (1975). Maternity nursing stops too soon. *American Journal of Nursing, 75,* 1680–1684.

Salk, L. (1972). *What every child would like his parents to know.* New York: David McKay Co.

Sanford, S. (1979). Promoting rest and sleep. In K. Sorensen & J. Luckmann (Eds.), *Basic nursing.* Philadelphia: Saunders, pp. 540–547.

Schmidt, J. (1978). Using a teaching guide for better postpartum and infant care. *Journal of Obstetric, Gynecologic, and Neonatal Nursing, 7,* 23–25.

Sharman, A. (1953). Postpartum regeneration of the human endometrium. *Journal of Anatomy, 87,* 1–10.

Sheehan, F. (1981). Assessing postpartum adjustment: A pilot study. *Journal of Obstetric, Gynecologic, and Neonatal Nursing, 10,* 19–23.

Shereshefsky, P. (1973). Summary and integration of findings. In P. Shereshefsky & L. Yarrow (Eds.), *Psychological aspects of a first pregnancy and early postnatal adaptation.* New York: Raven Press, pp. 237–251.

Smith, D., & Smith, H. (1978). Toward improvements in parenting: A description of prenatal and postpartum classes with teaching guide. *Journal of Obstetric, Gynecologic, and Neonatal Nursing, 7,* 22–27.

Smith, E. (1978). Group process and childbirth education: A position paper. *Journal of Obstetric, Gynecologic, and Neonatal Nursing, 7,*(4), 51–54.

Sonstegard, L., & Egan, E. (1976). Family-centered nursing makes a difference. *MCN: The American Journal of Maternal Child Nursing, 1,* 249–255.

Spock, B. (1976). *Baby and child care, revised.* New York: Pocket Books.

Storr, G. (1978). Postpartal assessment. *Canadian Nurse,* May, 35–37.

Stranik, M.K., & Hogberg, B.L. (1979). Transition into parenthood. *American Journal of Nursing, 79,* 90–93.

Sullivan, D., & Beeman, R. (1981). Satisfaction with postpartum care: Opportunities for bonding, reconstructing the birth and instruction. *Birth and the Faily Journal, 8,* 153–159.

Sumner, G., & Fritsch, J. (1977). Postnatal parental concerns: The first six weeks of life, *Journal of Obstetric, Gynecologic, and Neonatal Nursing, 6,* 27–32.

Swanson, J. (1980). The marital sexual relationship during pregnancy, *Nursing, 9,* 267–270.

Sweet, P. (1979). Prenatal classes especially for children. *MCN: The American Journal of Maternal Child Nursing, 4,* 82–83. (a)

Sweet, P. (1979). Letters to the editor. *MCN: The American Journal of Maternal Child Nursing, 4,* 276, 319. (b)

Swendsen, L., Meleis, A., & Jones, D. (1978). Role supplementation for new parents—A role mastery plan. *MCN: The American Journal of Maternal Child Nursing, 3,* 84–91.

Tentoni, S., & High, K. (1980). Culturally induced postpartum depression: A theoretical position. *Journal of Obstetric, Gynecologic, and Neonatal Nursing, 9,* 246–248.

Timberlake, B. (1975). The new life center. *American Journal of Nursing, 75,* 1456–1461.

Tindall, V.R. (1968). Factors influencing puerperal thrombo-embolism. *Journal of Obstetrics and Gynecology of the British Commonwealth, 75,* 1324–1327.

Tolor, A., & DiGrazia, P. (1976). Sexual attitudes and behavior patterns during and following pregnancy. *Archives of Sexual Behavior, 5,* 539–551.

Trause, M.A. (1978). Birth in the hospital: The effect on the sibling. *Birth and the Family Journal, 5,* 207–209.

Turnbull, A. (1968). Puerperal thrombo-embolism and suppression of lactation. *Journal of Obstetrics and Gynecology of the British Commonwealth, 75,* 1321–1323.

Tyson, J., Carter, J., Andreassen, B., Huth, J., & Smith, B. (1978). Nursing-mediated prolactin and luteinizing hormone secretion during puerperal lactation. *Fertility and Sterility, 30,* 154–162.

Voherr, H. (1974). *The breast.* New York: Academic Press.

Wandersman, L. (1980). The adjustment of fathers to their first baby: The roles of parenting groups and marital relationship. *Birth and the Family Journal, 7,* 155–161.

Williams, B. (1967). Sleep needs during the maternity cycle. *Nursing Outlook, 15,* 53–55.

Williams, J. (1977). Learning needs of new parents. *American Journal of Nursing, 77,* 1173.

Williams, J.W. (1931). Regeneration of the uterine mucosa after delivery, with especial reference to the placental site. *American Journal of Obstetrics and Gynecology, 22,* 664–693.

Womack, W., Allen, G., Christensen, O., Hansen, I., & Gomez, A. (1962). A comparison of home therapies for suppression of lactation. *Southern Medical Journal, 55,* 816–820.

Woolery, L., & Barkley, N. (1981). Enhancing couple relationships during prenatal and postnatal classes. *MCN: The American Journal of Maternal Child Nursing, 6,* 184–188.

Zalar, M. (1976). Sexual counseling for pregnant couples. *MCN: The American Journal of Maternal Child Nursing, 1,* 176–181. (Also see four other related articles on sexuality in this issue.)

Ziegel, E., & Cranley, M. (1978). *Obstetric nursing* (ed. 7). New York: Macmillan, pp. 551–601.

Chapter 15

Framework for Facilitating Attachment: Newborn Assessment

Lula O. Lubchenco

CONVINCING ANIMAL DATA showing the importance of the period immediately after the birth, and the effect of separation at this time on the mother's ability to attach to her offspring, have been known and accepted for at least two decades, although they haven't been applied to humans until recently. It is not known whether this is due to a greater human potential for attachment and a longer period in which it can occur, or because the human mother can mask her feelings and present outward behavior to conform to social standards of motherhood.

Currently, parents are expressing their feelings about the birth process, and in response, obstetric and pediatric practices are being altered to provide the family with the experience they desire during pregnancy, labor, delivery, and the postpartum period. Klaus and Kennell (1982) have studied the behavior of mothers as they bond to their infants and the characteristics of the newborn that contribute to the bonding process.

It is not yet known how beneficial early mother–infant contact is for mothers who have negative attitudes about the pregnancy, or for unhealthy mothers or infants.

This chapter deals primarily with healthy mothers and infants, and those who want their babies. However, it is important to detect problems in the mother–infant relationship at an early stage; methods to accomplish this will be addressed.

PHYSIOLOGY OF TRANSITION

Although dramatic changes occur when the fetus becomes a newborn, and thus an independent person, the transition is not so abrupt as one might imagine.

The development of each major organ system is appropriate for the age of the fetus and compatible with intra-uterine existence and preparation for the event of birth.

The Respiratory System

The first major task of the newborn is to breathe. He must change his oxygen source from that of the placental circulation to his own lungs. If he does not accomplish this task, he will die. If he is born at term, his lungs have developed and matured and are adequate to this task. Surfactant has been produced and is present in the alveoli so that they remain open when he takes his first breath. He has made breathing movements for weeks prior to the big event, and these muscles are ready to go.

Many organ systems, like the lungs, seem to be programmed on a developmental time schedule. Others, such as the cardiovascular system, are developed only to a level compatible with intra-uterine life; but once birth occurs they respond appropriately. When comparing in utero physiological processes with the adaptation of the newborn, one must marvel at the appropriateness of his functions and behavior in each situation. He cannot be considered immature compared to an older child or adult, but must be considered uniquely adaptive to this period of life.

The Cardiovascular System

The cardiovascular system is the second major organ called upon to make acute change. Consider for a moment what would happen if the ductus arteriosus closed on a time schedule, rather than in response to birth. If this happened at forty weeks' gestation, regardless of birth, and the infant was still in utero, flooding of the unaerated lungs with blood would reduce the amount of blood perfusing the placenta, brain and other organs and would place the fetus in jeopardy for his life. On the other hand, if the infant was delivered at thirty-eight weeks, and the pulmonary arteries and arterioles of the lung remained in spasm, oxygenation and blood perfusion of the lungs would not occur. Actually, this situation does occur and is known as *persistent fetal circulation*—a severe and often fatal condition.

After the first breath, when the blood vessels of the lungs are usually filled with blood, the cardiovascular system has a little leeway in completing its other changes. The ductus can remain open for days without harmful effects.

Suppose also that the gastrointestinal tract, rather than waiting for birth, began functioning at thirty-eight weeks' gestation. The amniotic fluid would be filled with meconium, and the problems of meconium aspiration would become astronomical. Why the fetus does *not* pass meconium is a mystery, for it is known that he swallows amniotic fluid in utero and that the gastrointestinal tract is functional.

These illustrations serve to emphasize the unique qualities of the fetus that make the transition from intra- to extra-uterine life possible.

The Newborn's Response to Stress

The qualities that make the newborn different from the older child are essential to the successful transition from fetal to extra-uterine life. Stave (1970) has referred to this quality as "tolerance," but has described it in the newborn as an active withdrawal or nonreacting to the stresses of birth and not as a passive, uninvolved act. Brazelton (1973) has referred to this same behavior as "turning off" and has demonstrated the infants' ability to decrement his responses to visual, auditory, and tactile stimuli. Furthermore, Stave has shown that the premature infant possesses more tolerance to various stresses than does the full-term infant. There is sketchy evidence suggesting that the postterm infant has less tolerance for the birth process than does the term infant—a factor that may be involved in the dangers of postterm birth.

The diagnosis of illness in a newborn, and especially a premature newborn, is much more difficult than it is in an older child since the newborn's protective behavior to any stress is to withdraw—that is, not to react with symptoms. By the time symptoms appear the infant's ability to protect himself has been exceeded.

An illustration of this concept is apparent in Cornblath and Schwartz's (1966) study of hypoglycemia. They use a glucose level of 20 mg/dl for the preterm and 30 mg/dl for the term infant. The preterm infant does not show symptoms until his glucose level reaches about 20 mg/dl. The term infant tolerates a glucose level well below that of the older child, but reacts when it drops below 30 mg/dl; the postterm infant may not tolerate 40 mg/dl, and we, as adults, get pretty uncomfortable at 50–60 mg/dl.

This suggests that we need to look for different symptoms in the newborn population. How can one detect that the infant is withdrawing? He is quiet, maybe lethargic, his eyes remain closed and it is difficult to bring him into an alert state. When he is disturbed, he may become irritable rather than alert. It

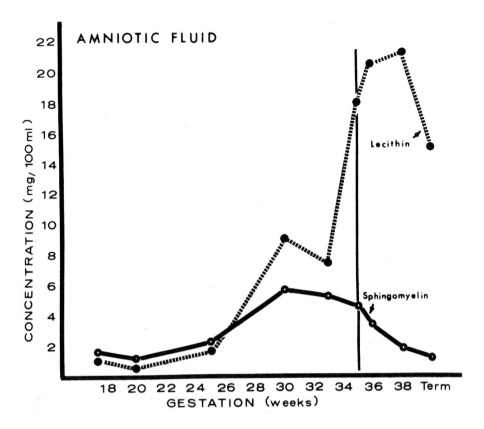

FIGURE 15-1   Mean concentration in amniotic fluid of sphingomyelin and lecithin during gestation. The acute rise in lecithin at thirty-five weeks marks pulmonary maturity. (From Gluck, L., Kulovich, M.V., Borer, W.N. (1971). Diagnosis of respiratory distress syndrome by amnioceutesis. *American Journal of Obstetrics and Gynecology, 109,* 440–445. With permission.)

usually follows that a "sleepy" infant does not nurse well, and physicians have often treated infants based on these symptoms alone.

Since the behavior of a stressed infant is similar for all stresses, neonatal laboratory screening becomes very important. Only with measurements of glucose, hematocrit, blood count, and cultures can one identify the exact cause of the stress. Vital signs checked routinely help identify pulmonary or vascular system disorders. Assessment of gestational age, birth weight, and classification of newborn infants can suggest only likely morbidities.

Adaptation During the Transition Period

The Lungs

The lungs begin as "outpocketings" of the gut in embryonic life and progress to the formation of bronchi and bronchioles by twenty-four weeks' gestation. By twenty-eight weeks alveoli are distinct. New alveoli are produced even after term birth, which makes possible the remarkable improvement of preterm infants with pulmonary disorders. The production of surfactant, necessary to maintain alveolar stability, does not usually appear until twenty-six to twenty-eight weeks' gestation. There are three types of epithelial cells identified in the alveoli: one produces osmiophilic inclusions, one produces connective tissue, and the other produces macrophages. The osmiophilic granules appear to be precursors of surfactant. Tracheobronchial fluid is excreted into the amniotic fluid and contributes, among other substances, lecithin and sphingomyelin. Since lecithin is the primary constituent that increases toward term, and sphingomyelin remains fairly constant throughout gestation, the ratio between the two (the L:S ratio) is used to determine lung maturity (Figure 15-1).

At term there are adequate alveoli, a good supply of surfactant, and well-defined evidence of "breathing" in utero. A great deal of research has attempted to determine the precise trigger that initiates the first breath. One of the important factors is body cooling. The wet

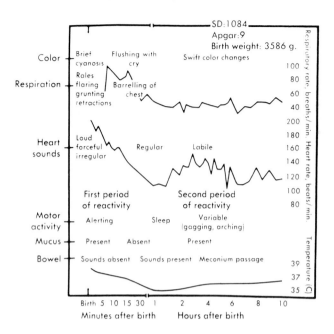

FIGURE 15-2 Desmond's chart: a summary of the physical findings noted during the first ten hours of extra-uterine life in a representative high-Apgar-score infant delivered under spinal anesthesia without prior medication. (From Desmond, M.M., Rudolf, A.J., & Phitakspraiwan, P. (1966). The transitional care nursery. *Pediatric Clinics of North America, 13,* 651–668. With permission.)

infant, born into a cooler air environment, gasps, and with this first breath most of the alveoli are opened. Successive breaths complete the process, and within minutes the lungs appear radiolucent on x-ray. Continued cooling is not beneficial, and in fact an energy source is required to maintain body temperature.

As illustrated in Figure 15-2 (Desmond's chart), one realizes that pulmonary adjustment may take some time. The respiratory rate is accelerated (60–80 breaths/min) for thirty to sixty minutes; there may be barrelling of the chest, indicating over-expansion of the lungs or the presence of extra alveolor air. By one to two hours after birth the rate is down although not stable.

This critical vital sign is usually overlooked, as it is not apparent unless the respiratory rate is actually counted. The infant's behavior to birth stress, described earlier, tends to distract one from his difficulty: for the most part he is lying quietly, usually in a flexed position, alert, eyes open and searching. One does not appreciate his distress until the process has advanced to the stage when he can no longer tolerate it and becomes obviously ill.

Cardiovascular System

The cardiovascular system is also uniquely suited to the fetus, yet is prepared to adapt to extra-uterine function once birth occurs. The heart begins to beat about three weeks after conception and by five weeks, the circulation is established. A large amount of the blood is in the placenta so that preterm birth poses a problem to the infant, either with hypovolemia if the cord is clamped immediately or hyperviscosity if clamped late and the infant is held below the placenta so that a large placental transfer of blood occurs.

During fetal development, oxygenated blood from the umbilical veins is shunted across the foramen ovale to the left atrium and ventricle, permitting the better oxygenated blood to perfuse the brain. Blood coming into the right atrium from the superior vena cava is less saturated with oxygen. A small amount goes from the ventricle to the lungs, the rest is then shunted via the ductus arteriosus to the descending aorta, the limbs, and via the umbilical arteries to the placenta.

The foramen ovale does not grow in size as gestation progresses, therefore more and more blood is left in the right atrium, preparing the fetus for the important task of filling the pulmonary vessels with blood at the time of birth.

As shown in the heart rate tracing of a normal high Apgar infant in Figure 15-2, this is not an easy task. At birth the sounds are loud, forceful, and irregular. The rate is 160–180 beats/min and falls over the next hour to a labile 100–140 range. The murmur of the ductus arteriosus is not heard at this time, either because the ductus is so large that the flow does not produce a murmur, or because it becomes functionally closed when the pulmonary artery pressure equals the aortic pressure. However, if one listens to the heart frequently over the next two to three days, a typical to-and-fro murmur is often heard.

Temperature Regulation

Heat production is not of great concern to the fetus, who lives in a carefully controlled environment. He begins laying down fat at about thirty-five weeks and by term is fairly well insulated against the temperature changes he will experience at birth. However, heat loss does occur at birth via conduction, convection, and evaporation.

In order to maintain a body temperature of 37°C in a cooler atmosphere, the infant must utilize available endogenous nutrients. Oxygen consumption studies indicate that there are thermal neutral zones in which infants expend the least amount of energy to maintain

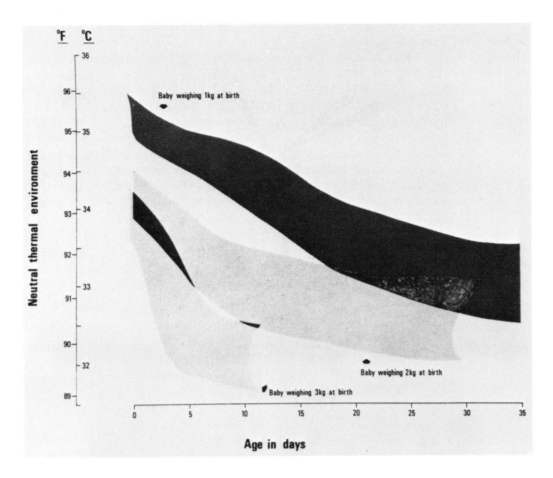

FIGURE 15-3 The range of temperatures needed to provide neutral environmental conditions for a baby lying naked on a warm mattress in draft-free surroundings at 50% humidity. (Adapted from Hey, E.N., & Katz, G. (1970). The optimum thermal environment for naked babies. *Archives of Diseases of Childhood, 45,* 328–334. With permission.)

body temperature, depending on birth weight and days after birth (Figure 15-3). Energy sources include glycogen stores, fats, and even proteins stored in muscles. Exogenous sources (food or parenteral supply) are necessary since the infant utilizes his stores of glycogen very quickly; once this occurs he may become hypoglycemic and eventually hypothermic. The infant generates very little heat through shivering, but does have a layer of brown fat around vital organs and in the region of the neck. This fat is metabolically active and locally warm.

It is clear from these data that a newborn infant needs a warm environment and early feeding soon after birth.

Gastrointestinal System

During fetal life, essential nutrients for growth are provided by the mother via the placenta. The growth and development of the gastrointestinal tract has been described, but characteristics of cells and morphology are not clearly related to nutrition. Neither the prematurely born infant nor the term infant has much, if any, difficulty in absorbing nutrients from the gastrointestinal tract. Sucking and swallowing occur in utero, and by about thirty-four weeks' gestation are sufficiently developed to make nipple feeding possible.

It has become increasingly clear that human milk is the nutrient of choice for the term infant. Not only is the overall composition of fats, carbohydrates, and protein ideal, but there are immunological factors vital to the well-being of the infant. Even substances once thought to be deficient in human milk, such as iron, are now found to be quite adequate because the newborn exhibits enhanced utilization of the amounts present (McMillan et al., 1976).

Some workers believe, however, that human milk is inadequate in calories, protein, and calcium for the

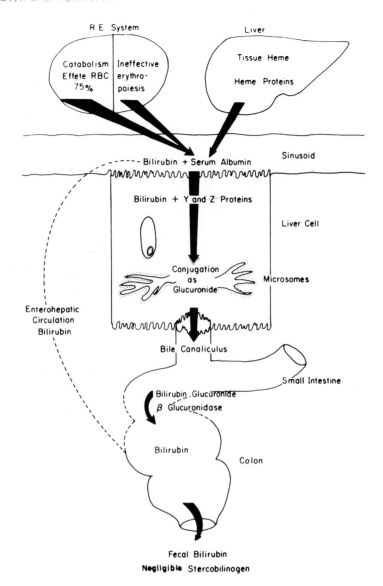

FIGURE 15-4   Bilirubin metabolism. (From Maisels, M.J. (1972). Bilirubin: On understanding and influencing its metabolism in the newborn infant. *Pediatric Clinics of North America, 19,* 447–501. With permission.)

preterm infant because of his increased need of these substances during rapid growth.

Renal Function

The term infant has limited renal function compared to the older child and adult, but experiences difficulty with renal function only under unusual conditions of water deprivation, water overload, or administration of a large load of solutes. The preterm infant is even more compromised, since the concentrating capacity of the kidney is less than that in the full-term infant. Renal maturity can be measured during fetal development by the amount of creatinine found in the amniotic fluid. Glomerular filtration rate seems to be related to blood pressure and blood flow through the kidneys. Tubular function is adequate for the term infant but is less developed than glomerular function.

Bilirubin Metabolism

This complex neonatal function is best explained visually (see Figure 15-4). It was once thought that conjugation of bilirubin in the liver began only after birth, but is now known to occur during fetal life. The term newborn is capable of conjugating at least two-thirds to three-fourths of the load presented to the liver.

The problem is not so much with conjugation of a "normal" load as it is with an extra amount of bilirubin. Conditions surrounding birth, which accentuate bilirubin accumulation, include an overload of bilirubin from the breakdown of extravasated blood (cephalhematoma). Just as important is the enterohepatic recirculation of bilirubin. Meconium is rich in bilirubin and if not excreted promptly may become hydrolyzed to the original unconjugated form, absorbed into the blood stream, taken to the liver, and conjugated a second or multiple times. Fetal distress, hypoxia, or a delay in provision of glucose may also reduce liver function.

When infections occur in the newborn, bilirubin levels increase. Jaundice accompanying sepsis may be due to hemolysis or toxicity to liver cells, plus decreased mobility of the gastrointestinal tract.

Immunological Maturity

The newborn is immunologically deficient. Low or deficient levels of immune substances (IgA, IgM) can be demonstrated in the newborn's plasma and numerous clinical examples of susceptibility to infection—primarily to gram-negative organisms—are known.

If the infant is fed breast milk in adequate amounts from his own mother, he becomes immunologically competent. Early, or first, contact with the mother serves to colonize the baby with organisms best tolerated by him—i.e., those for which the mother has made antibodies and has transferred some of these to the infant via IgG.

There are several factors in human milk that help to protect the newborn from infection: IgA, which coats the gastrointestinal tract; lysozyme, a nonspecific antibacterial substance; and lactoferrin, which inhibits the growth of microorganisms by chelating iron (see Chapter 17). The predominant organism in the gastrointestinal tract of breast-fed infants is *Lactobacillus bifidus.* The pH of the gastrointestinal tract is acid in breast-fed infants, allowing for growth of the *Lactobacillus* organism and decreasing the colonization of the intestine with enteric pathogens, especially gram-negative organisms. Living cells (leukocytes and phagocytes) from ingested milk further assist the newborn's fight against infection.

If breast milk is collected and then boiled, many of these substances are destroyed. Freezing is less destructive but does result in killing live cells and reducing some of the immunological properties. Obviously, the ideal feeding method is directly from the breast of the baby's own mother.

Central Nervous System

The brain and spinal cord develop early in embryonic life and are large enough to account for the gross appearance of the embryo during the early weeks. Reflex movement to tactile stimuli is apparent early in fetal life; the responses are incomplete, due more to lack of development of muscles and tendons than to sensory awareness.

Development of muscle tone and reflexes during the last trimester has been detailed and is basic to the determination of gestational age (see section on Gestational Age Assessment). Neurological development progresses in the same manner whether the fetus remains in utero or the infant is born prematurely.

Our understanding of the development and function of sensory organs is not yet complete, nor is our knowledge of sleep states and other behaviors, but the term infant possesses amazing qualities of awareness and ability to interact.

Vision has received a great deal of attention following Klaus and Kennell's (1979) observations on mother–infant interaction and Brazelton's (1973) documentation of the term infant's ability to fix and follow an object. Hearing, likewise, is obvious and discriminatory in the newborn. Sensitivity of the infant to touch is known but has not been studied as much as vision and hearing. The senses of smell and taste also need further research.

The Infant's Contribution to the Bonding Process

How can one analyze the appeal or the fascination of a newly born infant? Much depends on adult attitudes, customs, and culture, but the average person finds the event of birth a stirring time.

During birth the primary feelings are of concern, even of life or death: Will the mother be all right? Will the baby survive? Only vaguely, if at all, does one think about whether the baby is a boy or girl, how large he is, or what color his eyes are. But immediately after the baby is born, there is the realization that this infant is a new, unique individual, with physical characteristics unlike anyone else.

A frequent delivery room scene goes like this: "It's a boy!" "Our boy!" The first cry is met with smiles by the parents and often short comments such as "Listen to him, he's yelling his head off." Then attention to his eyes—"They're wide open." If the baby is on the mother's abdomen or in her arms, comforting measures, caresses, stroking the face, holding the hands occur. Mother and father talk to the infant—often unaware of the presence of anyone, save the baby. When delivery of the placenta is imminent, the father may take the baby and frequently becomes engrossed in the infant to the exclusion of the mother. Once out of the delivery room mother and father uncover the infant and examine him from head to toe, usually talking all the time. He is then bundled up and at this point often shared with family and friends. At about 1 hour of age the infant shows increasing hand to mouth behavior and sucking on his fists. Breast- or bottle-feeding at this time is usually successful. Shortly after the feeding both mother and infant fall asleep.

This first hour, including caretaking measures and feeding, is part of the birth process and is important to complete before the mother and infant go to sleep. Klaus and Kennell (1982) have described, as species specific, maternal behavior on first contact with her infant. The mother touches the extremities first with her fingertips, then goes to the rest of the body, and finally uses the palm on the baby—all within a few minutes.

The term infant possesses amazing qualities of awareness and ability to interact. He is small yet has distinctive human physical features including a relatively large head and wide open eyes. He is soft, cuddly, and cute. He moves his arms and legs and responds with movement to being touched. This muscle tone is synonymous with being alive. Somehow the baby's strength of movement tends to dispel fears of his being so very fragile.

Primitive Reflexes

Cry   The first cry has particular meaning in assuring the parents that their infant has survived the birth process. Further cries are interpreted to indicate needs of the infant and are compelling signals of distress.

Root and Suck   The root and suck instincts are basic to survival. The infant opens his mouth when there is contact with his cheeks or lips; once an object such as a nipple is in the mouth, strong sucking movement occurs. Nutritive sucking has a different pattern from nonnutritive sucking, which is more often the infant's means of quieting himself. Nutritive sucking occurs in steady sucks at about one per second and is associated with swallowing. Nonnutritive sucking is characterized by bursts and rest periods. Nutritive sucking is usually developed sufficiently so that oral feedings will sustain the infant at about thirty-four weeks' gestation.

Moro (Startle) Reflex   The Moro reflex occurs spontaneously, especially during non-rapid-eye-movement (NREM) sleep, and in response to loud noises, dropping sensation, or other jarring movement during the awake state.

Grasp Reflex   Both the fingers and toes exhibit the grasp reflex. The hand-grasp is especially meaningful to parents, who interpret this response as reciprocation by the baby. The grasp at term is sufficiently strong to lift the infant from the bed.

Crossed Extension   Crossed extension begins with flexion then extension of the free leg when the other is restrained and the sole of the restrained leg is stimulated. By full term, the free leg also adducts as it extends and crosses to the restrained leg as though trying to remove the undesired stimulus.

"Walking"   Automatic walking motions occur as a result of the reflex that prompts extension of the leg and body when the sole of the foot is stimulated. If one sole then the other is stimulated, walking results.

Other Reflexes   Reflex smiling and, in the boy, erections, are other reflexes. Reflex smiling occurs in REM sleep or drowsy states. It is interesting that reflex smiling occurs more frequently in the preterm period, with the highest incidence being in the very early gestation ages. Reflex smiling occurs twice as often in girls as in boys. Erections occur most often in REM sleep but do occur with crying in awake states. Males startle more than females but the mean rate for spontaneous behaviors is the same in both sexes if erections are excluded.

Sensory Organs

Vision   The retina is remarkably well developed in the newborn and visual pathways are intact. Vision is much more advanced than originally thought, but the lens is nearly spherical the infant is myopic with a focal length of about 8–12 inches. It has been demonstrated that the newborn will fix on inanimate objects and can follow them briefly. He can discriminate between simple and complex patterns and prefers the complex ones. The strongest stimulus for the newborn is that of a face. The eye-to-eye contact between parent and newborn appears to be one of the most significant processes in the bonding experience. The newborn is unusually alert and wide-eyed for the first one to one and a half hours after birth.

Hearing The newborn's sense of hearing has also been underestimated. He not only hears, but discriminates between a higher-pitched voice, which he prefers, and a lower-pitched one. He becomes attentive, opens his eyes, and can turn his head toward the voice.

Touch Tactile responses or touch are well developed and account for many of the reflexes described above. The desirability of skin-to-skin contact of mother and her baby is still in the investigative stage, but appears to be important to the bonding process.

Smell and Taste The sense of smell is probably as important as the other senses, but little is known about how this affects bonding or caretaking behaviors. It has been shown that the infant can discriminate between his own mother's milk and that of another woman. Whether smell is as significant as taste in this is uncertain. Very little is known about these two senses, but further research is warranted.

Other Behaviors

Intelligence in the newborn is difficult to assess although various behaviors requiring cortical control are beginning to be recognized.

The study of sleep states is especially important since more of the interaction between brainstem and cortex takes place during quiet sleep. Prechtl and Beintema (1964) and Brazelton (1973) stress the importance of specific sleep states in testing various neurological functions.

Personality traits of the newborn are also of great interest, especially as they may enhance or retard meaningful interaction between mother and infant. These behaviors distinguish between the active, hungry, demanding type and the quiet, calm, or placid baby. Some are cuddly; others resist being held. Some are easily consoled when disturbed; others continue to cry.

The ability of the infant to quiet himself has taken on additional meaning. It tells one something about the baby's neurological organization and intrinsic methods he uses to deal with stress. Habituation or response decrement to stimuli similarly give one insight into the infant's ability to respond to the environment.

Evaluation of Maternal–Infant Attachment

Klaus and Kennell (1982) have conceptualized a variety of conditions and situations that affect bonding of the mother and infant. Such items as socioeconomic conditions and education of the parents, the mother's own experiences as a child, and her emotional status are included. Many of these factors are considered "fixed" whereas items such as hospital practices might be altered to enhance or inhibit maternal bonding. Harmon and others believe that pregnancy and birth of the child provide an opportunity for mother and father to "rework" old conflicts and establish new relationships with their own parents and with each other (see Chapter 16).

It is necessary to identify problems in the mother that may inhibit bonding to her infant. A simple tool has been given by Prugh (1982) in the form of five questions to ask the mother on the second or third postpartum day:

1. *How are you (feeling)?* This question uncovers complaints of a physical nature (pain, headache, cramps, and other discomforts). The mother who is excited about the birth and baby, even though uncomfortable, rarely mentions them. *How is the baby?* Occasionally, the mother points out blemishes and the like.

2. *Do you have a name for the baby? What did you select for the other sex? For whom is the baby named? When was the name chosen?* If after the baby is born, the parents do not have a name for the baby, one needs to pursue the reasons. If only one sex was acceptable and the infant is unnamed, one should be concerned for the "unwanted" infant.

3. *How did you react to fetal movements when you first noticed them?* Most mothers say that they were excited and that they realized the infant was alive and well. But some complain that the movement was disagreeable, it kept them awake, and so on.

4. *Who will help you at home?* This question opens the way for a discussion of the relationship of the mother and her own mother. Since mothers tend to raise their children as they were raised, it is especially important information.

5. *Most mothers expect that they will feel warmly maternal immediately upon the birth of their baby. Some find that it does not occur right away. How was it with you?* This question gets at emergence of warm feelings toward the baby. A

lag in maternal feelings was quite prevalent a decade ago but is not frequently encountered today, perhaps due to changing hospital practices. It is all the more significant today when it does occur.

When problems are uncovered, one must provide the help necessary. It may be as simple as listening and interpreting the feelings of the mother. At other times professional services may be indicated, such as involvement of a social worker, psychiatrist, or in extreme cases the child protection team.

The father is much more involved emotionally during the pregnancy than was previously thought. Fathers tend to talk more with their own mothers during this time and to modify and add a new dimension to their relationships with their wives, to the extent that the family unit becomes established. This is not to the exclusion of the couple's own relationship but rather to the formation of a new dimension.

PHYSICAL ASSESSMENT OF THE NEWBORN

Physical examination of the newborn is not a single examination, but a series of examinations and observations over a two- to three-day period. Each evaluation is geared toward obtaining specific information necessary to care for the infant in an optimal manner without disrupting his process of adaptation to extra-uterine life, or his relationship to his parents.

Four separate time periods for observation and examination are identified in the full-term infant:

- *Immediately after birth,* usually in the delivery room. The examination is aimed at identifying life-threatening conditions or abnormalities that need immediate attention. A "complete" examination at this time is inappropriate, as it is during the second period.
- *The transition period,* which may last one to four hours after birth. Most of the observations made at this time can be made with minimum disturbance and in the mother's presence. These include the monitoring of vital signs during his adaptation to extra-uterine life, plus certain measurements needed to predict or anticipate specific morbidities (weight, length, head circumference, gestational age, glucose and hematocrit).
- *Twelve to twenty-four hours after birth* and preferably two hours after a feeding. This is when the third and most complete examination should be made.

- *When discharged.* This examination need not be so thorough. It is aimed more at detecting neonatal problems, such as jaundice and feeding difficulties, and should be in the presence of the mother. This situation affords an opportunity to discuss her concerns and observe her relationship to the infant.

The Initial Examination

Even before the Apgar score at sixty seconds, one should observe the presence of meconium in amniotic fluid, be familiar with the mother's obstetrical history, observe the course of labor, and note color, vernix, and heart rate of the infant at birth. The onset of crying and character of breathing are then observed and the Apgar score is obtained. The five-minute Apgar is scored similarly to the one-minute Apgar and indicates the ability of the infant to adapt to extra-uterine life, having either recovered from brief birth asphyxia or having suffered residual effects from severe asphyxia.

Between the one- and five-minute scores, the infant is examined for problems or abnormalities that require immediate attention.

General Appearance The sex, size, amount of vernix, and development in relation to gestational age are all noted as soon as the baby is delivered. One is surprised, at times, when a "term" infant is born small and immature, an undiagnosed twin, or one who is small for gestational age.

Breathing Problems associated with establishing respiration are obviously the most urgent ones and are clearly life-threatening. One does not wait for the one-minute Apgar score to assist the apneic infant. If meconium is present in the amniotic fluid, vigorous suction of the nasopharynx before the first breath will prevent most cases of meconium aspiration (see Chapters 8 and 9).

Congenital Anomalies Anomalies with immediate needs include diaphragmatic hernia associated with an "empty" scaphoid abdomen and beginning respiratory distress. Open myelomeningocele, anencephaly, or omphalocele require immediate attention. Tracheoesophageal fistula is often suspected in the delivery room because of perfuse and persistent oral secretions. Choanal atresia becomes an urgent problem since newborns are obligate nasal breathers. One can check for patency of the nares by closing the infant's mouth, rather than passing catheters. (Trauma to the nasal mucous membranes may result from routine passage of catheters and result in problems similar to choanal atresia). Chromosomal trisomies and other syndromes are best left for later diagnosis.

Skin   Color, appearance, and abnormalities include cyanosis, petechiae, ecchymoses, jaundice, plethora, and pallor. Cyanosis can be related to a falling body temperature or to pulmonary or cardiac problems. If jaundice is present, immediate work-up for isoimmunization or other hemolytic process is indicated. Pallor is equally significant—an acute or chronic bleed must be considered. It is essential to maintain blood pressure, but acute and chronic anemia require different treatments. Petechiae and ecchymoses may indicate birth trauma but may be related to underlying disorders, such as isoimmunization, low platelets, disseminated intravascular coagulation, or thrombocytopenia from other causes such as congenital infection.

Abdomen   This examination needs further mention. The scaphoid or "empty" abdomen alerts one to the presence of a diaphragmatic hernia. Respiratory distress beginning or increasing shortly after birth supports this impression and immediate work-up and treatment can be life-saving. A distended abdomen may indicate ascites—possibly chylous ascites—and may require early aspiration. Continued pulsation of umbilical vessels is an indication of continuing hypoxia.

Fetal Adnexa   The fetal intra-uterine supporting systems are often ignored in the excitement of the birth of the infant. However, this examination can be of equal importance to that of the infant.

AMNIOTIC FLUID   The color, appearance, and estimate of volume are important when assessing the amniotic fluid. It is usually straw colored and slightly turbid from vernix. If it is bright yellow, bilirubin may be present, as in hemolytic disease. A bright red color indicates fresh blood, and chocolate color indicates old blood. Meconium staining may be dark green or greenish yellow. Polyhydramnios occurs with intestinal obstruction or anencephaly (swallowing inhibited). Oligohydramnios occurs with renal agenesis, premature rupture of amniotic membranes, or postterm birth.

UMBILICAL CORD   The diameter of the umbilical cord reflects the size of the placenta. If the infant is small for gestational age, the umbilical cord is often thin and stained yellow. Meconium staining usually indicates prior fetal distress. Insertion of the cord is near the center of the placenta. If it is on the edge (velamentous)

there is increased risk of fetal hemorrhage. An unusually short cord can result in rupture of the cord or abruptio placentae. An unusually long cord may loop around the body or neck. However, loops around the neck are rarely a cause for asphyxia. A single umbilical artery, present in about one percent of births, portends the possibility of hidden anomalies.

PLACENTA   The size and appearance of the placenta need to be noted. The weight of the placenta is related, in general, to the weight of the infant. A large infant must have a large placenta, but when one finds a small infant with a large placenta, one should look for congenital anomalies or a diseased placenta. In case of twins, the examination may help differentiate single- or double-ovum twins.

The Transition Period Examination

The physical examination during this period is aimed at observing the infant's adaptation to extrauterine life and at assessing the risk of neonatal morbidity. The examination, then, consists of monitoring vital signs, determining gestational age, and obtaining certain laboratory procedures.

This period, from one to one and a half hours after birth, is also very important for maternal–infant interaction; the routines set up by individual nurseries must keep this in mind. The ideal situation might be a "birthing center" where the infant is not removed, or a "common recovery room" for mother and infant, where the pediatric-obstetric team cares for both. Other arrangements in conventional obstetric services include a brief evaluation of the infant while the mother delivers the placenta, receives sutures, and is cleaned up; mother and infant are reunited shortly after the mother leaves the delivery room. The physical arrangement is not as important as is the attitude and understanding of personnel (medical and nursing in both osbstetrics and pediatrics).

Vital Signs   Blood pressure, temperature, respiratory and cardiac rate, color of skin and awake–sleep state of the infant (see Figure 15-2) must be monitored.

Characteristics of normal adaptation include a falling respiratory rate if it was unusually high initially. Barrelling of the chest could indicate extravasated air, hyperexpansion of lungs, mediastinal emphysema, or pneumothorax. Associated cyanosis or restlessness would suggest that prompt recovery might not occur. Palpation of the stump of the umbilical cord for pulsation gives further evidence for or against persistent

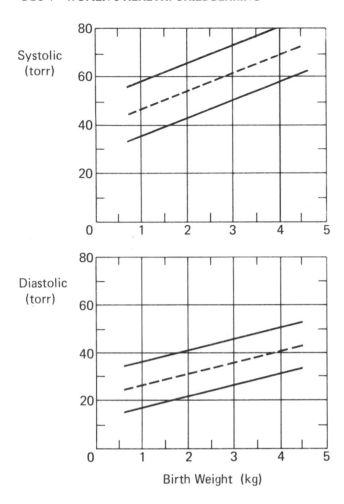

FIGURE 15-5 Linear regressions (broken lines) and ninety-five percent confidence limits (solid lines) of systolic and diastolic aortic blood pressures on birth weight in sixty-one healthy infants during the first twelve hours after birth. (From Versmold, H.T., & Kitterman, J.A. (1981). Aortic blood pressure during the first 12 hours of life in infants with birth weight 610 to 4220 grams. *Pediatrics, 67,* 607–613. Copyright American Academy of Pediatrics 1981. With permission.)

hypoxia, since the newborn often uses fetal responses, such as persistent umbilical artery pulsation during periods of hypoxia.

A decreasing cardiac rate, fluctuating between 100–140 beats/min, is to be expected in the normal infant. Blood pressure taken soon after birth can identify "shocky" infants, such as those who have lost blood acutely or have had fetal to maternal transfusions. Blood pressures have been established for newborns (Figure 15-5).

A fall in body temperature is not desirable and depends largely on environmental temperatures.

Newborns show lability of color, especially during the first six to twelve hours. Plethora is noted with crying, but there is prompt return. Plethora that decreases slowly and continues on to pallor with or without cyanosis should warn of the presence of polycythemia. Pallor is significant whenever noted.

The awake–sleep states of the infant have been carefully documented. The normal, full-term newborn is remarkably alert during the transition period with eyes wide open and searching. It has been shown that the newborn can fix and follow—especially a face—even minutes after birth. One becomes concerned about the newborn who is asleep at ten to fifteen minutes. Maternal analgesia, fetal distress, or other illness should be considered.

Determination of Gestational Age Gestational age is as necessary as birth weight in assessing risk of the infant for various morbidities. These two parameters, together give information neither alone can provide. The ability to assess gestational age of the infant after birth has opened a new era in anticipating morbidity and preventing many illnesses of newborns. Since gestational age is not always accurate, based on the mother's menstrual history, the age based on physical characteristics and neurological development has filled a most important gap. It is well to remember that the clinical findings are, at best, plus or minus two weeks compared to the gestational age based on accurate menstrual dates. A discrepancy between the mother's dates and the clinical examination should not be assumed unless the difference between the two is at least three weeks.

There are several scoring systems available to aid one in arriving at gestational age. The best known is that of Dubowitz et al. (1970). When all items are scored (eleven external and ten neurological criteria), the error in predicting gestational age is only plus or minus one week (Table 15-1 and Figure 15-6). The objections to the Dubowitz system are two: First, the gestational age is needed as soon after birth as possible and it does not seem appropriate to make twenty-one observations, however quickly they can be done, on the newborn during the stress of adapting to extra-uterine life. The second reason is more objective. When one looks at a weighted score such as in the Dubowitz system, one cannot equate a score with actual age. Does a 4 mean thirty-six or forty-two weeks?

I prefer to extract the items that require minimal manipulation and thus can be used in the first hours after birth (Figure 15-7). The longer list, which consists mainly of neurological testing, can be used later to confirm the gestational age of the infant (Figure 15-8).

TABLE 15-1 Scoring system using external criteria for estimating gestational age of newborns

External Sign	Score*				
	0	1	2	3	4
Edema	Obvious edema of hands and feet; pitting over tibia	No obvious edema of hands and feet; pitting over tibia	No edema		
Skin texture	Very thin, gelatinous	Thin and smooth	Smooth; medium thickness; rash or superficial peeling	Slight thickening; superficial cracking and peeling, especially of hands and feet	Thick and parchmentlike; superficial or deep cracking
Skin color	Dark red	Uniformly pink	Pale pink; variable over body	Pale; only pink over ears, lips, palms, or soles	
Skin opacity (trunk)	Numerous veins and venules clearly seen, especially over abdomen	Veins and tributaries seen	A few large vessels clearly seen over abdomen	A few large vessels seen indistinctly over abdomen	No blood vessels seen
Lanugo (over back)	No lanugo	Abundant; long and thick over whole back	Hair thinning, especially over lower back	Small amount of lanugo and bald areas	At least half of back devoid of lanugo
Plantar creases	No skin creases	Faint red marks over anterior half of sole	Definite red marks over more than anterior half of sole; indentations over less than anterior third	Indentations over more than anterior third of sole	Definite deep indentations over more than anterior third of sole;
Nipple formation	Nipple barely visible; no areola	Nipple well defined; areola smooth and flat; diameter <0.75 cm	Areola stippled, edge not raised; diameter <0.75 cm	Areola stippled, edge raised; diameter >0.75 cm	
Breast size	No breast tissue palpable	Breast tissue on on one or both sides; diameter <0.5 cm	Breast tissue on both sides; one or both 0.5–1.0 cm diameter	Breast tissue on both sides; one or both >1 cm diameter	
Ear form	Pinna flat and shapeless, little or no incurving of edge	Incurving of part of edge of pinna	Partial incurving of whole of upper pinna	Well-defined incurving of whole of upper pinna	
Ear firmness	Pinna soft, easily folded; no recoil	Pinna soft, easily folded; slow recoil	Cartilage to edge of pinna, but soft in places; ready recoil	Pinna firm, cartilage to edge; instant recoil	
Male genitals	Neither testis in scrotum	At least one testis high in scrotum	At least one testis right down		
Female genitals (with hips half abducted)	Labia majora widely separated, labia minora protruding	Labia majora almost cover labia minora	Labia majora completely over labia minora		

From Dubowitz, L.M.S., Dubowitz, V., & Goldberg, C. (1970). Clinical assessment of gestational age in the newborn infant. *Journal of Pediatrics, 77,* 1–10. With permission.
*If score differs on two sides, take the mean.

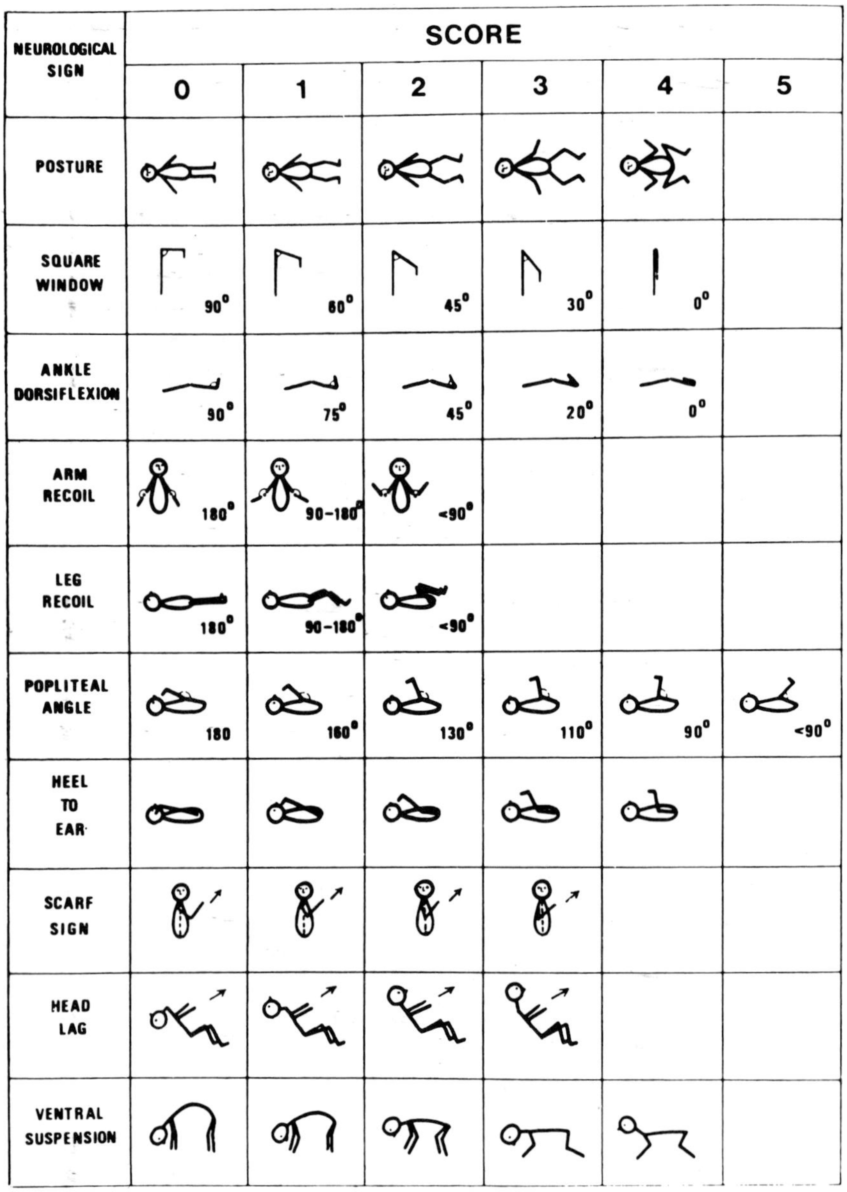

NEUROLOGICAL SIGN	SCORE					
	0	1	2	3	4	5
POSTURE						
SQUARE WINDOW	90°	60°	45°	30°	0°	
ANKLE DORSIFLEXION	90°	75°	45°	20°	0°	
ARM RECOIL	180°	90–180°	<90°			
LEG RECOIL	180°	90–180°	<90°			
POPLITEAL ANGLE	180	160°	130°	110°	90°	<90°
HEEL TO EAR						
SCARF SIGN						
HEAD LAG						
VENTRAL SUSPENSION						

FIGURE 15-6 Scoring system for neurological criteria (From Dubowitz, L.M.S., Dubowitz, V., & Goldberg, C. (1970). Clinical assessment of gestational age in the newborn infant. *Journal of Pediatrics, 77,* 1–10. With permission.)

The items are placed in relation to gestational age so that one might learn fetal development as one uses the various items. A byproduct of this approach has been the recognition that discrepancies in individual items frequently follow a pattern based on the intra-uterine environment.

Details of the examination during the first hour follow.

VERNIX One of the advantages of the perinatal approach to maternity care is that this item is being observed more frequently. The amount and distribution of the vernix must be noted as the baby is being born since he is usually wiped dry quickly after delivery. Vernix appears at about twenty to twenty-four weeks' gestation and becomes very thick over the entire body. Toward term, about thirty-eight weeks, it disappears

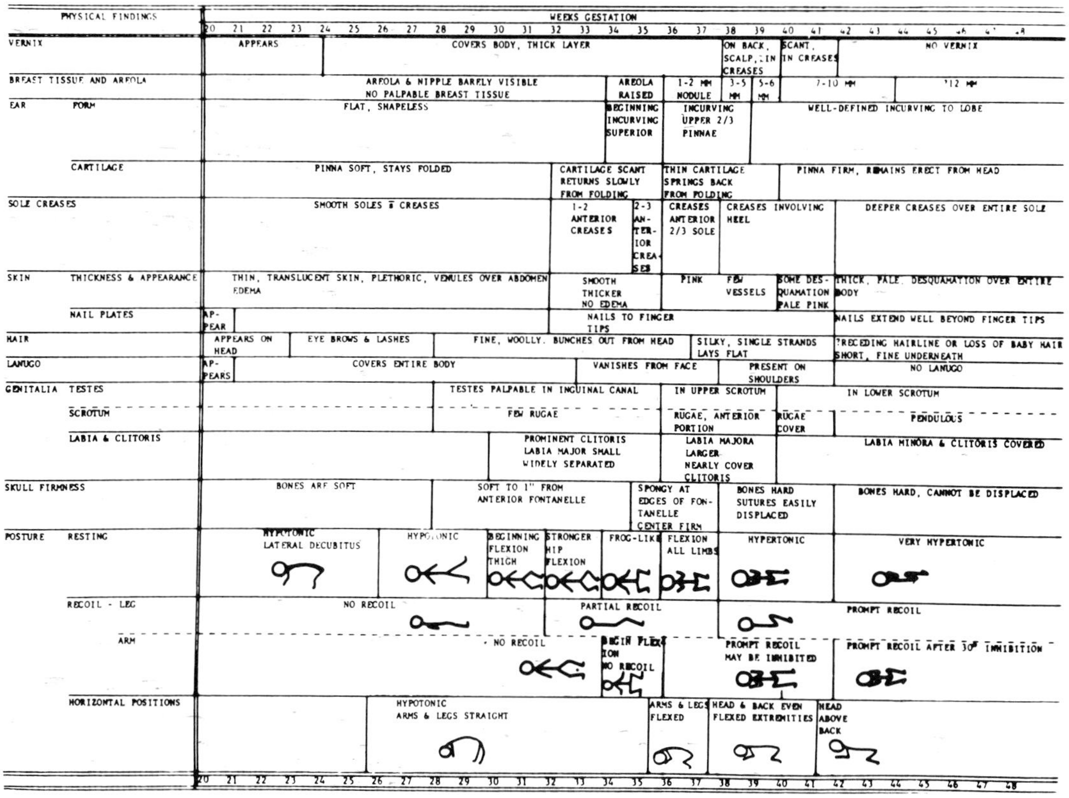

FIGURE 15-7 Clinical estimation of gestational age—external criteria, first-hour examination. (Adapted from Brazie, J.V., & Lubchenco, L.O. (1974). *Current pediatric diagnosis and treatment* (ed. 3). Los Altos, Ca.: Lange Medical Publications, p. 40. With permission.)

from the face and extremities and is found chiefly on the back, scalp, and in the creases. By forty-one weeks only scant amounts are present in the creases, and after forty-one weeks vernix is virtually absent.

BREAST TISSUE AND AREOLA About two weeks before any breast tissue is palpable, one notes a slightly raised areola. At thirty-six weeks a tiny nodule of breast tissue can be felt, which enlarges a millimeter or two each week, and by term the nodule is 7–10 mm in size. The nodule is best measured by rolling the forefinger over the nodule and making note of the size in relation to the finger. (A preformed model is useful in learning the estimate nodule size.)

EAR FORM AND CARTILAGE Each pinna begins as a double-thickness fold of skin without cartilage and rigor, and if folded, will stay in this position. As cartilage begins to form, at about thirty-two weeks, the pinna stiffens and there is resistance to folding. At term

the pinna is firm and returns promptly to its original position, which is erect and apart from the head.

Early in gestation, between thirty-three and thirty-four weeks, incurving of the outer edge of the pinna occurs. This incurvation progresses toward the lobe and is complete by forty weeks. ·

SOLE CREASES As vernix decreases, wrinkling of the skin occurs. Whether this accounts for sole creases is not certain, but it appears coincidentally. The sole is smooth until thirty-two weeks, when one or two anterior creases appear. These horizontal lines increase in number until they cover the anterior two-thirds of the sole by thirty-seven weeks. At this time the heel is still smooth. By thirty-eight to forty weeks the heel shows creases, and after forty-two weeks the entire sole is covered.

SKIN The skin of the premature infant is thin and transparent. Nail plates are present. As gestation ad-

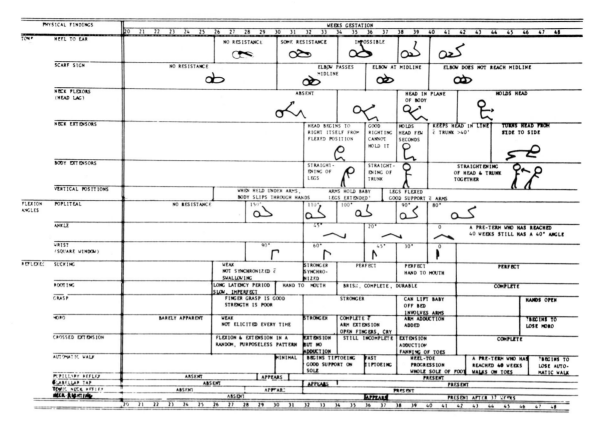

FIGURE 15-8 Clinical estimation of gestational age—neurological criteria, twenty-four hour examination. (Adapted from Brazie, J.V., & Lubchenco, L.O. (1974). *Current pediatric diagnosis and treatment* (ed. 3). Los Altos, Ca.: Lange Medical Publications, p. 40. With permission.)

vances, edema disappears and the skin becomes thicker and pale pink in appearance. Nails are apparent to the finger tips. After term the skin is pale and desquamation occurs. Nails become longer and extend beyond the finger tips.

HAIR Hair appears early in gestation. By twenty weeks eyebrows, lashes, and head hair are present. The hair is very fine at first and has a matted, wooley appearance (thirty to forty weeks). After thirty-six to forty weeks it becomes silky and lays flat except for the top and occiput. After term "baby hair" begins to disappear and a receding hairline becomes apparent.

Lanugo also appears early (twenty weeks) and covers the entire body by thirty-three to thirty-four weeks. It vanishes from the face and by term is only present on the shoulders. No lanugo is seen after forty-one to forty-two weeks.

GENITALIA Both male and female genitalia change with gestational age. Female genitalia appearance is more dependent on intra-uterine nutrition than male.

Testes can be felt in the inguinal canal at about twenty-eight weeks' gestation. By thirty weeks they have descended to the level of the scrotum and from thirty-seven to forty-one weeks are definitely within the scrotal sac. By term scrotal rugae are numerous. Testes and scrotum appear pendulous in the postterm infant.

The female genitalia depend on fat accumulations for appearance of maturity. The labia major are small and widely separated at thirty to thirty-four weeks' gestation. As they enlarge they begin to cover the labia minora and clitoris. By term only the labia major are evident.

SKULL FIRMNESS Skull bones are soft and easily displaced until twenty-eight to thirty weeks' gestation. Bone firmness begins in the central portion of the bone; the outer edges are soft, giving the sutures an exaggerated effect of being open. At term the sutures are still easily displaced and may be overriding immediately after birth.

NEUROLOGICAL FINDINGS It is a strange phenomenon that muscle tone appears first in the lower extremities and progresses cephalad, since most embryological

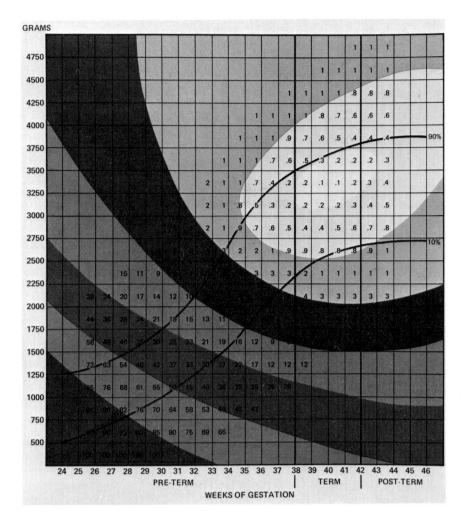

FIGURE 15-9 Newborn classification and neonatal mortality risk by birth weight and gestational age. (Interpolated data based on mathematical fit from original data gathered from University of Colorado Medical Center newborns between July 1, 1958, and July 1, 1969.) (From Lubchenco, L.O., Searls, D.T., & Brazie, J.V. (1972). Neonatal mortality rate: Relationship to birth weight, and gestational age. *Journal of Pediatrics, 81,* 814–822. With permission.)

development progresses from head to toe. At twenty to twenty-four weeks the postnatal premature has little tone and lies in a lateral decubitus position. By twenty-eight weeks some flexion of the ankles occurs, and by thirty weeks flexion of the thighs can be seen. At approximately two-week intervals, increased tone can be demonstrated by hip flexion, then arm flexion and evidence of recoil when the legs are extended. Finally, flexion of upper extremities and recoil appear. The postterm infant is hypertonic, tightly flexed, and recoil of extremities is prompt, even after inhibition.

Muscle tone can also be observed if the infant is held, abdomen down, in horizontal suspension (as when lifted to obtain a weight). The preterm infant is hypotonic. The body of the near term infant is also limp, but the arms and legs are flexed. By term the trunk is held horizontally, and the head is in line with the body. The postterm infant tends to raise the head above the body.

Prediction of Neonatal Illness Mortality risk is obtained from plotting the baby's birth weight and gestational age (derived from the mother's dates) on the chart. Both the gestational age determined from the mother's menstrual history and the gestational age determined from the clinical examination are useful. The mortality risk is determined from the mother's dates (Figure 15-9). Important data will be lost if only the clinical examination estimate is used, since infants with discrepant findings usually have a higher mortality rate.

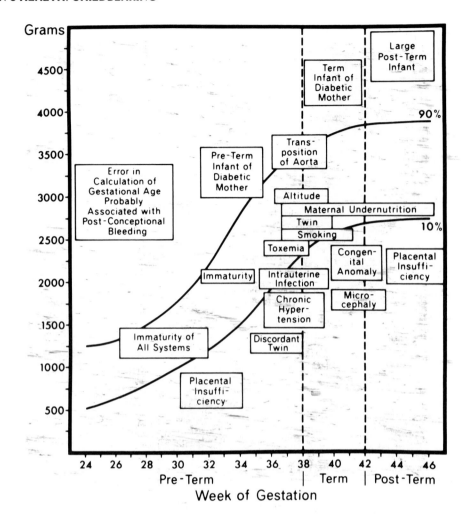

FIGURE 15-10 Specific morbidity in infants with deviations of birth weight for gestational age. (Adapted from Lubchenco, L.O., Hansman, C., & Backstrom, L. (1968). Factors influencing fetal growth. In J.H.P. Jonxis, H.K.A. Visser, and J.A. Troelstra (Eds.), *Aspects of prematurity and dysmaturity*. Leiden, Holland: H.E. Steinfert Kroese N.V. With permission.)

For example, the dates may indicate a preterm infant if the mother had postconceptional bleeding, whereas the clinical examination might indicate that the infant is term or near term. The mortality is increased in this condition and the infant should be considered at risk even though he appears mature. It is not clear what the morbidity is in this situation.

On the other hand the clinical examination is used to dictate nursery care. If the clinical examination suggests preterm birth, one is concerned about feeding, jaundice, respiratory problems, and other problems typical of the preterm infant. If the clinical examination is clearly term or postterm and the infant is small for gestational age then hypoglycemia, polycythemia, and other problems of the small-for-gestational-age baby are anticipated.

Infants with deviations of birth weight for gestational age from the standard scale have a high risk of specific morbidity as shown in Figure 15-10.

In addition to birth weight, measurement of length and head circumference are helpful in predicting neonatal morbidity (Figure 15-11). Relative percentile standings of birth weight, length, head circumference, and weight:length ratio can be obtained.

If all dimensions are proportional, one is not as concerned about the infant being abnormal as when discrepancies occur. For example, the most common pattern of intra-uterine growth retardation is a low weight with length and head circumference being unaffected. Even if length is affected, head circumference may continue to grow in the otherwise normal infant. If small-for-gestational-age infants are small

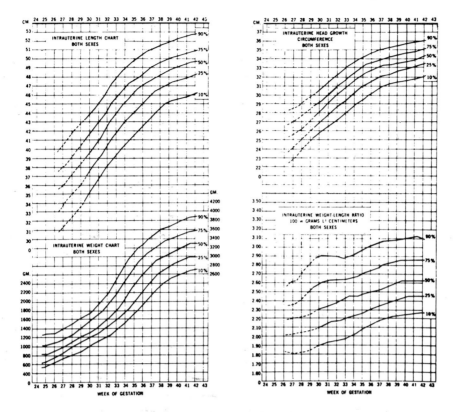

FIGURE 15-11 Colorado intra-uterine growth charts. (From Lubchenco. L.O., Hansman, C., & Boyd, E. (1966). Intrauterine growth in length and head circumference as estimated from live births at gestational from 26 to 42 weeks. *Pediatrics, 37,* 403–408. Copyright American Academy of Pediatrics 1966. With permission.)

because of congenital anomalies or congenital infection, the head circumference percentile is often lower than length percentile. Appropriate for gestational age infants may have a low weight:length ratio, indicating some intra-uterine growth retardation. These infants, like those small for gestational age, often do not tolerate labor very well, may have low Apgar scores, and are susceptible to cold stress and hypoglycemia.

Laboratory Screening Because of the difficulty in determining illness or its cause in newborns (see section on The Newborn's Response to Stress), laboratory documentation is necessary. Hypoglycemia is frequent and when found in the small-for-gestational-age infant or in an infant with a low weight:length ratio, the need for supplemental glucose is urgent. The large-for-gestational-age infant with abundant stores of glycogen and fat is not in as much danger from hypoglycemia, since he has energy sources he can mobilize.

Polycythemia is much more frequent than previously thought, and although treatment is not clearly defined, the symptomatic infant will benefit from partial plasma exchange transfusion. Hematocrit is best determined within four to eight hours after birth. Blood typing and Coombs'; bilirubin; PKU, or amino acid screen; and galactose in blood or urine are other frequently needed laboratory screening procedures.

The Complete Examination

This examination—the most important one in early life—can be postponed until about twenty-four hours after birth, when the examiner has sufficient time to do a thorough evaluation. It may be necessary to complete the examination in several stages.

Although the write-up is logical and follows a head-to-toe sequence, the actual examination begins with the items that least disturb the infant and proceeds to the more disturbing procedures.

Because items such as birth measurements, gestational age, and screening procedures have been carried out during the transition period, the complete examination builds upon those earlier observations and findings.

The examiner will learn a great deal about the newborn if he or she will take a couple of minutes to watch the clothed, sleeping infant. Periodic breathing may be observed; resting pulse taken; and jerks or twitches, skin color at rest, and so on noted.

Heart, lungs, and abdomen are then examined. Warm hands and instruments are essential at this point. If the baby comes to the alert state, the examination can be finished with a pacifier; talking to the infant; comforting strokes to the body, head, extremities; or gentle restraint of arms.

The neurological exam (except for moro and other disturbing procedures) can be carried out next, followed by percussion of heart, lungs, liver, and abdomen.

Manipulative procedures—including examination of ears, nose, throat, and eyes; and moro reflex testing—are the last items. Since the examiner obviously cannot explain the procedures as to an older child, he or she should talk to the infant and hold or cuddle him until he is quiet.

Vital signs and physical measurements should be reviewed prior to the examination. They frequently require repeating.

General Appearance Size and maturity, nutritional status, abnormalities and facies, as well as the state of well-being, should be noted. The words used to describe the appearance of the infant should be original and vivid as an aid in later visualizing the infant. Abbreviations, such as "WD, WN, NB ♂" could apply to the majority of admissions but a description such as the following is helpful: "This chubby, little, blonde boy with a squashed nose is in the twenty-fifth percentile for weight and length, but the head circumference is on the fiftieth percentile. A large caput extends over the left parietal area and edema is present in the left upper eyelid. He is remarkably alert."

Skin Color and appearance of the infant's skin should be checked; plethora or pallor, as well as cyanosis and jaundice should be noted. Distribution of jaundice is helpful in the first few days in estimating level of bilirubin. Jaundice occurs first on the face and trunk, then extremities, and finally on the palms and soles. Meconium staining pigmentation, moles, or hemangiomas are described. Erythema toxicum, milia, Mongolian spots, and petechiae should be looked for.

Head Size, shape, symmetry, molding, and caput succedaneum are mentioned. Cephalohematoma can be distinguished from a caput at twenty-four hours by its location (limited by individual skull bones). The size of the fontanelles is given and specific mention of a third fontanelle made. Separation or overriding of sutures should be checked for. Craniosynostosis may be suspected if the sutures are delineated by a ridge and are immobile. Increased intracranial pressure in the newborn results in a full or bulging anterior fontanelle and separation of sutures.

Face General appearance, symmetry, localized swellings, redness, or ecchymoses are noted. Facial nerve palsy is observed if one side of the mouth is drawn to one side when the infant cries, or if one eye is more open than the other. Odd facies often alert the examiner to the presence of a congenital abnormality or syndrome. One should especially note the shape and position of eyes, nose, upper lip, ears, and hairline.

Eyes The eye examination includes the periorbital structures, nerve function, and vision. General appearance, size of lid opening, eyebrows and eyelashes, epicanthal folds and size of the eye itself are checked. Proptosis or micropthalmia are apparent if present. Movement of eyes and lids is observed. Occasional uncoordinated eye movements are common, but persistent ones are indications for further evaluation. Conjunctivitis, or conjunctival hemorrhage can be seen. Hemorrhage in the anterior chamber is significant. Unusual findings in the iris include colobomas and brushfield spots. Ophthalmoscopic examination through undilated pupils is worth the effort. If a pacifier is given, the infant opens his eyes. If one can see retinal vessels clearly, one can be sure that no lens opacity exists and probably no vitreous hemorrhage has occurred. Other indications, such as congenital infection or hemorrhage, will dictate the need for dilation of pupils or ophthalmological consultation.

Ears Shape, size, and position of the ears are noted. Malformation of the pinnae is often associated with renal abnormalities and other syndromes. Patency, shape, and size of external auditory canal are looked at and tympanic membranes examined. Otitis media is not rare in the newborn.

Nose Shape and size of the nose can alert the examiner to possible congenital anomalies; however, deformities are common from intra-uterine pressures, especially of a limb in the vicinity of the face. Choanal atresia can be ruled out if one nostril and the mouth are held closed.

Mouth Lips and mucous membranes are usually pink. Pallor or cyanosis are identified early in these locations. Epithelial pearls are retention cysts along the gum margins and at the junction of hard and soft palates. A high, arched palate frequently accompanies abnormal facies. Cleft lip and palate, including submucous cleft, should be observed. Although small mandibles are frequently seen in newborns, unusually small ones are associated with several syndromes.

Neck Position, symmetry, and range of motion must be checked. Webbing of the neck suggests Turner's syndrome. Sinus tracts may be remnants of brachial clefts. Occasionally, the thyroid gland is enlarged. Torticollis occurs if the sternocleidomastoid muscle is shortened or in spasm. A very short neck may be associated with vertebral anomalies. A persistent tonic neck reflex is cause for careful neurological examination.

Cry A high-pitched cry suggests brain damage; a hoarse cry, hypothyroidism or vocal cord damage. The "cats cry" is typical of the chromosomal anomaly in which there is deletion of part of the short arm of chromosome 5. A weak cry occurs in preterm and sick infants. Expiratory grunting is common with respiratory distress syndrome. Inspiratory stridor results from a soft collapsible larynx or partial upper airway obstruction.

Thorax On inspection, one determines if both sides are symmetrical and notes the development of nipples and areola, the presence of superficial veins, and character and rate of respirations. "Fullness" of the chest occurs with overexpansion of the lungs or pneumomediastinum. Fracture of one or both clavicles can be detected because of pain on motion or pressure over the clavicle and later, by a nodule after callus formation occurs. Absent clavicles permit unusual flexion of the shoulders.

Lungs Percussion of the lungs must be very light, often with one-finger percussion. A hyperresonant note indicate overexpansion. A dull note occurs over the heart and liver. In order to outline the border of the heart, one should start at the anterior axillary line on the left and percuss medially until dullness is heard (and felt). Similarly, the right border is outlined. For liver size, percussion begins anteriorly in the mid-clavicular line and proceeds downward until dullness is heard, then continues to the abdomen until resonance reappears. Percussion has limited usefulness in the newborn examination, although a difference in percussion noted on the two sides of the chest is usually significant.

On auscultation, the normal breath sounds are bronchovesicular; both inspiration and expiration are heard equally well. Diminished breath sounds are found in most pathological pulmonary conditions in newborns. When pneumothorax occurs, both breath sounds and heart sounds are distant. There is decreased air entry with respiratory distress syndrome. Râles are rarely heard after the initial expansion of the lungs.

Heart Blood pressure (if necessary, in all extremities), heart rate, and rhythm are recorded. Inspection for pulsations in the apical area and neck, and for distended veins over chest, are helpful. Palpation for apical, femoral, radial, and dorsalis pedis pulses is part of the cardiovascular examination. Murmurs can often be felt, as well as heard. Coarctation of the aorta must be ruled out if femoral pulses are absent. Bounding pulses suggest patent ductus arteriosus. Auscultation should include evaluation of first and second heart sounds, with note of character of A_2 and P_2 at the base. Rhythm, especially in relation to respiration, should be noted, since sinus rhythm (sinus arrhythymia or childhood rhythm) is a healthy finding. Description, intensity, and location of murmurs must be carefully recorded. Newborn infants, however, may have serious congenital heart defects without murmurs, or a murmur that does not necessarily mean pathology. When one is evaluating cardiac function, signs of early congestive heart failure must be sought. Whenever heart disease is suspected, laboratory confirmation is essential.

Abdomen By twenty-four hours, the abdomen is slightly full in appearance. The scaphoid abdomen associated with a diaphragmatic hernia, omphaloceles, absent abdominal muscles, and hernias has already been discovered. The umbilical cord has also been described. Redness around the base should be noted. Abdominal distention is a serious finding and indicates the need for further diagnostic measures to rule out congenital defects, infection, necrotizing enterocolitis, or other irregularities.

Palpation for organs or masses needs to be done with a light touch, warm hands, and smooth, unhurried movements. The liver is usually palpable 1–2 cm below the costal margin. If the examiner begins at the costal margin and works down with fingertips, the edge will be recognized. The spleen is quite far laterally and is felt in the same manner. If the bladder is distended, it may

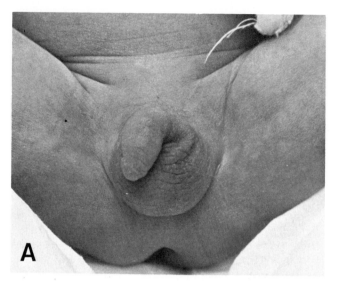

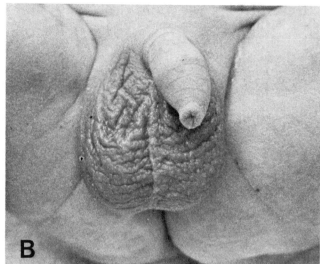

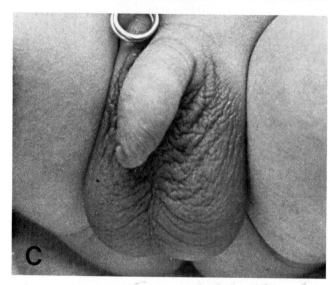

FIGURE 15-12 Male genitalia. (A) Immature, thirty-five to thirty-six week's gestation. (B) Mature, thirty-nine week's gestation. (C) Postmature, forty-two week's gestation. (Courtesy of Phil Stietenroth, University of Colorado Health Sciences Center.)

be seen and felt as a ballotable cystic mass above the symphysis pubis. Deep, firm pressure reaching the flank is necessary to feel kidneys. If they are felt easily after twelve to twenty-four hours, they may be enlarged. The right kidney is slightly lower than the left.

Genitalia Male and female genitalia show characteristics specific for gestational age (Figures 15-12 and 15-13). The testes are descended into the pendulous scrotum, and rugae completely cover the sac. In addition, the foreskin completely covers the glans and is adherent to it. Only a small area surrounding the urethra should be visible when the foreskin is retracted. The size of the phallus varies greatly among newborn infants. Hypospadius results in a loose foreskin with the urethral opening somewhere below the glans, or even onto the shaft of the penis.

Infants with ambiguous genitalia require prompt attention. Adrenal hyperplasia may be a medical emergency. Also, there is a need to establish sex for the parents' benefit.

Female genitalia are affected by intra-uterine growth retardation with less deposit of fat in the labia majora, and the appearance of being preterm. Occasionally, the hymen protrudes from the vagina, and a skin tag is suspected. It is not uncommon for a little bleeding to occur in newborn females on the second or third day.

Anus and Rectum The anus is sometimes very close to the vagina. Patency of the gastrointestinal tract is established if meconium has been passed. If it has not, a soft catheter or little finger should be inserted. Sometimes a meconium plug will be found to explain the obstruction—or, if it is not patent, consultation is required.

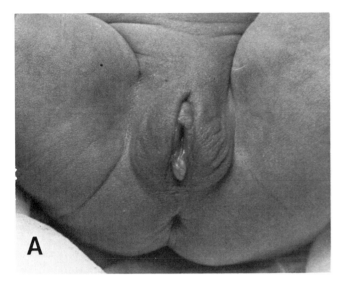

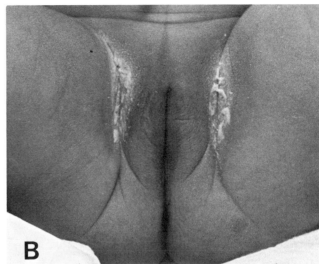

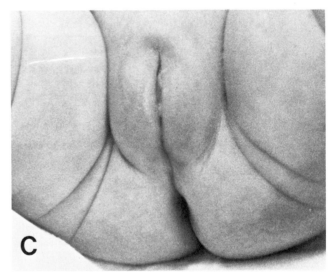

FIGURE 15-13 Female genitalia. (A) Very immature, twenty-eight week's gestation. (B) Immature, thirty-five week's gestation. (C) Mature, thirty-eight to forty-two week's gestation. (Courtesy of Phil Stietenroth, University of Colorado Health Sciences Center.)

Extremities and Back The arms and legs are normally flexed, have good tone, and move freely. Major anomalies, including club foot, should be obvious. Even minor anomalies are quite significant in identifying chromosomal or other syndromes (short, long, or fused digits; dermatoglyphics; excessive or limited movements of joints; etc.). Hip dislocation is suspected when a click is felt on abduction of the thigh (Ortolani's maneuver). Palsies or fractures are recognized by limited movement or evident pain.

The back is observed for curvature, and spinal defects such as myelomeningocele. Dimples or sinuses at the base of the spine are found in pilonidal cysts.

Neurological Examination There are three neurological examinations of the newborn currently in use. The neurological examination of the newborn described by the French neurologists Dargassies and Amiel-Tison (St. Anne-Dargassies, 1955) is largely of normal neurological development; as such it forms the basis for the estimation of gestational age. The one published by Prechtl and Beintema (1964), is aimed at detecting central nervous system pathology in the infant. The most recent examination is that of Brazelton (1973), who incorporates many items from Prechtl and Beintema, but adds items to examine higher central nervous system function. He also describes many personality items. Prechtl and Beintema and Brazelton all stress the importance of awake–sleep states and the effect these have on the examination.

The neurological examination for gestational age is done about twenty-four hours after birth to eliminate the transient effects of labor and birth that may skew the findings. The neurological examination confirms the initial examination, which is based primarily on overt physical characteristics. It is dependent on muscle tone, primitive reflexes, and flexion angles, which may be independent of muscle tone.

Muscle tone decreases the limit to which extremities can be extended; as muscle tone increases these angles become smaller, as seen in the popliteal angle.

Often included in these angles are wrist and ankle flexion. It has become apparent that these joints depend more on hormonal influences than muscle maturity, since they develop in opposite directions. It has long been known that maternal joints are made more mobile by pregnancy; fetal joints seem also to be affected. Thus, the wrists and ankles are more flexible as the baby reaches term, permitting the fetus to mold more easily to the restricted uterine space. These items are detailed in Figure 15-8.

MUSCLE TONE If there is little muscle tone, the heel can easily be placed to the infant's ear (heel-to-ear maneuver). As muscle tone increases it becomes progressively more difficult to accomplish this maneuver, and at term the leg can scarcely be extended to 90°.

Tone in the arms lags behind leg tone, but is clearly related to gestational age. At term the arm can be pulled across the body only to the extent that the elbow remains at midline (the scarf sign).

Neck flexors and neck extensors are tested by the pull-to-sit maneuver. The amount of head lag can thus be observed. Once the infant is upright the ability to hold the head in this position is noted. The head is allowed to fall forward and with slight stimulation of the lips the infant will reerect his head using the extensor muscles.

Body extensor muscles are noted when the feet are placed on a table, or the soles are stimulated. Straightening of the leg occurs as early as thirty-two to thirty-four weeks' gestation. By forty weeks the trunk is also straightened.

DORSIFLEXION OF FOOT AND WRIST FLEXION These two important tests indicate joint mobility. At thirty to thirty-two weeks the wrist is relatively stiff and flexion of the wrist on the arm is about 90°, making a "square window" with the hand. The angle decreases as mobility increases; the angle is approximately 60° at thirty-two to thirty-five weeks, 45° at thirty-six to thirty-seven weeks, and is almost obliterated by term or postterm.

Ankle mobility parallels wrist mobility. The foot is at right angles to the leg early in gestation with increasing flexion after thirty-two weeks, until no angle exists at term.

It is interesting that the premature infant does not follow the same sequence postnatally. The ankles remain relatively stiff, making him "walk" on his toes rather than flat on the sole at term. Muscle tone, on the other hand, continues to develop out of the uterus as it would have in utero.

REFLEXES The appearance of various reflexes has been used to determine gestational age, as seen in Figures 15-7 and 15-8.

• *Sucking and rooting:* Sucking is weak and not synchronized with swallowing until thirty-four weeks' gestation. By this age nipple feeding is possible. Additional information on patterns of nutritional versus nonnutritional sucking is needed to determine whether such a tool could be of value in defining gestational age.

Rooting is barely noted until thirty weeks, but appears to be established soon after thirty-four weeks. Hand-to-mouth activity is noted by thirty-four weeks.

• *Grasp:* Finger grasp is an early reflex, occurring by twenty-six weeks, but strength of the grasp is dependent on muscle tone. At term the grasp is sufficiently strong that the baby can be lifted.

When doing this test, as in many other neurological items, it is important to keep the head in the midline. Otherwise the asymmetrical tonic reflex may be stimulated, and one hand will open while the other is closed.

• *Tonic neck reflex:* As early as twenty-eight weeks' gestation, the tonic neck reflex appears. It is noted consistently after thirty-two weeks. At term it is common but the infant is not "locked into" the position for more than a few seconds.

• *The Moro, or startle, reflex:* This is barely apparent until twenty-six to thirty weeks. It becomes stronger in succeeding weeks, and by thirty-four weeks is complete with extension of arms, open fingers, and a cry. At term arm adduction is added. The Moro may be obtained by using the head drop maneuver (Prechtl & Beintema, 1964), dropping the head of the bassinet a few inches, suddenly slapping the side of the bed, or making a loud noise. Response to a loud noise, however, is said to cause involvement of legs as well as arms and may not test the same response.

• *Crossed extension:* When one leg is held extended and a disagreeable stimulus is applied to the sole of the foot, the free leg flexes, then extends freely from twenty-six to thirty-two weeks. From thirty-two to thirty-eight weeks there is extension of the leg and no adduction. Complete crossed extension is apparent only at term when the free leg adducts to "remove" the noxious stimulus.

• *Automatic walk:* This occurs when the leg and body extensors, via the sole, are stimulated alternately. It may be seen as early as thirty to thirty-two weeks. The

EXHIBIT 15-1   Performing the neurological examination: Reflexes

Muscle tone: In contrast to the observations and tests for gestational age, one is looking for increased or decreased tone or asymmetrical tone in the extremities. Tests for recoil of arms and legs is helpful, as are flexion and extension of various joints—neck, trunk, shoulders, elbows, wrist, knees, and ankles.

One method for testing tone is flopping the hand at the wrist and the foot at the ankle. A full-term infant resists the flopping approximately equal to the relaxation. (The head must be kept in the midline.) Unequal tone may be detected also.

The hypertonic baby tends to be jittery, startles easily, and exhibits tightly flexed extremities and closed fists. The hypotonic or lethargic infant is more likely to be floppy, "sleepy," and have poor head control.

Sucking reflex: The sucking reflex can be determined by placing a finger in the baby's mouth and noting the vigor of the movements and the amount of suction produced.

Rooting reflex: The rooting reflex is obtained by stroking the corners of the mouth or lips. The infant responds by opening his mouth and turning toward the stimulus. This reflex develops early in gestation and is a strong one. Its absence is usually significant, unless it is tested for immediately after a feeding.

Traction response, head flexion and extension: The infant's hands and wrists are grasped, and he is pulled gently to a sitting position. In the term infant, there is at first a head lag, and then active flexion of the neck muscles so that the head and chest are in line when the infant reaches the vertical position. He maintains his head in the upright position for a few seconds, and the head then falls forward. He will then raise his head again, either spontaneously or following a slight stimulus such as stroking the upper lip.

Grasp reflex: (1) If the palm is stimulated with a finger, the infant will close his fingers on it. The grasp should be sufficiently strong in the term infant so that he can be lifted from the table by holding onto the examiner's finger. (2) Pressing the ball of the foot elicits a definite and prompt toe flexion.

Biceps, triceps, knee and ankle tendon reflexes: These are best elicited with the finger rather than a percussion hammer. The infant must be relaxed.

Ankle clonus: Two or three jerks are normally present in the newborn; sustained clonus is uncommon.

Incurvation of the trunk: The infant is lifted up and held over the hand in a prone position. The amount of flexion of the head and body is noted for an additional estimate of tone. The incurvation reflex is obtained by stroking or applying intermittent pressure with the finger parallel to the spine, first on one side and then the other, watching for a movement of the pelvis to the stimulated side.

Righting reaction: When the infant is lifted from the table vertically, he will usually flex his legs. If the soles of the feet then touch the table, he will respond with the righting reflex; i.e., first the legs will extend, then the trunk, and the head.

Placing: The baby is held vertically with his back against the examiner and one leg held out of the way. The other leg is moved forward so that the dorsum of the foot touches the edge of the examining table. The baby should flex the knee and bring his foot up as though he were trying to step onto the table.

Automatic walking: Following the preceding tests, the ability to perform automatic walking movements is evaluated. The baby is inclined forward to begin automatic walking. When the sole of one foot touches the table, he tends to right himself with that leg and the other foot flexes. As the next foot touches the table, the reverse action occurs. Term infants will walk on the entire sole of the foot, whereas preterm infants often walk on their toes.

Moro (startle) reflex: When the Moro response is elicited, the arms, hands, and cry are observed. The arms show abduction at the shoulder and extension of the elbow, followed by abduction of the arms in most infants. The hands show a prominent spreading or extension of the fingers. Any abnormality in the character of the movements should be noted, such a jerkiness or tremor, slow response, or asymmetric response. A cry follows the startle and should be vigorous. The nature of the cry is important: absent, weak, high-pitched, or excessive. The Moro reflex may be elicited in several ways:

- The baby's hands are held and his body and neck (but not his head) are lifted off the examining table and quickly let go.
- The infant is held with one hand supporting his head and the other supporting his body; the head is allowed to drop a few centimeters rather suddenly.
- The infant is held in both hands, which are lowered rapidly a few centimeters so that he experiences a sensation of falling.
- If the baby is quiet in the bassinet, the head of the bassinet is lifted a few centimeters and allowed to drop.

If one observes abnormal findings during the examination it is well to check these again at a different time before embarking on an extensive work-up for illness.

premature infant walks on tiptoe from thirty-two weeks on, whereas the infant born at term walks on the full sole.

• *Neck righting:* At thirty-four weeks neck righting may appear, but it is consistently present after thirty-seven weeks. Pupillary reflex and glabellar tap response appear so early in gestation that they are of no use in determining gestational age.

Especially significant in the neurological examination aimed at detecting central nervous system pathology (Prechtl and Beintema, 1964) are discordant movements of one limb, opisthotonus, tremors, or jerks (Exhibit 15-1). Seizures may take the form of localized jerks, rolling of the eyes or staring, or continuous sucking or chewing movements.

Resting position, asymmetry of face and skull, or odd facies are noted. It should be stressed again that the head should be in the midline for evaluation of symmetry of movements or tone, since turning the head to the side invokes the tonic neck reflex and will give extension of limbs on the face side and flexion on the occipital side.

The Discharge Examination

At the present time, mother and baby leave the hospital about three days after birth. Many alternative patterns of maternity care are being proposed, some of which may alter the sequence of neonatal evaluation, but the basic information presented in the preceding examinations, plus the discharge examination, are necessary for optimum care of the infant. Discharge at forty-eight to seventy-two hours makes it impossible to evaluate problems related to jaundice, neonatal infection, or adequacy of breast-feeding. Earlier discharge (e.g., six to eight hours after birth) may be another trend that makes follow-up of mother and baby in the home a prime requisite. Early discharge, rather than home delivery, is to be commended and alternative methods to evaluate and protect the infant must be sought.

The following are appropriate when the discharge of the infant is at seventy-two hours after birth:

The discharge examination is done at the mother's bedside or on her bed, so that she can see the behavior and physical characteristics that the examiner checks.

Since the infant's behavior, as pointed out by Brazelton (1973), may influence maternal behavior, the items requiring sleep states are done first. These include response decrement to light, sound, and touch (carried out with the infant in state 2 or 3). Ability to turn off these stimuli is discussed with the mother.

Once the infant is in the alert state, his ability to fix on a face, and to follow, are demonstrated. Attention to a voice and turning toward it, especially the mother's, is discussed.

At this point, the infant is undressed, and his reaction to being undressed and examined are noted. At some point, the baby is disturbed enough to cry and his ability to quiet himself is noted. This behavior is observed as the infant responds to an adult who makes efforts to console the infant by first showing his or her face, then speaking to the baby, placing a hand on the abdomen, loosely restraining one and then both arms, and finally picking him up. Thus, the mother observes the ease or difficulty encountered in consoling the baby as progressively more effort is exerted in helping him quiet himself.

Once picked up, the baby's ability or lack of desire to be cuddled is noted. His tendency toward irritability or calm can be pointed out and helpful suggestions given so that mother and infant may start off a relationship with the best chance for success and mutual satisfaction.

Once the infant is undressed, the examiner notes any previous findings that may have been of concern. Skin color, especially jaundice, is noted, and if follow-up is needed, this is explained to the mother. Plethora, pallor, or cyanosis should have been observed previously and investigated. Condition of the umbilical cord and management at home are discussed.

If circumcision was requested (which should have been discussed previously in light of the repeated publications (American Academy of Pediatrics, 1971; Committee on the Fetus and the Newborn, 1975) stating it is not medically indicated), then care of the penis and foreskin at home is discussed. If circumcision is not desired, it is well to remind the parents that no treatment is indicated and that toward the end of the first year, the foreskin usually begins to separate from the glans.

Muscle tone, alertness, suck and vigor need to be noted. If a murmur was heard previously, this should be checked. If abdominal distention is present, associated problems should be sought. Feeding and weight gain are noted. Type of stools is checked and discussed if indicated.

Breast-feeding discussion may be especially important at this examination, since success or failure will occur over the next few days.

Also important at this examination is an evaluation of mother–infant attachment. Some of the Prugh questions (see pp. 307–308) may already have been asked. This is an ideal time to ask them or repeat some.

REFERENCES AND ADDITIONAL READINGS

Brazelton, T.B. (1973). A neonatal behavioral assessment scale. In *Clinics in developmental medicine* (No. 50). Philadelphia: Lippincott; London: Spastics International Medical Publications.

American Academy of Pediatrics. (1971). *Standards and recommendations for hospital care of newborn infants* (ed. 5). Evanston, Il.: American Academy of Pediatrics, p. 110.

Committee on the Fetus and Newborn. (1975). Report of the Task Force on Circumcision. *Pediatrics, 56,* 610–611.

Cornblath, M., & Schwartz, R. (1966). *Disorders of carbohydrate metabolism in infancy.* Philadelphia: Saunders.

Desmond, M.M., Rudolf, A.J., & Pineda, R.G. (1970). Neonatal morbidity and nursery function. *Journal of the American Medical Association, 212,* 281–287.

Dubowitz, L.M.S., Dubowitz, V., & Goldberg, C. (1970). Clinical assessment of gestational age in the newborn infant. *Journal of Pediatrics, 77,* 1–10.

Klaus, M., & Kennel, J. (1979). Care of the parents. In M. Klaus & A. Fanaroff (Eds.), *Care of the high risk neonate.* Philadelphia: Saunders, pp. 146–172.

Klaus, M., & Kennell, J. (1982). *Parent–infant bonding.* St. Louis: Mosby.

Lubchenco, L.O. (1976). *The high risk infant.* Philadelphia: Saunders.

McMillan, J.A., Landau, S.A., & Oski, S.A. (1976). Iron sufficiency in breast-fed infants and the availability of iron from human milk. *Pediatrics, 58,* 686–691.

Prechtl, H.F.R., & Beintema, D. (1964). *The neurological examination of the full-term newborn infant.* London: Heinemann/Spastics International Medical Publications.

Prugh, D.G. (1982). *Psychosocial aspects of pediatrics.* Philadelphia: Lea & Febiger.

St. Anne-Dargassies, S. (1955). La maturation neurologique du premature. *Etudes Neo-Natales, 4,* 71.

Stave, U. (1970). *Physiology of the perinatal period* (Vols. 1 & 2). New York: Appleton-Century-Crofts.

Chapter 16 | Infant Behavior and Family Development

Robert J. Harmon

INTEREST IN THE HUMAN NEWBORN and newborn behavior has grown tremendously in the last twenty years. As Emde and Robinson (1979) point out in a recent review, it is almost as if the human newborn is a new species under study. This recent burgeoning of research on the newborn infant points out infant capabilities and capacities that were not appreciated previously. Major interests are *how* the infant influences his or her parents and caretakers, and reorganization of the family system in which the infant plays a major role.

There are many biases influencing the view of the newborn infant (Emde, et al., 1976; Emde & Robinson, 1979); three such biases are issues of passivity, lack of differentiation, and drive reduction, all of which have resulted from the theoretical viewpoints of developmental psychology and psychoanalysis. Influences from ethology, embryology, and other disciplines have resulted in a new look at the human infant. As Wolff (1966) has so well described, a number of discrete state-related behaviors are rhythmic, and show some degree of predictability. In addition, there are endogenously controlled rhythms of sleep, wakefulness, and activity (Emde et al., 1975; Gaensbauer & Emde, 1973; Kleitman & Engelmann, 1953; Sander, 1969, 1975). A newborn will interrupt a feeding in order to look at a novel stimulus; wakefulness can be prolonged by such a stimulus. The infant will cease fussing and become quietly alert when presented with an interesting stimulus (Wolff, 1959, 1965, 1966): Korner and Thoman (1970, 1972) have shown that the infant will be alert and quiet and will begin scanning the environment when picked up by the mother and placed on her shoulder. Thus, the infant can no longer be viewed as a passive, unorganized organism attempting to discharge tension, but rather is seen as an endogenously organized organism, ready to act as well as react, and to seek stimulation from his or her environment.

PERINATAL INFLUENCES ON THE FAMILY

Recently, there has been a major focus by professionals and consumers on maternal–infant bonding and the critical importance of the early hours for mothers and babies to be together: The recent changes in hospital practice that allow parents to experience the birthing process in a humane and dignified way are certainly to be applauded and encouraged. Although early contact between parents and their infants would seem to be beneficial, particularly for high-risk families, and is certainly described as enjoyable by most families, the

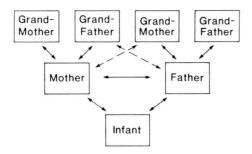

FIGURE 16-1 Perinatal influences within the family. (From Coppolillo, H.P. (1978). A conceptual model for study of some abusing parents. In E.J. Anthony, C. Koupernik, & C. Chiland (Eds.), *The child and his family: Vulnerable children* (Vol. 4). New York: John Wiley & Sons, pp. 231–238. With permission.)

role of the pregnancy and delivery and the psychological impact of parenthood on family members have been underemphasized.

Benedek (1952, 1956, 1962) was one of the first to describe that, during pregnancy, a mother reexperiences her own feelings of being mothered. This provides her with the opportunity of recreating that relationship with her own mother. This allows the new mother to relive unconsciously a period of her life that was potentially intensely gratifying (Coppolillo, 1979). In addition, in those cases in which the experience of having been mothered actually was a gratifying one, the new mother is able to use the experiences as a model for her own behavior, and also as a source of support for caring for her own child. In effect, if she has felt a sense of gratification in being mothered, she will find it easier to invest the tremendous amount of energy in the nurturance necessary to effectively mother her own child. This has led to the well-known notion that how one is mothered is an important predictor of one's ability to mother. This work has been further supported by that related to child abuse (Coppolillo, 1975, 1978; Steele & Pollock, 1968), in which it has been documented that battering mothers were often themselves battered as infants, and that these mothers have reexperienced crucial aspects of their own mothering as they mother their infants.

Harlow and Harlow (1965) and others working with monkeys have shown further evidence of the importance of being mothered in order to be a mother: they demonstrated that monkeys who had been raised with surrogate mothers were unable to engage in normal sexual behavior, and more important, when artificially inseminated, were unable to care for their young, and in fact often killed them.

The pregnancy and delivery experience itself may serve as another mechanism for the mother to rework and redefine her relationship with her own mother, often in a way that is more adaptive and gratifying for both of them. This relationship may become creatively restructured as a result of the birth process, such that not only is a baby born, but the relationship of the mother and her mother is re-created; it is no longer the same. This effect by the infant on the mother is an indirect, but very important, one (see the case study below).

During his wife's pregnancy, an expectant father may also reexperience certain crucial events in his own upbringing, and one often sees that a husband will become concerned about his wife's condition, and will, in effect, "mother" her. Research (Arnstein, 1972; Josselyn, 1956; Liebenberg, 1967) has demonstrated that during his mate's pregnancy, a man not only becomes increasingly concerned about her condition, but also seems to need more contact with his own mother. Fathers-to-be were shown to have increased contact with their mothers by phone or letter, underscoring the fact that the pregnancy experience has a crucial impact on the fathers as well.

Coppolillo (1978) has interpreted these data as suggesting that during the later stages of the woman's pregnancy and the early months of the child's life, the father becomes "motherly," and becomes concerned about his wife's health and general welfare. Although this has been considered by some (Arnstein, 1972) as a life crisis, it is clear that a shift in the father's role often does occur at this time. The importance of a nurturant role for the father, as a support system for the mother, is graphically illustrated in Figure 16-1.

What happens if a father is excluded from the pregnancy and birthing process that his wife is involved in, and, as dictated by society and custom, is restricted in his expression of feelings the impending birth has aroused in him? For example, is the well-documented observation that a man will often have his first extramarital affair during his wife's pregnancy related to his inability to share the events of the pregnancy with his wife? That inability may stem from societal exclusion of fathers from the pregnancy and birthing process, and from traditional medical practice, in which a woman often shares her feelings and concerns about her pregnancy with someone else—her obstetrician. This may be complicated by the fact that the obstetrician is commonly another man. Lamaze classes have served as an important catalyst for change for the better, as have our changing societal views of the role of the father in the family. Perhaps support for childbirth preparation classes of all kinds has come not only from the frustrated needs of mothers, but from similar frustrated needs of fathers.

Although both the mother and the father must design and develop their roles as parents, the marital relationship itself must not be neglected. In Solomon's (1973) description of stages of family development, the second stage is the birth of the first child. Within this stage are two tasks that the husband and wife must accomplish. First, they need to redefine their marital relationship. In effect, they must institutionalize their marriage so that it is understood as something separate from their roles as mother or father.

In addition, both parents must design and develop their new roles as parents. That is, they must define for themselves what it means to be a mother and a father. Too often, this is the only stage of the two-part process that is addressed. Crucial to this stage of development is the notion that the parental role and the role assigned to the child are *in addition to* the existing marital partner roles. Families in which the parents only develop their roles as parents are often the families that have later marital difficulties, especially during the adolescence of their last child, when, not seeing their marital relationship as something separate from their role as parents, they will flounder when their last child leaves home.

Often, when a couple is unable to deal with issues in their marital relationship, they will decide to have a child as a way of solidifying the marriage. This often leads to their assuming only the stereotypical role of mother (nurturer), or father (breadwinner), rather than dealing with each other as man and woman within their marriage. The negotiation that takes place between parents is not something that can be clearly defined or easily seen. However, health professionals working with parents of newborns can explore these issues with them by asking about their motivation for the pregnancy, their feelings about their parental roles, and their view of their marital relationship. In talking with parents about these issues, an appreciation of their developing sense of parenthood can be assessed.

Related to the issue of redefining the marital relationship is the support that the husband can give to his wife in her new role as mother. Although often overlooked, the support that the new mother receives from her family and friends may be a critical variable in how adequate she will feel as a mother. Coppolillo (1978) for example, has described the importance of support of the

father and the maternal grandmother, as well as the importance of feedback from the infant in helping a mother feel adequate about her caretaking ability (Figure 16-1). This notion can be broadened to include the reworking of the relationships described above. Additional evidence of the importance of the father's role can be found in a study of premature infants. Herzog (1977) has shown that when the father primarily attaches only to the infant, and does not support his wife in her role as mother, a destructive competition may ensue, such that difficulties in the marital relationship may arise. In his work relating to the follow-up of families who have a premature infant, Herzog found that in many cases the father became more attached to the infant than the mother did, leading to marital disharmony and eventual divorce. In some cases, custody of the child was awarded to the father. In our premature nursery, similar instances can be described. This is particularly the case if the infant is transported from one hospital to another, without the mother, and if the father accompanies the infant. Often, it is days to weeks later before the mother is physically able to visit by which time the father feels comfortable with the intensive care setting and with the health care professionals involved, and the potential for a destructive competitive seems clear. In working with these families, it is important to support the mother in her beginning attachment to her infant.

This is not to say that fathers cannot or should not attach to their infants, but emphasizes the point that this attachment should not be in lieu of their providing a support system for their wives, who are struggling with their new roles as mothers. Neither does this imply that shared parenting (Lerner, 1974, 1978) cannot or should not occur. Implicit in shared parenting is a notion of mutual support and respect for each partner's parental role. Lerner (1978), in discussing non-sex-stereotyped shared parenting, gives the example of a child being reared by two mature parents who are not in conflict over their gender identity. If these parents do not see their role in the family along traditional lines, the child is able to receive considerable psychological benefit. Thus, if both parents share authority, and household and professional tasks, the child is able to develop a definition of him- or herself incorporating a wide range of behaviors, feelings, and experiences rather than sex stereotyped ones.

The infant's indirect role in serving as a catalyst for major reorganization of family relationships is clear, but direct effect of the infant on his or her parents also needs to be emphasized. The infant is an active partici-

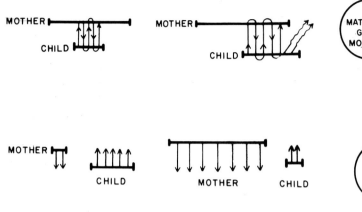

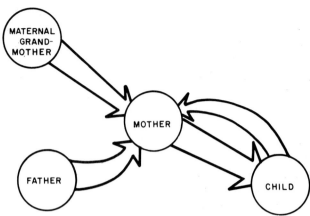

FIGURE 16-3   Mothering behavior. (Reprinted with permission from *Addictive Diseases: An International Journal,* *2*(1), 201–208, H.P. Coppolillo, Drug impediments to mothering behavior. (Reprinted with permission from *Addictive Diseases: An International Journal,* *2*(1), 201–208, H.P. Coppolillo, Drug impediments to mothering behavior. Copyright 1975, Pergamon Press, Ltd.)

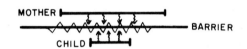

FIGURE 16-2   Mother–infant dyad. (From Coppolillo, H.P. (1978). A conceptual model for study of some abusing parents. In E.J. Anthony, et al. (Eds.), *The child and his family: Vulnerable children* (Vol. 4). New York: John Wiley & Sons, pp. 231–238. With permission.)

pant in his environment and has a wide variety of responses to exhibit, which allows for the mutual adaptation of the mother–infant dyad (Figure 16-2).

Before these infant characteristics are described, a case study will be presented that illustrates how the dynamic interactional model described above actually works. (See Figure 16-3 for an illustration of this model.)

Case Study

The mother of a premature male infant had become upset at a parents' meeting, during which some of the problems associated with the prematurity had been discussed. Because she became so upset, the nursery neonatologist referred her for psychiatric consultation. When seen by the psychiatrist (the author), both she and her husband talked about not being able to live together, and were considering divorce. They were seen three times during the infant's hospitalization; the major stresses under which they were living were discussed, and some problem solving with regard to their marriage was undertaken.

After the infant was transferred to a local hospital, the family was contacted for follow-up to see how they were doing. During this follow-up visit, the mother described a fascinating process that had occurred between her, her husband, and her parents (the maternal grandparents). The infant's parents had hoped that the baby would be home for

Christmas, since the grandparents were to visit during the holiday. Several weeks before the visit, the grandparents called with several complaints about the household pets and about an older sibling not being toilet-trained. Needless to say, the mother was devastated by her parents' call. However, unlike any other time in their marriage, the father called his in-laws and said, "We would like you to come visit, but we don't want you complaining about us, or the way we live our lives." This is an example of redefining the marital relationship.

After the grandparents' initial shock at being told by their son-in-law not to be critical of their daughter, they still agreed to come for the visit. As it turned out, the infant was discharged in time for the holiday, and it became clear that the real issue was the grandparents' fears concerning the young infant. They had adopted the mother when she was 18 months old, and were feeling uncertain and frightened about such a small baby. During the visit, the grandmother held the infant, and was able to express her own disappointment at never having had a little baby of her own. The grandmother and her daughter were able to talk about their relationship and what it had meant to both of them. The mother spontaneously said, "My mother and I have never been closer; I feel so much better about myself, and about myself as a mother." This illustrates the reworking of the maternal–grandmother relationship, and its potential beneficial effects on the mother's feeling about her abilities as a mother.

This case illustrates the tremendous stress that the birth of a premature infant can place on a marital relationship. For this couple, the birth had brought major disorganization to their marriage, and the stress had kindled certain intrapsychic conflicts for both of them. The mother became significantly depressed, and although the couple was contemplating divorce, it should be noted that a rather minor intervention—three contacts with a psychiatrist—had a major impact both on their marital relationship and on other issues with which they were dealing. This emphasizes an important point; that is, the period around the time of the birth of an infant is one in which major reorganization in a number of relationships can occur more readily than they would normally occur at other times. The work which this mother was able to do concerning her feelings about her own mother (the grandmother) and about her own mothering capabilities, was not something we would expect to have accomplished in a few brief contacts with a psychiatrist, or through a simple visit by the grandmother. The perinatal period may be a crucial one for appropriate preventive psychiatric intervention, if the health care professionals involved with the family are able to understand the dynamic processes involved. Recent research (Caplan et al., 1965; Kaplan & Mason, 1960; Leiderman et al., 1973; Leifer et al., 1972) has shown an increased rate of divorce in families with premature infants, especially if the parents are not allowed to visit the nursery. However, visiting alone should not be considered the only factor in family outcome, but as one of a number of factors to be evaluated in assessing families at risk (see later section on Psychosocial Conferences).

In addition, this case illustrates the importance of the parents' understanding of their infant (infant effects). This particular infant had intracranial bleeding and was somewhat irritable. The infant was given a Brazelton Neonatal Examination (see below) just prior to transfer, and was noted to be easily consoled when held, and to be alerted by the human face. After this infant went home, he was an extremely irritable baby, but could be soothed when held. This mother and child were able to work out a mutually adaptive relationship in spite of the many difficulties the child had. This is an example that when things go well, roles can be redefined in the whole family system, and because of this redefinition, the mother may be able to respond to the positive aspects of her infant, in spite of negative aspects.

THE CONCEPT OF STATE

As mentioned previously, the newborn infant is seen as an active participant in his interaction with the environment. In the newborn, the concept of *state* is a crucial one. State, as defined by Prechtl (Hutt et al., 1969; Prechtl et al., 1968), refers to certain patterns of psychological variables or patterns of behavior, which are repetitive and appear to be relatively stable. Wolff (1960) emphasized both the usefulness and the limitations of the concept of state. Another definition of state (Emde et al., 1976) refers to a group of variables at a given point in development that can define readiness to act on the one hand, and readiness to react on the other, again emphasizing the active role of the infant.

There are a number of descriptive systems for describing newborn behavioral states (Anders et al., 1971; Brazelton, 1973; Emde & Koenig, 1969b; Prechtl, 1974; Wolff, 1966). These systems recognize two qualitatively distinct sleep states. One is *active sleep*, which includes irregular respiration, rapid eye movements (REM), and behavioral activity. The other is *quiet sleep*, with no REM, very regular respiration, and little behavioral activity, except for occasional startles. Wakefulness is also divided into two states. The first, quiet wakefulness, or *quiet alert*, is a state in which the infant's eyes are wide open, there is little spontaneous movement, and the infant is able to follow visual objects and alert to sounds. The second state of wakefulness is active wakefulness, or *active alert*, in which the infant's eyes are wide open, and the infant is physically active and less likely to follow visual or auditory stimuli. In addition to the states of sleep and wakefulness, these systems describe crying. (See Exhibit 16-1 for Brazelton's (1973) description of infant states. Some researchers (Anders et al., 1971; Emde & Koenig, 1969b; Wolff, 1966) have further subdivided infant states. (See Exhibit 16-2 for Emde and Koenig's (1969b) description of states.)

The concept of state is helpful in predicting what behaviors to expect in a given state. Thus, Wolff (1966) described a number of discreet state-related behaviors that were rhythmic and showed some degree of predictability. For example, during non-rapid-eye-movement (NREM) sleep, the infant shows little or no behavioral activity except for occasional startles, or nibbling mouth movements. On the other hand, REM sleep often is interpreted by inexperienced mothers as being wakefulness; that is, the infant is so active and exhibits such a repertoire of "spontaneous" behaviors, that many mothers believe the baby to be awake. During REM sleep, the infant has many arm and leg movements, neck stretches, and many facial behaviors. In particular, during this state, infants are seen to frown and to smile in addition to other facial grimaces which are harder to categorize. During quiet wakefulness, the infant is most receptive to external stimulation. It is

EXHIBIT 16-1   Brazelton Neonatal Examination: Infant states, order of presentation, and general procedure

State

An important consideration throughout the tests is the state of consciousness or "state" of the infant. Reactions to stimuli must be interpreted within the context of the presenting state of consciousness, as reactions may vary markedly as the infant passes from one state to another. State depends on physiological variables such as hunger, nutrition, degree of hydration, and the time within the wake-sleep cycle of the infant. The pattern of states as well as the movement from one state to another appear to be important characteristics of infants in the neonatal period, and this kind of evaluation may be the best predictor of the infant's receptivity and ability to respond to stimuli in a cognitive sense. Our criteria for determining state are based on our own experiences and on those of others, and are comparable with the descriptions of Prechtl and Beintema (1964). A state is achieved if the child is in the particular state for at least fifteen seconds.

Sleep States

1. Deep sleep with regular breathing, eyes closed, no spontaneous activity except startles or jerky movements at quite regular intervals; external stimuli produce startles with some delay; suppression of startles is rapid, and state changes are less likely than from other states. No eye movements.
2. Light sleep with eyes closed; rapid eye movements can be observed under closed lids; low activity level, with random movements and startles or startle equivalents; movements are likely to be smoother and more monitored than in state 1; responds to internal and external stimuli with startle equivalents, often with a resulting change of state. Respirations are irregular, sucking movements occur off and on.

Awake States

3. Drowsy or semi-dozing; eyes may be open or closed, eyelids fluttering; activity level variable, with interspersed, mild startles from time to time; reactive to sensory stimuli, but response often delayed; state change after stimulation frequently noted. Movements are usually smooth. Fussing may or may not be present.
4. Alert, with bright look; seems to focus attention on source of stimulation, such as an object to be sucked, or a visual or auditory stimulus; impinging stimuli may break through, but with some delay in response. Minimal motor activity.
5. Eyes open; considerable motor activity, with thrusting movements of the extremities, and even a few spontaneous startles; reactive to external stimulation with increase in startles or motor activity, but discrete reactions difficult to distinguish because of high activity level. Fussing may or may not be present.
6. Crying; characterized by intense crying which is difficult to break through with stimulation.

Order of Presentation and General Procedure

The assessment of the infant should preferably be carried out in a quiet, dimly lit room, but, if this is not possible, disturbing aspects of a noisy, brightly lit room must be noted as part of the stimulation to which the infant might be reacting.

The examination itself usually takes between twenty and thirty minutes, and involves about thirty different tests and maneuvers. These should be performed in the following order:

1. Observe infant for two minutes—note state
2. Flashlight (three to ten times) through closed lids
3. Rattle (three to ten times)
4. Bell (three to ten times)
5. Uncover infant
6. Light pin-prick (five times)
7. Ankle clonus
8. Plantar grasp
9. Babinski response
10. Undress infant
11. Passive movements and general tone
12. Orientation, inanimate: visual and auditory
13. Palmar grasp
14. Pull to sit
15. Standing
16. Walking
17. Placing
18. Incurvation
19. Body tone across hand
20. Crawling—prone responses
21. Pick up and hold
22. Glabella reflex
23. Spin—tonic deviation and reflex
24. Orientation, animate: visual, auditory, and visual and auditory
25. Cloth on face
26. Tonic neck response
27. Moro response

From Brazelton, T.B. (1973). *Neonatal behavioral assessment scale*. London: William Heinemann Medical Books Ltd.; Philadelphia: J.B. Lippincott Co. With permission.

EXHIBIT 16-2 Neonatal smiling, frowning, and REM states

Sleep NREM
Eyes closed; face appears relaxed; no REMs.

Sleep REM
Eyes close; REMs are seen under eyelids; occasional transient (one second) eyelid opening during large upward-rolling eye movements.

Drowsy NREM
Eyes appear "glassy" and are open for more than thirty seconds of a one-minute observation; occasional to frequent eyelid blinking; face immobile; no REMs.

Drowsy REM
Same criteria as for drowsy NREM, except REMs are seen and facial expression often is fixed with a "strained," wide-eyed appearance.

Sucking NREM
At least half of a one-minute observation involves sucking; no REMs.

Sucking REM
Same as sucking NREM, except REMs are seen during sucking as well as during pauses.

Fussy-awake
Expiratory whimpers occurring more than three times but occupying less than ten seconds of a one-minute observation.

Fussy REM
Same criteria as for fussy-awake, except REMs are seen under closed eyelids. This state usually interrupts an ongoing sleep–REM state.

Crying-awake
Expiratory whimpers and/or frank crying for more than ten seconds of a one-minute observation.

Crying REM
Same criteria as for crying-awake, except REMs are seen under closed eyelids. This state usually interrupts an ongoing fussy-REM or sleep–REM state.

Alert-inactive
Less movement; eyes are "bright"; eyes pursue a slow-moving object for a brief period.

Alert-active
During the one-minute observation there is gross movement of two extremities, or of one exremity with much head movement.

From Emde, R.N., & Koenig, K. (1969). Neonatal smiling and rapid eye movement states. II. Sleep-cycle study. *Journal of the American Academy of Child Psychiatry, 8,* 637–656. Copyright 1969, American Academy of Child Psychiatry. With permission.

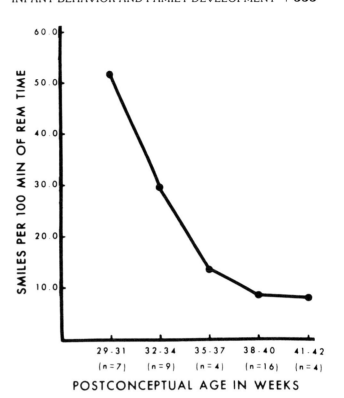

FIGURE 16-4 Premature infants have more REM smiling than full-term infants. (From Emde, R.N., McCartney, R.D., & Harmon, R.J. (1971). Neonatal smiling in REM states. IV. Premature study. *Child Development, 42,* 1657–1667. With permission.)

culty at times distinguishing between alert states and active REM sleep, the newborn's cry provides a clear message that an immediate, if not sooner, response is required, and that a diaper change, feeding, rocking, or some other soon-to-be-discovered soothing behavior needs to be put into motion.

Early Affect Expressions

Many psychiatrists have been interested in early crying and the REM-related affect expressions of smiling and frowning (Emde & Harmon, 1972; Emde & Koenig, 1969a, 1969b; Harmon & Emde, 1972; Wolff, 1966). In particular, these investigators were interested in the relationship between early affect expressions and later affect expressions, to which one could attribute feeling states. A relationship was sought between REM-related smiles and later social smiling, and between REM-related frowning and later crying. In the early studies (Emde & Koenig, 1969a, 1969b), it became clear that the spontaneous frowns and internal tension were, in fact, related. The frequency of frowning during any

during this state that newborns will follow brightly colored objects, although the most potent elicitor of following behavior is the human face and voice. Infants will turn toward a sound stimulus and search for it with their eyes.

Although less experienced parents may have diffi-

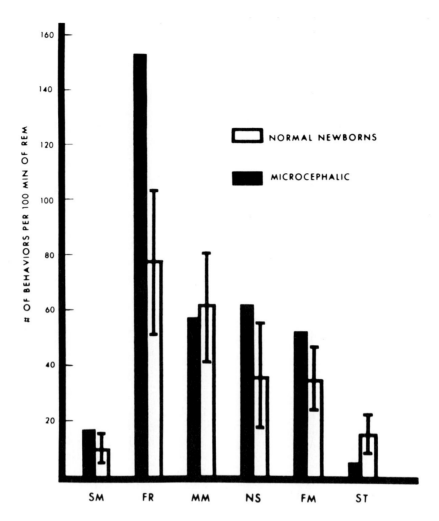

FIGURE 16-5 A comparison of the frequency of REM state behaviors between normal newborns and microcephalic newborns. Brackets indicate standard deviations from the normal population. SM, smiles; FR, frowns; MM, mouth movements; NS, stretches; FM, finger movements; ST, startles. (Reprinted with permission of authors and publishers from: Harmon, R. J., & Emde, R. N. Spontaneous REM behaviors in a microcephalic infant. PERCEPTUAL AND MOTOR SKILLS, 1972, 34, 827–833, Figure 1.)

given REM period remained the same until the last REM period, at which time there was a marked increase in the number of frowns, suggesting that the infant was beginning to feel internal distress before awakening to feed. On the other hand, there was no such support for a relationship between endogenous smiling and later social or exogenous smiling (Emde & Harmon, 1972). Emde and Harmon had originally hoped that REM smiling might indicate discharges in parts of the central nervous system, such as the limbic system, which would later become associated with feeling states. However, two additional studies made them realize that this was not the case. First, Emde and his co-workers (1971) found that premature infants had more REM smiling than full-term infants (Figure 16-4). In the second study (Harmon & Emde, 1972), it was found that a microcephalic infant, with anatomically verified impairment of both the cerebral cortex and limbic system, not only demonstrated spontaneous REM-related smiling but many other appropriate REM-related spontaneous behaviors as well (Figure 16-5). From this work, it was concluded that endogenous smiling is organized and mediated within the brainstem, along with the other REM-related behaviors, and that it is through later, neurological inhibition related to maturation of the cerebral cortex, that causes these behaviors to disappear during the first year of life. Of additional note; although mothers have suggested that the spontaneous REM

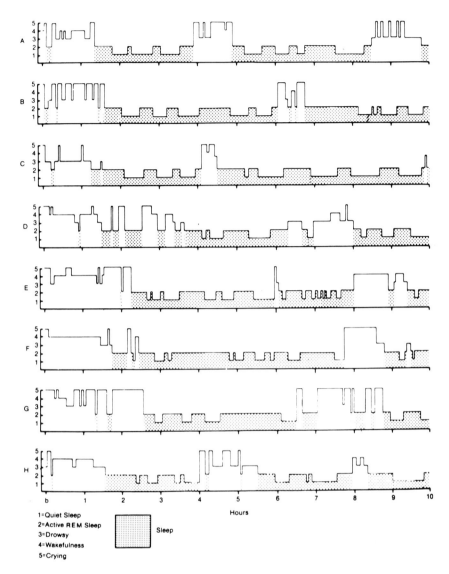

FIGURE 16-6 Behavioral cycles of sleep–wakefulness and rest–activity in eight newborns observed for ten hours following birth. Graphs A through D are for infants whose mothers received sedative medication. Graphs E through H are for infants born to unmedicated mothers. (From Emde, R.N., Swedberg, J., & Suzuki, B. (1975). Human wakefulness and biological rhythms after birth. *Archives of General Psychiatry, 32,* 780–783. Copyright 1975, American Medical Association. With permission.)

smiles are due either to gas or to "talking with angels," there was no evidence to support this as a gas-related behavior (Emde & Koenig, 1969a, 1969b). These investigators were unable to confirm or deny the second hypothesis.

Infant Sleep

The newborn spends approximately two-thirds of the day asleep. In spite of this, it is only recently that the study of sleep in infancy has held much interest.

According to Freud (1900), sleep was a "natural state of rest" and therefore of little interest. However, with the discovery by Aserinsky and Kleitman (1955) that infants alternated between an active form of sleep (REM sleep) and quiet sleep (NREM sleep), that sleep research was stimulated. Roffwarg et al. (1966) reviewed the research findings concerning the ontogenetic development of these types of sleep. They explained that sleep is not static, but shows rapid developmental change. For example, fifty percent of the newborn's total sleep is REM sleep; whereas sleep in the 1-year-old child is

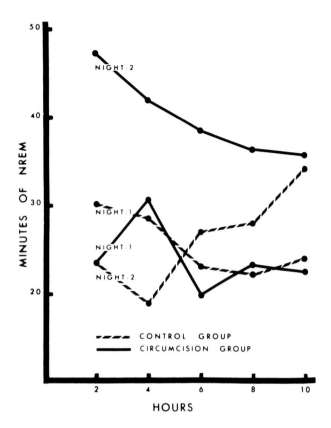

FIGURE 16-7 Circumcision results in an increased amount of NREM sleep. (From Emde, R.D., McCartney, R.D., & Harmon, R.J. (1971). Neonatal smiling in REM states. IV. Premature study. *Child Development, 42,* 1657–1661. With permission.)

thirty percent REM; and in the adolescent, it is twenty percent. They postulated that the high percentage of REM sleep in the neonate is important for neural growth. This "ontogenetic hypothesis" suggested that REM sleep, with its high amount of behavioral activity and neurophysiological activation, serves to provide a source of endogenous afferentation needed for central nervous system growth. Recently, there has been increasing interest in NREM or quiet sleep. Unlike REM sleep, which decreases in amount during the first year, NREM sleep evidences qualitative change during the first year (see Emde et al., 1976, for a review).

The human infant is born with well-organized and stable states, which cycle (Emde & Koenig, 1969a, 1969b) throughout the twenty-four hours. This cycling of states, or rhythmicity, is probably a manifestation of a more fundamental physiological rhythm, which has been termed the basic rest–activity cycle (BRAC), (Kleitman, 1963). The length of this cycle in the adult is

ninety minutes, while in the newborn, it is approximately forty-five minutes (Sterman & Hoppenbrouwers, 1971). This basic cycle is most prominently seen in sleep, through the alternation of REM and NREM cycles. Emde and his colleagues (1975) have shown that the BRAC is first in evidence in the early hours after birth, beginning following the one- to two-hour postbirth wakeful period that is typically seen in the unmedicated infant (Figure 16-6). In their study, they found this first basic cycle to be approximately three and a half hours during the first postnatal day and to be synchronous with feeding in the demand-fed, untraumatized infant. What, however, are the effects of maternal medication or trauma at birth?

Effects of Maternal Medication

Recently, the effects of maternal medication have been increasingly appreciated and often debated. Such effects as decreases in the extent of infant alertness (Stechler, 1964), increases in infant sucking (Brazelton, 1970; Kron et al., 1966), decreases in the number of spontaneous REM bahaviors (Emde & Koenig, 1969a), and on the amount of wakefulness (Brazelton, 1961; Emde et al., 1975) have had an impact on hospital practices. Although these studies have all shown effects on the newborn for several days after birth, a few studies (Aleksandrowicz & Aleksandrowicz, 1974; Bowes et al., 1970; Standley et al., 1974) have found effects beyond the neonatal period. There has been a controversy in the popular press (Kolata, 1979) with regard to some of the follow-up studies by Brackbill, where drug effects have been described into early childhood. Analgesics, local and general anesthetics, minor and major tranquilizers have all been implicated, as well as self-administered drugs of abuse (Standley et al., 1974).

Effects of Circumcision

Another factor that may affect the infant's state organization and his ability to interact with his mother is routine circumcision. In one study (Emde et al., 1971), it was found that routine circumcision, using the plastibel ligature technique of circumcision, resulted in an increased amount of NREM sleep as well as a decrease in the latency to the first NREM sleep period (Figure 16-7).

Other studies have also found dramatic effects of circumcision on the state of the newborn, but these were in the direction of prolonged wakefulness and crying. Although in the first study the results seemed to support the idea that a continuous painful stimulation may cause the infant to withdraw and go into the deepest state of consciousness possible (NREM sleep)—a view consistent with the conservation-withdrawal hypothesis of Engel (1962a, 1962b)—the other studies documented this procedure as a disruptive one, causing increased crying. The different results of these two groups of studies may well be the result of differing circumcision techniques (plastibel versus Gomko) rather than being contradictory.

An argument against the need for routine circumcision (American Academy of Pediatrics, 1971) would certainly be supported by these studies. Routine circumcision may result in decreased mother–infant interaction; a certain potential for negative feelings that parents might have about their male infants could well be reinforced in this early period by the state disruption. Kirya and Werthmann (1978) have suggested the use of penile-dorsal nerve block in neonatal circumcision to eliminate the pain associated with the procedure, and to potentially decrease state disruption and provide emotional relief for concerned parents. Although they describe that in all but two of fifty-two infants there was an absence of the usual clinical picture of crying, detailed behavioral studies using the methodologies described above would seem to be a useful step in assessing the effectiveness of the procedure.

Effects of Demand or Schedule Feeding

A third influence on neonatal state regulation is schedule versus demand feeding. In two studies (Emde et al., 1975; Gaensbauer & Emde, 1973), it was shown that during the first postnatal days, most infants have a basic endogenous sleep and wake cycle of approximately three and a half hours duration. There were no differences found between schedule-fed and demand-fed infants in the amount of wakefulness, but there was a difference in the patterning of the distribution of wakefulness in relation to feeding (Figure 16-8). Demand-fed infants had higher amounts of wakefulness prior to feeding, while schedule-fed infants had a higher amount of wakefulness during feeding and in the first hour after feeding. However, of greater importance is the fact that although all infants spent approximately the same amount of time in sleep and wakefulness regardless of feeding method, there was a tremendous amount of variability in the basic rest–activity cycle of infants in the demand-fed group. Although the demand-fed infants in general awoke on a four-hour basis, a large number of infants did not fit into a regular nursery schedule, due to a shorter or longer cycle. It is suggested that wakefulness is not only a function of

Mean Values of States*		
State	**Demand-Fed Infants**	**Schedule-Fed Infants**
Sleep-REM	46.08	47.95
Sleep NREM	20.60	18.91
Drowsy	8.27	8.11
Fussy & crying	11.27	10.25
Wakefulness	6.64	7.72
Nutritional sucking	6.61	7.05
Basetime	212.2 min	232.8 min

* Values expressed as % of observation time.

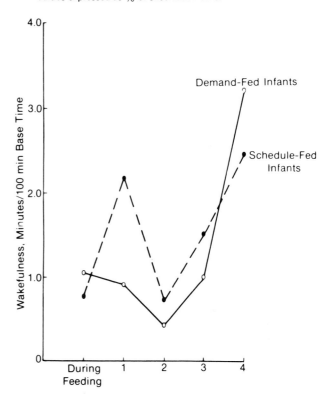

FIGURE 16-8 Amounts of wakefulness in schedule-fed and demand-fed infants. (From Gaensbauer, T.J., & Emde, R.N. (1973). Wakefulness and feeding in human newborns. *Archives of General Psychiatry, 28,* 894–897. Copyright 1973, American Medical Association. With permission.)

increased hunger, but is more likely the result of an independent sleep–wake rhythm in the basic rest–activity cycle.

Another issue with regard to schedule versus demand feeding is whether an infant is bottle- or breast-fed. Some pediatricians (Klaus & Kennell, 1976) have suggested that due to the lower fat content in human breast milk, infants should probably be fed more continuously than every 3 to 4 hours. Although this view of breast-feeding is at present a controversial one, demand in a breast-fed baby may differ from that in a bottle-fed baby. Most breast-feeding mothers are well aware that it usually takes longer for their infants to begin sleeping through the night than for bottle-fed infants; this is probably the result of the lower fat content and the lower calories in breast milk. It seems clear, however, that the many advantages that breast-feeding provides more than outweigh the increased number of feedings a breast-fed infant may require. The important issue seems to be education of the mother, regardless of whether she is breast- or bottle-feeding, as to the "appropriate" demand schedule that her infant will probably develop.

INNATE INFANT CAPACITIES AND CAPABILITIES

Not many years ago, pediatric textbooks asserted that a newborn infant could neither fix on a visual stimulus nor track a moving stimulus. Although this was asserted with great certainty, if one talked to parents, they would often describe their newborn's ability to follow parents' eyes and faces. In 1961, Fantz reported that the human newborn will look preferentially at a facial pattern. This research has been followed by other work (see review by Haith, 1975), which has shown that there is a pupillary light reflex present in full-term and premature infants. Although there is a great deal of controversy concerning infants' ability to accommodate (Haith, 1973; Haynes et al., 1965), it has been shown that the newborn is capable of attaining a focused retinal image. In addition, the newborn can discriminate brightness intensities, is sensitive to visual movement, and can track a moving stimulus (Emde & Robinson, 1979; Haith, 1973).

The newborn infant is also able to hear, and seems to come into the world preadapted to the environment in which he will be interacting. The newborn seems to be most responsive to sound frequencies found in human speech (Eisenberg, 1965, 1969). Some research has even shown that infants prefer speechlike sounds (Eimas et al., 1971; Hutt et al., 1969; Trehub & Robinovitch, 1972). Even more provocative are the findings of Condon and Sander (1974) on entrainment to the human voice. This rhythmic movement by the infant to his mother's voice is difficult to explain, but is impressive nonetheless. The infant's visual perception and preference, his auditory capabilities, and this entrainment to the human voice are beautifully reviewed in the movie *The Amazing Newborn* (Ross Laboratories, Columbus, Ohio).

The other senses have been less well studied in the newborn. Although it is clear that the infant is able to differentiate smells, temperatures, and tastes, little research has been done in this area (Emde & Robinson, 1979). One intriguing finding, however, is that of MacFarlane (1975), in which it was shown that 6-day-old infants can differentiate between their own mother's breast pad and that of another mother.

Assessment Scales

The most popular scale for assessing behavioral activity in the neonate is the Brazelton Neonatal Assessment Scale (1973). This assessment tool was preceded by several others (Graham, 1956; Graham et al., 1962; Rosenblith, 1961), but at present, the Brazelton is probably the most widely used. Although it was originally hoped that the scale would provide a screening test for predicting later pathological outcome as well as serve as an important research tool, it has become clear that its primary usefulness is in demonstrating to the mother the capabilities and capacities that her newborn infant possesses. In particular, it allows her an opportunity to see that her infant does see, can hear, and has individual charcteristics such as degree of cuddliness or ease of soothability. Thus, Brazelton (personal communication, 1976) strongly recommends that the examination be administered in the mother's presence. For this purpose, the whole examination or selected items from it can be used. A recent monograph (Sameroff, 1978) reviews the complicated issues with regard to use of the Brazelton examination for predicting later outcome and its limitations as a research instrument.

Reciprocal Influences

Klaus and Kennell, in their book, *Parent–Infant Bonding* (1982), have described certain processes by which the mother influences the infant, and the infant influences the mother. They described nine interactions, originating with the mother, that affect the infant; and six interactions originating with the infant, that affect the mother (Figure 16-9). A characteristic touching pattern has been described in human adults (Klaus et al., 1970; Lang, 1972; Rubin, 1963). When presented with their newborn infant, mothers begin fingertip touching the extremities, followed by massaging and palmar contact of the trunk. Klaus and Kennell (1976) suggest that this may be a species-specific behavior of adults elicited by the presence of a human newborn.

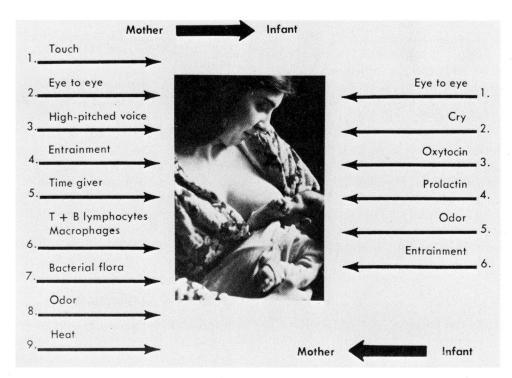

FIGURE 16-9 Mother–infant interactions. (From Klaus, M.H., & Kennell, J.H. (1982). Labor, birth, and bonding. In M.H. Klaus & J.H. Kennell (Eds.), *Parent–infant bonding* (ed. 2). St. Louis: The C.V. Mosby Company. With permission.)

The human newborn is able to see and follow at birth during the alert and active state. Mothers find looking into their infant's eyes to be a very rewarding and interesting behavior (Klaus et al., 1970; Robson, 1967). Many mothers have claimed that they did not know their infants until they were able to gain eye-to-eye contact in the enface or face-to-face position.

Infants prefer a high-pitched female voice at birth and in the early days of life. It has been an interesting observation that many mothers use a higher-pitched voice in addressing their infants than they do in normal conversation, a behavior that would enhance their infant's interest in them.

Condon and Sander (1974) have described the entrainment of bodily movement to human speech. Using microanalysis of sound film, they found that both speaker and listener move in rhythm to the words that are spoken. They then studied the human infant, and, in detailed behavioral analyses, demonstrated that the human newborn moves in time with adult speech, although disconnected vowel sounds or other sounds or noises do not effect this degree of entrainment. This phenomenon was found using either English or Chinese, and was not specific to the ethnic background of the infant. Sander (personal communication, 1978) has

noted further than an infant who has spent time in a nursery where English is spoken, has a difficult time when exposed to the very different rhythm of Chinese and may even find it distressful.

Sander has also described the important role of the mother as time-giver to the infant. In careful studies (Sander et al., 1970), he has elucidated the role of the mother in the establishment of the infant's biorhythmicity. He demonstrated that the intra-uterine rhthmicity, which the baby establishes to the mother's sleep–wake cycle and daily routine, is disrupted by the birth process; this disruption lasts through the first week of life. However, Sander (Sander, 1975; Sander & Julia, 1966) has shown that an infant can adapt its diurnal rhythm of sleep and wakefulness to its caregiver by 10 days of age. By this same age, infants who are cared for by a consistent caregiver show a disruption in their biorhythmic patterns when transferred to a new caregiver. In addition, Sander has shown an increase in the amount of time an infant is in an alert state when held by the mother from the second day (twenty-five percent) to the eighth day (fifty-seven percent). These findings have positive implications for the use of rooming-in, to allow a mother–infant dyad to begin developing their mutual biorhythmic pattern.

Parents have commented that following discharge, from the premature-infant nursery, the sleep–wake and feeding patterns that the nurses described as being typical of their infants were quite different from what was experienced by the parents in the home. Clearly, these infants had entrained to patterns in the nursery and to hospital routine, and not to the more typical diurnal home pattern. Nurses and physicians now explain this phenomenon to parents who are taking their infants home after a long stay in the hospital, in an attempt to help them adjust to the differences between their own, and their infant's routines.

The mother also imparts lymphocytes, macrophagias and antibodies to her infant through her breast milk. This may help protect the infant against infection. In addition, the mother's strains of respiratory organisms will populate the infant's respiratory and gastrointestinal tracts if she is allowed to be in contact with her baby. There is evidence that this also helps protect the infant from infection.

The fact that the infant can, by the fifth day of life, discriminate his mother's breast pad from that of another mother, has already been described, but the importance of the odor of the mother, as well as her ability to give heat and keep the infant warm, are the last two elements outlined in Figure 16-9.

Many of the six interactions that originate with the infant are reciprocal to those just described for the mother. The importance of eye-to-contact, and the ability of the eyes of the mother to serve as a "super stimulus" for infant visual fixation and following, have been described. In addition, the infant's crying has been demonstrated (Lind et al., 1973) to induce lactation and encourage nursing in mothers. Many nursing mothers report lactation at the sound of a crying baby, although some mothers report they are only affected by their own infant's cry.

A breast-fed infant will stimulate the secretion of oxytocin and prolactin in the mother. One could speculate that immediate breast-feeding following delivery might help uterine contraction and reduce bleeding, and it has been proposed (Klaus & Kennell, 1976) that the release of prolactin may enhance mother–infant attachment through a mechanism as yet not well delineated.

Just as infants are able to discrimnate between their mother's breast pad and that of another, some mothers report differences in their infants' odors.

Entrainment of the infant to the mother's voice and to her biorhythms is important for the infant in his or her adaptation to the new environment. Equally important are the infant responses that the mother finds rewarding, and which help to ensure the interlocking of mother and infant into a reciprocal interactional system.

APPLICATION TO CLINICAL PRACTICE

Understanding the human newborn and his or her effect on the family can be used in several ways in the hospital nursery, and regarding hospital practice. One of the best methods for attuning parents to the remarkable capacities of their infants is through the Brazelton neonatal examination, as discussed earlier. For research purposes, it is important to be trained and have one's reliability checked at one of the Brazelton examination centers.

Psychosocial Conferences

Another useful hospital practice can be a weekly psychosocial conference, in which the coping strategies of the families who have infants on the unit can be discussed. At the University of Colorado Health Sciences Center, we currently have weekly psychosocial rounds on all of our pediatric units, to discuss the emotional needs of children and their families, their needs for services, and how they are coping with the hospitalization. These rounds are coordinated by the nursing staff and are attended by a child psychiatrist, the social worker providing service to the unit, the public health nurse coordinator, a nutritionist, and other appropriate allied health professionals who provide services for the particular age group staying on the unit.

The format of the rounds varies according to the neonatal unit on which they are held. In the normal-newborn nursery and rooming-in nursery, where the hospital stay is generally two days, only those infants and their families who seem to be having difficulty are brought to the attention of the consulting team. A great deal of time has been spent in helping the nursing staff become aware of psychosocial problems and dynamic interactional issues that may be occurring in the families with which they are working. To facilitate this awareness, there are weekly teaching rounds, during which a mother and her newborn infant are interviewed using the Five-Question Approach of Prugh (1982) to elicit a range of normal and potentially high-risk responses from mothers in the nursery. This has been useful in helping the nursing staff and the pediatric housestaff become aware of the wide range of feelings and plans that parents have before, during, and after the birth of their child.

In the intensive-care premature nursery and the medium-risk nursery, rounds are structured so that each infant and his or her family are discussed weekly. Attention is paid to visiting patterns, or, as is often the case if the family lives a great distance from the hospital, the number of times which they call the unit to check on their infant. During these rounds, we discuss each family, not on the basis of their contact or lack of contact with their infant, and not as to whether they are "bonded"; rather, we use the dynamic inter-actional model proposed earlier in our assessment of their coping strategies. Some families, whose infant may be close to death or have a physical anomaly, may need time in order to grieve and work through these issues. We attempt to "titrate" the degree of closeness or contact with the infant dependent on the emotional needs of the parents. Our philosophy is to examine the factors that may be influencing the parents, rather than looking simply at their visiting or calling patterns.

In addition, we also discuss the family's needs for services; referrals are made on all patients to public health nurses for pre- as well as postdischarge visits. We are then able to use information gleaned from the public health nurse's visits in the home to help us in our total assessment of the family. In addition, referrals to social agencies, handicapped children's programs, or other appropriate agencies are made when they are relevant. These rounds also serve as a referral source for our Child Psychiatry Fellows, who can work with families who aren't coping well with the stresses they are facing during their infant's hospitalization. In general, the social worker on the unit attempts to evaluate all families in order to facilitate referrals and to offer supportive therapeutic counseling. From all of this input, we are able to develop intervention strategies for those families who need them, and monitor how well these strategies are working.

REFERENCES

Aleksandrowicz, M.K., & Aleksandrowicz, D.R. (1974). Obstetrical pain-relieving drugs as predictors of infant behavior variability. *Child Development, 45,* 935–945.

American Academy of Pediatrics. (1971). *Hospital care of newborn infants* (ed. 5). Evanston, Il.: Committee of Fetus and Newborn.

Anders, T., Emde, R., & Parmelee, A. (Eds.). (1971). *A manual of standardized terminology, techniques and criteria for scoring states of sleep and wakefulness in newborn infants.* Los Angeles: UCLA Brain Information Service, NINDS Neurological Information Network.

Arnstein, H. (1972). The crisis of becoming a father. *Sexual Behavior, 2,* 42.

Aserinsky, E., & Kleitman, N. (1955). A motility cycle in sleeping infants as manifested by ocular and gross bodily activity. *Journal of Applied Physiology, 8,* 11–18.

Benedek, T. (1952). *Psychosexual functions in women.* New York: Ronald Press.

Benedek, T. (1956). Toward the biology of the depressive constellation. *Journal of the American Psychoanalytic Association, 4,* 389.

Benedek, T. (1962). The psychobiologic approach to parenthood. In E.J. Anthony & T. Benedek (Eds.), *Parenthood: Its psychology and psychopathology* (Part II). Boston: Little, Brown. pp. 109–206.

Bowes, W.A., Brackbill, Y., Conway, E., & Steinschneider, A. (1970). The effects of obstetrical medication on fetus and infant. *Monographs of the Society for Research in Child Development, 35*(4, Serial No. 137).

Brazelton, T.B. (1961). Psychophysiologic reaction in the neonate. II. Effects of maternal medication on the neonate and his behavior. *Journal of Pediatrics, 58,* 513–518.

Brazelton, T.B. (1973). *Neonatal behavioral assessment scale.* London: Heinemann; Philadelphia: Lippincott.

Caplan, G., Mason, E., & Kaplan, D.M. (1965). Four studies of crisis in parents of prematures. *Community Mental Health Journal, 1,* 149–161.

Condon, W.S., & Sander, L.W. (1974). Neonate movement is synchronized with adult speech: Interactional participation and language acquisition. *Science, 183,* 99–101.

Coppolillo, H.P. (1975). Drug impediments to mothering behavior. *Addictive Diseases: An International Journal, 2*(1), 201–208.

Coppolillo, H.P. (1978). A conceptual model for study of some abusing parents. In E.J. Anthony, C. Koupernick, & C. Chiland (Eds), *The child and his family: Vulnerable children,* (Vol. 4). New York: Wiley, pp. 231–238.

Coppolillo, H.P., (1979). A conceptual model for some abusing parents. (Unpublished manuscript).

Eimas, P.D., Siqueland, E.R., Jusczyk, P., & Vigorito, J. (1971). Speech perception in infants. *Science, 171,* 303–306.

Eisenberg, R.B. (1965). Auditory behavior in the neonate. I. Methodologic problems and the logical design of research procedures. *Journal of Auditory Research, 5,* 159–177.

Eisenberg, R.B. (1969). Auditory behavior in the human neonate. *International Audiology, 8,* 34–45.

Emde, R.N., Gaensbauer, T.J., & Harmon, R.J. (1976). Emotional expression in infancy: A biobehavioral study. *Psychological Issues Monograph Series* (Monograph 37). New York: International Universities Press.

Emde, R.N., & Harmon, R.J. (1972). Endogenous and exogenous smiling systems in early infants. *Journal of the American Academy of Child Psychiatry, 11*(2), 177–200.

Emde, R.N., & Koenig, K. (1969). Neonatal smiling and rapid eye movement states. *Journal of the American Academy of Child Psychiatry, 8,* 57–67. (a)

Emde, R.N., & Koenig, K. (1969). Neonatal smiling and rapid eye movement states. II. Sleep-cycle study. *Journal of the American Academy of Child Psychiatry, 8,* 637–656. (b)

Emde, R.N., McCartney, R.D., & Harmon, R.J. (1971). Neonatal smiling in REM states. IV. Premature study. *Child Development, 42,* 1657–1661.

Emde, R.N., & Robinson, J. (1979). The first two months: Recent research in developmental psychobiology and the changing view of the newborn. In J. Noshpitz & J. Call (Eds.), *Basic handbook of child psychiatry,* New York: Basic Books.

Emde, R.N., Swedberg, J., & Suzuki, B. (1975). Human wakefulness and biological rhythms after birth. *Archives of General Psychiatry, 32,* 780-783.

Engel, G.L. (1962). Anxiety and depression-withdrawal: The primary affects of unpleasure. *International Journal of Psychoanalysis, 43,* 89-97. (a)

Engel, G.L. (1962). *Psychological development in health and disease.* Philadelphia: Saunders, pp. 384-388. (b)

Fantz, R.L. (1961). The origin of form perception. *Scientific American, 204,* 66-72.

Freud, S. (1900). The interpretation of dreams. In *The complete psychological work of Sigmund Freud* (standard eds. 4 & 5). London: Hogarth (published in 1953).

Gaensbauer, T.J., & Emde, R.N. (1973). Wakefulness and feeding in human newborns. *Archives of General Psychiatry, 28,* 894-897.

Graham, F.K. (1956). Behavioral differences between normal and traumatized newborns. I. The test procedure. *Psychology Monographs, 70,* 1-16.

Graham, F.K., Ernhard, C.B., Thurston, D., & Craft, M. (1962). Development three years after perinatal anoxia and other potentially damaging newborn experiences. *Psychological Monographs, 76*(3), 1-53.

Haith, M. (1973). Visual scanning in infants. In L.J. Stone, H.T. Smith, & L.B. Murphy (Eds.), *The competent infant.* New York: Basic Books.

Harlow, H.F., & Harlow, M.K. (1965). *The affectional systems.* In A.M. Schrier, H.F. Harlow, & F. Stollnitz (Eds.), *Behavior of Non-Human Primates* (Vol. 2). New York: Academic Press.

Harmon, R.J., & Emde, R.N. (1972). Spontaneous REM behaviors in a microcephalic infant. *Perceptual and Motor Skills, 34,* 827-833.

Haynes, H., White, B.L., & Held, R. (1965). Visual accommodation in human infants. *Science, 148,* 528-530.

Herzog, J.M. (1977). Patterns of parenting. Paper presented at the meeting of the American Academy of Child Psychiatry, Houston, October 21, 1977.

Hutt, S.J., Lenard, H.G., & Prechtl, H.F.R. (1969). Psychophysiological studies in newborn infants. In L.P. Lipsitt & H.W. Reese, (Eds.), *Advances in child development and behavior* (Vol. 4). New York: Academic Press, pp. 127-172.

Josselyn, I. (1956). Cultural forces, motherliness and fatherliness. *American Journal of Orthopsychiatry, 26,* 264.

Kaplan, D.N., & Mason, E.A. (1960). Maternal reactions to premature birth viewed as an acute emotional disorder. *American Journal of Orthopsychiatry, 30,* 539-552.

Kirya, C., & Werthmann, M.W. (1978). Neonatal circumcision and penile dorsal nerve block—A painless procedure. *The Journal of Pediatrics, 92,* 998-1000.

Klaus, M.H., & Kennell, J.H. (1976). *Maternal-infant bonding: The impact of early separation or loss on family development.* St. Louis: Mosby.

Klaus, M.H., & Kennell, J.H. (1982). *Parent-infant bonding* (ed. 2). St. Louis: Mosby.

Klaus, M.H., Kennell, J.H., Plumb, N., & Zuehlke, S. (1970). Human maternal behavior at first contact with her young. *Pediatrics, 46,* 187-192.

Kleitman, N. (1963). *Sleep and wakefulness.* Chicago: University of Chicago Press.

Kleitman, N., & Engelmann, T.G. (1953). Sleep characteristics of infants. *Journal of Applied Physiology, 6,* 269-282.

Kolata, G.B. (1979). Scientists attack report that obstetrical medications endanger children. *Science, 204,* 391-392.

Korner, A., & Thoman, E. (1970). Visual alertness in neonates as evoked by maternal care. *Journal of Experimental Child Psychology, 10,* 67-78.

Korner, A., & Thoman, E. (1972). The relative efficacy of contact and vestibular proprioceptive stimulation in soothing neonates. *Child Development, 43,* 443-453.

Kron, R.E., Stein, M., & Goddard, K.R. (1966). Newborn sucking behavior affected by obstetric sedation. *Pediatrics, 37,* 1012-1016.

Lang, R. (1972). *Birth book.* Ben Lomond, Ca.: Genesis Press.

Leiderman, P.H., Leifer, A.D., Seashore, M.J., Barnett, C.R., & Grobstein, R. (1973). Mother-infant interaction: Effects of early deprivation, prior experience and sex of infant. *Early Development* (Research Publication of the Association for Research in Nervous and Mental Disease), *51,* 154-175.

Leifer, A.D., Leiderman, P.H., Barnett, C.R., & Williams, J.A. (1972). Effects of mother-infant separation on maternal attachment behavior. *Child Development, 43,* 1203-1218.

Lerner, H.E. (1974). Early origins of envy and devaluation of women: Implications for sex role stereotypes. *Bulletin of the Menninger Clinic, 38*(5), 538-553.

Lerner, H.E. (1978). Adaptive and pathogenic aspects of sex-role stereotypes: Implications for parenting and psychotherapy. *American Journal of Psychiatry, 135,* 48-52.

Liebenberg, B. (1967). Expectant fathers. *American Journal of Orthopsychiatry, 37,* 358.

Lind, J., Vuorenkoski, V., & Wasz-Hackert, O. (1973). In N. Morris (Ed.), *Psychosomatic medicine in obstetrics and gynaecology.* Basel: Karger.

MacFarlane, J.A. (1975). In *Parent-infant interaction* (CIBA Foundation Symposium 33). Amsterdam: Elsevier.

Prechtl, H.F. (1974) The behavioral states of the newborn infant (a review). *Brain Research, 76,* 185-212.

Prechtl, H.F., & Beintema, D. (1964). *Neurological examination of the full-term newborn infant: Clinics and developmental medicine.* London: Heinemann.

Prechtl, H.F., Akiyama, Y., Zinkin, P., & Grant, D.K. (1968). Polygraphic studies of the full-term newborn. I. Technical aspects and qualitative analysis. In M.C. Bax & R.C. MacKeith (Eds.), *Studies in infancy.* London: Heinemann, pp. 1-25.

Prugh, D. (1982). *Psychosocial aspects of pediatrics.* Philadelphia: Lea & Febiger.

Robson, K.S. (1967). The role of eye-to-eye contact in maternal-infant attachment. *Journal of Child Psychology & Psychiatry, 8,* 13-25.

Roffwarg, H.P., Muzio, J.N., & Dement, W.C. (1966). Ontogenetic development of the human sleep-dream cycle. *Science, 152,* 604-609.

Rosenblith, J.F. (1961). The modified Graham Behavior Test for neonates. *Biology of the Neonate, 3,* 174-192.

Rubin, R., (1963). Maternal touch. *Nursing Outlook, 11,* 828-831.

Sameroff, A.J. (1978). Organization and stability of newborn behavior: A commentary on the Brazelton Neonatal Behavior Assessment Scale. *Monographs of the Society for Research in Child Development, 43*(5,6), 1-138.

Sander, L. (1969). Regulation and organization in the early infant-caretaker system. In J. Robinson (Ed.), *Brain and early behavior.* London: Academic Press, pp. 311-332.

Sander, L. (1975). Infant and caretaking environment: Investigation and conceptualization of adaptive behavior in a system of increasing complexity. In E.J. Anthony (Ed.), *Explorations in child psychiatry.* New York: Plenum Press, pp. 129-166.

Sander, L., & Julia, H. (1966). Continuous interactional monitoring in the neonate. *Psychosomatic Medicine, 28,* 822–835.

Sander, L.W. Stechler, G., Burns, P., & Julia, H. (1970). Early mother–infant interaction and 24-hour patterns of activity and sleep. *Journal of the American Academy of Child Psychiatry, 9,* 103–123.

Solomon, M.A. (1973). A developmental conceptual premise for family therapy. *Family Process, 12,* 179–188.

Standley, K., Soule, A.B. III, Copans, S.A., & Duchowny, M.S. (1974). Local-regional anesthesia during childbirth: Effect on newborn behaviors. *Science, 186,* 634–635.

Stechler, G. (1964). Newborn attention as affected by medication during labor. *Science, 144,* 315–317.

Steele, B.F., & Pollock, C. (1968). Psychiatric study of abusing parents. In R.E. Helfer & C.H. Kempe (Eds.), *The battered child.* Chicago, London: The University of Chicago Press, p. 103.

Sterman, M.B., & Hoppenbrouwers, T. (1971). The development of sleep-waking and rest-activity patterns from fetus to adult in man. In M.B. Sterman, D.J. McGinty, & A. Adinolfi (Eds.), *Brain development and behavior.* New York: Academic Press, pp. 203–227.

Trehub, S.E., & Robinovitch, M.S. (1972). Audiolinguistic sensitivity in early infancy. *Developmental Psychology, 6,* 74–77.

Wolff, P.H. (1959). Observations on newborn infants. *Psychosomatic Medicine, 21,* 110–118.

Wolff, P.H. (1960). The developmental psychologies of Jean Piaget and psychoanalysis. *Psychological Issues Monograph Series* (Monograph 5). New York: International Universities Press.

Wolff, P.H. (1965). The development of attention in young infants. *Annuals of the New York Academy of Science, 118,* 815–830.

Wolff, P.H. (1966). The causes, controls, and organization of behavior in the neonate. *Psychological issues monograph Series* (Monograph 17). New York: International Universities Press.

Chapter 17 | Infant Nutrition

Karren Mundell Kowalski

ISSUES OF INFANT FEEDING are laden with emotion. It is only in the last 100 years that society has concentrated such extensive energy on the bearing and rearing of children. In earlier periods, children were either ignored or viewed as physically smaller adults (Aries, 1962). A brief examination of the history of infant feeding provides a perspective for current controversies and some guideposts for future direction.

HISTORICAL BACKGROUND

Primitive Societies

In hunter–gatherer societies, infant feeding is surrounded by ritual and taboo. Many tribes allow several days to pass before the infants are put to their mothers' breasts. Due to this taboo against colostrum, infants are suckled by other women in the tribe during this interum period. The average duration of lactation is three to four years (Wickes, 1953a). It's possible that some future historian of infant feeding will view such recent practices as feeding schedules and giving babies nothing by mouth for twelve to twenty-four hours as ritualistic and taboo laden.

Although we think of bottle-feeding as a technological invention of the twentieth century, artificial feeding vessels appeared shortly after humans moved into herding–agrarian lifestyles. Animal milk and grains were then available as substitutes for human milk (Jelliffe, 1968).

Ancient Cultures

The first positively identified infant feeding vessels are from Egyptian tombs of the era 2500 B.C. Clay vessels in Greek settlements from the third century B.C. contain inscriptions indicating their use (Phillips, 1976).

The first written evidence of wet-nurses appears in the Hammurabi Code (2250 B.C.) of ancient Babylon. They were defined as women who suckled infants for monetary gain; the code specified amputation of a breast as punishment for allowing the infant to die and substituting another infant (Davidson, 1953).

During the Homeric period in Greece, infants whom the parents wished to survive were maternally breast-fed. Exposure of unwanted or weak infants was commonly accepted; they were often flung on a dung heap where they might be retrieved by a benevolent person who would arrange for a wet-nurse and raise them as slaves. Those less fortunate were devoured by dogs and wild animals. Infants of the more well-to-do Athenians were wet-nursed by slaves, captives, or free women. Large numbers of feeding "bottles" or receptacles have been found in infant graves from this period, indicating widespread artificial feeding (Davidson, 1953).

The Talmud (536 B.C.) instructed Hebrew parents to put the child to breast immediately after birth, even prior to cutting the umbilical cord. In addition to colostrum, honey was given to promote evacuation of meconium. Infants were suckled by their mothers for eighteen to twenty-four months. Babies were loved and had high status, and large families were considered a blessing from God. Wet-nurses, usually slaves, were used only as a necessity. While they nursed, they could do no other work nor nurse another child including their own. If the wet-nurse was competent, she was treated as a member of the family.

In contrast, the Roman civilization used artificial feeding and wet-nurses extensively, much after the Greek model. However, because large families were valued, there was very little infanticide, particularly of male infants.

The Mohammedan ethics seemed to be more closely patterned after the Talmud. The Koran directed mothers to suckle their young for two years. Family units were strong, and the Koran severely threatened those who practiced female infanticide, which was very common in many societies of the time.

Middle Ages

Due to the advent of Christianity, provisions were made by the Church for protection of abandoned infants. The first large home for foundlings was begun in Milan in 787 A.D. Soon there were foundling homes all over Europe. In the 1200s, Pope Innocent III was shocked by the number of infants found in the Tiber River and dedicated a large section of the Santa Maria Hospital to care for abandoned infants. During this period, wet-nurses were employed only in necessary situations, such as in foundling homes or in cases where the mother was sick or dying. Artificial feeding was unknown.

Renaissance

During this period, wet-nurses gained renewed popularity. Guillemean's *The Nursing of Children* (1612) makes the same recommendations about wet-nurses as the ancients did: A wet-nurse should be of healthy lineage, physically healthy, and have a rosy complexion and white teeth. She should exhibit good behavior, be even tempered (redheads were unacceptable!), happy, chaste, wise, discreet, careful, observant, understanding, and always willing to give the breast. She should have broad, yet not pendulous, breasts with good nipples; she should play with the infant and

change him often (Wickes, 1953b). It was believed that the characteristics of the nurse were passed to the infant through her milk. The wet-nurse held such an enviable position (well fed and well paid for comparatively little work) that poor young girls often became pregnant and then overlayed, or suffocated, their own infants before seeking employment. Perhaps this is a source of the old wives tale against a mother bringing a baby into her bed.

Dry-nursing, the feeding of paps and gruels, also gained in popularity. Wealthy ladies, and those of the nobility, did not breast-feed because it was considered unfashionable, injurious to their health, and ruinous to their figures. But most of all, breast-feeding interfered with social activities and responsibilities. Infants were sent to the country to wet-nurses, with disastrous results. These nurses frequently had more infants than they could provide for and infant mortality was very high. It is difficult for us to understand how parents could send infants into such situations.

> It is essential to take into account the social conditions of the times when considering the history of infant feeding, for they have a profound bearing upon the whole problem. Many infants fared badly and died simply because their lives were valued so cheaply that in many instances no food at all was given, the unwanted infant thus swelling the ranks of stillborns, the over-layed, and those dying from want of breast milk.*

This attitude toward children was prevalent until the mid-1800s.

Unwanted infants were sent to foundling homes. At one such home, 100 infants arrived each day. Of some 15,000 infants, more than 10,000 died soon after their arrival. The general public was not outraged because this human wastage was considered part of the imperfect workmanship of nature. Furthermore, it was assumed (rightly or wrongly) that these infants were the offspring of harlots and that death was a justifiable fate that prevented the children from perpetrating the sins of their mothers.

In Paris in 1780, the records show approximately 21,000 live births. About 700 of these infants were nursed by their biological mothers; another 700 were wet-nursed by surrogate mothers in the homes of the infants' biological parents. Two or three thousand were placed in homes in the Paris suburbs, where the wet-nurses were closely supervised by these well-to-do parents and where they could be assured of the nurses'

---

*From Wickes, I.G. (1953). History of infant feeding—Part I. *Archives of Disease in Childhood, 28,* 232–340. With permission.

integrity. The remaining eighty percent of these infants (nearly 17,000) were subjected to incomprehensible abuses and crimes, including abandonment in foundling hospitals and baby farms. Abandonment of infants in alleys and sewers became so common that there was hardly any notice taken of such incidents. Sometimes these infants were found and mutilated by beggars who wished to gain sympathy by providing the illusion that they had these pitiful infants and children who needed care (Davidson, 1953).

In the Dublin Foundling Hospital between 1775 and 1796, the mortality was 99.6 percent, and the most often cause of death recorded in the hospital ledger was "death from want of breast milk." Interestingly, during the seige of Paris (1870–1871) the total population death rate doubled while the infant rate actually decreased. It is speculated that when mothers could not obtain artificial food or wet nurses they were forced to breastfeed, and the infant mortality rate declined (Davidson, 1953).

Artificial Feeding

At the close of the eighteenth century, four principal methods of infant feeding existed: (1) breast-feeding by the biological mother, (2) breast-feeding by a wet-nurse, (3) feeding with animal milks, and (4) the use of pap and panada. Pap was a mixture of flour or bread cooked in water. Panada was a mixture of flour, cereal, or bread cooked in broth that was usually combined with butter or sometimes animal milk (Davidson, 1953). Other substances reportedly used included biscuits, rice, and barley as the starch base and beer or wine as the added liquid (Phillips, 1976). These were the forerunners of the early cereal feeding.

The paps and panada did not contain enough calories for the babies and were thinned so they could be taken by infants. The quantity of the feeding in a twenty-four-hour period might, therefore, be 1½–2 quarts. This resulted in terrible bloating and the development of diarrhea or "the watery gripes."

Cow's milk frequently came from animals kept in crowded, underground hovels where animal fodder and excreta were most likely not kept separate and where ventilation was practically nonexistent. Needless to say, disease was rampant and the milk yield was poor. Frequently, water, which was contaminated due to lack of sanitation, and chalk were added to this already poor-quality milk to increase the yield. This was fed to newborn infants. Infants who didn't die from malnutrition probably died of gastroenteritis of various causes.

The industrial revolution also affected this situation.

Women moved from the country to the city and worked twelve to sixteen hours per day in the factories to maintain a substandard level of existence. These women, who could not afford wet-nurses, had little choice but artificial feeding or baby farms. Obviously infant mortality in this group was extremely high.

Modern Scientific Technology

The evolution of "modern" artificial feeding methods began in 1835 when Newton produced the first dehydrated milk. In 1847, Grimsdale patented evaporated milk, and in 1866, Nestle's produced the first condensed milk in "tin boxes." Parallel to these developments in processing and storing milk were developments in prepared infant foods. In 1883 there were twenty-seven brands of infant foods with bases of wheat, barley, or potato flour. At that time, there was inadequate knowledge of vitamins; thus, none were added to infant foods or processed milk, creating the marked increase in the incidence of scurvy and rickets.

Philippe Bieslert (1847–1916) analyzed the composition of human and cow's milk and discovered that cow's milk casein is less digestible for human infants than human milk whey. Due to this amazing discovery, he suggested that graduated mixtures of cow's cream, water, and milk sugar be used in artificial feeding (Davidson, 1953).

Pierre Budin (1846–1907), a French obstetrician, began the first infant-welfare center before the turn of the century. Regular attendants were employed, infants were weighed, and infant nutrition was studied. Through trial and error, Budin arrived at accurate food requirements for infants and laid the foundation for modern infant-feeding practices. He emphasized breastfeeding and employed wet-nurses for the preterm infants who stayed at the center. If breast milk was unavailable he, as a student of Pasteur, supplied sterile undiluted cow's milk in individually sealed bottles. He disagreed with the commonly held assumption that heat totally destroyed properties in the milk (Jelliffe, 1968; Wickes, 1953c).

Even fanatical breast-feeding proponents, such as Fredrick Truby King of New Zealand, who developed the slogan "breast-fed is best fed," were caught in the extensiveness of problems created by overfeeding with artificial preparations (Wickes, 1953e). He, like others, assumed the breast-fed infant could also be overfed. Thus, rigid every-four-hour feeding schedules evolved for breast-fed infants. These schedules provided too little sucking time and too few feedings, and resulted in lack of stimulation of an adequate milk supply. It is ironic that these avid physician proponents of breast-feeding created situations for mothers in which following the physicians' directions doomed them to almost certain failure.

Clearly, the infant feeding controversy is an old one. The primary choice of infant-feeding method seems to cycle from natural to artificial and back again.

THE CURRENT CONTROVERSY: BREAST VERSUS BOTTLE

This controversy is fraught with bias and prejudices. Many busy male physicians have neither the patience nor the knowledge of how to support women attempting to breast-feed for the first time. Their emersion in science and technology gives them the perspective that technology is best, besides which, they know how to help with feeding problems if the baby is bottle-fed; there are so many unknowns in breast-feeding. Many nurses also put their faith in modern technology and medicine. In addition, helping with bottle-feeding requires considerably less time from busy nurses—it's easier.

On the other hand, those who are pro breast-feeding are often fanatical in their commitment and have little tolerance for professionals or mothers who bottle-feed. I must confess that I am a breast-feeding advocate. In spite of cracked and bleeding nipples with my first baby, I was a breast-feeding fanatic. However, after the second baby, which was physically a much better experience, I was able to identify the emotional strain of early breast-feeding. Professionals rarely prepare new mothers for the limited mother-specific responses a newborn provides. No one discusses the strain of being up much of the night and feeling as though the baby views its mother only as a giant breast. Because of these feelings, I understand for the first time, why women choose to bottle-feed and why many mothers give up breast-feeding soon after leaving the hospital.

Although I remain a strong proponent of breast-feeding, I now know that how mothers feel about their babies and how they interact with them is more important than how they feed them. The responsibility of professionals is to facilitate a loving, happy, communicative relationship between parents and infants. A mother who is firm in her decision to bottle-feed and understands how and why she reached that decision needs support from the nurse.

At the same time, mothers who are uncertain about a feeding choice need accurate information to make a decision. Scientific data are now available to substantiate that "breast is best." Bottle-feeding is not "just as good." It is only a reasonable alternative when there are good psychological or physiological reasons for not breast-feeding. There are numerous situations, such as among poor women in third-world countries, where bottle-feeding is not even a safe alternative.

Reasons for Artificial Feeding

There are many reasons artificial feeding is selected by mothers. Many of these reasons are legitimate and appropriate; some are questionable.

The second half of the nineteenth century had a grave impact on women. The major function of middle- and upper-class women was to look beautiful, procreate male heirs, and provide status for upwardly mobile husbands. This type of existence encouraged them to relinquish responsibility and control of their lives to men, including fathers, husbands, and physicians. Because of these influences, women allowed "the scientific method," as exemplified by physician mandates, to influence childrearing. Male physicians told women, who had shouldered this responsibility for thousands of years, how to rear infants and children. Many women had so little self-confidence that they listened. When physicians decided that "hand-fed" infants were overfed (which they were) and that every-four-hour feeding schedules should be instituted, they applied the same schedule to breast-fed infants. Their science was not advanced enough to analyze all the differences between breast milk and animal milks. Because of the fat content of human milk, this kind of schedule doomed breast-feeding mothers to failure, forcing babies to go hungry due to inadequate stimulation of milk production. Thus, new mothers would say, "I tried to breast-feed, but I didn't have enough milk." If a mother bottle-fed, she knew, in the scientific fashion, the exact quantity of milk her baby consumed and could thus be reassured that the infant did not cry from hunger. This is one reason Niles Newton (1971) describes the initiation of bottle-feeding as the least stressful to new mothers. This is because we scientific professionals have shattered women's confidence in their childrearing ability. These are certainly questionable reasons at best for selecting artificial feeding.

Bottle-feeding is much more expedant for professionals. It requires less time to teach and less problem solving. A nurse frequently spends thirty to sixty minutes with a breast-feeding mother. Bottle-feeding teaching is considerably shorter, and formula preparation classes are usually held in groups. There is not nearly the amount of ongoing consultation with the bottle-feeding mother as there is with the breast-feeding mother. Frequently, when nursing mothers call physicians or nurses for help with feeding problems, the professional advice is to give up breast-feeding rather than to support, encourage, and problem solve (Clausen et al., 1973).

There seems to be a phenomenon in Western culture that has identified the breast as a sexual symbol, the exclusive property of the husband (Bentovim, 1976; Gunther, 1976; Pryor, 1973). Because the breast is viewed as a genital or reproductive organ and "nice" women don't show their genitals in public, many women feel they could never nurse a baby in public. Breast-feeding isn't an advisable option for these women.

Partly because there is so much emphasis placed on "successful" mothering, partly because women are prone to deny maternal instincts or mothering suggestions from other women in deference to scientific-technological advice, and partly because women living in their isolated suburban houses lack the self-confidence in their own caretaking skills, support for their feeding decisions from their husbands, mothers, and friends is very important. Therefore, a woman who decides to breast-feed when her husband, family, and friends are not supportive of breast-feeding is not acknowledging reality. She will feel better about herself as a successful mother and caretaker if she bottle-feeds.

Some women do not wish to be "tied down" to a baby. They wish to resume activities that they believe require leaving an infant at home. They will probably be much more comfortable, will feel better about themselves, and better about their babies if they bottle-feed. Many working mothers see no options other than bottle-feeding. Some women see the bottle as a symbol of emancipation from old stereotypical female roles, while others are likely to put a breast-fed baby in a pouch tied to their chest and attend an ERA rally or provide two days of professional consultation in a distant city.

There are some women, probably less than one percent, who are physically unable to breast-feed. This may be due to severely inverted nipples, a true insufficient milk supply, or stress. Hytten (1976) discusses nipple changes in pregnancy and the important modification to the connective tissue anchorages of the nipple sufficient to allow for nipple mobility. The anchor substance absorbs water and becomes softer, thus the connective tissue becomes more elastic. This is true of pelvic joints and the cervix as well as the nipples. Because these nipple changes are cumulative, a woman has fewer problems with each successive breast-feeding experience. This mobility is crucial to successful breast-feeding because the infant must be able to suck the nipple into the back of his or her mouth. Although most women spontaneously undergo a positive change in nipple protraction during pregnancy, some can benefit from antepartum exercises, which will be discussed below. A few women are not able to overcome the problems of inverted nipples.

Hytten (1976) also discusses a small group of women who have little or no glandular component to the breast. For these women, the breast seems to be made up of fat, fibrous tissue, and dilated ducts. The amount of functional tissue has no correlation to the size of the breast. Sufficient glandular tissue to allow adequate lactation is genetically transmitted and would not be eliminated in one generation of artificial feeding.

Stress is an important factor due to the psychological influences on the "let-down" reflex. An example of mild temporary stress would be an argument with someone important to the mother. A severe stress could be lack of support for breast-feeding by husband or family, and the subsequent sabotage of the new mother's confidence in her abilities. A specific case of severe stress is a patient whose husband was killed in a plane crash about ten days after the birth of her child: her milk supply simply disappeared.

There are certain maternal disease processes that may preclude breast-feeding, such as active tuberculosis or organ transplants. There are also many medications that, when taken by the mother, are excreted in breast milk and to which babies should not be exposed. Diuretics, cortosone, anticoagulants, and radioactive preparations are some examples.

Anatomical and physiological factors that mandate bottle-feeding probably occur in less than one percent of the population. Therefore, the majority of factors influencing a mother to bottle-feed are still psycho-sociocultural factors.

Reasons for Breast-Feeding

Data from the National Center for Health Statistics (Hendershot, 1980; Hirshman & Hendershot, 1979) indicate that the number of breast-fed infants is increasing. From 1973 to 1975, the number of women with high school education or less who chose to breast-feed increased from 19.2 to 28.2 percent; for women with more than twelve years of education, the increase was from 42.2 to 51.9 percent. It seems as though these figures continue to increase.

There are many psychosocial factors that are beneficial to infants and influence mothers to breast-feed.

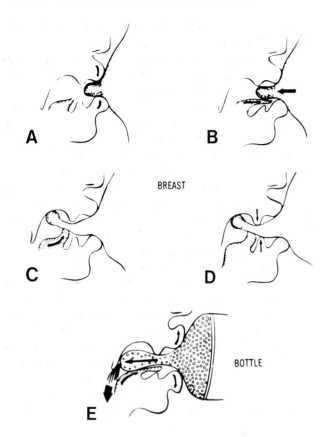

BREAST

BOTTLE

FIGURE 17-1 Oral mechanisms for breast- and bottle-feeding. (A) Notice how the lips clamp a "C" shape in the nipple-areolar concave junction, fitting like a glove. The cheek muscles contract. (B) The tongue thrusts forward to grasp the nipple and areola. (C) The nipple moves against the hard palate, as the tongue whips backward, bringing the areola into the mouth. *Negative* pressure is created by the tongue and cheeks against the nipple. A suction effect results. (D) The gums compress the areola, squeezing milk into the back of the throat where suction occurs against the nipple. Milk flows against the hard palate from the high-pressure system to the negative pressure at the back of the throat. (E) The large rubber nipple strikes the soft palate (with gagging) and displaces proper tongue action. The tongue moves forward with an "anterior tongue thrust" against the gums to control milk overflow into the esophagus. The lips flange an "O" shape. Compression does not occur. The cheek muscles relax. (From Applebaum, R. (1975). The obstetrician's approach to the breasts and breast feeding. *The Journal of Reproductive Medicine, 14*(3), 110. With permission.)

However, there are even more physiological benefits to infants. These can be summarized in such old sayings as "human milk is best for human infants and cow's milk is best for calves." There are many biochemical factors pertinent to breast-feeding, as well as nutritional, immune, and nonallergenic factors. These will be discussed in some detail later.

Physiological Benefits

Breast-feeding is beneficial to tooth and jaw development in the infant. Until let-down occurs, the nursing infant uses up to sixty times as much energy to obtain food as does the bottle-fed infant. To accomplish this work, the newborn's jaw muscles are, relative to those of adults, three times as strong. Well-formed jaws and straight, healthy teeth are encouraged by the extensive sucking exercise. Many fewer breast-fed babies than bottle-fed babies have "tongue thrust," an abnormal swallowing pattern that can lead to speech problems and dental malformations such as malocclusions or protruding front teeth. The bottle-fed infant needs to suck only lightly because milk flows so freely from rubber nipples. The infant actually pushes his tongue forward against the nipple to decrease the milk flow and prevent choking. On the other hand, the breast-fed infant moves his jaw back and forth to start the flow of milk; he pushes his tongue upward against the palate to hold the nipple in his mouth and then sucks the milk down his throat (Applebaum, 1975; Eiger & Olds, 1972; Pryor, 1973) (Figure 17–1).

There are many benefits in breast-feeding for the mother. The first benefit relates to the mother's health. Breast-feeding mothers experience involution of the uterus more rapidly, due partially to the release of oxytocin during nursing. Most nursing mothers experience uterine contractions while nursing their infants, as will be discussed in the section on Anatomy and Physiology of Lactation.

Economic Factors

The economical benefits of breast-feeding are frequently cited in the literature. It is generally accepted that pregnant women lay down 3.5–4.0 kg of fat, primarily in the area of hips, thighs, and abdomen to prepare the human body for lactation (Jelliffe, 1976; McKigney, 1971; Widdowson, 1976). Therefore, the nutritional requirement estimates of 1000 cal/day over the nonpregnant requirement, which were used as guidelines in the 1960s, are now thought excessive. The actual requirement is closer to 600 cal/day (Table 17-1).

Obviously, these estimates are general and do not reflect differences between women. However, discrepancies of as much as 400 cal/day make a significant difference in computing economic comparisons between the costs of breast-feeding and artificial feeding. McKigney (1971), in comparing costs of breast-feeding and artificial feeding in the Washington, D.C. area, found the costs to be about equal at the lowest cost level (the basic cheapest foods for breast-feeding women and the evaporated milk–sugar–ascorbic acid tablet regimen for artificially fed infants). At the "liberal" level

TABLE 17-1 Dietary recommendations for lactating women and their importance

Daily Dietary Requirements	Importance
2500–2600 cal	For energy production. Weight reduction is not recommended. If caloric intake is reduced, maternal body fat is mobilized and quantity of breast milk is reduced.
66 g protein	If restricted, there is no effect.
1200 mg calcium	If restricted, there is a depletion of maternal bone and teeth.
1200 mg phosphorus	Unknown.
450 mg magnesium	Unknown.
6000 IU vitamin A 400 IU vitamin D 15 IU vitamin E	Administration of these fat-soluble vitamins does not alter their amounts in breast milk.
1.4 mg vitamin B_1 1.9 mg vitamin B_2 2.5 mg vitamin B_6 0.4 mg vitamin B_{12} 18.0 mg niacin	Level of intake is directly related to level in breast milk.

Courtesy of Ede Burger, R.N., M.S., Loma Linda University.

for both lactation-supporting maternal nutrition and bottle-feeding formulas, the artificial feeding methods were nearly one and a half times more expensive than breast-feeding. With the addition of any prepared baby foods, the cost increases.

Jelliffe and Jelliffe (1977) report that in developing nations, adequate amounts of formula to artificially feed infants would require the expenditure of twenty to fifty percent of their families' entire income. In developed countries, artificial feeding is two to three times as expensive as breast-feeding.

The Recommended Dietary Allowances, upon which all these computations are based, are not minimum requirements but, instead, exceed the daily requirements of most individuals so that the needs of all can be met. It is also pertinent to note that the dietary allowances for infants are estimated on the intakes of breast-fed babies with an additional safety factor to allow for differences in the complex biochemical interactions of each between prepared formulas and breast milk. In the end analysis, it appears that breast-feeding is less expensive than artificial-feeding methods.

Emotional Factors

There is a substantial emotional aspect to breast-feeding. A closeness exists between mother and infant that is difficult to imagine with bottle-feeding. There is a giving of oneself in providing nourishment. A mutual stroking and touching occurs between mother and infant as the mother holds a bare baby foot or strokes a leg while the infant suckles, touches the breast, holds his mother's fingers, or reaches for her mouth as he stares into her eyes and then smiles as he lets go of the nipple for the briefest of moments. N. Newton (1971) reports that significantly more breast-feeding mothers slept or rested in bed with their babies than did bottle-feeding mothers. Significantly more mothers who were greatly pleased at the first sight of their babies wanted to breast-feed, as compared to mothers who were indifferent or disgusted in the delivery room. Bottle-feeding was significantly correlated with mother-centered reasons for feeding choice, while breast-feeding mothers gave infant-welfare-centered reasons for feeding choice.

Sosa et al. (1976) discovered that mothers in Guatemala City breast-fed nearly twice as long if they had contact with their infants in the first twelve hours of life, compared with mothers who had no infant contact for the first twelve hours. These data do not preclude strong emotional ties between mothers and their bottle-fed infants, they only indicate these behaviors are less likely in the bottle-feeding "couple." It is very easy to prop a bottle when a mother is busy, and soon the infant assuages his own discomforts and fears through an inanimate object—the bottle.

Unrestricted Breast-Feeding There can be great emotional gratification for the infant in breast-feeding. In what Niles Newton (1971) calls *unrestricted breast-feeding,* which has no rules restricting suckling, the breast is given whenever the infant cries or fusses. In this way, the breast is associated with comfort as much as it is associated with food, and the infant has mouth-nipple contact *and* body contact with her mother to assuage all types of discomforts and fears. Unrestricted breast-feeding has traditionally occurred in preindustrial and preliterate cultures. For the first weeks after birth, this usually means as many as ten or more feedings each day with nursing as frequently as every two hours.

Token Breast-Feeding In contrast, *token breast-feeding* is characterized by "rules restricting the number of feedings, and the amount of mother-baby contact that stimulates the urge to suck" (N. Newton, 1971, p. 994). The infant and mother frequently sleep in separate rooms, and sleeping with the mother is considered dangerous. The infant learns bottle-sucking techniques and frequently has supplemental artificial feedings of water, glucose, formula, and semisolid foods. These infants are usually totally weaned in a few weeks. Token breast-feeding mothers tend to hold infants only for feedings, and thus the infant doesn't receive the same emotional gratification of her discomforts and fears.

Convenience: The Double-Edged Sword

Convenience of breast-feeding is stressed by all breast-feeding authors (Thompson, 1971). No bottles or formulas have to be carried on trips and outings; no formula needs preparation; and no refrigeration is needed to prevent spoilage of formula. Bottles do not have to be heated in the middle of the night while the baby screams. On the other hand, convenience is a double-edged sword. If mother is working or has other commitments that take her away from the infant for more than two hours, she must make extensive plans, which may include hand expression of breast milk so that the infant will have a feeding while she is out, as well as arranging to express while she is away so that she doesn't leak into her clothes. In addition, there is the psychological worry: Did she leave enough milk? Is the baby hungry? Does the infant need suckling for comfort? If the mother takes the infant with her, she faces the possibility of negative comments and inuendoes because she dares to flaunt tradition and the current cultural norm by feeding her baby "in public."

Is breast-feeding a convenience? It depends on the priorities of the individual mother.

Other Factors

If a mother or father are aesthetically inclined, one of the benefits of breast-feeding is the mild odor of stools and regurgitated breast milk. As long as the infant is fed only breast milk, inoffensive odor remains. The situation changes markedly as soon as other foods or formula are introduced.

A definite advantage of breast-feeding is the decreased likelihood of overfeeding the infant. Breast-fed babies stop suckling or fall asleep when they are full. There is no temptation to persuade the infant to "finish the bottle," because the mother is not certain how much he has consumed. There has been considerable controversy about obesity as an infant leading to obesity as an adult. Thus, the recommendation has been made that solids not be introduced before the infant is 5 to 6 months old and has more control over the amount of food he takes in (Fomon et al., 1979).

However, the total decision-making process of breast-feeding versus bottle-feeding rests with the values of the mother. Guthrie and Kan (1977) have found that many women develop strong convictions about an early feeding method several years prior to planning a pregnancy or conception. Hospital personnel seem to function primarily in a supportive role for the decision already made by the mother. If the mother is undecided at delivery, then the attitudes of those close to her become influential. The timing, length, and quality of her first contacts with the infant can also be very influential. Because of the importance of early influence on decision making, Guthrie and Kan (1977) recommend widespread adolescent educational programs about infant feeding, which should also include boys, since as husbands and fathers they will become extremely important in supporting the woman's decision.

For all women, it is most important that they make an educated infant-feeding decision, with full awareness of the latest infant-feeding research. The breast *is* best, but for some women, the bottle is better. Women must understand *why* they make the decision they do, and feel good about that decision.

ANATOMY AND PHYSIOLOGY OF LACTATION

The anatomical development and the physiological functioning of the mammary gland is an intricate and delicately balanced process. The progressive development of the gland from the nonpregnant state to full lactation is illustrated in Figure 17-2. In pregnancy, the glandular growth and development are thought to be

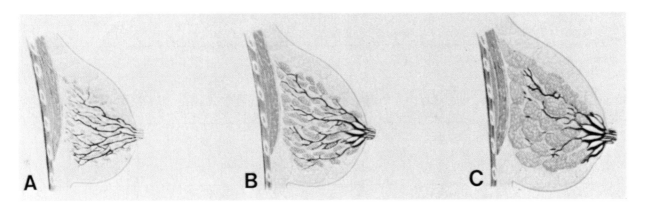

FIGURE 17-2   Mammary glands. (A) Nonpregnant. (B) During pregnancy. (C) During lactation. (Courtesy of Ross Laboratories, Columbus, Ohio.)

the result of the progressively higher levels of human placental lactogen (HPL), as well as to increasing levels of prolactin (Figure 17-3). There is abundant evidence on postmenopausal women, nonpregnant women, and even men that milk production can be stimulated by the prolactin release achieved from sucking alone (Hytten, 1976). Obviously, this group has no HPL. There are numerous cases of lactation being initiated by adoptive mothers with such devices as a Lact-Aid.*

One can see in Figure 17-4 that the epithelial or milk-secreting alveolar cells discharge their product into the lumen of the alveoli. The aveolar cells are surrounded by myoepithelial cells, which contract and express the milk into the capillary milk ducts. From the milk duct, other muscle cells in the duct lining contract to force the milk into the intralobar ducts and on to the sinuses (Catz & Giocoia, 1972; Speroff et al., 1978).

In milk production, there are two distinct processes functioning: the manufacture of milk in the alveolus, which is controlled by prolactin, and the delivery of milk to the sinuses by the neurohormonal reflex involving oxytocin. In the actual manufacture of milk at the intracellular level (Figure 17-5), the milk proteins are assembled in the ribosomes of the endoplasmic reticulum. Glycoproteins are formed after the carbohydrate compliment is added, which occurs when the milk protein is transferred to the Golgi apparatus (Catz & Giocoia, 1972). The glycoproteins are contained in transfer vesicles until they reach the apical membrane of the alveolar cell and empty their contents into the lumen. Lactose, the predominant carbohydrate, is syn-

thesized in the Golgi apparatus by the enzyme lactose synthetose. Fat is present as a membrane-wrapped droplet. Upon reaching the apex of the cell, the droplet becomes completely surrounded by cellular membrane and is then "pinched off," sliding into the lumen. This is not the mechanism for excretion of drugs into the milk. Other mechanisms are probably in operation, including active transport, passive diffusion, or attachment to protein-containing vesicles (Catz & Giocoia, 1972).

The neurohormonal reflex is illustrated in Figure 17-6. Optimum quantity and quality of milk are dependent on the appropriate functioning of the pituitary, thyroid, pancreas, adrenals, and the ovaries and placenta. Although all the hormones necessary for milk production are present during pregnancy, only colostrum, which is formed by desquamated epithelium and transudate, is produced prior to delivery. Lactation is thought to be prevented at the sight of production in the alveoli by the presence of estrogen, which stimulates the increase in prolactin production while inhibiting its effects (see Figure 17-3). The rapid decrease in estrogen after delivery stops the inhibiting effect on prolactin. Sucking elicits transitory rises in prolactin levels, and milk is produced. This was the basis for administering estrogen to suppress lactation, but in actuality, its effect was to simulate continued pregnancy (Hytten, 1976). Consequently, lactation was merely delayed until after the patient went home, and the chances of complaining to the obstetrician about engorgement were decreased.

It appears that sucking suppresses the formation of prolactin-inhibiting factor (PIF). During pregnancy, PIF suppresses secretion of prolactin into the cardiovascular system. When PIF is not present, prolactin is secreted. Therefore, sucking effects lactation in two ways: it causes the breast to eject or "let-down" milk, and it stimulates the replacement of milk by prolactin

---

*The Lact-Aid Nursing Supplementer delivers supplemental liquid food to the infant while nursing. This helps provide needed stimulation for inducing or enhancing lactation. For further information write to Lact-Aid, Box 6861, Denver, CO 80206.

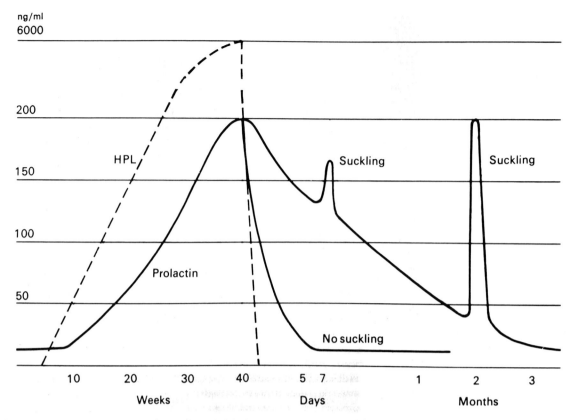

FIGURE 17-3 Pregnancy and milk secretion. Weeks: weeks of pregnancy; days: days postpartum; months: months postpartum; HPL: human placental lactogen. (From Speroff, L., Glass, R.H., & Kase, N.G. (1978). *Clinical gynecologic endocrinology and infertility*. Copyright 1978, The Williams & Wilkins Co., Baltimore. With permission.)

production. It appears that prolactin production is also influenced by the prolactin-releasing factor (PRF). This process is not yet well understood, but the releasing factor seems to suppress the prolactin-inhibiting factor (Catz & Giocoia, 1972; Speroff et al., 1978).

The infant does not obtain milk from the breast, because his sucking produces a negative pressure. Instead, the sucking stimulates tactile sensors in the areola that actuate an afferent sensory neural arc, which stimulates the hypothalamus to synthesize oxytocin, transport it to the posterior pituitary, and then out of the posterior pituitary. The efferent arc includes the oxytocin traveling through the circulatory system to the myoepithelial cells surrounding the alveolar glands. Upon reaching the myoepithelial cells, the oxytocin stimulates the cells to contract, ejecting milk into the ducts and lactiferous sinuses beneath the areola (Speroff et al., 1978). This is called *milk let-down*. The stretching of the ducts causes a tingling sensation in the breast.

The ejection reflex can also be conditioned. Some women experience let-down when they think about their infant or when they hear other infants cry.

Epinephrine inhibits oxytocin release. Such feelings as pain and anxiety, which stimulate epinephrine, are powerful inhibitors and can seriously disrupt milk ejection and thereafter breast-feeding (Hytten, 1976).

When suckling stops, lactation is gradually terminated. Milk let-down reflex is lost as the afferent sensory neural arc and the efferent arc are no longer stimulated and oxytocin is not released. With milk accumulating in the alveoli and no sucking occurring, the engorged alveoli depress milk formation. PIF production resumes and inhibits prolactin production. In mothers who nurse their infants fewer than four times a day, prolactin does not seem to be a factor because it has returned to prepregnant levels. Delvoye et al. (1977) found that the serum prolactin level does not decline significantly in mothers who nurse their infants more than six times a day. Within a week of no suckling, lactation has largely ceased. However, many women can still express a few drops of milk even months later.

Weaning is best done gradually by decreasing one feeding every few days. It is least traumatic both for mother and infant. Many mothers like to wean from the

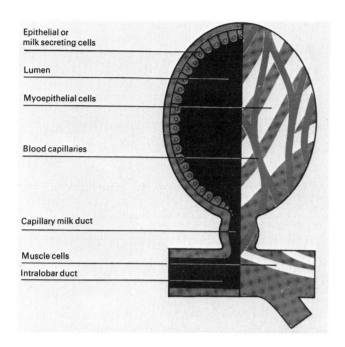

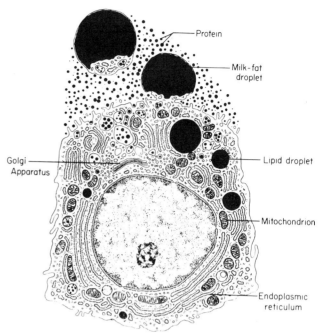

FIGURE 17-4 Cross section of the milk gland, showing the interior of the gland and the criss-crossing mantle of contractile myoepithelial strands, the capillary milk duct, and the intralobular collecting duct. (From Speroff, L., Glass, R.H., & Kase, N.G. (1978). *Clinical gynecologic endocrinology and infertility.* Copyright 1978, The Williams & Wilkins Co., Baltimore. With permission.)

FIGURE 17-5 Alveolar cells of the mammary gland and the synthesis of milk. (From Catz, C., & Giacoia, G. (1972). Drugs and breast milk. *Pediatric Clinics of North America, 19* (1), 152. With permission.)

breast straight to the cup. This can usually be done when the infant is between 9 and 12 months old. Until recently, there have been negative comments about infants nursing much longer than twelve months. However, in many primitive societies, infants nurse two years and some as long as four or five years. It is important that the mother and the child feel good about the decision to wean and that the issue does not turn into a battle.

NUTRITIONAL AND BIOCHEMICAL CONSIDERATIONS

The recommended daily nutritional allowances for infants are not minimum requirements. They compensate for individual variation in activity, sex, body size, genetic makeup, and environment by exceeding the minimal needs of most infants (Alfin-Slater & Jelliffe, 1977). In addition, these requirements are based on breast-feeding even though various nutrients vary significantly from mother to mother, from feeding to feeding, and even within feeds.

Water content should be 175.5 ml/kg body weight

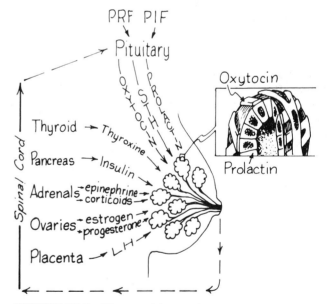

FIGURE 17-6 Hormonal interactions contributing to lactogenesis. The insert illustrates the alveolar and myoepithelial cells and their specific response to oxytocin and prolactin. PRF, prolactin-releasing factor; PIF, prolactin-inhibiting factor; LH, luteinizing hormone; STH, somatotropic (growth) hormone. (From Catz, C., & Giacoia, G. (1972). Drugs and breast milk. *Pediatric Clinics of North America, 19* (1), 153. With permission.)

TABLE 17-2 Energy and nutrient content of 100 ml of average human milk (colostrum, transition, and mature) versus 100 ml of bovine milk

	Energy (kcal)	Protein (g)	Fat (g)	Carbohydrate (g)	Vitamin A (g)	Vitamin C (mg)	Vitamin D (IU)
Human milk							
Colostrum	57	—	—	—	151	5.9	—
Transition	63	—	—	—	88	7.1	—
Mature	65	0.9	3.8	7.0	75	5.0	5.0
Bovine milk	67	3.4	3.7	4.8	41	1.1	2.5

	Na (mg)	K (mg)	Cl (mg)	Mg (mg)	P (mg)	Fe (μg)	Cu (μg)	Ca (mg)
Human milk								
Colostrum	48	74	85	4	14	70	40	39
Transition	29	64	46	4	20	70	50	46
Mature	15	57	40	4	15	100	40	35
Bovine milk	58	145	108	12	120	70	14	130

Data from Lawrence (1980).

from birth to 6 months. When considering special formulas, it is important to calculate solute load, since high-solute formulas place infants at risk for such problems as hypernatremia. The caloric intake for infants up to 6 months should be 117 kcal/kg body weight. It decreases to 108 kcal/kg body weight for the second half of the first year. Standard formulas of 20 kcal/oz meet this requirement. The calories should be supplied in a ratio of thirty to fifty-five percent fat, thirty-five to sixty-five percent carbohydrate, and seven to sixteen percent protein. Breast milk provides approximately fifty-five percent fat, thirty-eight percent carbohydrate, and seven percent protein (Alfin-Slater & Jelliffe, 1977).

Composition of Breast Milk and Formulas

During the previous two generations, it has been conveyed to parents that human milk and cow's-milk-based formulas are basically biochemically and nutritionally alike. Recently, however, infant-feeding experts have begun to inform the public that the constitutents of human milk and cow's milk are dissimilar in nearly every respect except water content and lactose (Jelliffe & Jelliffe, 1977) (Table 17-2). Analysis shows the protein composition, as well as the casein systems, of the two milks to be different. The cholesterol levels

and the fatty acid spectrums of lipids appear to be species-specific and very different for humans and cows, as well as being somewhat dependent on maternal diet. Breast milk has higher taurine and cystine levels and lower tyrosine and phenylalanine levels than cow's milk. An additional complicating factor is the interaction and independent qualities of the various milks. There are at least 157 known elements in human milk (Applebaum, 1975), all of which are balanced to effectively compliment one another and to facilitate maximum efficient utilization of each element.

The first marketed milks were dried or evaporated cow's milk. These were diluted with boiled water, and sucrose was added to ensure the energy value of the preparation. Next, vitamins A, C, and D were added to formulas. Then iron was added to protect against anemia. Currently, milk is skimmed and the butter fat is replaced with vegetable oils (Darke, 1976). With each biochemical or nutritional discovery about breast milk, formula makers attempt additional formula modifications—and appropriately so—for the benefit of babies who must be nourished with formula. However, it is important to recognize the vast difference between current cow's-milk-based formulas and actual cow's milk. Additive substances in formulas include emulsifiers, thickening agents, pH adjusters, and antioxidants. Various formulas have altered the cow's milk base by such techniques as electrodialyzing whey; defatting cow's milk and replacing it with oils such as coconut, soy, corn, or safflower; and adding lactose, vitamins, and minerals (Jelliffe & Jelliffe, 1977). By adjusting the amounts of the various oils, manufacturers have attempted to replicate the fatty acids of human milk. They are successful in duplicating the amount of fatty acids but find it much more difficult, if even possible, to achieve the same fatty acid pattern found in human milk, let alone to achieve the changing fat composition as it occurs throughout a feed (Darke, 1976).

There are numerous examples of biochemical and nutritional differences between cow's milk and human milk. (Continue referring to Table 17-2.) The amino acid patterns in cow's milk and human milk protein are not the same, so any reduction in cow's milk protein (3.3 g/100 ml) to more closely resemble human milk protein (1.2 g/100 ml) must be carefully controlled to assure the presence of all essential amino acids. As an example, the enzyme cystathionase is absent in the liver of the fetus and premature infant, and therefore the newborn cannot convert the amino acid methionine to cysteine. There is two to five times more methionine in cow's milk than in breast milk, which has more cysteine (Gyorgy, 1971).

Fatty Acids

Studies on newborn rats have shown that a diet too low in fat intake affects cerebral function, causing poorer memory traces; the rats had difficulty remembering their way through a maze. Research has shown that monoglycerides with the fatty acid in the 2-position (breast milk has palmitic acid in the 2-position) is absorbed by the newborn as it is. In cow's milk, palmitic acid is most likely to be found in the 1- or 3-position. In cow's milk, lipase interacts with palmitic acid in the 1-or 3-position and frees it from the monoglyceride. Free palmitic acid precipitates with calcium in the intestine and is excreted as calcium-palmitate soap. Breast-fed infants absorb almost all fat in human milk, while only two-thirds of the fat in cow's milk is absorbed, leading to loss of fat and calcium (Gyorgy, 1971). Some claim that the differences in the fatty acid pattern of human and cow's milk may be important, as these lipids are utilized in the development of the central nervous system and the myelinization of the brain (Darke, 1976; Gyorgy, 1971).

Iron

Iron sufficiency in infant nutrition has been a controversial issue. Term infants have iron stores from intra-uterine life that will maintain them until their birth weight is doubled. After that time, dietary iron must be adequate or the infant can develop a hypochromic, microcytic anemia. Iron in breast milk is attached to a protein called lactoferrin. This carrier-protein facilitates absorption of virtually all the iron in human milk, and also prevents pathogenic organisms from using the iron for growth (Rolles, 1976).

Studies by McMillan et al. (1976), indicate that it is possible for infants to remain iron sufficient on a breast-milk diet until they have tripled their birth weight, even if the mothers receive no vitamin or iron supplements. Although both cow's milk and human milk contain approximately the same amount of iron, there is increased iron availability in the human milk for reasons that are not completely understood. McMillan et al. (1976), hypothesized the following possibilities:

- Iron absorption is greater in the presence of lower percentages of animal protein; human milk has a lower percentage of protein.
- Lactose, as compared to other sugars, increases iron absorption; breast milk has more lactose.
- Large amounts of phosphorus decrease iron absorption; cow's milk is high in phosphorus.
- Ascorbate is a catalyst in the absorption of iron; breast milk is much higher in vitamin C than cow's milk.

Evidence is accumulating that indicates the amount of iron in food is much less important than the kinds of foods eaten together. From their work, McMillan and Oskie recommend the following:

1. An infant who is exclusively breast fed during the first six months of life requires no supplemental source of iron.
2. Infants who are exclusively breast fed for periods up to one year of age probably do not require a supplemental source of iron.
3. When solid foods are introduced into the diet after six months of age an effort should be made to select foods that are a good source of iron. The best sources are iron enriched cereals and meats.
4. When breast feeding is discontinued prior to a year the infant should receive an iron fortified formula and not whole cow's milk.*

Cholesterol

There are other health promotion factors that may be important indicators for breast-feeding. One of these is cholesterol. Human milk contains six to ten times more

---

*From McMillan, J.A., & Oski, F.A. (1977). Iron nutrition in the breast-fed infant. *Keeping Abreast, Journal of Human Nurturing,* Jan.–March, pp. 33–35. With permission.

cholesterol than formulas prepared with vegetable oil fats. Of course, adult elevated cholesterol levels and coronary artery disease are a concern, and efforts to prevent these adult problems are important, but cholesterol plays an important part in the infant's synthesis of bile acids, steroids, and myelin (Fomon, 1974). In addition, studies by Reiser (Reiser, 1971; Reiser & Sidelman, 1972) suggest that cholesterol levels also play an important role in the development of enzymes that will influence the adult serum cholesterol homeostatis. For example, piglets fed on low cholesterol formula had higher cholesterol levels at 17 months of age than piglets suckled on the high cholesterol natural milk. Epidemiologically, striking increases in coronary artery disease have paralleled the extensive use of artificial low-cholesterol feedings.

In examining the nutritional values of human milk, as shown in Table 17-2, Rolles (1976) believes it to be important to remember the source of the figures: they are an average; it has been known for some time that human milk varies from week to week. It is a dynamic substance that changes literally throughout a given twenty-four-hour period, and even within one feeding. Does this mean that Mother Nature is inefficient? Or could it be that the variation is just what the infant needs? To give a different perspective, Rolles examined the infant feeding of the red kangaroo, which suckles young of three different ages simultaneously with three separate pairs of teats. Each pair of teats produces milk that is specific for the age of the offspring, beginning with a protein-rich colostrumlike substance, then going to a more mature milk, and finally a more dilute milk for the oldest baby kangaroo. Perhaps the lower fat content and increased volume found in human milk produced for the second six months of the infant's life is exactly what the baby needs, as opposed to the 3.3 percent fat in formulas (Rolles, 1976). Perhaps the change in milk composition within a given feeding is a cue for the infant to stop feeding, serving as an appetite control mechanism and preventing obesity (Hall, 1977).

Anti-Infective Properties

The anti-infective, or immune, properties of breast milk are an extremely important aspect of human milk, particularly in areas of this country and the world where good sanitation is marginal or nonexistent. Host resistance factors such as immunoglobulins and the *Lactobacillus bifidus* factor will be discussed in more detail. *L. bifidus* quickly colonizes the intestines of newborns who are breast-fed. Because of the lactic acid produced by the *L. bifidus,* the breast-fed infant's stools have an acidic pH. Artificially fed infants have a neutral

or alkaline pH. The breast-fed infant's acid intestinal environment evidently inhibits the growth of such organisms as *Shigella, Escherichia coli,* and yeast (Mata & Wyat, 1971). In the acidic environment of the large intestine, acetic acid serves as an acetate buffer, exerting a bacteriostatic effect on these gram-negative and putrefactive organisms (Bullen et al., 1977). There is apparently a specific *L. bifidus* growth-promoting factor in human milk that is a nitrogen-containing polysaccharide. This factor is negligible in bovine milk (Goldman & Smith, 1973). Gyorgy (1971) also believes that the bifidus factor may interfere with influenza viruses. Whatever the multiple influences and interactions may be, they vary greatly from infants fed on cow's milk. Bullen et al. (1977) have substantiated that when supplemental formula feedings were given to breast-fed infants during the first seven days of life, the establishment of the strongly acidic environment was delayed. In fact, in comparison to breast-milk-only infants, the potential for a strong acidic intestinal environment never materialized.

Human milk contains all classes of immunoglobulins, although their levels are highest in colostrum. There are five major classes of immunoglobulins: IgG, IgM, IgD, IgE, and IgA. Each class has a specific function, three of which have known importance in breast milk. IgG, which destroys particular viral agents, appears early in the immune response. IgE serum levels are increased in persons who have allergies, thus connecting IgE in some way to allergic disease, although the connection is not yet clearly understood. The IgA class of immunoglobulins has been divided into two types: serus IgA and secretory IgA. While both are antiviral, secretory IgA is the type found in saliva, tears, colostrum, milk, and the various respiratory, genitourinary, and gastrointestinal secretions (Gordon, 1974; Grams, 1978).

Antibodies to organisms such as *Clostridium tetani, Hemophilus pertussis, Dipplococcus pneumoniae, Staphylococcus, Streptococcus, Corynebacterium diphtheriae,* enteropathogenic *E. coli, Salmonella, Shigella,* polio viruses 1, 2, and 3, Coxsackie virus, ECHO viruses 6 and 9, and influenza viruses, are found in breast milk. Table 17-3 describes the host resistance factors in human milk (Goldman & Smith, 1973). This antibody action is thought to take place primarily within the intestinal tract of the newborn. Until the recent research findings on immunoglobulins, it was believed that the infant received all his protection transplacentally, as an infusion of IgG. However, it is now understood that the newborn receives an initial bolus of secretory IgA in colostrum, and subsequently IgG, IgA, and IgM are received in colostrum and milk. Gerrard (1974) reports the findings of an *E. coli*

TABLE 17-3 Host resistance factors in human milk

Components	Proposed Mode of Action
Growth factor of *Lactobacillus bifidus*	*Lactobacillus bifidus* interferes with intestinal colonization of enteric pathogens.
Antistaphylococcal factor	Inhibits staphylococci.
Secretory IgA and other immunoglobulins	Protective antibodies for the gut and respiratory tract.
Complement proteins 3 and 4 (C_3, C_4)	C_3 fragments have opsonic, chemotactic, and anaphylotoxic activities.
Lysozyme	Lysis of bacterial cell wall.
Lactoperoxidase–hydrogen peroxide–thiocyanate	Kills streptococci.
Lactoferrin	Kills microorganisms by chelating iron.
Leukocytes	Phagocytosis; cell-mediated immunity production of IgA, C_4, C_3, lysozyme, and lactoferrin.

From Goldman, A., & Smith, W. (1973). Host resistance factors in human milk. *The Journal of Pediatrics,* *82*(6), 1086. With permission.

TABLE 17-4 Anti-infective properties of breast milk

Factor	Shown In Vitro To Be Active Against	Effect of Heat
Antiviral		
Secretory IgA	Polio types 1, 2, 3; coxsackie virus types A9, B3, B5; Echo types 6, 9; Semliki Forest virus; Ross River virus; rotavirus	Stable at 56°C for 30 min; some loss (0%–30%) at 62.5°C for 30 min; destroyed by boiling
Lipid (unsaturated fatty acids and monoglycerides)	Herpes simplex; Semliki Forest virus; influenza; dengue; Ross River virus; murine leukemia virus; Japanese B encephalitis virus	Stable to boiling for 30 min
Nonimmunoglobulin macromolecules	Herpes simplex; vesicular stomatitis virus	Destroyed at 60°C; stable at 56°C for 30 min; destroyed by boiling for 30 min
Milk cells	Rotavirus	Unknown
	Induced interferon active against Sendai virus; sensitized lymphocytes? phagocytosis?	Destroyed at 62.5°C for 30 min
Antibacterial		
L. bifidus growth factor	Enterobacteriaceae; enteric pathogens	Stable to boiling
Secretory IgA	*Escherichia coli; E. coli* enterotoxin; *Clostridium tetani; Corynebacterium diphtheriae; Dipplococcus pneumoniae; Salmonella; Shigella*	Stable at 56°C for 30 min; some loss (0%–30%) at 62.5°C for 30 min; destroyed by boiling
C_1–C_9	Effect not known	Destroyed by heating at 56°C for 30 min
Lactoferrin	*E. coli; Candida albicans*	Two-thirds destroyed at 62.5°C for 30 min
Lactoperoxidase	*Streptococcus; Pseudomonas; E. coli; Salmonella typhimurium*	Not known; presumably destroyed by boiling
Lysozyme	*E. coli; Salmonella; Micrococcus lysodeikticus*	Stable at 62.5°C for 30 min; activity reduced 97% by boiling for 15 min
Lipid (unsaturated fatty acid)	*Staphylococcus aureus*	Stable to boiling
Milk cells	By phagocytosis: *E. coli, C. albicans;* by sensitized lymphocytes: *E. coli*	Destroyed by 62.5°C for 30 min

From Welsh, J., & May, J. (1979). Anti-infective properties of breast milk. *Journal of Pediatrics,* *94*(1), 3, 5. With permission.

epidemic that occurred in a Belgrade nursery. All the babies who died had received boiled breast milk rather than fresh breast milk, thus indicating that the protective aspect in milk was destroyed by heat. Table 17-4 delineates antiviral and antibacterial factors in breast milk and the effects of heat on these factors (Welsh & May, 1979).

From studies of calves and piglets, it has been discovered that daily injections of immunoglobulins that provide systemic protection are not adequate. Colostrum feeding, followed by four to six weeks of suckling are needed to provide adequate protection. Gerrard (1974) believes that the human infant also requires colostrum plus suckling to be spared gastrointestinal infections. Breast-feeding, which provides infant protection from the maternal antibodies that are transmitted, permits the gradual development of the infant's own immune system. While he is gradually losing maternally derived protection (at about 6 months of age), he is gradually acquiring his own.

There are several epidemiological studies comparing mortality and morbidity rates in breast-fed and bottle-fed infants. Newman in 1906 reported that the frequency of infant diarrheal deaths in Great Britain was six times greater in artificially fed infants than in breast-fed infants. In the 1930s, Grulee et al. studied 20,061 babies in Chicago. Gastrointestinal and respiratory infections, as well as unclassified infections, were significantly higher in infants not given breast milk. Death rates were also significantly higher (Gerrard, 1974). In 1951, Robinson of Great Britain found that mortality and morbidity rates in 3226 children were highest in artificially-fed infants and lowest in breast-fed infants. The breast-fed infants who were supplemented with bottles fell around the mean (Goldman & Smith, 1973). Most recently, from a middle-class patient population at Kaiser Permanente in California, only 1 of 107 infants admitted to the hospital with acute gastroenteritis was breast-fed. The data in this study indicate that breast-feeding plays a major role in protection against intestinal infections even in middle-class communities with excellent sanitation (Larsen & Homer, 1978). The implication is clear: breast-feeding is not *only* for developing nations where sanitation is poor.

Allergy Factors

One of the most frequently discussed rationales for breast-feeding is decreased incidence or avoidance of allergic disorders. The National Institutes of Health estimate approximately thirty-one million persons (fifteen percent of the U.S. population) suffer from allergic

disorders, which are a major source of chronic illness in all age groups (Committee on Nutrition of the Mother and Preschool Child, 1978). The most common food allergen in newborns is β-lactoglobulin, which is a protein found in cow's milk. Large amounts of this allergen are absorbed directly through the newborn intestinal wall while it is still relatively "open" to absorption of foreign protein macromolecules. Breast milk has no allergens and, in addition, provides the protection of the antiabsorptive effect of secretory IgA (Jelliffe & Jelliffe, 1977).

As Rolles (1976) describes, a drop of fresh breast milk examined under the microscope reveals 1500–3000 polymorphs. The polymorphs are alive and active phagocytes. An equivalent number of lymphocytes are present, active and capable of stimulating production of antibodies. In this one drop of breast milk there are almost as many white cells as in the peripheral blood. It is clear that the various biochemical and nutritional components of breast milk make it a very special, valuable, species-specific substance. Until about seventy-five years ago, the survival of the species depended on human milk, and the species has done remarkably well. It is difficult to imagine even the complete duplication of this complex intradependent substance. It is important that work continue to constantly improve artificial feedings, since there will always be a need for them. However, it is just as important to encourage the more than ninety percent of women who could breast-feed to do so.

ANTEPARTUM BREAST PREPARATION

History Taking

A usual question asked during the antepartum history is, "Do you plan to breast or bottle feed?" It would be more appropriate to ask a women what thoughts she has had about infant feeding and what questions she has. It might be helpful to know how she was fed as an infant, how the women she knows have fed their babies, and what her husband thinks about a feeding method. These kinds of questions help in assessing the woman's exposure to breast-feeding, what kind of support she might receive, and whether she has a good chance of success in breast-feeding. It isn't reasonable to encourage breast-feeding if the woman's peer group all bottle-feed and her husband thinks breast-feeding is disgusting. If, in spite of such circumstances, a woman is committed to attempting to breast-feed, the nurse can help her look at building a support system. If she is uncertain, or hasn't thought about infant feeding, the nurse can proceed with an educational program.

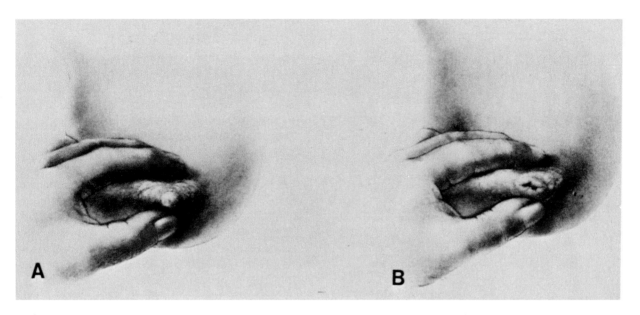

FIGURE 17-7 Nipple examination. (A) The normal nipple when stimulated. (B) The inverted nipple when stimulated. (From Lawrence, R.A. (1980). *Breast-feeding: A guide for the medical profession.* St. Louis: The C. V. Mosby Co., p. 112. With permission.)

Breast Examination

An examination of the breasts is an important part of the prenatal examination not only because it is part of a complete physical examination, but also because it is an integral part of preparation for breast-feeding. The nurse responsible for this education should repeat the examination if it has been done by a physician, so that breast-feeding education can be incorporated.

With the woman in the sitting position, the nurse notes the following:

- *Size and symmetry.* Some assymmetry is common. The amount of mammary tissue is not correlated with milk production. Women with small breasts merely have less fat pad and are quite successful at breast-feeding. These women often enjoy having large breasts during pregnancy and lactation.
- *Breast contour.* Lumps or masses that might need treatment should be looked for.
- *Breast texture.* Texture should be assessed by palpation. The inelastic breast, which is more prone to engorgement, is firmly knit together, and the skin is taut and firm so that it cannot be picked up. The elastic breast is loose and the overlying skin is free and can easily be picked up between the thumb and forefinger. Inelastic breasts appear to be helped by antepartum massage and careful attention to prevention of engorgement postpartum (Lawrence, 1980).

- *The areola and nipple.* Gross malformations and obvious inversion of the nipple should be checked for. In addition, the normal appearing nipple should be stimulated or grasped between thumb and forefinger to be certain it everts. Occasionally nipples that appear normal will invert or retract when gentle pressure is applied (Figure 17-7). Neither inverted nor flat nipples preclude breast-feeding, but it is essential that antepartum preparation be done.

Breast Preparation

Antepartum preparation consists of nipple preparation and breast massage. Nipple preparation includes nipple exercise and the use of breast shields. As shown in Figure 17-8, the nipple is gently pulled outward between thumb and forefinger, while the breast is supported, until there is discomfort, then it is released. This exercise is done five or six times several times a day. Other exercises include Hoffman's exercise (Applebaum, 1975) and nipple rolling, which is similar to the exercise described above except that the nipple is rolled between finger and thumb in an effort to break up adhesions. Inverted nipples respond best to the use of a shield. These plastic cups with a large hole on the breast side fit inside a brassiere. The most common ones are Woolrich or Eschmann Shields and can be found in most drugstores or ordered through the La Leche

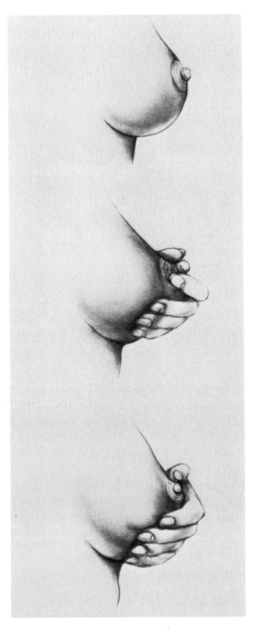

FIGURE 17-8 Nipple rolling. (From Lawrence, R.A. (1980). *Breast-feeding: A guide for the medical profession.* St. Louis: The C. V. Mosby Co., p. 115. With permission.)

League. The constant pressure promotes the eversion of the inverted nipple through the hole. These shields can be worn daily for the last several weeks of pregnancy. They are very successful in breaking down adhesions and allowing the nipple to evert so that the baby can suck it into his mouth.

Breast massage (Figure 17-9) is helpful in increasing the elasticity of the breast so that engorgement is not such a problem. There has been considerable discussion of antepartum manual expression of colostrum. The latest thinking is that it may stimulate uterine contractions and contribute to premature labor. Occasionally, antepartum mastitis has been attributed to manual expression. Of course, the expressed colostrum is lost to the infant. Consequently, the risks seem to far outweigh any possible benefits (Lawrence, 1980).

Regular bathing should continue during pregnancy, but no soap should be used on the nipples as it removes the sebasious secretions of the Montgomery glands, which lubricate the areola and nipple. Other drying agents such as alcohol or tincture of benzoin should never be used as they predispose the nipples to cracking.

There is still considerable debate over the effectiveness of nipple "toughening" through gentle rubbing with a soft turkish towel. Some data demonstrate less nipple tenderness with such treatment and other data show no difference. It may be that wearing bras protects nipples while wearing loose clothes and no bras, as is the custom in some other cultures, toughens the nipples so there are significantly fewer problems with nipple tenderness.

There is a psychological aspect of breast preparation that bears consideration. Due to the cultural value placed on modesty, many women in this society have never touched or carefully examined their breasts. They may be self-conscious, and breast preparation provides an opportunity to overcome these feelings prior to putting their newborn to breast. If the nurse is very matter of fact, yet sensitive, when discussing breast-feeding, performing the breast examination, and offering the breast preparation education, she can help the woman to discuss feelings and concerns as well as facilitate an appropriate infant-feeding decision and prepare the woman to do breast self-examination in the future. (For further information on this essential aspect of health care, see "The Breast," *Women's Health: Ambulatory Care.*)

HELPING MOTHERS WITH BREAST-FEEDING

The Initial Feedings

First feedings are extremely important, especially psychologically. Unless the mother has severe complications in the recovery room, or the infant is sick or severely depressed, the mother and baby need to be together during the first approximately ninety minutes, which is a time of quiet alert state for most infants as described by Harmon (see Figure 16-2 in Chapter 16).

EXHIBIT 17-1 Breast-feeding guidelines for mothers

General Principles

- Breast-feeding should begin within the first ninety minutes after birth and should proceed on demand during the first twenty-four hours to stimulate milk coming in early and decrease the severity of engorgement.
- Feed the baby on demand, but do not allow the baby to go longer than five or six hours between feedings. Expect every-three-hour feedings to be a normal average, with feedings two hours common at some times during a twenty-four-hour period.
- Nurse at all feedings, particularly after the first twenty-four hours following delivery and the first night if desired. *Do not* let the baby sleep through the night for the first four to six weeks because this can lead to inadequate weight gain due to decreased caloric intake. This makes pediatricians hysterical and can begin the formula supplement cycle, leading to "failed" breast-feeding.
- It is not necessary to clean the nipples before or after nursing, although cold water will stimulate the nipple to become erect. A daily shower or bath using only water on the nipples is all that is required.
- Don't use ointments or soap on the nipples
- Alternate starting breasts at each feeding. (If you wear a bra, a safety pin on the starting side for next feeding will help you remember the starting side.)
- Nurse from both breasts at each feeding.
- Air dry the nipples ten minutes following each feeding.
- Bras are encouraged *only* if you have *very* large, pendulous breasts. Keep flaps *down* so no moisture collects against the nipple. Trapped moisture causes sore and cracked nipples.
- If engorgement occurs (it will frequently be avoided with sufficient nursing and stimulation during the first twenty-four hours, as described above), remove milk and colostrum by hand expression or with a breast pump until the area is soft and the nipple stands out so the baby can grasp it. Hot showers or hot towels applied to the breasts will help you relax, stimulate let-down, and relieve the pain of engorgement.
- Don't use breast shields.
- Wash your hands before beginning to nurse.

Putting the Baby to Breast

- Before putting the baby to breast, express a few drops of colostrum or milk from each nipple. This is sometimes difficult in the beginning so be careful not to traumatize the nipple. This hand expression will make the nipples stand out so the baby can hold the nipple well back in his mouth. It also provides an encouraging taste for the baby.
- You can stroke the baby's cheek with the nipple as you hold him in your arms. He should turn toward the nipple and open his mouth. Guide the nipple and the darkened area behind the nipple into his mouth as he does this. He should begin sucking. (This is the rooting reflex–clamp-down–suck response.) If the baby misses the nipple and areola, begin the process from the root reflex. It is ineffective to try and pry the mouth open or stuff areola into the sucking mouth. To encourage suction, gently bump him under the chin. Don't stroke his cheek again because he will turn away from the breast and lose his grasp of the nipple.
- Length of nursing recommended:
  Five to ten minutes on each breast at every feeding during the first twenty-four hours
  Ten to fifteen minutes on each breast at every feeding the second twenty-four hours
  Fifteen to twenty minutes on the first side and as long as the baby is hungry on the second side; usually ten to twenty minutes from then on. The objective is to be certain to empty the first breast completely.
- When taking the baby off the breast, break suction by putting a finger in the corner of the baby's mouth or by pushing down on the chin or by pushing in on the breast tissue.

Many breast-fed infants who are truly on a demand schedule may at times nurse as often as every one and a half hours. It is certain they will want to nurse that frequently when they are in growth-spurt periods. In fact, there is a current controversy over the possibility of human infants being continuous feeders, like some other mammals. Therefore, demand feeding, which is crucial to successful breast-feeding, can be very demanding on women.

Demand feeding is also vital to the establishment of a good milk supply (Applebaum, 1977; Leighton, 1978). If infants are put to the breast more frequently in the immediate period after birth, the more frequent sucking will keep the prolactin levels higher and peaking more frequently (see Figure 17-3), and the milk will let-down more rapidly. As the infant continues to empty the breasts, there will be much less, if any, engorgement (Applebaum, 1977; Rees, 1976).

Time-Restricted Suckling

The standard instructions to new mothers have been to nurse for two to three minutes on each side the first day; three to five minutes the second day; five to seven

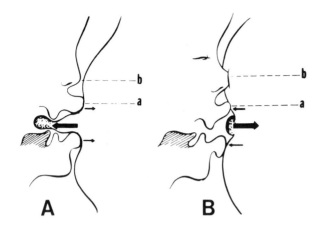

FIGURE 17-10 Infant suckling at normal and engorged breast. (A) Normal breast. The infant's jaws compress the areola and fit like a glove in the concave pocket of the nipple-areolar junction ("well" area) (a), while pulling the nipple back into the mouth. Breathing space is present (b). (B) Engorged breast. If the breast engorges, the nipple-areolar junction becomes convex (a), and the infant's jaws attempt to suck the inverted nipple, causing soreness and damage to the nipple epithelium. Breathing space is closed (b). Preventing engorgement will help prevent nipple soreness by encouraging proper nursing grasp. (From Appelbaum, R. (1975). The obstetrician's approach to breasts and breast feeding. *The Journal of Reproductive Medicine, 14*(3), 111. With permission.)

minutes the third day; and seven to ten minutes the fourth day. The rationale has been that gradually increasing suckling will prevent sore nipples. This logic has been highly questioned. When suckling is restricted to two to three minutes, the infant is removed from the breast before the milk let-down reflex is activated, thus preventing the baby from obtaining the majority of the colostrum and, later, the milk which is in the breast. The substances remaining in the breast then produce a back pressure, which interferes with the circulating blood and, in turn, hinders the neural-hormonal arc that controls the milk let-down and milk production. Thus begins the vicious cycle of engorgement. Of course, the breast becomes more and more rigid so the infant has difficulty getting the nipple to protract, and he subsequently has difficulty suckling. The hungry baby then bites down with his gums in his attempt to get some part of the nipple in his mouth (Figure 17-10). This causes the mother pain, which further inhibits let-down and leads to sore nipples (Applebaum, 1977; Rees, 1976).

If, instead, the infant suckles for a *minimum* of five minutes at each breast every time he nurses for the first

twenty-four hours; a *minimum* of ten minutes on each breast at every feeding in the second twenty-four hours; and a *minimum* of fifteen minutes on each breast for the third twenty-four hours, the breasts can be emptied and engorgement will be minimal or absent.

Breast Support

Traditionally, snug, well-fitting nursing bras with paper liners have been recommended for the new mother to wear essentially all the time. The rationale has been that good support will prevent the breast structures from excessive stretching, and thus prevent sagging after weaning.

It is now believed that the significant stretching of breast structures occurs antepartally as a result of the normal, hormonally induced breast enlargement of pregnancy. If true, this eliminates the rationale for bras. In addition, there is a notable problem associated with postpartum bra wearing. With or without liners, bras trap moisture from leaking nipples and hold it close to the areola and particularly the nipple. This can lead to soreness, cracking, and bleeding. I now recommend no bra except for those women with exceptionally large, pendulous breasts. However, if a mother has difficulty going braless altogether, she can wear a bra when she leaves the house or has company. Women who feel they must wear bras should leave the flap down so that nipples stay dry. The following vignette is an example of these problems.

Jean, an exceedingly fair-complexioned redhead, followed the standard breast-feeding instructions with her first infant: two to three minutes every three to four hours for the first twenty-four hours, etc. She experienced severe engorgement. She wore a bra all the time, and her nipples became so macerated, sore, cracked, and bleeding that she thought she might have to give up breast-feeding. Instead, she put Woolwich shields inside her bras so that milk leaking from her nipples would collect in the bottom of the shield and her nipples would stay dry. Then she adopted a "grin and bear it" attitude and kept nursing. After all, it had to get better. And it did.

However, with her second child, Jean decided to do things differently. She began nursing at the birth, to the astonishment and stern disapproval of the pediatrician. She continued nursing on demand with a twenty-four-hour rooming-in situation. Usually, the baby nursed ten minutes on the first side (beginning sides were alternated at each feeding) and as long as the baby wanted on the second side. Jean experienced no engorgement, no cracked or bleeding nipples, and only slight tenderness with each feeding for the first ten to fifteen seconds as the milk let-down. This tenderness lasted a couple weeks but was only a trifle bothersome instead of terribly traumatic as it was with her first infant. Jean wore no bra in the hospital and no bra at home for the first three weeks and had no additional breast-feeding problems.

Although subsequent breast-feeding experiences are commonly easier than the first experience, this is an area in need of further research. It is unlikely that women could have a worse experience with immediate demand feeding than the negative experiences many women have had with the traditional hospital procedure.

Breast-Feeding Problems

Sore Nipples

Sore nipples are often a result of rigid every-four-hour feeding schedules, restricted feeding time immediately postpartum, and engorgement. Sometimes, in spite of every preparation and precaution mothers still have sore nipples. The best plan for sore nipples is prevention: education and preparation of the mother antepartally; education of hospital staff to provide flexible routines, demand feeding, rooming-in, and lots of support; and assuring that mothers use correct basic breast-feeding skills (Rees, 1976).

If, in spite of all the above efforts, a mother develops sore nipples, the nurse should attempt to determine the cause. If engorgement is the problem, the mother can manually express some milk to soften the breasts before encouraging the infant to nurse (Applebaum, 1975). Manual expression and massage is illustrated in Figure 17-9. It will be much easier for the infant to suck the entire nipple and much of the areola into his mouth if the breasts are soft. To decrease edema of breast tissue, ice packs can be used. Hot packs do not decrease edema, but hot showers frequently relax the mother and stimulate blood flow and the let-down reflex, which in turn softens the breast by releasing milk.

If nipple stress seems to be the primary cause, the mother should feed in alternating positions so that primary stress lines on the nipple are rotated. One feeding could be sitting with the infant's feet and legs across the abdomen and his nose at one o'clock. The next feeding could be reclining so the infant is parallel to the mother and his nose is at twelve o'clock. The third position could be a football hold with the infant's legs off to the mother's side and under her arm; the infant's nose would be at eleven o'clock. The use of these positions in a rotating system could more evenly distribute the stress points over the nipple (Applebaum, 1975; Dutton, 1979). To further decrease stress to the nipple, the mother should be discouraged from putting the baby on and off the breast. Rather, she should put

him on the breast and leave him for the entire feeding time. The nurse can demonstrate how to break the suction correctly when taking the baby off the breast, and can caution the mother to avoid letting the baby fall asleep at the breast, which maintains prolonged negative pressure on the nipple. Feeding should begin on the breast that is least sore so that the let-down reflex will be in effect by the time the second, more sensitive breast is used. Only water should be used to cleanse the nipples—no soap or abrasives. If a bra is being worn, the nurse can ascertain whether the nipple ever sticks to the inside of the flap. Should this be the case, the mother can be directed to moisten the flap prior to pulling it away from the nipple. If she cannot dispense with the bra, then she must leave the flaps down. Air and heat seem to be the best treatment for sore nipples; leaving them open to the air to dry or using a dry heat such as a heat lamp will heal them probably much faster than ointments or creams.* Plastic breast cups may also be used so that the milk will leak into the cup rather than stay on the nipple.

If the let-down response is implicated as a problem, the nurse should make certain the infant is nursing at least five to ten minutes on each breast, so there is adequate sucking to stimulate the prolactin and oxytocin. Other let-down inhibitors include pain, anxiety, fear, and fatigue. For pain, whether it is from sore nipples, episiotomy, surgery, or uterine cramping, appropriate pain medication can be given twenty to thirty minutes before the feeding. Chances for an effective let-down reflex are much improved if the mother is comfortable. For anxiety, fear, or stress, a hot shower or a half glass of wine or beer can relax a mother enough to allow the milk to be ejected out of the alveoli and into the sinuses. Oxytocin nasal spray can be prescribed by the physician and will help stimulate let-down in some patients.

Fatigue

Fatigue is a very important factor—particularly when the mother goes home believing she needs to wash, iron, cook, clean, and entertain visitors while she is sleep-deprived from being up at night with her newborn. When I receive phone calls describing the newborn as crying all the time and hungry, I recommend complete bed rest for seventy-two hours (unless

---

*A heat lamp can be made at home by using a cylinder such as a large oatmeal box with both ends removed. Place a 15-watt light bulb in a lamp in one end and the breast at the other, minimum of 12 inches apart. (See: Mini sauna for sore nipples. *Keeping Abreast, Journal of Human Nutrition,* 1(2), 147.)

there is a toddler and *no* help), with the infant in bed with the mother or in a bassinet along side, and pitchers of fluids to be certain intake is adequate. She should get up only to go to the bathroom—no cooking meals or other household chores. She should suckle the baby whenever he wakes and seems hungry, should nap a lot, and play with her new baby.

Is There Enough Breast Milk?

One of the most stressful aspects of breast-feeding is knowing the baby is getting enough to eat. There is the old standby of six to eight wet diapers per day. And, obviously, if the baby gains weight, that is reassuring. I strongly discourage weighing after feedings because of the anxiety it causes the mother and the serious question regarding its accuracy. If the baby nurses for ten to twenty minutes at each breast and seems content, he is getting enough. What does content mean? If one watches infants at breast, they seem to begin the feeding very tense with their hands clinched into fists. As they nurse and burp, they seem to relax, close their eyes, and almost nap; their hands unfold and their whole bodies seem to go limp. Infants will often fall asleep at the breast. That is a picture of a contented baby. I suggest mothers should *not* allow babies to sleep through the night for the first three to six weeks because of lack of stimulation in milk production, because of engorgement, and because of the possible decrease in total caloric intake by the infant. Babies who drop below the tenth percentile often have supplementation encouraged by the physician; this decreases the breast milk, which in turn increases supplements and further decreases breast milk supply, and a vicious cycle develops. Although the problem of inadequate weight gain in infants is a complex one, the common solution, use of formula, often is the beginning of the end of the breast-feeding experience. Hopefully, we can soon find better solutions to these kinds of breast-feeding problems.

Stasis

For some reason, such as incomplete ejection reflex for a few feedings, milk may fail to flow from one section of the breast and stasis, or "clogged ducts," sets in. Mothers usually notice an area of the breast that is hard and somewhat tender to touch. Statis can lead to mastitis. It is, therefore, important that the mother institute treatment immediately to relieve the statis. A hot towel or washcloth can be placed over the affected area fifteen to twenty minutes prior to nursing. The infant should be encouraged to nurse longer and more frequently on that breast to help with the ejection reflex. It sometimes requires twelve hours or more to relieve all the stasis in the affected ducts. Additional treatment measures include: (1) changing nursing positions with each feeding; (2) being sure the bra is not too tight and is not pressing on the affected ducts; (3) hand expressing milk after each feeding to be certain the breast is as nearly empty as possible; and (4) offering the affected breast first to the infant (Eiger & Olds, 1973; Pryor, 1973).

Mastitis

With true mastitis, the mother will be able to palpate a hard, extremely tender area that is inflamed, red, and warm to touch. The mother may also be febrile and have a headache, generalized aching, and other flulike symptoms (M. Newton, 1971). Immediate treatment with antibiotics and bed rest is indicated. Analgesics and ice bags can be used for pain. Again, a significant component of treatment is to keep the breast empty, and this is most efficiently done by the baby.

Mastitis may progress to localized infection containing purulent material—an abscess. Occasionally, it will heal with antibiotics. However, it may require incision and drainage. This can usually be done in the doctors office and subsequent healing is rapid. The infant may be taken off the breast for twenty-four to forty-eight hours but should not be weaned. The affected breast can be emptied with a hand pump (Eiger & Olds, 1973; Marshall et al., 1975; M. Newton, 1971).

Other Medical Issues

Over the years, a common belief has evolved that only mothers who are at low risk and experience normal vaginal deliveries can breast-feed. Nothing could be farther from the truth. There are *very* few mothers who cannot breast-feed for medical reasons. For example, most diabetic mothers who breast-feed are in better control on lower amounts of insulin than they have been in years. Cesarean mothers who have had regional anesthesia can breast-feed in the recovery room, and many do. Since the breasts don't know how many babies there are, mothers of twins and even triplets can breast-feed successfully. Twins are frequently nursed simultaneously, one on each breast (La Leche League, 1963). Premature and sick infants can be breast-fed, or milk can be expressed and fed to the infant by gavage feeding. A milk supply can thus be maintained until the infant can suckle effectively.

One of the major questions about breast-feeding is the use of various drugs during lactation. An extensive listing of drugs, whether they are excreted in breast milk, and the subsequent effect on the infant can be found in Lawrence's *Breast Feeding*. Lawrence (1980) also provides an excellent overview of the major drugs and indicates those which should be avoided by lactating women. Others, including Catz and Giacola (1972) have reviewed various drugs and conclude that certain drugs should not be taken at all. These include radioactive drugs, anticoagulants, iodides, antimetabolites, most cathartics, and specifically tetracycline, ergot, atropine, and thiouracil. Other drugs may be taken only if mother and infant are monitored closely by the physician. These agents include sulfonamides, steroids, reserpine, diuretics, barbiturates, codeine cough medicines, and contraceptives (Applebaum, 1977; Brown, 1976).

Drug lists can give a false sense of security because they quickly become outdated. If there are questions, the baby should be watched closely. Maternal blood and milk levels should be monitored, as should infant blood levels when indicated.

The Roles of Professionals

The roles of physicians and nurses are vitally important to breast-feeding mothers. A study reported by Joseph and Peck (Clausen et al., 1973) at a major university teaching hospital indicated that thirty-four percent of new mothers, in a primarily indigent clinical population, chose to breast-feed their infants. A one-month follow-up showed only half of these mothers were still breast-feeding. Of the women who were still nursing, over half of them had nursed a prior infant. Of the mothers who stopped nursing, it is significant that one-third did so at the ill-considered advice of a physician. Although sixty-nine percent of all the mothers had chosen rooming-in, neither this nor breast-feeding instruction seemed to influence breast-feeding success. In contrast, forty-three consecutive patients in a private practice had a success rate of ninety-four percent at one month. The private physician in this study was a strong advocate of breast-feeding, while the residents providing care for the clinic group had a variety of beliefs.

In a study by Hall (1978), a control group of breast-feeding patients received routine postpartum care. The first experimental group received routine care and breast-feeding teaching, which included a slide tape series and a pamphlet; the second experimental group received the same teaching as the first experimental group plus nursing support (consisting of the nurse being present during at least one feeding, daily visits while in the hospital, and two follow-up phone calls within first week to ten days). The control group and the first experimental group had a fifty percent success rate (mothers who were still breast-feeding) at six weeks. The second experimental group had an eighty percent success rate, indicating the value of a strong support person. Mothers indicated it was important to be prepared for the possibility of problems with breast-feeding. Both of these studies indicate the powerful influence of doctors and nurses either in a supportive or negative way.

A major concern of breast-feeding mothers is all of the different, and even conflicting, advice they receive from nursing personnel. Because of traditional staffing patterns new mothers might see minimally one postpartum nurse and one nursery nurse on each shift. One alternative staffing pattern being used is primary nursing, in which one nurse is assigned to care for the family unit of mother and infant. When one person is responsible for coordination of care for both mother and infant, much of the fragmentation, confusion, and inconsistency in both support of and teaching of breast-feeding mothers can be avoided.

Nurses have considerable influence over policies for the hospital and can either promote or limit the flexibility necessary to successful breast-feeding.

FATHERS AND BREAST-FEEDING

The support of the father for the breast-feeding mother is pivotal for success. Education of the father about the value of breast-feeding and the fact that "breast is best" for the newborn is of paramount importance. If the father is involved in the pregnancy from the beginning of antepartum care, he is much more apt to be knowledgeable and supportive of breast-feeding. From their research, Guthrie and Kan (1977) recommend that adolescent boys as well as girls receive factual breast-feeding information as part of the parenting–family life–sex education program in the school systems. Young people form opinions early in life, and the male is very influential on the female's decision. If her male is negative, or is adamently opposed to breast-feeding in spite of the educational process, that is a legitimate reason not to encourage the mother to nurse. Encouraging nursing in this situation is encouraging conflict and maternal feeding failure.

Although many authors talk about creative fathers finding alternative interactions with their infants other than feeding, developing a strong paternal–infant relationship requires energy. It is crucial that the father's contact with his child be expanded beyond "the baby's fussy and mother can't think of anything else to quiet him; it's Dad's turn." Because fathers don't feed babies, they need more than diaper changing and crying. They need to feel like an active participant in child care. Although some fathers view breast-feeding as a reason for them to be up less at night with the baby, others get up and change diapers and bring the infant to the mother in bed. Both mothers and fathers need to evolve a "shared" parenting role, while maintaining their spouse roles and individuality (see Chapter 16.)

WORKING MOTHERS AND BREAST-FEEDING

Women who are attempting to combine careers and motherhood, or who must work to support the family, often believe their only feeding option is the bottle. This is not true. They can breast-feed and manually express milk, save it, and take it to the day care setting, provided the milk can be refrigerated. Or they can discard the breast milk and provide formula for the time they are away from the infant. It is possible to arrange that the baby be hungry when he is picked up from the day care provider, so that mother and infant can come home, lay down, and have an extended feeding session. This provides time for the mother to rest in a horizontal position, for the infant to nurse, and for both to touch and stroke and communicate with one another. Some working mothers believe the most valuable gift they give their babies is the continuation of breast-feeding. There is never the temptation, or the actuality, of a "propped bottle."

A very small number of working mothers find a day care setting in which the day care mother is also nursing an infant. A question may arise concerning wet-nursing the infant. Although this is a common practice in many areas of the world, it is rarely practiced in Western cultures today. There are no medical contra-indications, providing the mother who is wet-nursing is healthy and is taking no medications (Lawrence, 1980). The main concerns are psychological and social. A woman might have a difficult time adjusting to another woman suckling her infant. However, it could be helpful for a mother of a premature infant to have a strong sucking infant to help in establishing a milk supply. For the working mother, it could be comforting to know that her baby could receive solice suckling, in addition to the nutrition of the expressed milk she could leave for the infant. A special bond seems to develop between a suckling infant and the woman who feeds him. The working breast-feeding mother might receive great comfort from knowing her child is getting this special kind of care.

Societal support for nursing mothers who work is sadly lacking in our society. Such support is strongly needed, including longer maternity leaves, adequate child care near the place of employment, lactation breaks to nurse or express, and refrigeration available for mothers who express and save milk. Many other countries have these kinds of facilities.

NURSING MOTHER SUPPORT GROUPS

One of the best support systems for nursing mothers is La Leche League. A mother can share problems and successes with other breast-feeding mothers; and this group is unfailing in their support of women who have severe problems. Group members accept phone calls for help at practically any time. They will even come into the home to help on occasion. A few professionals have been alienated because some members can be overly enthusiastic and underinformed. However, the major-ity of the group are sincere, dedicated, knowledgeable, and supportive. A professional who uses this group, or groups like them, to help patients will profit in every way.

BOTTLE-FEEDING

The single greatest problem of bottle-feeding is over-feeding. Mothers and grandmothers across the nation, from all socioeconomic groups, have equated feeding with love and subsequently with good parenting. In bottle-fed infants, it is quite easy to force-feed an infant until he "finishes" the bottle. Breast-fed infants stop when they are full and the mother has no measure—no endpoint to which the infant must go. Slattery (1977) stresses how important it is for maternal–child nurses to stress factors *other* than weight gain to reinforce good parenting. For example, the nurse could devote time to discussing how the parent plays with the baby, stim-ulates the baby, and soothes the baby with behavior *other* than feeding.

Mothers who choose bottle-feeding also need support for their feeding decision, and support to feel good about their parenting ability. They have problems associated with their feeding choice just as breast-feeding mothers do. For example, they will probably experience slower uterine involution than breast-feeding mothers, and it may be difficult for them to lose the fat stores that were accumulated during pregnancy to assure the fat content of their breast milk.

All commercially prepared formulas are fortified in most all nutrients to meet the Recommended Dietary Allowances of the Food and Nutrition Board. Some, however, may not have iron unless specified, and supplemental iron is important for bottle-fed infants (American Academy of Pediatrics, 1971). Table milks, both skimmed milk and two-percent milk, are inappropriate to feed during the first year of life. They provide insufficient calories in proportion to excessive amounts of protein, low fat content, and inadequate fatty acids (Fomon, 1974). The American Academy of Pediatrics, based on work by Fomon et al. (1979) suggests that formula or breast milk should be fed for the entire first year of life.

Slattery (1977) discusses extensively the dilemma of what to teach mothers about formula preparation. Ideally, terminal sterilization or the aseptic single-feeding method should be used at home. In the United States, all milk produced for infant consumption is heat treated. Refrigeration is readily available, and adequate sanitation and safe water supplies can be obtained by nearly everyone. Fomon et al. (1979) have determined that gastrointestinal disorders in infants can rarely be traced to contaminated formula, probably because of the infrequency with which enteric pathogens are found in the environment. Consequently, it seems appropriate to teach a good, "clean" formula preparation technique, which people would be more apt to use than sterilization.

When the above conditions are in effect, control of bacterial growth is dependent on the use of clean bottles and nipples (automatic dishwashers are very effective if available) and storage of prepared formula at temperatures less than 50°F (10°C). One bottle at a time is the safest method of clean-formula preparation. Thus, bottle-feeding and formula preparation are not an option for feeding infants of poor families in developing nations where sanitation is inadequate, the water supply is contaminated, and there is no refrigeration.

Mothers have many concerns about bottle-feeding their infants. The baby eats too slow or too fast, he works too hard, or he regurgitates what seems to them a large portion of the feeding. Guidelines for teaching mothers about bottle-feeding are shown in Exhibit 17-2. The most important things for bottle-feeding mothers to remember are not to overfeed, and to spend time holding, touching, and stroking the baby during feedings. They should be instructed not to prop bottles. If these suggestions are followed, the bottle-feeding mother can have a close relationship with her infant, similar to the breast-feeding mother.

EXHIBIT 17-2   Bottle-feeding guidelines

When teaching a mother to bottle-feed her infant, the nurse should devote an amount of time similar to that with the breast-feeding mother. The nurse should stay with the mother and talk about the following points:

- When feeding is begun the infant can be held away from the body so as not to stimulate the rooting reflex.

- The nipple should be pointed directly into the mouth rather than toward the top of the palate, and it should be on top of the tongue.

- The entire nipple should be full of milk at all times to avoid ingestion of air.

- As soon as the baby becomes accustomed to the bottle and nipple, he should be held close to the body and cuddled to facilitate eye-to-eye contact with the person who is feeding him. Stroking and talking to a baby during feeding promotes pleasure and relaxation for the baby as well as his parents.

- The nipple hole size should be big enough so that milk flows in drops when it is inverted. When the nipple hole is too large, the baby can eat too fast and regurgitate or overeat. Bottle-feedings should take twenty to thirty minutes, depending on how often the baby is burped.

- Babies swallow air when they cry, so it is occasionally necessary to burp a baby prior to beginning the feeding. Minimally, the baby should be burped at the middle and end of the feeding. Too frequent burping confuses the baby. The baby is held in an upright position (either sitting on a lap or over a shoulder), and his back is massaged or stroked.

- *Bottles should never be propped.* Positional otitis media can develop if milk and nasal mucus occlude the eustachian tube when the baby is lying in a horizontal position. In addition, if the nipple hole is large, the young baby can choke from too much milk and have difficulty getting the nipple out of his mouth.

- Caution should be used if warming bottles in microwave ovens; the liquid easily becomes too hot and the first couple of drops tested may not reflect the true temperature of the milk.

- Milk should not be saved for the next feeding if the baby doesn't empty the bottle. Organisms grow, and the baby can develop diarrhea. Leftover formula can be used for coffee or cooking.

REFERENCES AND ADDITIONAL READINGS

Alfin-Slater, R.B., & Jelliffe, D. (1977). Nutritional requirements with specific reference to infancy. *Pediatric Clinics of North America, 24*(1), 3-15.

American Academy of Pediatrics, Committee on Nutrition. (1971). Iron fortified formulas. *Pediatrics, 47,* 786.

Applebaum, R.M. (1975). The obstetrician's approach to the breasts and breast feeding. *The Journal of Reproductive Medicine, 14*(3), 98-116.

Applebaum, R. (1977). Breast feeding and drugs in human milk. *Keeping Abreast Journal, 2*(4), 292-293.

Arias, I., Gartner, L.M., Seifter, S., & Furman, M. (1964). Prolonged neonatal unconjugated hyperbilirubinemia associated with breast feeding and a steroid, pregnane-3 (alpha) 2-(beta) diol in maternal milk that inhibits glucuronide formation in vitro. *Journal of Clinical Investigation, 43,* 2037-2047.

Aries, P. (1962). *Centuries of childhood. A social history of family life.* New York: Vintage Books.

Bentovim, A. (1976). Shame and other anxieties associated with breastfeeding: A systems theory and psychodynamic approach. In *Breastfeeding and the mother,* Ciba Foundation Symposium 45 (new series). New York: Ciba Foundation, pp. 159-172.

Bertino, J.S. (1981). The pharmacology of human milk. *Birth and the Family Journal, 8*(4), 237-243.

Beske, E.J., Garvis, M.S., & Mullett, S.E. (1982). Important factors in breast-feeding success. *MCN, The American Journal of Maternal-Child Nursing, 7*(3), 174-178.

Blachman, L. (1981). Dancing in the dark. I. Romanticized motherhood and the breastfeeding venture. *Birth and the Family Journal, 8*(4), 271-279. (a)

Blachman, L. (1981). Dancing in the dark. II. Helping and not-so-helping hands. *Birth and the Family Journal, 8*(4), 280-286. (b)

Blackwell, A., & Salisbury, L. (1981). Administrative petition to relieve the health hazards of promotion of infant formulas in the United States. *Birth and the Family Journal, 8*(4), 287-296.

Bloom, M. (1977). Is Breast-feeding best for babies? *Consumer Reports,* March.

Bloom, M. (1978). Breast feeding and avoidance of food antigens in the prevention and management of allergic disease. *Nutrition Reviews, 36*(6), 181-183.

Bloom, M. (1981). The romance and power of breastfeeding. *Birth and the Family Journal, 8*(4), 259-269.

Brown, M.S. (1976). Drugs, contaminants, and nutrients in human milk. *Keeping Abreast Journal, 1*(1), 34-36.

Bullen, C.L., Tearle, P.V., & Stewart, M.G. (1977). The effect of "Humanised" milks and supplemented breast milk on the faecal flora of infants. *The Journal of Medical Microbiology, 10*(4), 403-413.

Catz, C.S., & Giocoia, G.P. (1972). Drugs and breast milk. *Pediatric Clinics of North America, 19*(1), 151-166.

Cerutti, E.R. (1981). The management of breastfeeding. *Birth and the Family Journal, 8*(4), 251-256.

Clausen, J.P., Flook, M., Ford, B., Green, M.M., & Popiel, E.S. (1973). *Maternity nursing today.* New York: McGraw-Hill.

Commitee on Nutrition of the Mother and Preschool Child, National Research Council. (1978). *A selected annotated bibliography on breast feeding 1970-1977.* Washington, D.C.: National Academy of Sciences.

Cone, T.E. (1976). *200 Years of feeding infants in America.* Columbus, Oh.: Ross Laboratories.

Darke, S.J. (1976). Human milk versus cow's milk. *Journal of Human Nutrition, 30*(4), 233-238.

Davidson, W.D. (1953). A brief history of infant feeding. *Journal of Pediatrics, 43,* 74-87.

Delvoye, P., Demaegd, M., Delogne-Desnoeck, J., & Robyn, C. (1977). The influence of the frequency of nursing and of previous lactation experience on serum prolactin in lactating mothers. *Journal of Biosocial Science, 9,* 447-451.

Dutton, M.A. (1979). A breast feeding protocol. *Journal of Obstetric Gynecologic and Neonatal Nursing, 8*(3), 151-155.

Eiger, M.S., & Olds, S.W. (1973). *The complete book of breast feeding.* New York: Bantam Books.

Ewy, D., & Ewy, R. (1975). *Preparation for breast feeding.* Garden City, N.Y.: Dolphin Books.

Fields, V. (1978). The Elizabethan wet nurse. *Nursing Times,* March 16, pp. 472-473.

Fomon, S.J. (1974). *Infant nutrition.* Philadelphia: Saunders.

Fomon, S., Filer, L.J., Anderson, T., & Ziegler, E. (1979). Recommendations for feeding normal infants. *Pediatrics, 63*(1), 52-59.

Gerrard, J.W. (1974). Breast feeding: Second thoughts. *Pediatrics, 54*(6), 757-764.

Goldman, A.S., & Smith, C.W. (1973). Host resistance factors in human milk. *The Journal of Pediatrics, 82*(6), 1082-1090.

Gordon, B.L. (1974). *Essentials of immunology,* (ed. 2). Philadelphia: Davis.

Grams, K.E. (1978). Breast feeding: A means of imparting immunity? *The American Journal of Maternal Child Nursing, 3*(6), 340-344.

Gunther, M. (1976). The new mother's view of herself. In *Breastfeeding and the mother,* Ciba Foundation Symposium 45 (new series). New York: Ciba Foundation, 145-152.

Guthrie, H.A., & Kan, E.J. (1977). Infant feeding decisions—Timing and rationale. *Journal of Tropical Pediatrics, 23,* 264-266.

Gyorgy, P. (1971). Biochemical aspects. *The American Journal of Clinical Nutrition, 24,* 970-975.

Hall, B. (1977). Changing composition of human milk and early development of an appetite control. *Keeping Abreast, Journal of Human Nurturing, 2*(2), 139-142.

Hall, J.M. (1978). Influencing breast feeding success. *Journal of Obstetric, Gynecologic and Neonatal Nursing, 7*(6), 28-32.

Hartmann, P.E., Kulski, J.K., Rattigan, S., Prosser, C.G., & Saint, L. (1981). Breastfeeding and reproduction in women in western Australia—A review. *Birth and the Family Journal, 8*(4), 215-226.

Hendershot, G. (1980). *Trends in breast feeding.* Advance data from vital and health statistics of the National Center for Health Statistics, No. 59, March, 28.

Hirschman, C., & Hendershot, G. (1979). *Trends in breast feeding among American mothers.* Vital and health statistics data from the National Survey of Family Growth, National Center for Health Statistics, Series, 23, No. 3.

Hytten, F.E. (1976). The physiology of lactation. *The Journal of Human Nutrition, 30*(4), 225-232.

Jelliffe, D.B. (1968). *Infant nutrition in the subtropics and tropics.* Geneva: World Health Organization.

Jellife, D., & Jelliffe, E.F.P. (1977). Current concepts in nutrition. *The New England Journal of Medicine, 297*(17), 912-915.

Jelliffe, E.F.P. (1976). Maternal nutrition and lactation. In *Breastfeeding and the mother.* Ciba Foundation Symposium 45 (new series). New York: Ciba Foundation, pp. 103-113.

Jensen, M.D., Benson, R.C., & Bobak, I.M. (1977). *Maternity care*. St. Louis: Mosby.

Johnson, J.D. (1975). Neonatal nonhemolytic jaundice. *The New England Journal of Medicine,* 292(4), 194-196.

Johnson, N. (1976). Breast feeding at one hour of age. *American Journal of Maternal Child Nursing, 1*(1), 12-16.

La Leche League. (1963). *The womanly art of breast feeding*. Franklin Park, Il.: La Leche League International.

Larsen, S.A., & Homer, D.R. (1978). Relation of breast versus bottle feeding to hospitalization for gastroenteritis in a middle class U.S. population. *The Journal of Pediatrics, 87*(3), 417-418.

Lawrence, R. (1980). *Breast feeding: A guide for the medical profession*. St. Louis: Mosby.

Leighton, N.S. (1978). Initiating and supporting the early breast feeding relationship. *Keeping Abreast, Journal of Human Nurturing, 3*(3), 214-219.

Maisels, M.L. (1981). Breastfeeding and jaundice. *Birth and the Family Journal, 8*(4), 245-249.

Marshall, B., Hepler, J., & Zirbel, C. (1975). Sporadic puerperal mastitis. *Journal of the American Medical Association, 233,* 1377-1379.

Mata, L.J., & Wyat, R.G. (1971). Host resistance to infection. *The American Journal of Clinical Nutrition, 24,* 976-985.

McKigney, J. (1971). Economic aspects. *The American Journal of Clinical Nutrition, 24,* 1005-1012.

McMillan, J.A., Landaw, S.A., & Oski, F.A. (1976). Iron sufficiency in breast-fed infants and the availability of iron from human milk. *Pediatrics, 58*(5), 686-691.

McMillan, J.A., & Oski, F.A. (1977). Iron nutrition in the breast fed infant. *Keeping Abreast, Journal of Human Nurturing, 2*(1), 33-35.

Newton, M. (1971). Mammary effects. *The American Journal of Clinical Nutrition, 24,* 987-990.

Newton, N. (1971). Psychologic differences between breast and bottle feeding. *The American Journal of Clinical Nutrition, 24,* 993-1004.

Phillips, V. (1976). Infant feeding through the ages. *Keeping Abreast, Journal of Human Nurturing, 1*(4), 296-300.

Pittard, W.B. (1981). Special properties of human milk. *Birth and the Family Journal, 8*(4), 229-235.

Pryor, K. (1973). *Nursing your baby*. New York: Pocket Books.

Rees, D. (1976). Sore nipples are a pain! *Keeping Abreast, Journal of Human Nurturing, 1*(2), 125-135.

Reiser, R. (1971). Control of serum cholesterol by the nutrition of the neonate: A progress report. *Circulation, 44* (Suppl. 2), 3.

Reiser, R., & Sidelman, Z. (1972). Control of serum cholesterol, homeostasis by cholesterol in the milk of suckling rat. *Journal of Nutrition, 102,* 1009-1016.

Rolles, C. (1976). Can we really mimic human milk? *Keeping Abreast, Journal of Human Nurturing, 13,* 216-221.

Roy, C. (1975). Nonhemolytic hyperbilirubinemia syndromes. In C.C. Roy, A. Silverman, & Cozzetto, F.J. (Eds.), *Pediatric clinical gastroenterology* (ed. 2). St. Louis: Mosby, pp. 451-465.

Savage, R. (1977). Drugs and breast milk. *Journal of Human Nutrition, 31,* 459-464.

Scahill, M. (1975). Helping the mother solve problems with feeding her infant. *Journal of Obstetrical, Gynecologic, and Neonatal Nursing, 4,* 51-54. March-April.

Simkin, P., Simkin, P., & Edwards, M. (1979). Physiologic jaundice of the newborn. *Birth and the Family Journal, 6*(1), 23-40.

Slattery, J.S. (1977). Nutrition for the normal healthy infant. *MCN, The American Journal of Maternal-Child Nursing, 2*(2), 105-112.

Smith, W.G., & Beer, A.E. (1976). Current concepts of reproductive immuno-biology. *Journal of Perinatal Medicine, 4,* 59-67.

Sosa, R., Kennell, J., Klaus, M., & Urrutia, J. (1976). The effect of early mother-infant contact on breast feeding, infection and growth. In *Breastfeeding and the mother*. Ciba Foundation Symposium 45 (new series). New York: Ciba Foundation, pp. 179-188.

Speroff, L. (1977). The breast as an endocrine target organ. *Contemporary OB/GYN, 9.*

Speroff, L., Glass, R.H., & Kase, N.G. (1978). *Clinical gynecologic endocrinology and infertility*. Baltimore: Williams & Wilkins.

Thompson, M. (1971). The convenience of breast feeding. *The American Journal of Nutrition, 24,* 991-992.

Welsh, J., & May, J. (1979). Anti-infective properties of breast milk. *Journal of Pediatrics, 94*(1), 1-9.

Wickes, I.G. (1953). History of infant feeding—Part I. *Archives of Disease in Childhood, 28,* 151-158. (a)

Wickes, I.G. (1953). History of infant feeding—Part II. *Archives of Disease in Childhood, 28,* 232-340. (b)

Wickes, I.G. (1953). History of infant feeding—Part III. *Archives of Disease in Childhood, 28,* 332-340. (c)

Wickes, I.G. (1953). History of infant feeding—Part IV. *Archives of Disease in Childhood, 28,* 416-422. (d)

Wickes, I.G. (1953). History of infant feeding—Part V. *Archives of Disease in Childhood, 28,* 495-502. (e)

Widdowson, E.M. (1976). Changes in the body and its organs during lactation: Nutritional implications. In *Breastfeeding and the mother*. Ciba Foundation Symposium 45 (new series). New York: Ciba Foundation, pp. 103-113.

Worthington, B., Vermeersch, J., & Williams, S. (1977). *Nutrition in pregnancy and lactation*. St. Louis: Mosby.

Index

b
3 c
4 d
5 e
6 f
7 g
8 h
9 i
8 0 j